Clinical Handbook of Assessing and Treating Conduct Problems in Youth

Clinical Handbook of

Assessing and Treating Conduct Problems in Youth

Edited by

Rachael C. Murrihy

University of Technology, Sydney, NSW, Australia

Antony D. Kidman

University of Technology, Sydney, NSW, Australia

Thomas H. Ollendick

Virginia Polytechnic Institute and State University, Blacksburg, VA, USA

Springer

Editors
Rachael C. Murrihy
Health Psychology Unit
University of Technology, Sydney
Sydney, NSW
Australia
Rachael.Murrihy@uts.edu.au

Antony D. Kidman
Health Psychology Unit
University of Technology, Sydney
Sydney, NSW
Australia
Tony.Kidman@uts.edu.au

Thomas H. Ollendick
Department of Psychology
Child Study Center
Virginia Polytechnic Institute
and State University
Blacksburg, VA
USA
tho@vt.edu

ISBN: 978-1-4419-6295-9 e-ISBN: 978-1-4419-6297-3
DOI: 10.1007/978-1-4419-6297-3
Springer New York Dordrecht Heidelberg London

Library of Congress Control Number: 2010930603

Printed on acid-free paper

Springer is part of Springer Science+Business Media (www.springer.com)

Preface

Identifying evidence-based treatments for youth with conduct problems is vitally important, not only because conduct problems are the most common of all youth mental health problems, but also because the impairment associated with conduct problems is so severe and pervasive, costly to society and, at times, life threatening. For an individual, antisocial and aggressive behavior interferes with the ability to reach optimal potential in academic, occupational, and social pursuits. Families suffer as they struggle to manage challenging behaviors, ensure their safety, and deal with the social alienation that frequently goes hand in hand with raising aggressive youth. School communities are also affected. Teachers managing sizeable classrooms face pressure, often in the absence of specialized training, to circumvent demanding behaviors and protect the learning environment and safety of other students. Ultimately, one needs only to look to the daily newspapers, to stories of unemployment, crime, and violence at home, in schools, and on the streets, to understand the far-reaching impact of conduct problems on society.

That said, the development of evidence-based treatments for youth with conduct problems has not been a simple or straightforward undertaking. Indeed, it can be argued that few greater challenges in clinical psychology exist than that of understanding conduct problems and developing comprehensive treatments. The reasons for this are many, but the main obstacle concerns the complex etiological mechanisms at play in youth with conduct problems and the impact of these complexities on assessment and treatment. These youth constitute a heterogeneous group, and, because of this diversity, conduct problems are thought to be the product of multiple developmental pathways – each pathway with its own unique causal factors. If we consider how clinical treatments are formulated, we see they are typically guided by an understanding of causal and maintaining factors, and they are frequently based on the underlying assumption that a single etiological pathway is present in all individuals with a specified disorder. For youth with conduct problems, however, this approach is overly simplistic as there is no single developmental pathway. With this in mind, it is clear why the identification of etiological mechanisms – the building blocks that inform the development of evidence-based treatment – has been such a complex undertaking. Although major advancements have been made (e.g., identification of broad risk factors), more remains to be achieved (e.g., the delineation of risk factors associated with specific developmental pathways).

Unraveling the etiology of conduct problems has not been the only challenge faced by researchers and clinicians in this field. Assessing and treating youth with conduct problems typically requires a systemic approach that relies on the cooperation of parents, the child or adolescent, and, sometimes, extended family and school staff. Maintaining the ongoing participation and cooperation of all parties, however, can be difficult. Therapy with this population is typically laden with therapeutic and familial process issues, which, if not handled well, can result in poor outcomes, including early drop out. In addition to delivering the "content" of treatment, practitioners in this field by necessity must direct much of their energy towards monitoring and managing these process and contextual issues.

Fortunately, the complexities inherent to this population have not deterred researchers and an impressive amount of research has amassed during the last quarter of a century. This has resulted in a wide range of available treatments – particularly so for children and preadolescents with conduct problems – that have been well established and tested across a variety of settings, countries, and populations.

The aim of this book is to integrate this considerable body of research into a practicable summary of epidemiology, assessment, and treatment models. We aim to provide the reader with a clear conceptualization of where the research currently stands, while highlighting future research pathways that will facilitate answers to the next generation of questions. In analogous terms, we are poised at the base camp on Everest, and as we look down we can see that huge gains have already been made in this field, primarily with regard to identifying broad risk factors and developing evidence-based treatments. Indeed, many comprehensive treatments are now available that target the wide range of risk factors associated with conduct problems and are tailored to the individual as much as possible. As we look upwards towards the summit, however, we consider whether treatments can be streamlined further. Can we divide this heterogeneous youth population into smaller groups, based on distinct developmental pathways and etiological mechanisms, enabling the development of subtype-specific treatment? Research has already commenced into this exciting arena and an overview of early subtypes is included within this volume. We hope that these discussions will stimulate further questions and encourage research into potential developmental pathways and matching treatment components.

We expect that those who will benefit most from reading this book will be researchers seeking a thought-provoking discussion of the latest knowledge in the field as well as clinicians, both expert and novice, who will find this book a useful reference because it provides both a summary of the current state of knowledge about conduct problems and an in-depth review of nine major evidence-based treatment interventions. It also includes case study discussions that illustrate practical approaches to treatments, including the management of complex process issues. Mental health specialists and researchers are not the only group, however, who may benefit from this book. It will also serve as a useful resource for policy makers in education and health who want to learn more about gold-standard interventions that may be applicable for them.

For this volume, we have brought together experts, widely considered to be the best thinkers in this field, to deliver state-of-the-art reviews in their respective areas of expertise. An international focus has seen authors enlisted from diverse locations, including Australia, the United Kingdom, and the United States. To have such outstanding authors contribute to this volume is an enormous privilege, and we thank them sincerely for their dedication and commitment to furthering knowledge in this field.

The volume has been divided into four parts. Part I offers the basic foundation for the subsequent three sections, covering the nature of conduct problems and providing an etiological explanation of these difficulties. In Chap. 1, Wolff and Ollendick offer a comprehensive introduction to the reader by discussing the phenomenology, classification, and epidemiology of conduct problems in youth. The next two chapters focus on etiological mechanisms underlying conduct problems, starting with larger societal explanations and moving through to more individualistic and family-based perspectives. Shoemaker, in Chap. 2, provides us with a sociological perspective on the cause of conduct problems, drawing attention to the many contextual factors (e.g., lack of community integration and stability) in societies that influence antisocial behavior. This reminder of the wider contextual forces at play is complemented by a more individualistic approach to explaining etiology in Chap. 3, in which Kimonis and Frick focus on biological, temperamental, and familial risk factors for the development of conduct problems. In addition, Kimonis and Frick provide an enlightening description of the currently proposed developmental pathways associated with conduct problems. Taken together, this etiological data guides the final chapter of this section by Rhodes and Dadds (Chap. 4), which outlines the assessment of conduct problems, including assessment strategies, tools, process issues, differential diagnosis, and functional analysis.

With this foundation laid, the second section of this volume outlines the evidence-based clinical treatment of conduct problems. In Part II, a loosely consistent format is adopted by all authors, whereby a general introduction about conduct problems is followed by a description of the key features of the treatment model, the content and format of the treatment approach, empirical evidence for the approach, and, lastly, a case study to illustrate the clinical application of the treatment. We start the treatment section by focusing on three evidence-based treatments for children that utilize parent management skills (among other skills) as a core component of treatment. In Chap. 5, Webster-Stratton and Reid give an overview of Incredible Years, a comprehensive treatment program that has developed and evolved over a 30-year period. Next, following a similarly long period of evolution, is Parent–Child Interaction Therapy, an intervention discussed in detail by Eyberg and Bussing in Chap. 6. Finally, in

Chap. 7, McMahon, Long, and Forehand offer an in-depth review of the Helping the Noncompliant Child treatment program.

Moving away from parent management training towards a collaborative problem-solving approach, Greene emphasizes how conduct problems result from poor compatibility or "fit" between a parent and child in Chap. 8. Much is known about parenting styles associated with conduct problems, but Greene makes an important addition to the literature by discussing socioemotional and cognitive deficits in children (e.g., emotional dysregulation, rigid thinking) that, when combined with certain characteristics (e.g., inflexibility) in a parent, may lead to the expression of conduct problems.

Group-based therapy for school children, based on the social cognitive model of aggression, is discussed by Lochman, Boxmeyer, Powell, and Wells in Chap. 9. The Coping Power program, initially devised for youth only, is now complemented by parent groups. The authors in this chapter provide insight into some of the process difficulties associated with group work in this population and how these issues may be overcome.

Next, we review the limited group of treatments that are suitable for older cohorts of youth with complex presentations. In Chap. 10, Alexander and Robbins discuss the clinical application of a family therapy approach, Functional Family Therapy. Similar to Chap. 9, much of the focus in this chapter is directed towards the management of process issues. In Chap. 11, Schaeffer, McCart, Henggeler, and Cunningham describe Multisystemic Therapy, the only therapy that has been validated for adolescents with serious conduct problems who are at risk for out-of-home placement. The authors explain the importance of taking an ecological, community-based approach to the assessment and treatment of serious conduct problems.

In Part III, we consider the effectiveness of treatment for youth with conduct problems, when implemented in three diverse settings. Murrihy, in Chap. 12, examines social competency programs for youth in alternative school settings. In Chap. 13, LeBuffe, Robison, and Chamberlin-Elliott review treatment for youth in their residential treatment centers; and, in Chap. 14, Coventry and Swanson consider the effectiveness of wilderness and boot camps for treating antisocial youth. Historically, these treatment options have attracted criticism for their lack of evidence base, but recent advances in research have added to existing knowledge and built evidence for these approaches. These authors analyze the latest evidence and share their conclusions regarding the effectiveness of interventions conducted in these settings. Part III concludes with a discussion by Smith and Coghill (Chap. 15) about the effectiveness of medications as a second-line treatment for the treatment of conduct problems and aggression.

In Part IV of this volume, we look to the future with a consideration of population level prevention strategies, multilevel treatment interventions, evidence-based therapies for minority youth, and program cost-effectiveness. In Chap. 16, the Conduct Problems Prevention Research Group reviews the Fast Track treatment program, a large-scale intervention differentiated by its longitudinal format (administered over 10 years), which blends universal and targeted interventions to prevent conduct problems in high-risk youth. Next, in Chap. 17, Sanders and Morawska discuss the Triple P program, another multilevel prevention program, which also emphasizes the importance of blended interventions. These authors argue that to lower the prevalence of conduct problems population level strategies must be adopted. Universal interventions, such as television documentaries on parenting, would enable widespread access to parenting knowledge and skills for the general population without the stigma associated with more intensive psychological treatments. In Chap. 18, Ho, McCabe, Yeh, and Lau consider whether standard evidence-based therapies can be used in minority populations or if treatments need to be culturally modified before doing so. Finally, Foster, in Chap. 19, argues that all interventions should be analyzed for cost-effectiveness, before going on to discuss the many issues associated with determining the feasibility of treatment programs.

We find ourselves in an enviable position. Practitioners in this field have at their disposal a wealth of evidence-based treatments. Moving forward, we can glimpse the possibility of tailoring these treatments even further, through the identification of distinct etiological pathways. The challenge remains that one day soon, subtypes will be identified and treatment components matched to these subtypes. This is a considerable task, but an exciting one, and one that we hope will propel researchers into action. We are honored to be a part of this process.

Sydney, Australia — Rachael C. Murrihy
Sydney, Australia — Antony D. Kidman
Blacksburg, VA — Thomas H. Ollendick

Acknowledgments

First and foremost, I (Rachael Murrihy) would like to acknowledge, with heartfelt gratitude, my family. With the arrival of a newborn (Thomas Elijah) during this process, it really did take a village to bring this book to fruition. Words cannot adequately express my thanks to my husband Gregory, mother Anne-Maree, and father Raymond. Without their patience, understanding, and cooperation, this book would not have been possible.

I (Antony Kidman) also wish to acknowledge a number of individuals whose contributions have made the book possible. Thank you to my wife, Janelle, my two children, and seven grandchildren, whose love and support has inspired me throughout this project.

Together, Rachael and I would also like to thank the talented and hardworking team of clinical psychologists at the Health Psychology Unit, especially Anna Dedousis-Wallace, Yael Perry, and Megan Varlow, who provided us with helpful feedback along the way. Lastly, and importantly, thanks go to our coeditor Thomas Ollendick. We value his collegiality and marvel at the depth of his knowledge in this field.

Lastly, I (Thomas Ollendick) wish to give thanks to Rachael and Tony who have really been the driving force behind this project and who invited me to coedit this book with them. I have greatly enjoyed, and benefited from, this joint venture. It has been a fun and rewarding project. I also wish to extend special thanks to my family as well. Mary, my spouse, has been a source of support, encouragement, friendship and love over the years we have been together. She has been a very important part of my (our) journey. Similarly, our daughters, Laurie Kristine and Kathleen Marie, have been a source of support, love, pride, and inspiration over the years. Their children (our grandchildren, Braden Thomas Perryman, Ethan Ray Perryman, Calvin David Perryman, and Addison Haley Smith) are also thanked as they keep us young and in touch with the realities of growing up in an exciting and ever-changing world.

Many other persons are to be thanked in a venture such as this. Collectively, we wish to thank the many children, adolescents, and families whom we have had the great pleasure of working with over the years. They have helped us grow as mental health professionals and taught us much more than they probably realize. Without them, the ideas for this book would not have evolved or its completion realized. We also wish to thank our many contributors – without whom this volume would have been only a vanishing vision on our part. Their collective expertise and wisdom make this volume what it is. We also wish to thank Judy Jones and Garth Haller at Springer for helping us realize our vision and bringing this project to fruition. We thank them for their invaluable assistance and dedication to this project.

Contents

SECTION II: EVIDENCE-BASED TREATMENTS OF CONDUCT PROBLEMS: AN APPLIED APPROACH FOR PRACTITIONERS

SECTION III: EVIDENCE-BASED TREATMENT OF YOUTH WITH CONDUCT PROBLEMS IN DIVERSE SETTINGS

Contributors

James F. (Jim) Alexander
University of Utah, & Functional Family Therapy (FFT Inc.), 4748 So Ichabod St, Salt Lake City, UT 84117, USA, jfafft@aol.com

Karen L. Bierman
The Conduct Problems Prevention Research Group, Department of Psychology, The Pennsylvania State University, University Park, PA 16802, USA, kb2@psu.edu

Caroline Boxmeyer
Center for the Prevention of Youth Behavior Problems, The University of Alabama, Box 870348, Tuscaloosa, AL 35487-0348, USA, boxmeyer@as.ua.edu

Regina Bussing
Departments of Psychiatry, Pediatrics, and Clinical and Health Psychology, University of Florida, Box 100234 UFHSC, Gainesville, FL 32610-0234, USA, rbussing@UFL.EDU

Davida J. Chamberlin-Elliott
Outpatient and Substance Abuse Services, Devereux Texas Treatment Network 1150 Devereux Drive, League City, TX 77573, USA, delliott@devereux.org

David R. Coghill
Centre for Neuroscience, Division of Medical Sciences, University of Dundee, Center for Child Health, 19 Dudhope Terrace, Dundee DD3 6HH, Scotland, d.r.coghill@dundee.ac.uk

John D. Coie
The Conduct Problems Prevention Research Group, Duke University, 1510 Franceschi Rd, Santa Barbara, CA 93103, USA, john.coie@duke.edu.

Garry F. A. Coventry
School of Arts and Social Sciences, Fellow Cairns Institute, James Cook University, Townsville, QLD 4811, Australia, garry.coventry@jcu.edu.au

Phillippe B. Cunningham
Family Services Research Center, Department of Psychiatry and Behavioral Sciences, Medical University of South Carolina, McClennan Banks Building 4th floor, 326 Calhoun St. STE MC406, Charleston, SC 29401, USA, cunninpb@musc.edu

Mark R. Dadds
School of Psychology, University of New South Wales, Sydney, NSW 2052, Australia, m.dadds@unsw.edu.au

Kenneth A. Dodge
The Conduct Problems Prevention Research Group, Center for Child and Family Policy, Sanford School of Public Policy, 302 Towerview Drive, Duke University, Durham, NC 27705, USA, Dodge@duke.edu

Sheila M. Eyberg
Department of Clinical and Health Psychology, University of Florida, Gainesville, FL 32610, USA, eyberg@PHHP.UFL.EDU

Rex L. Forehand
Department of Psychology, University of Vermont, Dewey Hall, Burlington, VT 05405, USA, rex.forehand@uvm.edu

E. Michael Foster
School of Public Health, University of North Carolina, Chapel Hill, Rosenau Hall, Campus Box# 7445, Chapel Hill, NC 27599-7445, USA, emfoster@unc.edu

Paul J. Frick
Department of Psychology, University of New Orleans, 2001 Geology & Psychology Bldg., New Orleans, LA 70148, USA, pfrick@uno.edu

Mark T. Greenberg
The Conduct Problems Prevention Research Group, Prevention Research Center, The Pennsylvania State University, HDFS–Henderson Building South Room 109, University Park, PA 16802, USA, mxg47@psu.edu

Ross W. Greene
Harvard Medical School, 246 Walnut Street, Suite 203, Newton, MA 02460, USA, DrRossGreene@gmail.com

Scott W. Henggeler
Family Services Research Center, Department of Psychiatry and Behavioral Sciences, Medical University of South Carolina, McClennan Banks Building 4th floor, 326 Calhoun St. STE MC406, Charleston, SC 29401, USA, henggesw@musc.edu

Judy K. Ho
UCLA Department of Psychiatry, Semel Institute Health Services Research Center, 10920 Wilshire Blvd. Suite 300, Los Angeles, CA 90095, USA, judyho@ucla.edu

Antony D. Kidman
Health Psychology Unit, University of Technology, Sydney, Royal North Shore Hospital, Sydney, NSW 2065, Australia, Tony.kidman@uts.edu.au

Eva R. Kimonis
Louis de la Parte Florida Mental Health Institute, Mental Health Law and Policy, University of South Florida, 13301 Bruce B. Downs Blvd. MHC 2639, Tampa, FL 33612, USA, ekimonis@fmhi.usf.edu

Anna S. Lau
UCLA Psychology Department, 1285 Franz Hall, Box 951563, Los Angeles, CA 90095-1563, USA, alau@psych.ucla.edu

Paul A. LeBuffe
Devereux Center for Resilient Children, 444 Devereux Drive, P.O. Box 638, Villanova, PA 19085, USA, plebuffe@Devereux.org

John E. Lochman
The Conduct Problems Prevention Research Group, Department of Psychology, Center for Prevention of Youth Behavior Problems, The University of Alabama, Box 870348, 348 Gordon Palmer Hall, Tuscaloosa, AL 35487, USA, jlochman@as.ua.edu

Nicholas Long
Department of Pediatrics, University of Arkansas for Medical Sciences, 1 Children's Way, Slot 512-21, Little Rock, AR 72202, USA, LongNicholas@uams.edu

Kristen M. McCabe
Rady Children's Hospital Child and Adolescent Services Research Center – San Diego, University of San Diego, 5998 Alcala Park, San Diego, CA 92123, USA, kmccabe@sandiego.edu

Michael R. McCart
Family Services Research Center, Department of Psychiatry and Behavioral Sciences, Medical University of South Carolina, McClennan Banks Building 4th floor, 326 Calhoun St. STE MC406, Charleston, SC 29401, USA, mccartm@musc.edu

Robert J. McMahon
The Conduct Problems Prevention Research Group, Child Clinical Psychology, Department of Psychology, University of Washington, Box 351525, Seattle, WA 98195-1525, USA, mcmahon@u.washington.edu

Alina Morawska
Parenting and Family Support Centre, School of Psychology, University of Queensland, Brisbane, QLD 4072, Australia, alina@psy.uq.edu.au

Rachael C. Murrihy
Health Psychology Unit, University of Technology, Sydney, Royal North Shore Hospital, Sydney, NSW 2065, Australia, Rachael.Murrihy@uts.edu.au

Thomas H. Ollendick
Child Study Center, Department of Psychology, Virginia Tech, Blacksburg, VA 24060, USA, tho@vt.edu

Ellen E. Pinderhughes
The Conduct Problems Prevention Research Group, Eliot-Pearson Dept. of Child Development, Tufts University, 105 College Avenue, Medford, MA 02155, USA, ellen.pinderhughes@tufts.edu

Nicole P. Powell
Center for the Prevention of Youth Behavior Problems, The University of Alabama, Box 870348, Tuscaloosa, AL 35487-0348, USA, npowell@as.ua.edu

M. Jamila Reid
Parenting Clinic, School of Nursing, University of Washington, 1107 NE 54th St, Suite 320, Seattle, WA 98105, USA, mjreid@u.washington.edu

Tracy E. Rhodes
Child Behavior Research Clinic, School of Psychology, University of New South Wales, Sydney, NSW 2052, Australia, trhodes@psy.unsw.edu.au

Michael S. Robbins
Oregon Research Institute, Functional Family Therapy Inc., 1901 NW 108 Avenue, Pembroke Pines, FL 33026, USA, mrobbins@ori.org

Suzanne Robison
Psychological Services and Human Development Center, 220 Commerce Drive, Fort Washington, PA 19034, USA, robison@pshdc.com

Matthew R. Sanders
Parenting and Family Support Centre, School of Psychology, University of Queensland, Brisbane, QLD 4072, Australia, m.sanders@psy.uq.edu.au

Cindy M. Schaeffer
Family Services Research Center, Department of Psychiatry and Behavioral Sciences, Medical University of South Carolina, McClennan Banks Building 4th floor, 326 Calhoun St. STE MC406, Charleston, SC 29401, USA, schaeffc@musc.edu

Donald J. Shoemaker
Department of Sociology, 512 McBryde Hall, Virginia Tech, Blacksburg, VA 24061, USA, shoemake@vt.edu

Helen L. Smith
Department of Psychiatry, Centre for Neuroscience, University of Dundee, Center for Child Health, 19 Dudhope Terrace, Dundee DD3 6HH, Scotland, H.Y.Smith@dundeee.ac.ak

Laura G. Swanson
Family Studies Clinic, Criminology, School of Arts and Social Sciences, James Cook University, Townsville, QLD 4811, Australia, laura.swanson@jcu.edu.au

Carolyn H. Webster-Stratton
Parenting Clinic, School of Nursing, University of Washington, 1107 NE 54th St, Suite 320, Seattle, WA 98105, USA, cws@u.washington.edu

Karen C. Wells
Duke University Medical Center, 718 Rutherford St, Durham, NC 27705, USA, wells020@mc.duke.edu

Jennifer C. Wolff
Rhode Island Hospital, Brown Medical School, POB 122, 593 Eddy Street, Providence, RI 02903, USA, jennifer_wolff@brown.edu

May Yeh
SDSU/UCSD Joint Doctoral Program in Clinical Psychology, San Diego State University, Child and Adolescent Services Research Center at Rady Children's Hospital-San Diego, University of California, San Diego, 3020 Children's Way (MC5033), San Diego, CA 92123, USA, myeh@sciences.sdsu.edu

About the Editors

Rachael C. Murrihy, PsyD. Dr. Murrihy is currently Senior Clinical Psychologist and Research Associate at the Health Psychology Unit, an adolescent-based unit, at the University of Technology, Sydney, Australia. Dr. Murrihy's specialty is in the area of clinical adolescent psychology. She has extensive experience lecturing, training, and supervising professionals in this field, including clinical psychologists, psychiatrists, family physicians, nurses, educators, and interns. She also provides mental health lectures for members of the general public. As a practicing clinician, Dr. Murrihy works with youth experiencing both internalizing and externalizing disorders across a diverse range of settings, including the university clinic, private practice, inpatient wards, and in mainstream and alternative schools. She has published research on adolescent mental health and has presented this work at conferences, both nationally and internationally. She has held research grants from the Australian Psychological Society, New South Wales (NSW) Department of Health, and the NSW Department of Education and Training. Her research and clinical interests include the assessment and treatment of youth with conduct problems, callous–unemotional traits in youth, cyber bullying and indirect bullying, and Cognitive Behavioral Therapy for early psychosis.

Antony D. Kidman, PhD. Dr. Kidman is a Clinical Psychologist and Director of the Health Psychology Unit of the University of Technology, Sydney, Australia. He has more than 140 scholarly publications to his name including seven books: *Tactics for Change*; *Managing Love and Hate*; *Family Life, Adapting to Change*; *Feeling Better, a Guide to Mood Management*; *From Thought to Action*; *Stress, Coping and Social Support in the Age of Anxiety*; and *Schizophrenia, a Guide for Families*. Dr. Kidman was a member of the National Executive of the Australian college of clinical psychologists for 10 years and was the founder and inaugural Editor for 6 years of the College's journal, *The Clinical Psychologist*. He is a Member of the Clinical College of the Australian Psychological Society, an Associate Fellow of the Albert Ellis Institute of Rational Emotive Therapy (NY), and a Fellow of the

International Academy of Cognitive Therapy. He has held research grants from the Australian National Health and Medical Research Council and the New South Wales Department of Health. Dr. Kidman has had a long-term clinical and research interest in adolescent mental health including anxiety, depression, and psychosis. He is a frequent guest speaker on radio and television and writes for the media on mental health. He was made a Member of the Order of Australia in 2005 for his contributions to clinical psychology.

Thomas H. Ollendick, PhD. Dr. Ollendick is University Distinguished Professor in Clinical Psychology and Director of the Child Study Center at Virginia Polytechnic Institute and State University, Blacksburg, VA, USA. He is the author of several research articles, book chapters, and books. His books include *Clinical Behavior Therapy with Children* (Plenum Press), *Child Behavioral Assessment: Principles and Procedures* (Pergamon Press), *Handbook of Child Psychopathology* (Plenum Press), *Developmental Issues in the Clinical Treatment of Children* (Allyn and Bacon) (Oxford), and the *Handbook of Interventions that Work with Children and Adolescents* (Wiley). He is the past Editor of the *Journal of Clinical Child Psychology*, past Associate Editor of the *Journal of Consulting and Clinical Psychology*, current Editor of *Behavior Therapy*, and founding Coeditor of *Clinical Child and Family Psychology Review*. In addition, he is Past-President of the Association for the Advancement of Behavior Therapy (1995), the Society of Clinical Psychology (1999), the Society of Clinical Child and Adolescent Psychology (2003), and is currently President of the Society for the Science of Clinical Psychology. A frequent speaker at national and international conferences, he is the recipient of several NIH grants. His clinical and research interests range from the study of diverse forms of child psychopathology to the assessment, treatment, and prevention of these child disorders from a social learning/social cognitive theory perspective.

Section I

An Introduction to Conduct Problems in Youth

1

Conduct Problems in Youth: Phenomenology, Classification, and Epidemiology

JENNIFER C. WOLFF and THOMAS H. OLLENDICK

Youth with conduct problems comprise a heterogeneous group of children and adolescents who engage in a broad array of problem behaviors ranging from defiance, argumentativeness, and temper outbursts to physical aggression, destructiveness, and stealing. Taken together, these problem behaviors continue to be the most frequent basis for child and adolescent referrals to mental health clinics and residential treatment facilities and are of great concern because of the high degree of impairment associated with them, their potential for persistence over time, and their association with negative life outcomes (Cohen et al., 1993; Lahey, Loeber, Quay, Frick, & Grimm, 1997; Loeber et al., 2000). Indeed, youth with clinically significant levels of oppositional and conduct problems often face a wide range of individual, family, and community-wide difficulties including interpersonal conflicts, violent behavior, delinquent acts, out-of-home placements, and involvement with the juvenile justice system. They are also estimated to be the most costly of all mental health problems in the United States (Cohen, 1998).

Although almost all children display some aggressive behavior at some point in their lives, these behaviors are considered to be indicative of a

JENNIFER C. WOLFF • Brown Medical School
THOMAS H. OLLENDICK • Virginia Tech

R.C. Murrihy et al. (eds.), *Clinical Handbook of Assessing and Treating Conduct Problems in Youth*, DOI 10.1007/978-1-4419-6297-3_1,

clinical syndrome when they are severe, persistent, and lead to significant impairment in psychosocial functioning (Frick, 1998a). The Diagnostic and Statistical Manual of Mental Disorders (DSM-IV; American Psychiatric Association (APA), 2000) includes two such clinical disorders in youth: Oppositional Defiant Disorder (ODD) and Conduct Disorder (CD). For the purposes of this book, the term "conduct problems" will be used to refer to this broad constellation of aggressive behaviors; however, DSM categorizations will be used in those instances when a formal diagnosis is being referenced or discussed. This chapter focuses on the classification, phenomenology, developmental course, and epidemiology of aggression and conduct problems in youth including subtypes, stability, and comorbid conditions.

CLASSIFICATION

The clinical diagnosis of conduct problems is rooted in a strong empirical foundation. Indeed, an impressive amount of information has established decision-making rules that serve as a framework for clinicians diagnosing these conditions. However, some debate continues over the exact nature of conduct problem disorders and how these behaviors should be classified. Many attempts have been made to classify these disorders and researchers continue to struggle with capturing the heterogeneous nature of these behaviors in extant diagnostic nomenclature.

DSM-IV Oppositional Defiant Disorder. ODD refers to a recurrent pattern of developmentally inappropriate levels of negativistic, defiant, disobedient, and hostile behavior toward authority figures. Behaviors associated with ODD include temper outbursts; persistent stubbornness; resistance to directions; unwillingness to compromise, give in, or negotiate with adults or peers; deliberate or persistent testing of limits; and verbal (and minor physical) aggression. In DSM-IV, four of these oppositional behaviors are required for at least a 6-month duration for the diagnosis to be warranted (see Table 1.1). The behaviors must have a higher frequency than is generally seen in other children of similar developmental level and age and these behaviors must lead to meaningful social, personal, and familial impairments. These behaviors are almost always present in the home and school, usually with individuals the child knows well, and often occur simultaneously with low self-esteem, mood lability, low frustration tolerance, and poor executive functioning.

Oppositional disorder was first introduced as a separate diagnostic category in 1980 as part of DSM-III (APA, 1980). The introduction of ODD into the diagnostic nomenclature was met with controversy because its distinctiveness from normal developmental stages was questioned and because it was unclear whether it was simply a mild form of CD (Rowe, Maughan, Costello, & Angold, 2005). Those in support of this new diagnostic category argued that the severity of CD symptomatology neglected important precursors to antisocial behavior in young children and failed to

Table 1.1. DSM-IV diagnostic criteria for oppositional defiant disorder and conduct disorder

DSM-IV criteria: oppositional defiant disorder

A. A pattern of negativistic, hostile, and defiant behavior lasting at least 6 months, during which four (or more) of the following are present:

1. Often loses temper
2. Often argues with adults
3. Often actively defies or refuses to comply with adults' requests or rules
4. Often deliberately annoys people
5. Often blames others for his or her mistakes or misbehavior
6. Is often touchy or easily annoyed by others
7. Is often angry and resentful
8. Is often spiteful or vindictive

DSM-IV criteria: conduct disorder

1. Often bullies, threatens, or intimidates others
2. Often initiates physical fights
3. Has used a weapon
4. Has been physically cruel to people
5. Has been physically cruel to animals
6. Has stolen while confronting a victim
7. Has forced someone into sexual activity
8. Has deliberately engaged in fire setting
9. Has deliberately destroyed others' property
10. Has broken into someone else's house, building, or car
11. Often lies to obtain goods or favors or to avoid obligations
12. Has stolen items of nontrivial value
13. Often stays out late without permission, starting before age 13
14. Has run away from home overnight at least twice
15. Is often truant from school, starting before age 13

recognize the clinical impairment associated with more mild forms of antisocial behavior. With subsequent research and revisions of DSM criteria, the legitimacy of this disorder has been established and the substantial psychosocial impairment evidenced in these youth is now more widely recognized (e.g., Greene et al. 2002).

DSM-IV Conduct Disorder. CD refers to a repetitive and persistent pattern of behavior in which the basic rights of others or major age-appropriate societal norms or rules are violated. It is also characterized by aggressive conduct that causes or threatens physical harm to other people or animals; nonaggressive conduct that causes property loss or damage; and deceitfulness or theft. To meet DSM-IV criteria for the disorder, at least three of 15 behavioral criteria (see Table 1.1) must have been present in the past 12 months, with at least one of the behaviors present in the past 6 months. The scope of severity in these behaviors (i.e., bullying versus forced sexual activity) contributes to high levels of heterogeneity in youth diagnosed with CD and the host of possible symptom profiles may reveal important distinctions in etiology, course, and treatment. In an effort to better categorize these behaviors, DSM-IV classifies symptoms according to four subcategories: aggression to people and animals, destruction of property, deceitfulness or theft, and serious violations of rules. The extent to which antisocial behaviors are sufficiently severe to constitute CD depends on the frequency, intensity, and chronicity of these behaviors, whether they are isolated acts or part of a larger syndrome with other deviant behaviors, and whether they lead to significant impairment of the child, as judged by parents, teachers, or others.

DSM-IV Subtypes of CD. DSM-IV distinguishes two types of CD. The childhood-onset subtype is defined by onset of at least one CD symptom prior to age 10, and the adolescent-onset type is defined by the absence of any CD symptoms prior to age 10. While the adolescent period is associated with general increases in rebelliousness and status offenses, conduct problems are evident in a small subset of adolescents who show more extreme or persistent forms of behavior problems. DSM-IV notes that subtyping on the basis of age of onset captures differential information about the likely nature of the characteristic presenting problems, developmental course, and prognosis.

Children showing the childhood-onset pattern display more severe behavior problems early in childhood that tend to worsen over development (Lahey & Loeber, 1994), and, compared to their adolescent-onset counterparts, these children are more likely to continue to show antisocial and criminal behavior well into adulthood (Frick & Loney, 1999). In addition, children in the childhood-onset group are characterized by more aggression, more cognitive and neuropsychological disturbances, greater impulsivity, greater social alienation, and more dysfunctional family backgrounds than are children in the adolescent-onset group (see Frick, 1998b; Moffitt, 1993; Moffitt et al., 1996).

ICD-10 Definition of Conduct Disorder. Whereas DSM-IV draws a distinction between conduct disorder and oppositional defiant disorder, ICD-10 defines conduct disorder as an amalgam of the two DSM-IV disorders. ICD-10 includes a symptom list similar to the combined symptom lists of DSM-IV ODD and DSM-IV CD, but divides this into 15 "more severe items" (corresponding with DSM-IV CD symptoms), and eight "less severe items" corresponding to the DSM symptoms of ODD. A diagnosis of CD is made similarly in both systems, with three or more of the "more severe items" being required in ICD-10. ODD, by contrast, is treated as a subtype of CD in ICD-10, and the diagnosis is made in the presence of four or more symptoms from the full list of 23, but where no more than two come from the list of more severe items. As a result, all children who receive a diagnosis on the DSM-IV scheme also receive an ICD-10 diagnosis, but a small number of children who meet ICD-10 criteria for CD (ODD sub-type) would not receive an ODD diagnosis in DSM-IV (Angold & Costello, 2001).

Reactive and Proactive Aggression. Due to the heterogeneous nature of youth displaying these behavior problems, various alternative classification schemes for aggressive symptoms have also been suggested. Along these lines, the study of aggressive behavior in humans and animals has revealed the existence of distinct subtypes of aggression including direct, physical, verbal, relational, indirect, and social aggression (Dodge & Coie, 1987; Poulin & Boivin, 2000; Vitiello & Stoff, 1997). Although different subtypes of aggression have been identified, they have typically been based upon the *forms* or expressions of aggression rather than the *functions* or purposes of the aggressive acts, the latter of which is useful for informing case conceptualization and determining treatment formulation (Polman, Orobio de Castro, Koops, van Boxtel, & Merk, 2007). A well-known approach that considers the *functions* of aggressive behavior is that which distinguishes between reactive and proactive aggression (Dodge & Coie, 1987).

Proactive aggression is described as aggression without immediate provocation that is used as a means of achieving some outcome. This function or purpose of aggression is less emotional in nature and more organized and goal-directed. It includes such forms of aggression as bullying, name-calling, coercion, and the breaking of rules (Price & Dodge, 1989). Reactive aggression, on the other hand, is an affect-laden, impulsive, and defensive reaction to a perceived threatening stimulus. This function of aggression is thought to be more emotional in nature and is viewed as a frustration response, driven by poor self-regulation, poor affective modulation, and intense physiological reactivity (Dodge, Lochman, Harnish, Bates, & Pettit, 1997; Hubbard et al., 2002). Reactive behaviors include expressions of anger, temper tantrums, and vengeful hostility. In addition, these reactions are often linked to hostile attribution biases (Dodge et al., 1997). It should be noted that "pure" proactive aggression is relatively rare and aggression in children typically has at least a partial reactive component (e.g., Dodge et al., 1997; Waschbusch, Willoughby, & Pelham, 1998). The validity of this distinction of aggression in children has been supported in both community and clinical samples (Coie, Dodge, Terry, & Wright, 1991; Crick & Dodge, 1996; Dodge et al., 1997; Ollendick, Jarrett, Wolff, & Scarpa, 2009; Waschbusch et al., 1998).

Given these fundamental differences in the functions of aggressive acts, it has been suggested that this is an important means of classification for the assessment and treatment of aggressive youth. More specifically, it has been suggested that children whose aggression is aimed more at securing rewards and other instrumental outcomes (i.e., proactive) may be more responsive to contingency management procedures, whereas children displaying reactive aggression may be more likely to respond to psychosocial treatments aimed at simultaneously increasing cognitive functioning and decreasing high-levels of hostility, impulsivity, and arousal (e.g., Crick & Dodge, 1996; Ollendick et al., 2009; Vitiello & Stoff, 1997; Wolff, Greene, & Ollendick, 2008). Thus, these differences in the function of aggression may be an important means of classifying children with conduct problems as they account for the psychological processes that precede aggressive behaviors.

Callous and Unemotional (CU) Traits. An additional method of classifying a subset of children with conduct problems is based on the earlier onset of temperamental-like traits related to the concept of psychopathy. CU traits found in youth consist of lacking sympathy and helpfulness, selfishness, diminished guilt, lack of empathy, reduced need for social affiliation and approval, and dampened emotional expression (Frick, O'Brien, Wootton, & McBurnett, 1994; Lahey, Waldman, & McBurnett, 1999). CU traits are suggestive not only of the onset of conduct problems, but also the increased severity and chronicity of these behavioral patterns once they are developed. For instance, those identified with CU traits tend to exhibit a greater number and variety of CD symptoms (Frick, 1998a). Twin studies have also revealed substantial genetic influences on the onset and course of CU traits (Larson, Andershed & Lichtenstein, 2006).

Many children with CU traits evidence lower behavioral inhibition, as manifested by increased thrill and adventure seeking, low fearfulness, and low autonomic reactivity on skin conductance measures (Frick et al., 1994). These characteristics suggest that conduct problem children with CU traits may show a temperamental style associated with low emotional reactivity to aversive stimuli that is characterized physiologically by under reactivity in the sympathetic arm of the autonomic nervous system and behaviorally by low fearfulness to novel or threatening situations and poor responsiveness to cues to punishment (Kagan & Snidman, 1991). The lower behavioral inhibition exhibited by a child with CU traits is related to increased dependence on rewards and decreased attention to punishments or consequences. This may help to explain why children with CU traits are less influenced and affected by the painful reactions and experiences of others as a function of their behavior.

In all, research suggests that the presence of CU traits in youth with conduct problems results in different patterns of aggressive behavior that tend to be more severe and chronic. Specifically, these youth have extreme files. Moreover, at least one study has shown that children with CU traits may not benefit from typical behavioral interventions which appear to work for most youth with CD (Hawes & Dadds, 2005), suggesting that this may be an important subtype for treatment planning. Although more longitudinal evidence is needed, the available evidence indicates that these traits suggest a relatively stable characteristic that predicts poorer outcomes. The use of these traits to subtype youth with conduct problems could help to integrate previous attempts at defining distinct groups of antisocial youth. However, some critics of the subtype argue that labeling children with CU traits may lead treatment professionals to conclude these youth are untreatable (Moffitt et al., 2008). Still, subtyping those with conduct problems on the basis of these traits has considerable potential for explaining the causes of the most severe and aggressive patterns of antisocial behavior in youth and the pathway to later psychopathy (Frick & White, 2008).

DEVELOPMENTAL PROGRESSION OF CONDUCT PROBLEMS

Recent research has helped to clarify the development of aggression and antisocial behavior from early childhood to adulthood. Although many questions remain unanswered, we now have a better understanding of the stability and prognosis of these disorders and factors which may be associated with later antisocial personality disorder. The developmental sequence of these disorders suggests a developmental and hierarchical pattern of behavioral problems of less severity that precedes more serious forms of aggression and delinquency, at least for some youth.

While considered independent diagnoses, researchers recognize the continuity between ODD and CD, such that the onset of ODD often occurs in the context of earlier forms of oppositional behavior whereas the onset of CD emerges subsequent to an existing ODD diagnosis. Follow-back studies show that most CD children were previously diagnosed with ODD and most adults with antisocial personality disorder (ASPD) were diagnosed with CD. Specifically, Loeber et al. (1995) found that 80% of boys who developed CD had a previous diagnosis of ODD at least 1 year earlier. Conversely, follow-forward studies reveal that most ODD children do *not* develop CD and most CD children do *not* develop ASPD (Moffitt et al., 2008). In fact, over two-thirds of children with ODD are not subsequently diagnosed with CD (Biederman et al., 1996; Hinshaw, Lahey, & Hart, 1993). Certainly a clear overlap has been established between CD and ODD, and there is evidence to suggest that ODD precedes CD in a most cases. However, a majority of children with ODD do not have CD and many ODD children evidence ongoing oppositional behavior without ever developing CD (Biederman et al., 1996; Lahey & Loeber, 1994; Nock, Kazdin, Hirpi, & Kessler, 2007).

Lahey and Loeber (1994) have shown that oppositional behavior tends to emerge in childhood, with some children progressing to "intermediate" CD behaviors (such as lying, fighting, and bullying), and a further subset developing "advanced" levels of CD (e.g., mugging, stealing, truancy). Children rarely commence conduct problems by evidencing the more severe behaviors from the onset. Instead, these problems develop in a predictable manner from oppositionality to more severe aggression. Those who develop these advanced problems are more likely to display antisocial characteristics in adulthood.

The pathway by which early forms of oppositionality lead to the emergence of less severe forms of conduct problems (i.e., ODD) and to the development of more severe manifestations (i.e., CD) is multifaceted. In general, the early age of onset for these disorders is usually related to a system of transacting individual and family environment risk factors, which take place early in life and prevent the child from developing the social skills and self-regulation required to prevent the onset of conduct problems (Moffitt, 1993). For example, oppositionality may contribute to impaired interpersonal relationships often starting in the home and then spanning to school and other community settings. Early oppositionality is also associated with increased peer rejection and decreased opportunity for classroom learning (Fergusson & Horwood, 1996; Lewin, Davis, & Hops, 1999). In addition to the impairment caused by the symptoms themselves, patterns of oppositional behavior are highly relevant in the prediction of later delinquency. Studies show that higher frequency and variety of early oppositional behavior, as well as the presence of problem behavior in multiple settings, increases a child's risk for later deviant outcomes (Loeber, 1990). Thus, not only the specific behaviors, but also the presentation of these behaviors is important in maintaining this cycle of escalating and transforming antisocial behavior. Thus, to the degree that the behaviors associated with ODD often precede more serious forms of psychopathology – including not only CD but also adult antisocial behavior (see Langbehn, Cadoret, Yates, Troughton, & Stewart, 1998) – the manifestation of these behaviors represents an important window of opportunity for prevention efforts (Loeber, 1990; Lynam, 1996).

EPIDEMIOLOGY

The prevalence of these disorders is estimated to be between 2% and 16%, depending on the population, ascertainment methods, and diagnostic measures used (Loeber et al., 2000; Maughan, Rowe, Messer, Goodman, & Meltzer, 2004). The National Comorbidity Survey Replication recently assessed prevalence of ODD and CD in a nationally representative sample of over 3,000 adults in the United States. On the basis of this survey, lifetime prevalence of ODD was estimated to be 10.2% (Nock et al., 2007) and the lifetime prevalence of CD was 9.5% (Nock, Kazdin, Hirpi, & Kessler, 2006).

As discussed below, prevalence rates have been shown to vary as a function of age and sex of the child, as well as the type of aggressive behavior. These rates also tend to vary based on the informants used to assess the disorders. For example, the prevalence rates of conduct and oppositional defiant disorders in community samples range from 1.6% to 10.2%, depending on whether parent or teacher ratings are relied on to classify disorder in the child or whether both are considered simultaneously (Offord et al., 1996). Prevalence of classification of disorder ranges widely in clinic samples as well.

Gender. From preschool age on, young boys tend to engage in significantly more aggressive and non-aggressive antisocial behavior than girls (Keenan & Shaw, 1997). This trend is also apparent in more serious manifestations of conduct problems. As it is currently defined in the DSM-IV, the prevalence of both CD and ODD is greater for males than for females. Further, severity ratings of CD symptomology are significantly higher for males, particularly those involving physical harm to others (Lahey et al., 2000). It is important to note, however, that this distinction in prevalence is less apparent by adolescence (APA, 2000).

A number of hypotheses have been generated to explain the gender specificity observed in the onset and phenomenology of these disorders. For example, one review of the literature (Keenan, Loeber, & Greene, 1999) suggests that young girls score higher on ratings of empathy as well as guilt and rumination about breaking rules and hurting others. These early factors may temporarily protect girls from engaging in early-onset antisocial behavior. However, one study has found that girls' guilt about aggressive behavior seems to decline with age (Keenan et al., 1999), perhaps helping to explain the relative absence of gender differences in conduct problems in adolescence. As such, an interaction between gender and age also warrants consideration. Additionally, there seem to be gender differences in the development of communication skills, such that girls may be more skilled at social interaction at an earlier age than boys (see Keenan & Shaw, 1997). There has also been some speculation regarding the role of gender-specific hormone levels (e.g., testosterone) in the onset of conduct problems, but findings are inconsistent (Steiner et al., 1997). Lastly, the development of conduct problems may be related to the interaction between gender and parental responses to behavior problems. Evidence suggests that parents may respond more strictly to temperamental traits and antisocial behaviors exhibited by girls than boys because of the perceived social unacceptability of these behaviors in girls (Keenan & Shaw, 1997). Thus, it is possible that both girls and boys have similar initial developmental trajectories in the development of conduct problems, but differential parental responses directly influence risk for diagnosis.

Despite recent advances in studying both girls and boys, data regarding gender differences in CD and ODD are relatively sparse. Additionally, debate exists as to the appropriateness of the current diagnostic nosology in these disorders (Moffitt et al., 2008). For instance, girls and boys tend to vary on the specific types of antisocial behavior exhibited. Girls tend to engage in more relational aggression (i.e., social exclusion, spreading rumors) and non-physical antisocial behavior whereas boys fit better into the mold of the standard DSM diagnosis, including overt physical features and delinquency. However, both boys and girls are clearly engaging in problematic social deviance and, upon follow-up, may meet criteria for CD or ODD. Thus, there is still much to discover about the role of gender in the risk for, as well as the emergence and expression of, conduct problems.

Age. It is widely recognized that the age at which conduct problems emerge critically influences the developmental course and phenomenology of these problems over time. In fact, as mentioned previously, this factor has formed the basis for a division in diagnostic subtypes of CD. In general, younger children are more likely to engage in oppositional behaviors, whereas older children and adolescents are more likely to engage in more covert behavior problems such as stealing. Although rates of seriously physically aggressive acts such as rape and robbery rise in adolescence (Maughan et al., 2004), numerous studies have shown that the more common forms of aggression (i.e., fighting) decline from childhood to adolescence (Lahey et al., 2000; Loeber et al., 2000; Tremblay, 2000). Most ODD behaviors emerge by the age of 6, but the majority of full-fledged CD behaviors usually do not appear before the age of 9–10 (Loeber, Green, Lahey, Christ, & Frick, 1992). DSM-IV specifies that CD may onset in children as young as 5 or 6 but usually onsets later. The question as to whether or not CD can be diagnosed in children younger than 5 has been a source of ongoing controversy (Moffitt et al., 2008).

Socioeconomic Status. Low socioeconomic status (SES) has also been associated with conduct problems in youth, as has low education, marital disruption, and urban residence (Loeber & Keenan, 1994; Nock et al., 2006). In one study, low SES was found in almost 60% of families of children with conduct disorders as opposed to about 24% of families with non-conduct disordered children (Loeber, Green, Keenan, & Lahey, 1995). Although DSM-IV specifies that the diagnosis of CD should not be made when behaviors are in reaction to the immediate social context, it is often hard to distinguish between internal dysfunction and external contextual factors (Loeber et al., 2000).

The exact nature of the association between conduct problems and SES remains a source of considerable debate. Researchers have found a direct relation with SES and specific conduct disorder symptoms, such as aggression (Loeber et al., 2000). Further, Lahey et al. (1995) suggest that SES is more reflective of other factors that give rise to conduct problems than it is a causal pathway in itself. In fact, low SES was related only to transient forms of antisocial behavior in the absence of other risk factors. As Frick (1998b) acknowledges, it is difficult to specifically identify which factors in a child's social ecology are related to the development of conduct problems. Children from families with low income may have an increased likelihood of exposure to high-crime neighborhoods, delinquent peers, parental stress and maladjustment, and reduced community and academic support. In many cases, low SES may serve as a risk factor for both parental dysfunction and child conduct problems, or, alternatively, as a consequence of parental dysfunction and a correlate of conduct problems. Additionally, Frick (1998b) asserts that wide variations found inside the same impoverished neighborhoods provide further evidence for the importance of other environmental and individual risk factors that exist within this context.

Comorbidity. The co-existence of conduct problems and other psychological conditions tends to be the rule rather than the exception (Ollendick, Jarrett, Grills-Taquechel, Seligman, & Wolff, 2008). Indeed, children with oppositional and conduct problems are at increased risk for manifesting a variety of other emotional and behavior disorders, including ADHD, anxiety, depression, and substance use. A meta-analysis of general population studies found that of those with ODD or CD, 3.1–41.0% had ADHD, 2.2–45.9% had depression, and 4.8–55.3% had a comorbid anxiety disorder (Angold, Costello, & Erkanli, 1999). More recently, the National Comorbidity Replication Survey found that of those with lifetime ODD, 92.4% meet criteria for at least one other lifetime *DSM-IV* disorder, including anxiety disorders (62.3%), substance use disorders (47.2%), mood disorders (45.8%), and ADHD (35.0% Nock et al., 2007). Similarly high rates of comorbidity have been reported for those with CD (Nock et al., 2006). In a clinic-referred sample, Greene et al. (2002) reported that over 80% of those diagnosed with a conduct problem disorder also had ADHD, approximately 50% met criteria for depression, and about 40% met criteria for an anxiety disorder. Thus, ODD and CD tend to co-occur with other childhood disorders at rates significantly greater than chance. The comorbidity of these disorders is an important factor to consider as it may have important ramifications for the onset, manifestation, and course of these disorders.

In comparison to youth with conduct problems alone, those with comorbid ADHD tend to be more deviant and aggressive, have an earlier onset of problem behavior, experience more peer rejection, and display greater persistence of social and academic difficulties (Abikoff & Klein, 1992; Lyman, 1998; Moffitt, 1990; van Lier, van der Ende, Koot, & Verhulst, 2007). Moreover, conduct problem children who exhibit comorbid hyperactivity and impulsivity are at greatest risk for chronic delinquency and recidivism, and it has been suggested that this comorbid presentation may be a premorbid indicator of adult psychopathy (Lyman, 1998).

The presentation and prognosis for children and adolescents with co-occurring conduct problems and internalizing disorders is somewhat less clear. For example, while many studies suggest that depression does not aggravate the severity of conduct problems (e.g., Ingoldsby, Kohl, McMahon, & Lengua, 2006), other studies reveal that suicidal ideation tends to be considerably higher in this comorbid group (Capaldi, 1992; Lewinsohn, Rohde, & Seeley, 1995). This comorbid group has also been shown to be more frequently angry and resentful, manifest more irritability, set more fires, have greater affiliation with antisocial peers and have more severe somatic complaints, anxiety, academic problems, and substance use (Capaldi, 1991, 1992; Ezpeleta, Domènech, & Angold, 2006; Fleming, Boyle, & Offord, 1993; Ingoldsby et al., 2006; Lewinsohn et al., 1995). Overall, the co-occurrence of these disorders has been shown to exacerbate emotional symptoms and functional impairment.

In terms of comorbid anxiety, many have suggested that significant levels of anxiety may serve as a protective factor against the development of conduct problems, while others have suggested that anxiety may exacerbate aggression (Loeber et al., 2000). In one study, Walker et al. (1991) found that this comorbid group had fewer police contacts, fewer school suspensions, and were rated as less aggressive by peers than children with conduct problems alone. However, others have shown that the overlap in these disorders escalates or magnifies the problems (e.g., Verhulst & van der Ende, 1993) or has no demonstrable effect whatsoever (Ollendick, Seligman, & Butcher, 1988). It has been suggested that different aspects or forms of anxiety may function in different ways such that some aspects ameliorate conduct problems and others exacerbate the manifestation of these problem behaviors. Along these lines, one study found that inhibition, but not withdrawal, served as a protective factor against delinquency while withdrawal was a risk factor for behavior problems (Kerr, Tremblay, Pagani, & Vitaro, 1997). Overall, however, studies of ODD or CD and comorbid internalizing disorders have yielded mixed results in terms of the clinical presentation of these youth.

Finally, high rates of substance use have been found in those with conduct problems. Epidemiological studies find that substance use among adolescents is more strongly associated with conduct problems than any other psychiatric disorder (Armstrong & Costello, 2002). Perhaps more importantly early use of alcohol has been found to exacerbate the course of conduct problems and accelerate the development of CD symptoms. For example, one study found that children aged 10–12 who used alcohol without parental permission had higher initial rates of CD symptoms and more rapid increases in symptoms (Johnson, Arria, Borges, Ialongo, & Anthony, 1995). Moreover, Loeber et al. (2002) found that repeated marijuana use in the adolescent years was the strongest predictor of the pathway from CD in adolescence to ASPD in adulthood.

In considering these comorbid conditions, it is important to reflect on the temporal ordering of conduct problems and other psychological conditions. Most often, the onset of ADHD occurs concurrently with aggression, and frequently before the age of 7. In contrast, anxiety disorders tend to have an earlier onset than conduct problems (Lahey & Loeber, 1994; Nock et al., 2007) whereas depression frequently follows the onset of conduct problems (Nock et al., 2007), and substance abuse tends to develop concurrently with conduct disorder in adolescence (Le Blanc & Loeber, 1998). Thus, the presence of conduct problems substantially increases the risk of developing a wide range of secondary conditions. The reasons for overlap in these disorders require further elucidation although several possibilities have been put forth. First, it is possible that conduct problems and other disorders have common causes including genetic vulnerability and psychosocial risk factors. Second, it is possible that conduct problems play a causal role in the development of subsequent disorders. Along these lines, it has been hypothesized that the progression of conduct problems into secondary disorders is related to the chain reaction of developmental failures experienced by these youths (Capaldi, 1991, 1992; Capaldi & Stoolmiller, 1999; Patterson, Reid, & Dishion, 1992). Specifically, the combination of lack of competence and negative reactions from others may result in pervasive failures in adaptation that subsequently contributes to a child's vulnerability to the onset of other psychiatric symptoms (Capaldi & Stoolmiller, 1999). For example, higher levels of conduct problems are associated with peer rejection, problems in the parent–child relationship, and failure to develop academic skills (e.g., Capaldi, 1991). Such consequences often affect social development, leading to negative attitudes and associations with deviant peers which may in turn contribute to depressed mood and substance use. Of course, the presence of these comorbid conditions may also exacerbate the course of conduct problems and it has been hypothesized that deficits in the domains of self-regulation and affective modulation (associated with both internalizing and externalizing disorders) may exacerbate aggressive behaviors (Greene & Doyle, 1999).

Still, research on the temporal ordering of these problems is not without its limitations as there are few longitudinal investigations of this topic and these studies have tended to cover a relatively brief period of time (Wolff & Ollendick, 2006). Moreover, studies of temporal ordering tend to focus on the onset of disorders without accounting for the emergence of early symptomatology. For example, a depressed child may begin to display temper outbursts, but may not meet full criteria for ODD. While the onset of a disorder serves as one marker of comorbidity, it may be useful for clinical purposes to consider co-occurring symptoms that subsequently develop into a second disorder. Research in this area has also failed to identify specific mechanisms for risk as well as moderators of this relationship. For example, severity of the initial disorder may be a primary predictor of which individuals subsequently develop a second disorder. Along these lines, Nock et al. (2006) found that conduct-disordered individuals with increased symptom number and severity were more likely to develop a second disorder. Further elucidation of such factors is needed.

Finally, it should be noted that while the risk of conduct problems in childhood for girls is lower than for boys, the risk for comorbidity for girls with conduct problems appears higher than for boys. Moreover, the severity of conduct problems in girls is exacerbated more than it is for boys when comorbid disorders are present (Loeber & Keenan, 1994). Still, when adolescent youth of either gender have a co-occurring disorder, the symptoms of each tend to be more severe and chronic, with poorer outcomes.

IMPLICATIONS FOR ASSESSMENT AND TREATMENT

The above review highlights the diverse and complex presentations of children and adolescents with conduct problems. The prevalence and nature of conduct problems have a high and enduring cost for children, their families, schools, communities, and society at large. Thus, the need for effective intervention programs is essential and a thorough comprehensive assessment is a critical first step in identifying factors that may serve to exacerbate or maintain these symptoms.

The primary areas to assess are child behavior, the context in which this behavior occurs, associated child characteristics and disorders, and familial or extra-familial (i.e., community, school) factors. To obtain this information, assessments should include multiple informants including the child, parent, teacher, and other relevant individuals. Multiple modalities should be used including the clinical interview, behavioral observations, situational analyses, behavior-rating scales, and cognitive or neuropsychological testing. Areas of focus include a history of the child's development (including temperament), academics, medical conditions, and previous treatment. Aspects of the child's social environment including parenting characteristics, parental stress, and marital discord as well as affiliations with deviant peers should be considered. Potential comorbid conditions and intellectual functioning should be evaluated and, finally, given the transactional nature of conduct problems, assessment of adult–child communication patterns and adults' reactions to, attributions about, and understanding of the child's difficulties would be crucial.

Following a thorough assessment of the factors that give rise to and maintain these disorders, a child's specific needs can be matched to a particular intervention that is best suited to address these deficits (Greene & Doyle, 1999). There are currently 16 empirically based treatments for disruptive behavior disorders (Eyberg, Nelson, & Boggs, 2008). Treatments for oppositional and conduct problems can be classified according to each treatment's focus on parent, child, or systemic characteristics (Nock, 2003). Subsequent chapters in this volume attest to the many effective interventions that have been developed and tested over the years. When these various treatments are matched to the multifaceted needs of a given child, parent, or group, the chances of successful outcomes are enhanced.

CASE STUDY

Many of the concepts reviewed in the present chapter can be illustrated in the case study of Michael, a 12-year-old boy who was brought to a community mental health clinic by his mother due to oppositionality, academic underachievement, fights at school, and recent suicidal ideation.

Michael lived with his biological mother, stepfather, and two siblings. The whereabouts of Michael's biological father were unknown, but his father reportedly had a history of substance abuse, affective lability, and criminal offenses. His mother had a history of depression. Michael's mother and stepfather reported high levels of stress related to working long hours on opposite shifts, financial strains, and difficulties related to parent–child conflict.

According to his mother, Michael had received psychological treatment since the age of 7 when she first noticed that he was hyperactive and had difficulty following through on tasks and completing school work. At that time, Michael reportedly often became oppositional when he was asked to complete work, failed to comply with his mother's requests, and he sometimes lied. He was prescribed stimulant medication to address his hyperactivity. An intellectual evaluation that was conducted when Michael was 9 revealed that his verbal intelligence was below average.

At the age of 12, Michael's oppositionality persisted. He refused to comply with his mother's requests, blamed others for his mistakes, and broke family rules. At school, Michael often had difficulty completing assignments and he was failing several subjects. His teachers indicated that Michael sometimes became overwhelmed when working on writing assignments which led to explosive outbursts. Michael had few friends and he was often teased by his peers. He was easily provoked and he sometimes retaliated with physical aggression. Michael often cried and he expressed some suicidal ideation although he had made no attempts. His mother was extremely frustrated with Michael's behavior and she was spending less time with him to avoid conflicts. His mother and stepfather often argued over the best way to handle Michael's behaviors. Behavior-rating scales (completed by Michael, his mother, and teacher) showed elevated oppositionality as well as the onset of some conduct problem behaviors including fighting, lying, and bullying. Following the assessment, Michael, his mother, and stepfather began attending therapy sessions to address his conduct problems and associated symptoms.

SUMMARY

Conduct problems represent a serious set of symptoms with significant personal and societal costs. The current chapter has presented major research developments that have been made in elucidating the complexity of these disorders and their associated characteristics. As discussed, diagnostic differences in ODD and CD have been well established and these disorders appear to be developmentally and hierarchically related. Research has also established factors which may be related to the onset, presentation, and stability of these disorders including age, gender, type of aggression, temperament, and comorbid conditions. The complex nature of conduct problems greatly impacts on both the assessment and treatment of this disorder. Identifying and achieving an understanding of such factors is essential to the development and implementation of effective prevention and intervention programs.

REFERENCES

Abikoff, H., & Klein, R. G. (1992). Attention-deficit hyperactivity disorder and conduct disorder: Comorbidity and implications for treatment. *Journal of Consulting and Clinical Psychology, 60,* 881–892.

American Psychiatric Association. (1980). *Diagnostic and statistical manual of mental disorders: Text revision* (3rd ed.). Washington, DC: American Psychiatric Press.

American Psychiatric Association. (2000). *Diagnostic and statistical manual of mental disorders: Text revision* (4th ed.). Washington, DC: American Psychiatric Press.

Angold, A., Costello, E. J., & Erkanli, A. (1999). Comorbidity. *Journal of Child Psychology and Psychiatry and Allied Disciplines, 40,* 57–87.

Armstrong, T. D., & Costello, E. J. (2002). Community studies on adolescent substance use, abuse, or dependence and psychiatric comorbidity. *Journal of Consulting and Clinical Psychology, 70,* 1224–1239.

Biederman, J., Faraone, S. V., Mick, E., Wozniak, J., Chen, L., Ouellette, C., et al. (1996). Attention-deficit hyperactivity disorder and juvenile mania: An overlooked comorbidity? *Journal of the American Academy of Child and Adolescent Psychiatry, 35,* 997–1008.

Capaldi, D. (1991). Co-occurrence of conduct problems and depressive symptoms in early adolescent boys: I. Familial factors and general adjustment at Grade 6. *Development and Psychopathology, 3,* 277–300.

Capaldi, D. (1992). Co-occurrence of conduct problems and depressive symptoms in early adolescent boys: II. A 2-year follow-up at Grade 8. *Development and Psychopathology, 4,* 125–144.

Capaldi, D., & Stoolmiller, M. (1999). Co-occurrence of conduct problems and depressive symptoms in early adolescent boys: III. Prediction to young-adult adjustment. *Development and Psychopathology, 11,* 59–84.

Cohen, M. A. (1998). The monetary value of saving a high-risk youth. *Journal of Quantitative Criminology, 14,* 5–33.

Cohen, P., Cohen, J., Kasen, S., Velez, C. N., Hartmark, C., Johnson, J., et al. (1993). An epidemiological study of disorders in late adolescence: I. Age- and gender-specific prevalence. *Journal of Child Psychology and Psychiatry, 6,* 851–867.

Coie, J. D., Dodge, K. A., Terry, R., & Wright, V. (1991). The role of aggression in peer relations: An analysis of aggression episodes in boy's play groups. *Child Development, 62,* 812–826.

Crick, N. R., & Dodge, K. A. (1996). Social information-processing mechanisms in reactive and proactive aggression. *Child Development, 67,* 993–1002.

Dodge, K. A., & Coie, J. D. (1987). Social information processing factors in reactive and proactive aggression in children's peer groups. *Journal of Personality and Social Psychology, 53,* 1146–1158.

Dodge, K. A., Lochman, J. E., Harnish, J. D., Bates, J. E., & Pettit, G. S. (1997). Reactive and proactive aggression in school children and psychiatrically impaired chronically assaultive youth. *Journal of Abnormal Psychology, 106,* 37–51.

Eyberg, S. M., Nelson, M. M., & Boggs, S. R. (2008). Evidence-based psychosocial treatments for children and adolescents with disruptive behavior. *Journal of Clinical Child and Adolescent Psychology, 37,* 215–237.

Ezpeleta, L., Domènech, J., & Angold, A. (2006). A comparison of pure and comorbid CD/ODD and depression. *Journal of Child Psychology and Psychiatry, 47,* 704–712.

Fergusson, D. M., & Horwood, L. J. (1996). The role of adolescent peer affiliations in the continuity between childhood behavioral adjustment and juvenile offending. *Journal of Abnormal Child Psychology, 24,* 205–221.

Fleming, J. E., Boyle, M. H., & Offord, D. R. (1993). The outcome of adolescent depression in the Ontario Child Health Study follow-up. *Journal of the American Academy of Child and Adolescent Psychiatry, 32,* 28–33.

Frick, P. J. (1998a). Conduct Disorders. In T. H. Ollendick & M. Hersen (Eds.), *Handbook of child psychopathology* (3rd ed., pp. 213–238). New York: Plenum.

Frick, P. J. (1998b). *Conduct disorders and severe antisocial behavior.* New York: Plenum.

Frick, P. J., O'Brien, B. S., Wootton, J. M., & McBurnett, K. (1994). Psychopathy and conduct problems in children. *Journal of Abnormal Psychology, 103*, 700–707.

Frick, P., & White, S. (2008). The importance of callous-unemotional traits for developmental models of aggressive and antisocial behavior. *Journal of Child Psychology and Psychiatry, 49*, 359–375.

Greene, R., Ablon, J., Monuteaux, M., Goring, J., Henin, A., Raezer, L., et al. (2004). Effectiveness of collaborative problem solving in affectively dysregulated youth with oppositional defiant disorder: Initial findings. *Journal of Consulting and Clinical Psychology, 72*, 1157–1164.

Greene, R., Biederman, J., Zerwas, S., Monuteaux, M., Goring, J. C., & Faraone, S. (2002). Psychiatric comorbidity, family dysfunction, and social impairment in referred youth with oppositional defiant disorder. *American Journal of Psychiatry, 159*, 1214–1224.

Greene, R. W., & Doyle, A. E. (1999). Toward a transactional conceptualization of oppositional defiant disorder: Implications for assessment and treatment. *Clinical Child and Family Psychology Review, 2*, 129–148.

Hawes, D., & Dadds, M. (2005). The treatment of conduct problems in children with callous-unemotional traits. *Journal of Consulting and Clinical Psychology*, 73, 737–741.

Hinshaw, S., Lahey, B., & Hart, E. (1993). Issues of taxonomy and comorbidity in the development of conduct disorder. *Development and Psychopathology, 5*, 31–49.

Hubbard, J. A., Smithmyer, C. M., Ramsden, S. R., Parker, E. H., Flanagan, K. D., Dearing, K. F., et al. (2002). Observational, physiological, and self-report measures of children's anger: Relations to reactive versus proactive aggression. *Child Development, 73*, 1101–1118.

Ingoldsby, E. M., Kohl, G. O., McMahon, R. J., & Lengua, L. (2006). Conduct problems, depressive symptomatology and their co-occurring presentation in childhood as predictors of adjustment in early adolescence. *Journal of Abnormal Child Psychology, 34*, 603–621.

Johnson, E., Arria, A., Borges, G., Ialongo, N., & Anthony, J. (1995). The growth of conduct problem behaviors from middle childhood to early adolescence: Sex differences and the suspected influence of early alcohol use. *Journal of Studies on Alcohol, 56*, 661–671.

Kagan, J., & Snidman, N. (1991). Infant predictors of inhibited and uninhibited profiles. *Psychological Science, 2*, 40–44.

Keenan, K., Loeber, R., & Green, S. (1999). Conduct disorder in girls: A review of the literature. *Clinical Child & Family Psychology Review, 2*, 3–19.

Keenan, K., & Shaw, D. (1997). Developmental and social influences on young girls' early problem behavior. *Psychological Bulletin, 121*, 95–113.

Kerr, M., Tremblay, R., Pagain, L., & Vitaro, F. (1997). Boys' behavioral inhibition and the risk of later delinquency. *Archives of General Psychiatry, 54*, 809–816.

Lahey, B. B., & Loeber, R. (1994). Framework for a developmental model of oppositional defiant disorder and conduct disorder. In D. K. Routh (Ed.), *Disruptive behavior disorders in childhood*. New York: Plenum.

Lahey, B., Loeber, R., Hart, E., Frick, P., Applegate, B., Zhang, Q., et al. (1995). Four-year longitudinal study of conduct disorder in boys: Patterns and predictors of persistence. *Journal of Abnormal Psychology, 104*, 83–93.

Lahey, B. B., Loeber, R., Quay, H. C., Frick, P. J., & Grimm, J. (1997). Oppositional defiant disorder and conduct disorder. In T. A. Widiger, A. J. Frances, H. A. Pincus, R. Ross, M. B. First, & W. Davis (Eds.), *DSM-IV sourcebook* (Vol. 3, pp. 189–209). Washington, DC: American Psychiatric Association.

Lahey, B., Schwab-Stone, M., Goodman, S., Waldman, I., Canino, G., Rathouz, P., et al. (2000). Age and gender differences in oppositional behavior and conduct problems: A cross-sectional study of middle childhood and adolescence. *Journal of Abnormal Psychology, 109*, 488–503.

Lahey, B. B., Waldman, I. D., & McBurnett, K. (1999). Annotation: The development of antisocial behavior: An integrative causal model. *Journal of Child Psychology and Psychiatry, 40*, 669–682.

Langbehn, D. R., Cadoret, R. J., Yates, W. R., Troughton, E. P., & Stewart, M. A. (1998). Distinct contributions of conduct and oppositional defiant symptoms to adult antisocial behavior. *Archives of General Psychiatry, 55*, 821–829.

Larson, H., Andershed, H., & Lichtenstein, P. (2006). A genetic factor explains most of the variation in the psychopathic personality. *Journal of Abnormal Psychology, 115*, 221–230.

Le Blanc, M., & Loeber, R. (1998). Developmental Criminology Updated. In M. Tonry (Ed.), *Crime and justice: A review of research, 23* (pp. 115–198). Chicago, IL: The University of Chicago Press.

Lewin, L. M., Davis, B., & Hops, H. (1999). Childhood social predictors of adolescent antisocial behavior: Gender differences in predictive accuracy and efficacy. *Journal of Abnormal Child Psychology, 27*, 277–292.

Lewinsohn, P. M., Rohde, P., & Seeley, J. R. (1995). Adolescent psychopathology: III. The clinical consequences of comorbidity. *Journal of the American Academy of Child and Adolescent Psychiatry, 34*, 510–519.

Loeber, R. (1990). Development and risk factors of juvenile antisocial behavior and delinquency. *Clinical Psychology Review, 10*, 1–41.

Loeber, R., Burke, J. D., & Lahey, B. B. (2002). What are the adolescent antecedents to antisocial personality disorder? *Criminal Behavior and Mental Health, 12*, 24–36.

Loeber, R., Burke, J., Lahey, B., Winters, A., & Zera, M. (2000). Oppositional defiant disorder and conduct disorder: A review of the past 10 years, Part I. *Journal of the American Academy of Child and Adolescent Psychiatry, 39*, 1468–1484.

Loeber, R., Green, S. M., Lahey, B. B., Christ, M. A. G., & Frick, P. J. (1992). Developmental sequences in the age of onset of disruptive child behaviors. *Journal of Child and Family Studies, 1*, 21–41.

Loeber, R., & Keenan, K. (1994). Interaction between conduct disorder and its comorbid conditions: Effects of age and gender. *Clinical Psyc Review, 14*(6), 497–523.

Lyman, D. R. (1998). Early identification of the fledgling psychopath: Locating the psychopathic child in the current nomenclature. *Journal of Abnormal Psychology, 107*, 566–575.

Lynam, D. R. (1996). Early identification of chronic offenders: Who is the fledgling psychopath? *Psychological Bulletin, 120*, 209–234.

Maughan, B., Rowe, R., Messer, J., Goodman, R., & Meltzer, H. (2004). Conduct disorder and oppositional defiant disorder in a national sample: Developmental epidemiology. *Journal of Child Psychology and Psychiatry, 45*, 609–621.

Moffitt, T. E. (1990). The neuropsychology of delinquency: A critical review of theory and research. In N. Morris & M. Tonry (Eds.), *Crime and justice Vol. 12* (pp. 99–169). Chicago, IL: The University of Chicago Press.

Moffitt, T., Arseneault, L., Jaffee, S., Kim-Cohen, J., Koenen, K., Odgers, C., et al. (2008). DSM-V conduct disorder: Research needs for an evidence base. *Journal of Child Psychology and Psychiatry, 49*, 3–33.

Moffitt, T. E., Caspi, A., Dickson, N., Silva, P., & Stanton, W. (1996). Childhood-onset versus adolescent-onset antisocial conduct problems in males: Natural history from ages 3–18 years. *Development and Psychopathology, 8*, 399–424.

Nock, M. (2003). Progress review of the psychosocial treatment of child conduct problems. *Clinical Psychology: Science and Practice, 10*, 1–28.

Nock, M., Kazdin, A., Hiripi, E., & Kessler, R. C. (2007). Lifetime prevalence, correlates and persistence of oppositional defiant disorder: Results from the National Comorbidity Survey Replication. *Journal of Child Psychology and Psychiatry, 48*, 703–713.

Nock, M., Kazdin, A., Hirpi, E., & Kessler, R. (2006). Prevalence, subtypes, and correlates of DSM-IV conduct disorder in the National Comorbidity Survey Replication. *Psychological Medicine, 36*, 699–710.

Ollendick, T. H., Jarrett, M. A., Grills-Taquechel, A. E., Hovey, L. D., & Wolff, J. (2008). Comorbidity as a predictor and moderator of treatment outcome in youth with anxiety, affective, AD/HD, and oppositional/conduct disorders. *Clinical Psychology Review, 28*, 1447–1471.

Ollendick, T. H., Jarrett, M. A., Wolff, J. C., & Scarpa, A. (2009). Reactive and proactive aggression: Cross-informant agreement and incremental validity. *Journal of Psychopathology and Behavioral Assessment, 31*, 51–59.

Ollendick, T. H., Seligman, L. D., & Butcher, T. (1999). Does anxiety mitigate the behavioral expression of severe conduct disorder in delinquent youths? *Journal of Anxiety Disorders, 13*, 565–574.

Patterson, G. R., Reid, J. B., & Dishion, T. J. (1992). *Antisocial boys*. Patterson, OR: Castalia.

Polman, H., Orobiao de Castro, B., Koops, W., van Boxtel, H. W., & Merk, W. W. (2007). A meta-analysis of the distinction between reactive and proactive aggression in children and adolescents. *Journal of Abnormal Child Psychology, 35*(4), 522–535.

Poulin, F., & Boivin, M. (2000). Reactive and proactive aggression: Evidence of a two-factor model. *Psychological Assessment, 12*, 115–122.

Price, K. F., & Dodge, K. A. (1989). Reactive and proactive aggression in childhood: Relations to peer status and social context dimensions. *Journal of Abnormal Child Psychology, 17*, 455–471.

Rowe, R., Maughan, B., Costella, E., & Angold, A. (2005). Defining oppositional defiant disorder. *Journal of Child Psychology and Psychiatry, 46*, 1309–1316.

Steiner, H., Dunne, J. E., Ayres, W., Arnold, V., Benedek, E., Benson, R. S., et al. (1997). Practice parameters for the assessment and treatment of children and adolescents with conduct disorder. *Journal of the American Academy of Child and Adolescent Psychiatry, 36*, 122–140.

Tremblay, R. E. (2000). The development of aggressive behavior during childhood: What have we learned in the past century? *International Journal of Behavioral Development, 24*, 129–141.

Van Lier, P., van der Ende, J., Koot, H., & Verhulst, F. (2007). Which better predicts conduct problems? The relationship of trajectories of Conduct Problems, with ODD and ADHD. *Journal of Child Psychology and Psychiatry, 48*, 601–608.

Verhulst, F., & van der Ende, J. (1993). "Comorbidity" in an epidemiological sample: A longitudinal perspective. *Journal of Child Psychology and Psychiatry, 34*, 767–783.

Vitiello, B., & Stoff, D. M. (1997). Subtypes of aggression and their relevance to child psychiatry. *Journal of the American Academy of Child and Adolescent Psychiatry, 36*, 307–315.

Walker, J. L., Lahey, B. B., Russo, M. F., Frick, P. J., Christ, M. A. G., McBurnett, K., et al. (1991). Anxiety, inhibition, and conduct disorder in children: I. Relations to social impairment. *Journal of the American Academy of Child and Adolescent Psychiatry, 30*, 187–191.

Waschbusch, D. A., Willoughby, M. T., & Pelham, W. E. (1998). Criterion validity and the utility of reactive and proactive aggression; Comparisons to attention deficit hyperactivity disorder, oppositional defiant disorder, conduct disorder, and other measures of functioning. *Journal of Clinical Child Psychology, 27*(4), 396–405.

Wolff, J. C., Greene, R. W., & Ollendick, T. H. (2008). Differential responses of children with varying degrees of reactive and proactive aggression to two forms of psychosocial treatment. *Child and Family Behavior Therapy, 30*, 37–50.

Wolff, J. C., & Ollendick, T. H. (2006). The comorbidity of conduct problems and depression in childhood and adolescence. *Clinical Child and Family Psychology Review, 9*, 201–220.

2

Conduct Problems in Youth: Sociological Perspectives

DONALD J. SHOEMAKER

INTRODUCTION

Within the field of sociology, conduct problems are often described in terms of *juvenile delinquency*. Juvenile delinquency is a legal term with social implications. Often, delinquent behavior represents an effort of a youth to handle a difficult situation in his or her life, but with behavior which has been proscribed by legislative action. Most legal definitions of delinquency include at least two concepts: (a) the commission of criminal behavior by youth; and (b) the commission of behavior which is unlawful for youth but not for adults. These latter offenses are termed *status offenses* (Shoemaker, 2009). Thus, juveniles can commit actions which would be a crime for anyone to commit, as well as behaviors which are prohibited solely because of underage status. Typically, the age of majority for establishing delinquency is age 18. The age of majority means when one becomes an adult in terms of legal responsibilities; that is, when one is legally an adult. One important benefit as a legal adult is the right to vote. Within this chapter, general patterns of crime and delinquency will sometimes be referred to as *criminality*. Studies of delinquency from sociological perspectives may include both formal assessments of delinquency, as represented by police, court, and institutional data, as well as informal accounts of delinquency, which include observational and self-report data.

Sociological explanations of behavior are typically classified as *macro* or *micro*. In both examples, an important goal is the understanding of patterns of behavior among people in different settings and from different backgrounds. That is, a sociological perspective attempts to identify and

---

DONALD J. SHOEMAKER • Virginia Tech

R.C. Murrihy et al. (eds.), *Clinical Handbook of Assessing and Treating Conduct Problems in Youth*, DOI 10.1007/978-1-4419-6297-3_2,

explain social order and disorder (Inkeles, 1964). A major interest is the explanation of how societies and social processes within societies are arranged or ordered, and how they may change, or become disordered. At first glance, social disorder may seem the proper focus of explanations of criminality, and indeed, there is much interest in the disordered nature of social behavior in the study of crime and delinquency. However, sociological observations of criminality also clearly indicate that there is *order* within the seemingly disordered expressions of crime and delinquency. Patterns of criminality often display logic and order among offenders, even if these are not consistent with the general patterns of logic and behavior established within "normal" components of society.

Macro-level theories focus on the rates of behavior as these are expressed across larger collectivities, such as communities or societies. One issue of interest to macro theories of criminality, for example, would be the differential distribution of crime rates between or among societies or between communities within a society. Micro explanations concentrate on individual behavior but from a societal or environmental point of view. Thus, micro-level explanations are also termed social psychological. Micro approaches to an understanding of crime or delinquency examine the impact on criminality of an individual's characteristics and attitudes as these are affected by social groups or environmental conditions. For example, a micro-level explanation of delinquency would examine not only how one's attitudes are related to crime and delinquency, but also how these attitudes are influenced by different social situations or across differing personal characteristics of individuals, such as race and ethnicity, age, or gender. The purpose of this chapter is to present a discussion of several sociological explanations of delinquency. Thus, the objective is to acquaint the reader with basic sociological explanations of crime and delinquency, including their assumptions and interpretations for youth. However, the comparative validity of these explanations, or their overall utility as explanations of delinquency, as well as policy implications of the explanations, will not be pursued in this chapter. Such would require a volume to do so (see Shoemaker, 2009). In addition, the discussion of sociological approaches to an understanding of delinquency will be presented from an historical perspective. Theories will be discussed as they originally developed and in terms of modifications and alterations over time.

BRIEF HISTORICAL BACKGROUND

Explanations of crime did not differentiate juveniles from adults until the early nineteenth century. Historically, juveniles were viewed as miniature adults (Aries, 1962; Grossberg, 2002). Early religious authority and English Common Law established criminal responsibility at the age of 7, and this age was adopted by most jurisdictions in the United States (Kerper, 1972; Postman, 1982). The use of the term, "delinquency," was not common until the end of the nineteenth century, when the first delinquency law was created in 1899 in the United States (Tanenhaus, 2002). While certainly juveniles have been misbehaving and otherwise creating problems for their elders and society for untold hundreds, and probably thousands, of years (Sanders, 1970), they were not legally referred to as "delinquents" until the passage of delinquency laws. In colonial times, for example, such children were often labeled as "stubborn" (Sutton, 1988).

Child reformers in the nineteenth century often associated juvenile misbehavior with one of two conditions: (a) criminogenic forces emanating from urban living conditions; and (b) parents who were unable to instruct and/or control their children (Grossberg, 2002; Tanenhaus, 2002). Often, and unfortunately, youth who were placed in institutions for juvenile corrections were sons and daughters of immigrant families who were thought to be living unrestricted lives in the streets of large cities. An illustration of this conceptualization is evident in the "orphan trains" of the mid-late nineteenth century. Orphan trains were literally trains which were used to transport miscreant youth from large urban areas, such as New York City, to families living in Midwestern states, such as Kansas or Nebraska. The person often associated with developing the notion of orphan trains was Charles Loring Brace, who founded the Children's Aid Society in New York in 1853. Although the supposed purpose of orphan trains was the rehabilitation of wayward urban youth, Brace's view of these children was not always favorable. It is argued he developed the phrase, "dangerous classes," to refer to these youth, along with the prediction that if they were not carted off somewhere for special attention and treatment; that is, "orphaned" to host families sometimes thousands of miles away in Midwestern towns, the result would be chaos and destruction for the people of New York and, presumably, other large cities (Grossberg, 2002).

In the United States, the number of delinquents has been declining since the 1990s. For example, the number of youth arrested in 2006 was approximately 24% lower than the number arrested in 1997. In addition, the number of youth confined in juvenile correctional facilities declined from 116,701 in 1997 to 109,225 in 2003 (Shoemaker, 2009).

Worldwide, rates of delinquency have also been declining or holding steady since the 1990s, although this decline is certainly not universal (Hartjen, 2008; Junger-Tas & Decker, 2006). In Japan, for example, juvenile crime increased from the mid 1946 to the early 1980s, but has been declining since that time (Elrod & Yokoyama, 2006). On the other hand, delinquency is thought to be increasing in Turkey (Atasoy, Baskan, & Ziyalar, 2006).

In some countries, increases in juvenile crime and delinquency may be attributed to increasing industrialization and significant socio-economic and political changes. However, in countries such as Japan, which has experienced significant industrial growth since World War II, the rate of delinquency has declined. Thus, it is difficult to explain historical trends and variations in delinquency across nationalities with a single explanation. The following discussion will focus on theoretical explanations of youth crime and delinquency informed by sociological conceptualization, rather than particular analyses of trends and variations of delinquency within any country.

MACRO SOCIOLOGICAL VIEWS OF DELINQUENCY

The early conceptions of delinquency identified above were decidedly sociological in nature. However, at that time, there were no sound sociological theories or principles to guide the development of these views. In their place, many biological and psychological explanations of delinquency surfaced and became popular in the latter part of the nineteenth century and into the first decade or two of the twentieth century. Some suggest that the creation of the juvenile courts and the further development of juvenile justice institutions were supported largely by individualistic views of delinquency, especially from a psychological perspective. As one social historian has noted, by the beginning of the 1920s, the juvenile court "idea" had been clearly established, along with a set of procedures and practices, such as probation and private records, and individual or clinical treatment (Tanenhaus, 2002).

Social Disorganization

One of the earliest sociological explanations of delinquency is named *social disorganization* theory. Basically, this explanation of delinquency focuses on the lack of community integration and stability as an important contributor to delinquency. The theory was developed by Clifford Shaw (one of the first probation officers in the United States), Henry McKay et al. (1929), and then refined in 1969 (Shaw & McKay, 1942, 1969). Although this explanation concentrated on gang delinquency, its scope can be applied to most forms of delinquent behavior. The theory of social disorganization offers a clear contrast to the personalized view of delinquency causation popular at that time, as indicated earlier. Shaw noted that many of the youngsters he supervised seemed to come from the same areas or neighborhoods, even after several years. Later, Shaw and McKay (1969) noted that patterns of delinquency seemed to occur regularly in some neighborhoods, "backward in time in an unbroken continuity" (p. 175).

An interesting feature of Shaw and McKay's studies of delinquency is the use of areas of residence as a key indication of both disorganization and delinquency. Social and economic features of a neighborhood, or area, were used to identify areas as disorganized. Similarly, rates of delinquency were developed based on where juveniles *lived*, not where their offenses occurred. This perspective clearly separated the social disorganization perspective from individualistic views of delinquency. The concept of social disorganization basically suggests that social control, both formal and informal, have been weakened, making it difficult for residents to solve problems, such as delinquency (Shoemaker, 2005; Thomas & Znaniecki, 1927). Formal social control is exemplified by the presence of police officers, while informal social control is often associated with supervision and control exercised by parents, neighbors, and institutional representatives in the community, such as teachers, ministers, and others.

Another feature of the studies of Shaw and McKay was the use of mapping to chart and analyze delinquency patterns. Utilizing previous depictions of growth patterns in Chicago, Robert Park and Ernest Burgess

(Park, Burgess, & McKenzie, 1925) analyzed delinquency by two-mile *concentric zones*. According to the concentric zone pattern of Chicago's growth, there were five zones: Zone I, or the central business district; Zone II, or the zone in transition; Zone III, or the zone of working-class homes; Zone IV, the zone of single-family and residences and upscale apartments; and Zone V, or the suburban zone.

One of the more common findings of Shaw and McKay's research was the pattern of delinquency by residential zones. Data from 1900 through the 1930s in Chicago consistently documented the regular decline in the percentage of males aged 10–16 petitioned (or referred) to juvenile court (as well as juveniles found in police and juvenile institutional records), from Zone 1 to Zone 5. Moreover, within zones with high rates of delinquency, especially Zones I and II, there were identified high *delinquency areas*. Often, these areas were found near sections of the city which had industrial and business activities (Shaw & McKay, 1969). Subsequent research, using samples of males and females and in cities other than Chicago, continued to support the conclusion that residential patterns of delinquency declined from the center of the city outward to its suburbs, although not all of this research used the concentric zone method of depicting city growth (Shaw & McKay, 1969).

In addition to displaying high rates of crime and delinquency, these areas also were characterized by high rates of mental illness, tuberculosis, and other "community problems" (Shaw & McKay, 1969). In addition, and perhaps most telling of all, the authors noted that the areas of the city which had the highest rates of crime and delinquency, especially from 1900 to 1933, also experienced a rapid turnover of the ethnic and racial composition of the population. Specifically, they observed that these areas went from predominantly English–Scotch, German and Irish populations in the early 1900s, to Polish and Italian by the 1920s, with African–American arriving in the 1930s (Shaw & McKay, 1969). This finding led Shaw and McKay to suggest that community-based problems, namely areas characterized by social disorganization, were responsible for consistently high rates of crime and delinquency, as opposed to cultural factors expressed through specific racial and ethnic composition.

Contemporary studies of social disorganization often attribute crime and delinquency to the lack of *collective efficacy*. Collective efficacy refers to the notion that people in a neighborhood share common concerns and expectations of neighbors' behavior, in particular the behavior of youth, and that they are willing to support each other in supervising and attempting to control youthful misbehavior (Sampson, 2006; Sampson et al., 1997; Sampson et al., 1999). Thus, areas of a community which are characterized by collective *inefficacy* are also representative of *social disorganization*; namely, the difficulty of area residents to identify and solve issues and problems in their neighborhoods and communities (Sampson, 2006).

In addition, contemporary conceptualizations of social disorganization incorporate the concept of *social capital* into their analyses. Social capital essentially refers to the collection of social ties or networks in a community or residential area. The closer or denser the social ties, the more social capital is thought to exist. The presence of social capital, or extensive and deep social networks, in turn, is thought to reduce the level of crime and delinquency in a neighborhood (Bursik, 1999; Coleman, 1988; Putnam, 2000; Sampson, 2006).

As noted, Shaw and McKay's studies indicated that high rates of delinquency persisted in certain areas or neighborhoods despite racial and ethnic turnover in those areas. This prompted them to suggest that conditions of the area, namely social disorganization, contributed significantly to patterns of delinquency. In contrast, other investigators have suggested that cultural factors are influential in the explanation of delinquency. Cultural values and norms can affect whether one is likely to engage in criminality. For example, some have observed that cultures which stress family ties and behavior which brings honor to one's family tend to have lower rates of crime and delinquency than do other societies (Braithwaite, 1989; Chambliss, 1974).

Others have proposed that *culture conflict* can create tensions and confusion which can contribute to criminality (Sellin, 1938). The theory of culture conflict and criminality argues that disagreements, or conflicts, between cultural conduct norms, or laws in many cases, can create confusion and anguish in people who have emigrated from one country to another. In most countries, it has been assumed that immigrants are often socially and politically less powerful than those representing the host country. Consequently, immigrants struggling to assimilate to the host country's cultural norms may express cultural conflicts in terms of crime and delinquency.

Research on this theory suggests that first-generation immigrants are somewhat insulated from the pressures and conflicts of different cultures. Perhaps this insulation derives from immigrants living in cultural enclaves where they receive support and assistance from those of the same ethnic background who have been in the host country for a longer period of time and have become more acculturated into the receiving country. However, it is with the second-generation immigrants, particularly the youth that behavioral problems resulting from cultural conflicts begin to appear in significant numbers. Second-generation youth reflect the conflicts between the customs and language of their parents, representing the immigrant country as well as the norms and values and language of the host country, primarily represented in the school and social groups (Hagan, Levi, & Dinovitzer, 2008; Sellin, 1938; Sheu, 1986; Shoemaker, 1995; Wong, 1997). However, studies clearly indicate that although second-generation immigrants have higher rates of crime and delinquency compared to their parents, their involvement in delinquency is lower than comparable populations of native-born youth. Thus, immigration *per se* does not contribute significantly to crime. Rather, the more likely contribution to crime among immigrant youth results from the experiences of subsequent-generation immigrants, experiences such as culture conflict as well as negative experiences from the process of cultural assimilation, including discrimination against immigrants (Hagan et al., 2008).

Anomie

Another macro level theory of crime and delinquency is based on the concept of *anomie*. Earlier discussions of anomie as a condition of society are often credited to a sociologist named Emile Durkheim. Durkheim noted that during times of social and economic change, societies go through transformations of their organizational states, particularly in regard to their division of labor. In a simpler state of organization, or mechanical solidarity, Durkheim posited that the division of labor was simple and people tended to interact on the basis of similarities and commonalities in terms of values and behavioral norms. As societies grow and become more complex, their organizational states and division of labor become more complex. This state of organization is called organic solidarity and it is characterized in part by interactions based on interdependence and mutual needs. During these periods of growth, societies can lose the ability to meet the needs and expectations of their people. In a sense, a state of "normlessness" develops. Expectations concerning goals and aspirations and behavioral expectations become less clear. This state of uncertainty and frustration is known as anomie. In advanced, organic societies, anomie can occur as the result of sudden and/or major changes in the society, such as major shifts in the economy. Although anomie is a condition of society, its consequences are often discussed in individual terms. Increased numbers of people commit suicide during times of economic crises and uncertainty (Durkheim, 1933, 1951; Vold et al., 2002).

Durkheim's ideas concerning crime, anomie, and social change have been examined in contemporary times in connection with the impact of modernization on crime rates. Much research supports the general conclusion that crime increases with modernization. However, this trend is most notable for property crimes, not violent crimes. Rather, if there is any trend regarding the connection between modernization and violent crime, it is that violent crimes *decline* with modernization (Shelley, 1989; Vold et al., 2002).

Durkheim's notions of crime and anomie, and the studies examining the relationship between crime and modernization, focused on society in general. However, a few decades after Durkheim, Robert Merton, proposed another sociological view of anomie. This newer interpretation of anomie and crime focused not just on crime, but on patterns of deviant behavior in general. In addition, this newer conceptualization of anomie addressed attention to the impact of anomie on crime and deviance primarily among those in the *lower social* class (Merton, 1957). Merton defined anomie as the structured, or more permanent, tension or strain, between achieving highly valued cultural goals and the availability of legitimate means for achieving those goals. For this reason, his theory is often called a means–end theory or a strain theory. For Merton, society, particularly American society, promotes economic success above other possible definitions of accomplishment. For the most part, individuals gain economic success through educational achievement and/or business acumen. For those who have less access to these legitimate avenues for success, other, more deviant or criminal pathways, are more likely to be chosen. When the pressures to succeed become too great in the mind of the individual, crime and/or deviance is more likely to result. As Merton put it, "It is only when a system of cultural values extols, virtually above all else, certain *common* success-goals *for the population at large* while the social structure rigorously restricts or completely closes access to approved modes of reaching these goals *for a considerable part of the same population*, that deviant behavior ensues on a large scale" (Merton, 1957, p. 146).

Based upon these notions, Merton constructed a theoretical series of five possible options, or responses, an individual may make to this situation of structured strain, or anomie. Each option is expressed in terms of accepting or rejecting the cultural value of economic success and the legitimate means of achieving this success. These are options, not individual expressions of personality, and they can change and/or be combined in a lifetime. The first option is considered the most common, and it is called *conformity*. Conformity results in accepting both the goal of success and legitimate means of achieving it. The next four responses are either criminal or deviant. *Innovation* involves accepting the goal of success but rejecting legitimate avenues for achieving success. This adaptation is more clearly connected with crime and delinquency, such as theft. *Ritualism* involves rejecting the goal of success, but accepting the means – a kind of deviant response often found among bureaucratic workers and primarily those in the lower middle class. To Merton, the least common response is *retreatism*, or dropping out of society. This response involves rejecting both means and goals. It may be exemplified by heavy drug use or addiction. The final response is *rebellion*, which involves not only rejecting means and goals but the desire to substitute new means and goals in their place (Merton, 1957). The essence of Merton's means–end or anomic theory of crime and deviance is that social and cultural structures are largely responsible for the creation of factors that may lead to crime. Merton clearly recognized that individual responses or adaptations to this structural situation played a major role in the actual commission of criminal behavior. This recognition is exemplified in the notion that the most common adaptation to anomie is conformity. Nonetheless, this explanation of criminality is considered more structural, or macro level, than individual, or micro level.

Others have offered refinements or modifications of this theory to further clarify the structural roots of crime and delinquency. For example, Richard Cloward (1959) argued that the availability of illegitimate means of success was not evenly distributed in society. Thus, those individuals facing the prospect of not having legitimate means for achieving success may not always be able to prevail on illegitimate means of success. Wanting to make money by selling drugs or robbing banks, for example, may be what one desires, but being able to accomplish these criminal tasks with any degree of success may not be possible for just anyone.

Another extension of this theory focuses on the institutionalized and pervasive influence economic success has had on American society, and the pursuit of "the American Dream," or the achievement of economic and material success through individual competition and abilities (Messner & Rosenfeld, 2001). Messner and Rosenfeld argue that this goal is emphasized in the basic fabric of American society, and promoted in institutions such as the family and schools. In addition, they argue that economic institutions dominate other institutions in society. Economic concerns, for example, often influence the daily schedules of families. Schools exist primarily to support the job market. Schools depend on the economic system for their operations. Although not specified by Messner and Rosenfeld, school schedules can also be influenced by the job market, as when schools modify opening and closing dates to accommodate summer job opportunities for students. When the economic institution contributes to criminal incentives, the entire society is affected. Thus, what Merton offered as an example of an anomic situation, which could promote crime and deviance (i.e., economic success for everyone), has been refashioned by Messner and Rosenfeld into an endemic criminogenic factor which has become a basic part of society, "a society organized for crime" (p. 1).

Both anomic explanations of crime have tended to focus on adult patterns of criminality, rather than juvenile crime. Theoretically, anomie can be used to explain crime among people of any age. The nature of the arguments, however, seems to address the experiences of adults, more so than juveniles. Nonetheless, there have been a couple of attempts to focus the issues of anomie theory on juveniles. In particular, researchers have adopted Merton's strain theory of anomie to juveniles, especially juvenile gangs or subcultures.

One of these efforts follows up on the argument that the distribution of access to illegitimate means of achieving success is not evenly distributed in society (Cloward & Ohlin, 1960). This view of gang delinquency maintains that gangs are primarily composed of youth from working and lower-class backgrounds. As such, these youth are exposed to the same pressures or strains to commit crime as are their adult counterparts. The assumption of this view is that youth aspire to gain economic success, as Merton suggested. Thus, the ultimate goal is to become economically successful. However, the particular expression of criminal activity depends upon the structure of the neighborhood in which a youth lives. In areas where there is the presence of adult criminal role models, specifically organized criminal activity, a *criminal gang* tends to emerge. This type of gang is focused on property crime. In neighborhoods where organized adult criminal activity does not exist, there tends to be less restraint placed on youth and violent or *conflict gangs* emerge. Another type of gang might appear in either type of neighborhood. This type of gang is named *retreatist*, because its members are drug users and the gang tends to be organized around drug activity. The members of this gang are considered double failures because they are dropouts from school and conventional society in general, as well as from other gangs, whose members rejected these *retreatists* because of their drug use. Attempts to examine this explanation have not typically discovered retreatist gangs (Shoemaker, 2005). In addition, some have suggested that a fourth type of gang can emerge in neighborhoods in which members of organized crime reside, a *racket gang*, which differs from the criminal gang .... (Spergel, 1964).

The view that juveniles, including gang members, are primarily motivated by economic concerns is not accepted by all scholars. For example, Albert Cohen (1955) developed an explanation of gang delinquency which posited that the primary source of social status for juveniles is found within the school setting. Juveniles are not as motivated to obtain a high-paying job as adults may be. In addition, juveniles are often brought together for significant amounts of time, particularly within the school setting, so their sources of social identity tend to come from this setting. In addition, Cohen maintains that most gang members are from the lower social classes, which is consistent with macro-level strain theories in general. Consequently, the argument is that class-based differences and strains, within the school setting, are the basis for delinquency, including gang delinquency, among youth in working and lower social classes.

Cohen makes the argument that all youth wish to succeed at school, at least in earlier years of education. However, an important impediment to academic success for lower-class youth is the existence of middle-class values which dominate the educational institution and which are expressed by teachers and school administrators. These values include a willingness to delay the immediate gratification of wants and desires for longer-term profits (delayed gratification), respect for the property of others, a desire to succeed in school, long-range plans, and self-control in relationships with others, especially resistance to the use of violence in interpersonal relationships. While one may quarrel with the view that these values are specifically middle-class values, they are an important component of Cohen's argument. Moreover, they are not values which are emphasized in lower-class settings. In essence, they are evaluated according to a *middle-class measuring rod*. Thus, lower-class youth learn early in their school careers that school work may involve activities and normative standards which they are not prepared to follow.

One consequence of this class-based system of strain, especially for a lower-class youth, is failure at school, failure which is interpreted by those leading the school system as individualized. Thus, the young student must learn to handle this failure, one way or another. Cohen hypothesizes that there are three major responses to this source of strain. One reaction is described as a *corner-boy* response. This adaptation to strain is basically conformist, and predicted by Cohen to be most dominant within the lower class. This response basically involves coming to terms with the situation and doing the best one can, given the circumstances. It may involve some delinquency, but typically not serious crime. A second mode of adapting to this strain is considered by Cohen to be the least common, the *college-boy* response. This reaction involves not only adjusting to class-based strains in the school system, but overcoming the sources of tension and excelling at school. Delinquency is rare with this response. The last reaction is considered the most serious and threatening to society and often associated with gang delinquency. It is called the *delinquent-boy* response. The delinquent boy is full of resentment at his situation, and comes to reject the school system in which he wished to succeed earlier in life, and the middle-class values it represents. He becomes "negativistic," "malicious," and "just plain mean" (Cohen, 1955). Thus, within the delinquent boy mentality, other students, especially those doing well in school, are to be terrorized and victimized. Symbols of success, including schools, are to be vandalized, and so on. Thus, while Cohen is definitely proposing what might be considered a psychological profile of a gang youth, the basic motivation for this behavior pattern is social-class strain within the school system.

Conflict Perspective

Both social disorganization and anomie theories suggest that there are commonly accepted norms and values which exist in society, and that delinquency in one way or another violates those basic norms. The conflict perspective, however, is based on the assumption that there are real and meaningful differences in society, created by various factors, and these differences are influential in shaping the behavioral patterns of people. One example of this view is the culture conflict theory, which is based on the assumption that there is a dominant value system which is expected to be honored and followed by immigrants, despite differences in their cultural norms and ideas. In addition, there are other conflict views which maintain that basic divisions in society are accountable for criminality more so than social forces which influence people to violate *commonly accepted* norms and values.

One conflict explanation of crime and delinquency has been termed the "radical" perspective, largely because its assumptions call for radical reorganization of social and economic structures for crime prevention. The radical view of criminality argues that the basic cause of criminal behavior is the capitalist system. In many ways, this perspective is based on the ideas of Karl Marx, even though Marx did not specifically develop a theory of crime (Shoemaker, 2005). One conflict proponent maintains that there are two kinds of crime: *crimes of domination and repression* and *crimes of accommodation* (Quinney, 1977). Crimes of domination and repression are committed by the ruling class, owners and managers of property and means of production, and constitute efforts to control and dominate the social, economic, and political institutions of society. These crimes include price fixing, environmental crimes, and white-collar crimes in general. Crimes of accommodation and resistance include common property and violent crimes, such as larceny and robbery, as well as rebellious activity. These crimes are committed in response to the efforts of the ruling class to control the economic and social lives of others.

While the radical or "Marxist" view of crime has achieved some measure of interest and support from criminologists, its basic tenets seem to apply more to adults than to juveniles. This view of criminality stresses economic issues. Juveniles, it would seem, are more concerned about social and peer issues, school-related problems, and other issues than jobs and economic problems. Some, however, suggest that the ideas of the radical view can be applied to juveniles. For example, developing the issue of economic concerns among juveniles, David Greenberg (1977) suggests that capitalist societies tend to prolong adolescence and extend schooling. These conditions result in an extended reliance on peer acceptance for social status and alienation, or at least separation, from the adult world of work and economic independence. To Greenberg, capitalism works better for adults than for juveniles and juveniles are relegated to lower social status and dependency as a result. Thus, the age and work structure of a capitalist society create conditions conducive to juvenile defiance and resistance to their low status. In addition, especially among lower-class males, anxiety may develop about supporting oneself and a family adequately because of low-paying jobs for young men, which can lead to violence committed by adolescent males from lower-class backgrounds.

In sum, macro-level explanations of criminality view the larger societal context as the proper focus of attention. As such, these explanations are better able to elucidate the origins of criminal behavior patterns, rather than the continuation of such patterns of behavior. In addition, macro-level theories typically do not address the manner in which individuals perceive and incorporate societal conditions into personal motivations for behavior. The personalization of societal conditions is often addressed by the next set of factors to be discussed; micro-level theories.

MICRO-LEVEL EXPLANATIONS

One of the troubling aspects of macro-level explanations of crime and delinquency is the difficulty in understanding how structural and cultural factors get "in the heads," so to speak, of individuals. In other words, while macro theories may offer reasonable explanations of the structural conditions under which crime and delinquency are *more likely* to occur, these views do not provide adequate explanations of how the structural conditions are interpreted and acted upon by individual people. This problem is no minor consideration. For example, in the Shaw and McKay research discussed above, only about 30% of youth living in high delinquency areas appeared in juvenile court data (Shoemaker, 2005). While it may be argued that substantially more youth are involved in criminal behavior than those who appear in juvenile court, the issue still remains, why are not more youth affected by generic structural factors with respect to committing delinquent behavior? In addition, advocates of anomie or strain theory, suggest that conformity, or involvement in low levels of criminality, are the *most common* reactions to anomie, as was indicated earlier. Again, these conditions do not affect all individuals the same way. Micro-level explanations of criminality have been offered in part to address this issue. While some advocate that these theories are substantially sufficient as explanations of delinquency in their own right, the argument that these explanations can serve as a link between structural conditions and individual behavior is persuasive.

Differential Association Theory

One of the more popular micro-level theories of delinquency is called differential association theory, originally proposed by Edwin Sutherland in 1939. One of the major assumptions of this explanation is that behavior, including delinquent behavior, is *learned*, not biologically inherited. While this assumption may seem almost mundane by today's standards, it was an important consideration 70 years ago, and it remains an important feature of most micro-level sociological views of crime and delinquency today. Over several years, Sutherland refined and modified this theory to ultimately include nine basic propositions:

1. *Criminal behavior is learned.*
2. *Criminal behavior is learned in interaction with other persons in a process of communication.*
3. *The principal part of the learning of criminal behavior occurs within intimate personal groups.*
4. *When criminal behavior is learned, the learning includes (a) techniques of committing the crime, which are sometimes very complicated, sometimes very simple, and (b) specific direction of motives, drives, rationalizations, and attitudes.*
5. *The specific direction of motives and drives is learned from definitions of the legal codes as favorable or unfavorable.*
6. *A person becomes delinquent because of an excess of definitions favorable to violation of law over definitions unfavorable to violation of law.*
7. *Differential associations may vary in frequency, duration, priority, and intensity.*
8. *The process of learning criminal behavior by associations with criminal and anti- criminal patterns involves all of the mechanisms that are involved in any other learning.*
9. *While criminal behavior is an expression of general needs and values, it is not explained by those general needs and values, since non-criminal behavior is an expression of the same needs and values* (Sutherland & Cressey, 1978, p. 80–83).

The contention that crime and delinquency are learned in primary group settings has attracted the attention of many researchers and has been examined most often with respect to delinquency (Vold et al., 2002). The group context of delinquency is clear from the behavior patterns of juvenile gangs. However, studies indicate that delinquency in general is often committed in a group context. As one commentator put it, "One of the most consistently reported features of delinquent behavior is its group nature" (Warr, 2002, p. 31). While the group context of delinquency alone does not "prove" the validity of differential association theory, the consistency of this pattern does lend credence to the theory.

Differential association theory assumes that delinquency is formed, perhaps shaped, by group involvement. An important issue here is the direction of the group influence. That is, do delinquent youth choose delinquent companions, or do delinquent groups create delinquency (Vold et al., 2002)? Studies concerning this question have concluded that the answer is both patterns exist. Some evidence suggests that delinquent youth seek out delinquent companions; whereas, other studies suggest that involvement in youth gangs contributes to delinquency of youth (Shoemaker, 2009). The most reasonable conclusion to this question, however, is that both patterns exist, and they exist in a reciprocal, bi-directional fashion. That is, regardless of one's past behavior, involvement with delinquent companions increases one's delinquency involvement, and one's delinquency increases associations with delinquent peers (Warr, 2002).

Another issue regarding differential association theory is the importance of group membership and participation. Does one have to be a member of a group, and participate in its activities, in order to be affected by the group? Some have suggested that individuals may be influenced by groups of which they are not true members but in which they *desire to belong*. One term used to express this situation is *differential identification* (Glaser, 1956). Others add that this concept identifies the importance of *reference groups* in the understanding of delinquency (Haskell, 1960). Studies of gangs further maintain that gangs are often admired by younger members of a neighborhood, who become *wannabes*, or aspirants for gang membership. These wannabes can be used to help gangs in the pursuit of criminal activities (Shoemaker, 2009). Their desire for acceptance by the gang can make them attractive to the gang for criminal purposes, such as serving as lookouts during a burglary, or helping out in times of gang fights, or rumbles.

General Strain Theory

Another attempt to bridge the gap between structural factors and individual-level responses to these macro conditions is the *general strain theory*, or GST (Agnew, 1992, 2006). The basic argument of GST is that juveniles are presented with stressful situations, sometimes reflecting structural conditions, such as poverty, racism, and so on, and sometimes more localized, such as bullying at school, or abuse in the home. The ability of the child to escape these stressful situations is limited, and may even involve illegal actions, such as running away or truancy. According to Robert Agnew, the developer of GST theory, there are three types of strain: "Individuals may (a) lose something they value, (b) be treated in an aversive or negative manner by others, and (c) be unable to achieve their goals" (Agnew, 2006). This latter example of strain theory is similar to Merton's anomie strain theory. The original version of the general strain theory was a more modest revision of anomie (Agnew, 1985). For juveniles, strains associated with family or school problems are thought to have the greatest impact on delinquency (Agnew, 2006). In general, strains that are more likely to result in criminality are those which are seen as unjust and salient to the individual, and among those with low levels of self-control (see the discussion below), and who feel "pressured" to respond in criminal ways (Agnew, 2006)

GST also includes a variety of social and individual, or emotional, reactions to strain, which definitely augments structural anomic or strain explanations of criminality. For example, Agnew discusses various individual "coping" mechanisms, or strategies, in response to strain, such as anger. More generally, the argument is that coping strategies can be divided into three categories; behavioral, cognitive, or emotional. Each of these three categories can be influenced in specific cases of individual coping by social psychological and environmental characteristics, such as social class, neighborhood context, and personality characteristics.

For example, individuals with low self-control, who are living in poverty and in neighborhoods with high crime rates, are more likely to respond to strain in criminal ways than are those who have ample economic resources, living in secure and stable neighborhoods, and with high levels of frustration tolerance (Agnew, 2006).

Control Theories

Control theories pose a different question than the other explanations considered so far. Instead of asking why people offend, control theories assume that the tendency to offend is common among humans. Thus, the more appropriate question to ask is why do people *not* offend more than they do? The answer to this question within the perspective of control theories is that some type of control prevents a person from offending. The nature of the control mechanism divides control explanations into personal or social controls. Both perspectives are properly categorized as micro-level explanations of crime and delinquency, but *personal* control theories focus on *internal* sources of control, such as self-concept. *Social* control explanations focus more on *external* sources of control, such as ties to family or school.

One example of a control theory is containment theory, proposed by Walter Reckless (Reckless, 1961, 1967). Containment theory is a broad multi-level explanation of criminality. It proposes that there are substantial pressures and pulls upon a youth which can result in delinquency. These pressures and pulls are both internal, such as deviant personality configurations, and external, such as delinquent peer groups. However, at the same time, there are numerous internal and external controls, or containments, which help prevent delinquency; external controls such as strong social institutions and internal controls such as a strong self-concept. Although the theory basically addresses external and internal sources and controls of criminality, Reckless and others have focused on the importance of internal controls as the major containment of delinquency. One reason for the focus on self-concept is the view that self-concept is more important as a control of crime and delinquency in modern industrialized societies, because in these societies, external sources of control, such as social institutions, are weaker (Shoemaker, 2005).

The basic prediction of this aspect of containment theory is that one's self-concept affects behavior. Specifically, the lower the self-concept, the more likely delinquency will occur. Delinquency, therefore, becomes a mechanism for improving self-concept, or at least for providing a behavioral outlet for those with low self-esteem. The relationship between self-concept and delinquency has been examined frequently, and, in general, the predicted relationship has been supported; that is, those with low levels of self-concept are more involved with delinquency than those with higher levels of self-esteem (Dinitz, Scarpitti, & Reckless, 1962; Reckless, Dinitz, & Murray, 1956; Reckless, Dinitz, & Kay, 1957; Schwartz and Tangri, 1965; Wells, 1978). In addition, some studies have shown that self-concept *increases* with delinquency, or at least with associating with delinquent peers (Kaplan, 1978; Jang and Thornberry, 1998), particularly for those with lower levels of self-esteem prior to delinquency involvement (Kaplan, 1980; Mason, 2001). While authors may use different names relating to self-concept, such as self-esteem, self-derogation, and self-enhancement, the conclusions seem generally the same; namely, those committing acts of delinquency tend to have initially lower levels of self-concept which are elevated through committing delinquency, or at least associating with delinquent others.

While most scholars agree that self-concept has some impact on delinquency, many now think that self-concept is not as strongly connected to youth deviance as are other constructs, such as peer associations or social bonds (Jensen, 1973; Rankin, 1977; see also Shoemaker, 2005). A modification of this view suggests self-concept should be combined with these other factors to enhance the delinquency explanatory model (Kaplan, Martin, & Johnson, 1986). In addition, some view the importance of self-concept as a mediating construct between these other factors and delinquency (Wells & Rankin, 1983). Thus, self-concept may either augment or reduce the impact of peers and social bonds on delinquency. Overall, self-concept or self esteem seems to be an important variable in the explanation of delinquency, but probably not the primary factor. Self-concept can be a moderator of other influences on delinquency, but a low self-concept, in the absence of other significant variables, is not likely to result in delinquency.

Social Bond

Another control variable which has been used to explain delinquency is social control, or the social bond theory. The main prediction in this explanation of crime and delinquency is that the stronger the bond between a juvenile and representatives of social institutions, the less the likelihood of a youth committing acts of delinquency. The developer of this explanation of delinquency, Travis Hirschi, conceptualized four major components of the social bond including attachment, belief, commitment, and involvement (Hirschi, 1969).

Attachment refers to emotional connection with someone who is significantly related to social institutions such as a parent, teacher, or minister. The bond, in this sense, is usually identified through feelings such as admiration, respect, trust, and so forth. *Belief* is the component of the social bond which involves acceptance of basic rules, laws, and policies, especially with regard to formal systems of social control, such as the police and courts. Belief is summarized by Hirschi in terms of moral values. If a person's moral values have been weakened or compromised, then "The probability that he will commit delinquent acts is therefore increased" (Hirschi, 1969, p. 26). *Commitment* includes investing time, money, or other personal sacrifices into something desired, such as an education or the development of a successful career. Consequently, acts of crime and delinquency are inversely connected to commitment in part because an individual wishes not to risk losing the gains made by these investments, or stakes in conformity (Toby, 1957). The more one has to lose, so to speak, the more he or she will consider the "costs" of committing crime.

The final component of the bond, *involvement*, is often associated with busy work, or doing things in connection with an institution. An example would be participating in extra-curricular activity at school, or serving on committees and boards in an organization. In the logic of the social bond theory, a juvenile who is kept busy with conventional activity has less time to commit delinquent acts. As Hirschi (1969) states, "The assumption, widely shared, is that a person may be simply too busy doing conventional things to find time to engage in deviant behavior" (p. 22).

Hirschi expressed the argument that all elements of the bond were uniformly and positively related (Hirschi, 1969). Thus, if one were committed to the rules and laws of society, then he or she would also express conventional beliefs, maintain positive attachments with conventional others, and be involved in conventional activities. These bonds, in turn, would logically predict, through the theory, that such individuals would be less likely to commit acts of crime and delinquency.

The social bond theory has received considerable attention in the study of delinquency. Some of this research has focused on the relationships between specific elements of the bond and delinquency. Other studies have examined the connection between the social bond, in general, and specific social institutions, such as religion, the family, and schools. For the most part, these attempts to examine the validity of the theory's assumptions have been supportive. Not only is there support for the direct contribution of a weak social bond to delinquency, but social bonds are often found to interact with other factors, such as delinquent peers, social disorganization, and low self-concept, to enhance the explanation of delinquency (Shoemaker, 2005).

Self-Control

Although the social bond theory has received general support in the literature, a revision of the theory was offered by Hirschi and Michael Gottfredson, which focused on the impact of low self-control as a major contributor to criminality. The basic argument with this explanation is that *low self-control* better explains or predicts delinquency, compared to a weakened social bond. Gottfredson and Hirschi further claim that the impact of low self-control is evident for general acts of crime and deviance and is so pervasive in the characteristics of offenders that it is appropriate to refer to low self-control as a *general* theory of crime (Gottfredson & Hirschi, 1990).

Gottfredson and Hirschi reason that the nature of low self-control "can be derived directly from the nature of criminal acts" (Gottfredson and Hirschi, 1990, p. 88). From their understanding of criminal traits, they posit that criminals are characterized by the following: inability to delay gratification of wants and desires; interest in short-term rather than long-term goals; lack of training or apprenticeship in manual skills; and insensitivity to pain and suffering especially among victims of crime. Thus, criminal activity is based on the satisfaction of short-term goals, needs, or desires, with little or no planning or concern for the harm inflicted on victims or society. The relationship between low self-control and crime is expressed in the following passage, "In sum, people who lack self-control will tend to be impulsive, insensitive, physical (as opposed to mental), risk-taking, short-sighted, and nonverbal, and they will tend therefore, to engage in criminal and analogous acts" (Gottfredson & Hirschi, 1990, p. 90).

In addition, according to Gottfredson and Hirschi, self-control is *a learned* trait, not inborn or inherited. Thus, the basic contribution to crime and delinquency is acquired, not innate. Thus, individuals who have been properly socialized tend to become more controlled in social settings, and thus less likely to commit criminal acts. Furthermore, the primary agent of socialization in society is the family. Other social institutional settings, such as the school, may have a significant impact on the levels of self-control among its members, but the family remains the primary setting in which self-control is or is not learned. Parents, or by implication, significant care-givers who do not properly socialize youth into conformist activity are considered ineffective and so "ineffective parenting" is thought to lead to low self-control and to crime. More particularly, ineffective parenting includes inadequate monitoring or supervision of youths' behavior, the lack of recognition of criminal or deviant behavior committed by their children, and the failure to punish transgressions among children.

The general theory of crime, in particular the connection between low self-control and criminality, has received considerable support in the criminological literature over the past 2 decades. While there is ample evidence to support a connection between low self-control and criminality, there have been many criticisms leveled at this theory as well (Gottfredson, 2006). There is the contention that self-control theory is tautological, especially since it assumes that characteristics of criminals identify causes of criminality. That is, the impulsive, short-sighted, uncaring nature of criminals is used to describe low self-control *as an explanation* of crime (see above). In addition, Gottfredson and Hirschi maintain that their general theory is a social explanation of criminality. Gottfredson (2006) further suggests that low self-control and the social bond are essentially control theories and are more similar than distinct. Thus, if anything, a social bond and self-control are different in that they occur along different points on a control spectrum. Despite these claims that self-control is a social construct, some have noted that the basic, underlying general trait ascribed to this theory, namely low self-control, is essentially a psychological construct (Shoemaker, 2005; Vold et al., 2002;). Still, most scholars of crime and delinquency place the theoretical context of this theory into a social psychological category, rather than a psychological field.

Gottfredson and Hirschi also claim that low self-control is not automatically followed by criminality. Indeed, they assume that many individuals with low self-control are able to construct a life without criminal activity. This contention is not remarkable in itself, since virtually all explanations of crime would allow for the nonobservance of criminality among individuals possessing traits or living in societal conditions which are thought to be conducive to crime. However, for a theory which purports to offer an explanation of crime and deviance in general, the claim that the primary contributor to criminality, low self-control, is not always followed by crime indicates recognition that low self-control is not a single, major impetus to crime.

Criminality, as recognized by Gottfredson and Hirschi, is a product of several contributing factors, often working in concert, or in an integrated fashion. Theoretical integration, or convergence, is a concept which will be discussed further below.

In sum, micro-level explanations posit that social psychological factors play an important role in the etiology of crime and delinquency. As such, these variables are conceptualized as lying between individual-level characteristics, such as biological and psychological factors, and larger structural and societal variables in the explanation of criminality. Micro-level explanations are better able to explain the continuation of criminal behavior patterns, than the origin of criminality. The combination, or integration of both levels of explanation, macro and micro, offers a more complete description and understanding of the origins and transmission of delinquency, from a sociological perspective.

OTHER CONSIDERATIONS

Besides the macro- and micro-level explanations of crime and delinquency discussed above, there are other perspectives which should be briefly noted, but which do not fall neatly into a macro or micro category. Two of these perspectives will be commented upon below, life-course and labeling.

Life-Course Perspective

The life-course perspective is based on the view that crime and delinquency are the results of dynamic patterns of events and traits which change over the life course. As noted above, a common finding in the literature on delinquency is that rates of crime and delinquency decline with age. Some have argued that these changes should be considered in connection with overall patterns of delinquency. In particular, Robert Sampson and John Laub have promoted the view that behavior patterns of delinquents can and do change not only over the course of adolescence, but also over a lifetime. Sampson and Laub have been studying the long-term behavior patterns of a sample of delinquent youth first studied by Sheldon and Eleanor Glueck in the 1930s and 1940s. This study examined the individual and social characteristics of 500 delinquent males, who had been incarcerated in Massachusetts' reform schools, compared to a control sample of 500 "non-delinquent" males from public schools in Boston. The non-delinquent youth were so designated because they had not been institutionalized and were not considered serious offenders. All of the youth were 10–17 years old, white, and lower-class with average IQs; enabling matched pair comparisons between delinquent and non-delinquent subjects.. The original sample of youth were restudied when they were 25 and then again at age 32. These two follow-up studies included 88% of both delinquents and controls (Sampson & Laub, 1993). The original study also included interviews with the youth, their parents, and school officials (Glueck & Glueck, 1950; Sampson & Laub, 1993).

Sampson and Laub re-analyzed the Glueck data, including their two follow-up studies, and then collected additional information on them up to age 45 (Sampson & Laub, 1993). They conducted a subsequent follow-up study of the sample at age 70 (Laub & Sampson, 2003). One of the findings of the follow-up studies was that 76% of the delinquent youth, compared to 20% of the non-delinquent youth, were arrested between ages 17 and 25. These differences were 61% versus 14% between ages 25 and 32, and 55% versus 16% between ages 32 and 45. In addition, 64% of the delinquent youth were charged with criminal behavior while in the military, compared to 20% of the control youth. Similar disparities appeared between the delinquent and control youth when considering parent and teacher self-reports of delinquency and disruptive behavior, as well as indications of early disruptive behavior in the youth, such as having tantrums. In addition, interviews of samples of the youth who became men suggested that behavioral patterns of delinquent youth transferred to more difficulties in marriage and work in adulthood, compared to the control sample (Sampson & Laub, 1993). Thus, one of the conclusions of the Glueck and Sampson and Laub studies was that patterns of offending among youth tend to persist and become generalized to other venues in life as individuals mature and become adults.

Further analyses of Sampson and Laub; however, suggest that an explanation for the persistence of delinquency, crime, and misfortune is the inability of delinquent youth to form and maintain strong social connections, or bonds as youth, especially in the family and school. These weak bonds carry over into adulthood. Thus, problems of delinquency generated in youth persist to additional legal and social problems in adulthood, as exemplified by continued patterns of arrest and incarceration, problems in military service, with marriage, and at work (Sampson & Laub, 1993).

However, the Sampson and Laub analyses also indicated that a significant number of the original delinquents did not continue to lead lives of crime and social disruption. Some were able to develop "turning points" in their lives, which tended to redirect their behavior patterns and lifestyles to conformist activities. Again, according to Sampson and Laub, these turning points were largely achieved through strong and stable marriages and employment histories, which were described in terms of "social capital" (Sampson & Laub, 1993).

Laub and Sampson continued their analysis of the Glueck data by examining arrest data for the original 500 delinquents and interviewing a sample of 52 of those still alive at age 70 (Laub & Sampson, 2003). Their analysis confirmed the general conclusions from the first study; namely, that most delinquents desist from criminal behavior, especially after age 16. In addition, again for older youth or young adults, significant turning points were responsible for much of the desistance from criminality. However, this analysis also indicated that individual will, choice, or agency (i.e., the desire and will to change) contributed to the pattern of desistance for many individuals (p. 249). These conclusions are based on a limited sample of the original 500 delinquents studied by the Gluecks, However, additional research and reflection on this perspective continues to identify social bonds as an important turning point, but underscores the importance of human agency as well (Laub, Robert, Sampson, & Sweeten, 2006).

The life-course perspective is part of a *social development* interest in theoretical explanations of crime and delinquency (Farrington, 2006; Laub & Sampson, 2003; Vold et al., 2002). Although social development has a long history in psychology, its use in sociology is more recent but becoming more commonplace. Often, a social development component is included in integrated theoretical perspectives (see discussion below). In addition, many social development views of delinquency incorporate aspects of social bond and social learning, along with a life-course view of delinquency (Huang, Kosterman, Catalano, Hawkins, & Abbott, 2001).

A relatively recent approach to the understanding of delinquency is the notion that delinquency is not just a common term, but involves more than one "pathway." Some, such as Terrie Moffitt and colleagues, suggest that there are two predominant pathways to delinquency, the "life-course persistent" pathway and the "adolescence-limited" pathway (Moffitt, 1993, 1997; see also Chap. 3 this volume). The life-course persistent pattern suggests that some juveniles become delinquent, or criminal, relatively early in life, sometimes before school age, and remain involved in criminality well into adulthood. The life-course persistent pattern of delinquency pathway is often associated with relatively few delinquents, typically less than 10% of a delinquent population. Moreover, this sample of delinquents is involved in a variety of delinquent activity, including serious violent crime. The adolescence-limited pattern usually begins in mid-adolescence, lasts 1 or 2 years, and involves relatively minor acts of crime, such as minor theft or status offending. This pattern of delinquency fits the typical age–crime relationship, which suggests that most delinquents cease delinquent activity around the age of 16 or 17. It also applies to the majority of delinquent offenders. Research continues to support these two pathways as major patterns of delinquency (Moffitt, 2006).

The life-course persistent and adolescence-limited pathways to delinquency are not the only pathway views of delinquent patterns. Some have suggested that there are three patterns of delinquency: "authority conflict," which involves status offending; "covert," which includes acts of theft; and "overt," which is considered the most serious pathway and involves violent crimes (Loeber, Farrington, Stouthamer-Loeber, Moffitt, & Caspi, 1998). Regardless of whether there are two, three, or more pathways to delinquency, the concept that not all youth are equally delinquent is informative, and likely to remain a key component of theoretical perspectives on delinquency.

Labeling Perspective

The labeling perspective has two primary concerns in connection with criminality. First is the issue of law making and enforcing. That is, this perspective questions the motives and intentions of law makers and enforcers. Key questions from this concern are who makes the laws and how are they enforced? The labeling perspective views these processes as potentially discriminatory, or at least in need of research (Shoemaker, 2005). The second concern of labeling theory is the impact of a label, typically a formal label applied by the police or courts, on the offender. Basically, labeling theory proposes that identifying one as an offender tends to separate him or her from the rest of society. The label becomes a stigma which is difficult to shed. One important result is the change in one's identity to that of an offender and subsequent behavioral changes conducted to conform to the label and one's identity (Shoemaker, 2005; Vold et al., 2002).

An important contributor to the development of the labeling theory was Edwin Lemert. As originally proposed, Lemert developed a perspective which applied to general patterns of deviance. However, the labeling theory has been applied to crime and delinquency as well. Lemert distinguished between *primary deviance* and *secondary deviance* (Lemert, 1951, 1967). Primary deviance is that which is not enhanced by the impact of a formal label. Its causes are many and varied, as seen in part by the theoretical overview presented in this paper. Secondary deviance occurs *after* a formal label has been applied, and ultimately results in a change of one's identification, to that of a delinquent. It is as if the offender now says, "since I am called a delinquent, I will act that way." In addition, the theory suggests secondary deviants begin to alter their behavior to accommodate the label and its consequences.

Of course, there has to be a reason for a label of delinquency to be applied in the first place, namely, an act of crime or delinquency, so in part, the rationalization implied with secondary deviance might be interpreted as a way of avoiding responsibility for wrongful acts. As mentioned earlier; however, the other concern of labeling theory rests with discriminatory or unfair labeling by criminal and juvenile justice authorities. Thus, in part, secondary deviance may be viewed as truly a reaction to being labeled through societal processes (Becker, 1973).

Of course, scholars recognize that the path from primary to secondary deviance is not as straightforward or inevitable as labeling theorists might suggest. In part, the theory seems to downplay the impact of human will, or agency, in the acceptance, or modification, of a label and its impact on one's self-concept and behavior (Akers, 1967; Shoemaker, 2005; Vold et al., 2001). However, Lemert suggested that the movement from primary to secondary deviance was a process which involved several steps, any one of which could be broken by intervening factors. In addition, this process is replete with efforts by the individual to resist, or at least manage, the label of deviant or delinquent (Lemert, 1967). Whether that secondary deviance, with its change in identity and behavior patterns, occurs at all seems to be more a product of strong social pressures, rather than unthinking willingness on the part of the offender to accept the label when first applied.

Efforts to examine, or test, labeling theory have not uniformly supported its tenets (Shoemaker, 2005). Besides mixed empirical results concerning deviant identities based on formal applications of labels, and the issue of human will (as discussed earlier), there is the difficulty of reconciling the implications of secondary deviance with the typical pattern of cessation of delinquency at mid-late adolescence. Despite these drawbacks and questions regarding the labeling theory, its assumptions appear to lie behind many current practices and policies in the juvenile justice in western societies, such as diversion, restorative justice and re-integrative shaming (Braithwaite, 1989; Braithwaite, Ahmed, & Braithwaite, 2006; Shoemaker, 2009). Thus, despite inconsistent evidence that the assumptions of labeling theory are accurate, considerations and modifications of labeling theory are likely to continue.

CONCLUDING COMMENTS

In this chapter, several sociological explanations of delinquency and youth misconduct have been identified. It should be emphasized, however, that this discourse has not included numerous variations and conditions which might specify or modify the theoretical links with delinquency. For example, no separate discussion of female or gang delinquency has been presented, although certainly there are explanations of these examples of youth misconduct which could go beyond the broad explanations presented. In addition, no separate considerations of race, ethnicity, social class (especially middle-class delinquency), geographical location, or international settings have been presented.

In addition, many have suggested that explanations of youth misconduct be refined to include integrated or combined interaction models (Elliott, Huizinga, & Ageton, 1985; Shoemaker, 2005; Vold et al, 2002). Combining or integrating different explanations of criminality is a challenging exercise, especially if the attempt includes micro and macro sociological explanations, and/or interdisciplinary perspectives. Often, integrated explanations of crime and delinquency include *interactions* between contributing factors and delinquency (Thornberry, 1987; Thornberry, Lizotte, Krohn, Farnworth, & Jang, 1994). For example, a weakened social bond may be an explanation of delinquency, but delinquency may also weaken the social bond between a child and his or her family. Or, family conflict may interfere with academic performance, which, in turn, may lead to further conflicts in the home, both of which may contribute to delinquency. Thus, "cause and effect" can be reciprocal.

Further, explanations of crime and delinquency may be linked, especially when considering micro and macro level theories. For example, social disorganization may well lead to weakened social bonds, which may be the more proximate contributing factor to crime and delinquency. The basic cause, which is social dislocation in a neighborhood, may thus be overlooked, or undervalued, as the explanation of youth misconduct because the concern is directed more at the proximate cause, that is, the relationship between the child and the family, or the school setting.

Thus, sociological explanations of crime and delinquency are considerably more detailed and integrative than this brief chapter can describe. In addition, modern explanations of crime and delinquency are becoming more interdisciplinary, encompassing biological, psychological, and sociological perspectives, rendering unique disciplinary efforts more difficult to establish. Nonetheless, it is anticipated that this overview of sociological explanations of youth crime and misconduct will enable the reader to appreciate the range of factors which can impact on delinquency.

REFERENCES

Agnew, R. (1985). A revised strain theory of delinquency. *Social Forces, 64*, 151–167.

Agnew, R. (1992). Foundation for a general strain theory of crime and delinquency. *Criminology, 30*, 47–87.

Agnew, R. (2006). *Pressured into crime: An overview of general strain theory*. Los Angeles, CA: Roxbury.

Akers, R. L. (1967). Problems in the sociology of deviance: Social definitions and behavior. *Social Forces, 46*, 455–465.

Aries, P. (1962). *Centuries of childhood: A social history of family life, translated by R. Baldick*. New York: Alfred A. Knopf.

Atasoy, S., Baskan, T. M., & Ziyalar, N. (2006). Juvenile justice in Turkey. In P. C. Friday & X. Ren (Eds.), *Delinquency and juvenile justice in the non-western world* (pp. 125–142). Monsey, NY: Criminal Justice Press.

Becker, H. M. (1973). *Outsiders*. New York: Free Press. First published in 1963.

Braithwaite, J. (1989). *Crime, shame, and reintegration*. Cambridge, MA: Cambridge University Press.

Braithwaite, J., Ahmed, E., & Braithwaite, V. (2006). Shame, restorative justice, and crime. In F. T. Cullen, J. P. Wright, & K. R. Blevins (Eds.), *Taking stock: The status of criminological theory, Volume 15, Advances in criminological theory* (pp. 397–417). New Brunswick, NJ: Transaction.

Bursik, R. J. (1999). The informal control of crime through neighborhood networks. *Sociological Focus, 32*, 85–97.

Chambliss, W. J. (1974). Functional and conflict theories of crime. *MSS Modular Publications, Module 17*, 1–23.

Cloward, R. A. (1959). Illegitimate means, anomie and deviant behavior. *American Sociological Review, 24*, 164–176.

Cloward, R. A., & Ohlin, L. E. (1960). *Delinquency and opportunity*. New York: Free Press.

Cohen, A. (1955). *Delinquent Boys: The culture of the gang*. New York: Free Press.

Coleman, J. S. (1988). Social capital and the creation of human capital. *American Journal of Sociology, 94*(Supplement), S95–S120.

Dinitz, S., Scarpitti, F. R., & Reckless, W. C. (1962). Delinquency vulnerability: A cross group and longitudinal analysis. *American Sociological Review, 27*, 515–517.

Durkheim, E. (1933). *The division of labor in society, translated by G. Simpson*. London: The Free Press of Glencoe. First published in 1893.

Durkheim, E. (1951). *Suicide, translated by J.A. Spaulding and G. Simpson*. New York: Free Press. First published in 1897.

Elliott, D. S., Huizinga, D., & Ageton, S. S. (1985). *Explaining delinquency and drug use*. Beverly Hills, CA: Sage.

Elrod, P., & Yokoyama, M. (2006). Juvenile justice in Japan. In P. C. Friday & X. Ren (Eds.), *Delinquency and juvenile justice in the non-western world* (pp. 211–228). Monsey, NY: Criminal Justice Press.

Farrington, D. (2006). Building developmental and life-course theories of offending. In F. T. Cullen, J. P. Wright, & K. R. Blevins (Eds.), *Taking stock: Advances in criminological theory, Volume 15, Advances in criminological theory* (pp. 335–364). New Brunswick, NJ: Transaction.

Glaser, D. (1956). Criminality theories and behavioral images. *American Journal of Sociology, 61*, 433–444.

Glueck, S., & Glueck, E. (1950). *Unraveling juvenile delinquency*. New York: The Commonwealth Fund.

Gottfredson, M. R. (2006). The empirical status of control theory in criminology. In F. T. Cullen, J. P. Wright, & K. R. Blevins (Eds.), *Taking stock: The status of criminological theory, Volume 15, Advances in criminological theory* (pp. 77–100). New Brunswick, NJ: Transaction.

Gottfredson, M. R., & Hirschi, T. (1990). *A general theory of crime*. Stanford, CA: Stanford University Press.

Greenberg, D. F. (1977). Delinquency and the age structure of society. *Contemporary Crises: Crime, Law, and Social Policy, 1*, 189–223.

Grossberg, M. (2002). Changing conceptions of child welfare in the United States, 1820–1935. In M. K. Rosenheim, F. E. Zimring, D. S. Tanenhaus, & B. Dohrn (Eds.), *A century of juvenile justice*. Chicago, IL: University of Chicago Press.

Hagan, J., Levi, R., & Dinovitzer, R. (2008). The symbolic violence of the crime-immigration nexus: Migrant mythologies in the Americas. *Criminology and Public Policy, 7*, 95–112.

Hartjen, C. A. (2008). *Youth, crime & justice: A global inquiry*. New Brunswick, NJ: Rutgers University Press.

Haskell, M. R. (1960). Toward a reference group theory of juvenile delinquency. *Social Problems, 8*, 220–230.

Hirschi, T. (1969). *Causes of delinquency*. Berkeley, CA: University of California Press.

Huang, B., Kosterman, R., Catalano, R. E., Hawkins, J. D., & Abbott, R. D. (2001). Modeling mediation in the etiology of violent behavior in adolescents: A test of the social development model. *Criminology, 39*, 75–107.

Inkeles, A. (1964). *What is sociology? An introduction to the discipline and profession*. Englewood Cliffs, NJ: Prentice-Hall.

Jang, S. J., & Thornberry, T. P. (1998). Self-esteem, delinquent peers, and delinquency: A test of self- enhancement theory. *American Sociological Review, 63*, 586–598.

Junger-Tas, J., & Decker, S. H. (Eds.). (2006). *International handbook of juvenile justice*. Dordrecht, The Netherlands: Springer.

Kaplan, H. B. (1978). Deviant behavior and self – enhancement in adolescence. *Journal of Youth and Adolescence, 7*, 253–277.

Kaplan, H. B. (1980). *Deviant behavior in defense of self*. New York: Academic Press.

Kaplan, H. B., Martin, S. S., & Johnson, R. J. (1986). Self-rejection and the explanation of deviance: Specification of the structure among latent constructs. *American Journal of Sociology, 92*, 384–411.

Kerper, H. B. (1972). *Introduction to the criminal justice system*. St. Paul, MN: West.

Laub, J. H., Robert, J., Sampson, R. J., & Sweeten, G. A. (2006). Assessing Sampson and Laub's life-course theory of crime. In F. T. Cullen, J. P. Wright, & K. R. Blevins (Eds.), *Taking stock; The status of criminological theory, Volume 15, Advances in criminological theory* (pp. 313–333). New Brunswick, NJ: Transaction.

Laub, J. H., & Sampson, R. J. (2003). *Shared beginnings, divergent lives: Delinquent boys to age 70*. Cambridge, MA: Harvard University Press.

Lemert, E. M. (1951). *Social pathology*. New York: McGraw-Hill.

Lemert, E. M. (1967). *Human deviance, social problems, and social control* (2nd ed.). Englewood Cliffs, NJ: Prentice-Hall.

Loeber, R., Farrington, D. P., Stouthamer-Loeber, M., Moffitt, T. E., & Caspi, A. (1998). The development of male offending: Key findings from the Pittsburgh Youth Study. *Studies in Crime and Crime Prevention, 7*, 141–171.

Mason, W. A. (2001). Self-esteem and delinquency revisited (again): A test of Kaplan's self-derogation theory of delinquency using latent growth curve modeling. *Journal of Youth and Adolescence, 30*, 83–102.

Merton, R. (1957). *Social theory and social structure*. New York: Free Press (revised and enlarged edition).

Messner, S. F., & Rosenfeld, R. (2001). *Crime and the American dream* (3rd ed.). Belmont, CA: Wadsworth/Thomson Learning.

Moffitt, T. E. (1993). "Life-course persistent" and "adolescence-limited" antisocial behavior: A developmental taxonomy. *Psychological Review, 100*, 674–701.

Moffitt, T. E. (1997). Adolescence-limited and life course persistent offending: A complementary pair of developmental theories. In T. Thornberry (Ed.), *Advances in developmental theory: Developmental theories of crime and delinquency* (pp. 11–54). London: Transaction.

Moffitt, T. E. (2006). A review of research ion the taxonomy of life-course persistent versus adolescence-limited antisocial behavior. In F. T. Cullen, J. P. Wright, & K. R. Blevins (Eds.), *Taking stock: The status of criminological theory, Volume 15, Advances in criminological theory* (pp. 277–311). New Brunswick, NJ: Transaction.

Park, R. E., Burgess, E. W., & McKenzie, R. D. (1925). *The city*. Chicago, IL: University of Chicago Press.

Postman, N. (1982). *The disappearance of childhood.* New York: Delacorte Press.
Putnam, R. (2000). *Bowling alone.* New York: Simon and Schuster.
Quinney, R. (1977). *Class, state, and crime: On the theory and practice of criminal justice.* New York: David McKay Company.
Reckless, W. C. (1961). A new theory of delinquency and crime. *Federal Probation, 25,* 42–46.
Reckless, W. C. (1967). *The crime problem* (4th ed.). New York: Appleton-Century Crofts.
Reckless, W. C., Dinitz, S., & Kay, B. (1957). The self component in potential delinquency and potential nondelinquency. *American Sociological Review, 22,* 566–570.
Reckless, W. C., Dinitz, S., & Murray, E. (1956). Self-Concept as an insulator against delinquency. *American Sociological Review, 21,* 744–746.
Sampson, R. J. (2006). Collective efficacy theory: Lessons learned and directions for future inquiry. In F. T. Cullen, J. P. Wright, & K. R. Blevins (Eds.), *Taking stock: The status of criminological theory, Volume 15, Advances in criminological theory* (pp. 149–167). New Brunswick, NJ: Transaction.
Sampson, R. J., & Laub, J. H. (1993). *Crime in the making: Pathways and turning points through life.* Cambridge, MA: Harvard University Press.
Sampson, R. J., Morenoff, J. D., & Earls, F. (1999). Beyond social capital: Spatial dynamics of collective efficacy. *American Sociological Review, 64,* 633–660.
Sampson, R. J., Raudenbusch, S. W., & Earl, F. (1997). Neighborhoods and violent crime: A multilevel study of collective efficacy. *Science, 277,* 918–924.
Sanders, W. B. (1970). *Juvenile offenders for a thousand years: Selected readings from Anglo-Saxon times to 1900.* Chapel Hill, NC: University of North Carolina Press.
Schwartz, M., & Tangri, S. S. (1965). A note on self-concept as an insulator against delinquency. *American Sociological Review, 30,* 922–926.
Sellin, T. (1938). *Culture conflict and crime.* New York: Social Science Research Council.
Shaw, C., & McKay, H. D. (1942). *Juvenile delinquency and urban areas.* Chicago, IL: University of Chicago Press.
Shaw, C., & McKay, H. D. (1969). *Juvenile delinquency and urban areas* (revisedth ed.). Chicago, IL: University of Chicago Press.
Shaw, C., Zorbaugh, F. M., McKay, H. D., & Cottrell, L. S. (1929). *Delinquency areas.* Chicago, IL: University of Chicago Press.
Shelley, L. (1989). *Crime and modernization.* Carbondale, IL: Southern Illinois University Press.
Sheu, C.-J. (1986). *Delinquency and identity: Juvenile delinquency in an American Chinatown.* New York: Harrow and Heston.
Shoemaker, D. J. (1995). Ethnic identity and delinquency among Filipino-American youth: A theoretical view. *Philippine Sociological Review, 43,* 95–114.
Shoemaker, D. J. (2005). *Theories of delinquency: An examination of explanations of delinquent behavior* (5th ed.). New York: Oxford.
Shoemaker, D. J. (2009). *Juvenile delinquency.* New York: Rowman & Littlefield.
Spergel, I. (1964). *Racketville, slumtown, and haulberg.* Chicago, IL: University of Chicago Press.
Sutherland, E. H., & Cressey, D. R. (1978). *Criminology* (10th ed.). New York: Lippincott.
Sutton, J. R. (1988). *Stubborn children: Controlling delinquency in the United States, 1640–1841.* Berkeley, CA: University of California Press.
Tanenhaus, D. S. (2002). The evolution of juvenile courts in the early twentieth century: Beyond the myth of immaculate construction. In M. K. Rosenheim, F. E. Zimring, D. S. Tanenhaus, & B. Dohrn (Eds.), *A century of juvenile justice* (pp. 42–73). Chicago, IL: University of Chicago Press.
Thomas, W. I., & Znaniecki, F. (1927). *The Polish peasant in Europe and America* (Vol. 2). New York: Knopf.
Thornberry, T. P. (1987). Toward an interactional theory of delinquency. *Criminology, 25,* 863–891.
Thornberry, T. P., Lizotte, A. J., Krohn, M. D., Farnworth, M., & Jang, S. J. (1994). Delinquent peers, beliefs, and delinquent behavior: A longitudinal test of interactional theory. *Criminology, 82,* 47–83.

Toby, J. (1957). Social disorganization and stake in conformity: Complementary factors in the predatory behavior of hoodlums. *Journal of Criminal Law, Criminology, and Police Science, 48*, 12–17.
Vold, G. B., Bernard, T. J., & Snipes, J. B. (2002). *Theoretical criminology* (5th ed.). New York: Oxford.
Warr, M. (2002). *Companions in crime: The social aspects of criminal conduct.* Cambridge, MA: Cambridge University Press.
Wells, L. E. (1978). Theories of deviance and the Self-concept. *Social Psychology, 41*, 189–204.
Wells, L. E., & Rankin, J. H. (1983). Self-concept as a mediating factor in delinquency. *Social Psychology Quarterlyy, 46*, 11–22.
Wong, S. K. (1997). Delinquency of Chinese-Canadian youth: A test of opportunity, control, andintergenerational conflict theories. *Youth and Society, 29*, 112–133.

3

Etiology of Oppositional Defiant Disorder and Conduct Disorder: Biological, Familial and Environmental Factors Identified in the Development of Disruptive Behavior Disorders

EVA R. KIMONIS and PAUL J. FRICK

Conduct problems are associated with a large number of biological, affective, cognitive, familial, and environmental risk factors. Further, research suggests that there may be multiple developmental pathways to conduct problems, each with their own unique constellation of risk and protective factors. Attempts at disaggregating youth into more homogeneous subtypes have uncovered groups of youth that show similar risk factors and distinct developmental trajectories. This chapter will provide an overview of these major subtypes of conduct disorder (CD) and the specific risk factors associated with each subtype. Assessment and treatment implications are discussed.

EVA R. KIMONIS • University of South Florida
PAUL J. FRICK • University of New Orleans

R.C. Murrihy et al. (eds.), *Clinical Handbook of Assessing and Treating Conduct Problems in Youth*, DOI 10.1007/978-1-4419-6297-3_3,

THE DIAGNOSTIC AND STATISTICAL MANUAL OF MENTAL DISORDERS

The DSM-IV/TR, now in its fourth edition, is the most widely adopted system for classifying psychological disorders (American Psychiatric Association, 2000). Beyond its utility for differential diagnosis in clinical settings, mental health researchers also use the DSM to guide their research studies. The DSM-IV/TR defines oppositional defiant disorder (ODD) as a pattern of negativistic, defiant, disobedient and hostile behavior toward authority figures, whereas the more severe disruptive behavior disorder (DBD), conduct disorder (CD), is defined as a repetitive and persistent pattern of behavior that violates the rights of others as well as major age-appropriate societal norms and rules. CD is operationalized as comprising four types of antisocial behaviors: aggressive conduct that threatens physical harm to people or animals, nonaggressive conduct that causes property loss or damage, deceitfulness and theft, and serious violations of rules (see Chap. 1). As is typical of other DSM-IV/TR definitions of mental disorders, these definitions are strictly behavioral in scope. That is, the current classification system does not specify causal factors in its conceptualization of DBDs.

DBDs are one of the most common reasons for referral of children and adolescents to outpatient mental health clinics and residential treatment centers (Frick & Silverthorn, 2001; Kazdin, 1995; Lynam, 1996). The behavior of youth with conduct problems causes significant disruption and distress to family members, peers, and school personnel, who must balance appropriately treating these youth with maintaining the safety of other students and teachers. In addition, their frequent contacts with law enforcement and juvenile courts, and greater rates of incarceration, are quite costly to society (Cohen, 1998; Loeber & Farrington, 2000; Zigler, Taussig, & Black, 1992).

The prevalence of DBDs varies across settings, ethnic groups, age groups, and gender. In community settings, the prevalence of ODD is estimated at 3–16%, and the prevalence of CD is estimated at 2–16%, although rates are significantly higher in clinical setting (Boylan, Vaillancourt, Boyle, & Szatmari, 2007; Loeber, Burke, Lahey, Winters, & Zera, 2000). With regard to race, research suggests that African–American youth show higher rates of conduct problems compared with Caucasian youth (Fabrega, Ulrich, & Mezzich, 1993; Lahey et al., 1995), although these differences have been attributed to the disproportionate experience of adverse environmental factors (e.g., poor neighborhoods with high crime rates and community violence) by ethnic minority youth (Lahey, Miller, Gordon, & Riley, 1999; Peeples & Loeber, 1994). Prevalence rates may also vary by age. For example, Loeber et al. (2000) found that whereas CD rates were similar for 7- and 11-year-old boys (5.6% versus 5.4%, respectively), they jumped to 8.3% for 13-year-old boys in a large urban area, demonstrating an increase in the rates of CD into adolescence. With regard to gender, prevalence rates for CD are roughly equivalent in boys and girls before age 5 (Keenan & Shaw, 1997), although they increase twofold to fourfold among boys in later childhood (Cohen et al., 1993; Loeber et al., 2000; Moffitt, Caspi, Rutter, & Silva, 2001; Offord et al., 1987). However, by adolescence, rates of conduct problems dramatically increase in girls, leading to a much smaller male predominance of CD (see Silverthorn & Frick, 1999 for a review). Also, during adolescence, boys and girls show equal rates of ODD, although prior to adolescence prevalence rates are significantly higher for boys than girls (Boylan et al., 2007).

PROACTIVE, REACTIVE, AND RELATIONAL AGGRESSION

Aggressive behavior constitutes a key class of symptoms used to diagnose CD. Although not included in the DSM-IV/TR, an important distinction has been made in the literature between children who show largely reactive forms of aggression (e.g., retaliatory and often in response to real or perceived provocation) and those who show both reactive and proactive forms of aggression (Poulin & Boivin, 2000; Salmivalli & Nieminen, 2002). Aggression that is proactive in form is premeditated and instrumental, such as to obtain goods or services, to obtain dominance over others, or to enhance one's social status. Although these two forms of aggression often co-occur in school-aged children, many studies have documented that they show distinct correlates (e.g., Brown, Atkins, Osborne, & Milnamow, 1996). For example, reactive aggression is associated with greater social isolation, peer rejection, social information processing deficits (i.e., social problem-solving deficits, hostile attributional bias to ambiguous provocation situations), and a temperamental propensity toward angry reactivity and emotional dysregulation (Crick & Dodge, 1996; Dodge, Lochman, Harnish, Bates, & Pettit, 1997; Dodge & Pettit, 2003; Hubbard et al., 2002). In contrast, proactively aggressive children show lower levels of anxiety and associate more positive outcomes with their aggressive behavior, compared with reactively aggressive children (Dodge et al., 1997; Price & Dodge, 1989; Schwartz et al., 1998).

A third type of aggression, relational aggression is a form of antisocial behavior that is more common among girls than boys (Coie & Dodge, 1998). Several studies have found that when girls behave aggressively, they are less likely to display physical or overt aggressive behaviors common to boys with CD, and are more likely to choose relational aggression as a strategy for use within the peer group (Crick, 1996; Crick, Casas, & Mosher, 1997; Crick & Grotpeter, 1995a; Ostrov & Keating, 2004). Relationally aggressive behaviors include gossiping and telling lies about others, spreading rumors, and actively excluding others from participation in social events or inclusion and acceptance into a peer group. These behaviors function to purposely damage another child's social relationships and friendships (Crick & Grotpeter, 1995a, 1995b; Crick et al., 1997; Crick et al., 1999). It should be noted that although relational aggression is more common in girls than boys, physical aggression is present in both girls and boys.

CHILDHOOD- VERSUS ADOLESCENT-ONSET CD

It has become increasingly clear that youth with CD constitute a heterogeneous group in ways other than types of aggression. As a result, there have been a number of attempts to define more homogeneous subgroups that share similar behavioral manifestations (i.e., type and trajectory of behaviors), common risk factors, and similar risk for future adjustment problems (see Frick & Marsee, 2006 for a review). At the crux of these approaches is the notion that there may be multiple developmental pathways to conduct problems, each with somewhat unique causal processes and etiological factors involved (Frick, 1998; Moffitt, 1993; Patterson, Reid, & Dishion, 1992a; Richters, 1997). The most widely accepted method for distinguishing between subtypes of youth with CD is based on the age of symptom onset. That is, the DSM-IV distinguishes between two subtypes of CD – childhood-onset and adolescent-onset – depending on whether a child begins showing severe behavior problems in early childhood or after the onset of adolescence. Longitudinal studies suggest that the proportion of youth with adolescent-onset CD is significantly greater than the proportion of youth with a childhood-onset to their conduct problems (Fergusson & Horwood, 2002; Lahey et al., 2006; Wiesner, Kim, & Capaldi, 2005), although this may not be the case in incarcerated samples where the proportion is more equal (Silverthorn, Frick, & Reynolds, 2001). Importantly, the distinction between childhood- and adolescent-onset CD is critical for identifying distinctions in causal mechanisms and developmental course and prognosis (Frick & Loney, 1999).

Adolescent-Onset CD

Youth with the adolescent-onset pattern of CD fail to show distinct temperamental or personality deficits prior to adolescence (Moffitt, 2003; Moffitt & Caspi, 2001; Moffitt, Caspi, Dickson, Silva, & Stanton, 1996). That is, they are less likely than children with childhood-onset CD to show elevated rates of family dysfunction, comorbid psychopathology, neurocognitive deficits, academic, and peer difficulties. Compared with childhood-onset CD, youth with adolescent-onset CD are less likely to show a family history of externalizing problems and the genetic contribution to their conduct problems is low (Moffitt, 2003, 2006). The emergence of serious antisocial behaviors for youth in the adolescent-onset pathway coincides with the onset of puberty. That is, youth with adolescent-onset CD do not typically show the less severe ODD behaviors earlier in development, but instead show a range of both ODD and CD behaviors coinciding with the onset of puberty (Moffitt, 2003).

Whereas the developmental process of identity formation and independence leads all adolescents to show some level of rebelliousness against parents and other authority figures (Brezina & Piquero, 2007), youth with adolescent-onset CD show an exaggeration of this normative process (Moffitt, 1993, 2003). Consistent with this model, youth with adolescent-onset CD score higher on measures of rebelliousness and authority conflict and are more rejecting of conventional values, compared with control children

(Dandreaux & Frick, in press; Moffitt et al., 1996). For youth with adolescent-onset CD, engagement in delinquent and aggressive behaviors seems to be a maladaptive and misguided attempt to obtain a subjective sense of maturity and adult status. Further, these youth are highly influenced by their associations with delinquent peers and they attempt to achieve social status within these peer groups by engaging in delinquent activities, which are encouraged and reinforced. Although youth with both a childhood- and adolescent-onset to their conduct problems show equally high levels of delinquent peer affiliation (Moffitt et al., 1996), this association provides a more direct causal link to the development of conduct problems in youth with adolescent-onset CD (Moffitt, 1993; Moffitt & Caspi, 2001; Moffitt et al., 1996). That is, for the adolescent-onset group, association with delinquent peers may be a critical factor in their extreme rebelliousness, rejection of authority, and rejection of societal norms.

Given that the antisocial behavior of the adolescent-onset group is believed to be an exaggeration of a process specific to adolescence, and not due to an enduring vulnerability, this behavior is less likely to persist beyond adolescence. Consistent with this notion, youth with adolescent-onset CD are less likely to show academic, occupational, social, or physical impairment in adulthood compared with youth with childhood-onset CD (Moffitt, 2003), although they are at greater risk for substance abuse problems (Odgers et al., 2007). For example, in a prospective study of the adult outcomes of a birth cohort in New Zealand, Moffitt, Caspi, Harrington, and Milne (2002) reported that the adolescent-onset CD group was 50–60% less likely to be convicted of an offense in adulthood, and their offenses tended to be less serious (e.g., minor theft, public drunkenness) and less violent (e.g., property offenses) than children whose chronic conduct problems started prior to adolescence.

Childhood-Onset CD

Youth with childhood-onset CD typically begin showing mild oppositional problems (e.g., argumentativeness, non-compliance) early in development, around ages 3 and 4, and these problems tend to increase in rate and severity over the course of development (Lahey & Loeber, 1994). Thus, ODD seems to be a developmental precursor to childhood onset CD in that oppositional symptoms often gradually progress into increasingly more severe types of conduct problems that are added to the youth's existing behavioral repertoire over the course of childhood (Hinshaw, Lahey, & Hart, 1993; Lahey & Loeber, 1994; Moffitt, 1993). In fact, ODD has been identified as one of the strongest predictors of the onset of CD (Loeber, Green, Keenan, & Lahey, 1995), and as many as 80% of boys with childhood-onset CD were previously diagnosed with ODD (Lahey & Loeber, 1997). However, it is important to note that a large number of children with ODD (40%) never progress to more severe conduct problems (Lahey & Loeber, 1994).

Dispositional risk factors. In contrast to the adolescent-onset subtype of CD, youth in the childhood-onset group show a number of distinct dispositional and environmental risk factors early in life that place them at risk for developing a more severe, stable, and chronic pattern of antisocial and aggressive behavior (Frick & Morris, 2004; Moffitt & Caspi, 2001). That is, childhood-onset CD is associated with neuropsychological (e.g., autonomic irregularities, executive functioning deficits, ADHD symptoms, emotional dysregulation, low IQ) and temperamental deficits (i.e., impulsivity). For example, youth with childhood-onset CD are at greater risk for comorbid psychopathology, such as Attention Deficit/Hyperactivity Disorder (ADHD) (Abikoff & Klein, 1992; Frick, 1998; Lilienfeld & Waldman, 1990; Lynam, 1996). In fact, in children with CD, rates of comorbid ADHD diagnosis range from 36% in community samples (Waschbusch, 2002) to as high as 90% in clinic-referred samples with severe conduct problems (Abikoff & Klein, 1992). The impulsivity associated with ADHD may also lead directly to some of the aggressive and other poorly regulated behaviors characteristic of children with CD (Frick & Morris, 2004).

Internalizing problems (i.e., anxiety, depression) are also highly comorbid in children with DBDs (Andershed, Gustafson, Kerr, & Stattin, 2002; Frick, Cornell, Bodin et al., 2003). An estimated 15–31% of community children with CD present with comorbid depression, and an estimated 22–33% present with a comorbid anxiety disorder (60–75% in clinic-referred samples) (Russo & Beidel, 1994; Zoccolillo, 1993). However, there is some suggestion that internalizing problems, especially depression, have their onset after CD symptoms and may be the result of interpersonal conflicts (e.g., with parents, peers, teachers, and police) and other stressors (e.g., family dysfunction, failure in school) experienced by youth with severe conduct problems (Capaldi, 1992; Frick, Lilienfeld, Ellis, Loney, & Silverthorn, 1999). There is also significant comorbidity between CD and learning disabilities (Cantwell & Baker, 1992), which may contribute to the academic problems found in children with severe conduct problems.

Environmental risk factors. Individual differences in susceptibility to antisocial behavior have both a heritable and an environmental component. Research suggests that genetic factors have a more substantial contribution to the development of childhood-onset CD (Eaves et al., 2000; Eley, Lichenstein, & Stevenson, 1999; Moffitt, 2005; Rhee & Waldman, 2002), whereas greater emphasis is placed on social causes for the adolescent-onset group. However, youth with childhood-onset CD are still at greater risk for experiencing several types of environmental risk factors, such as perinatal complications, severe family dysfunction, neighborhood disorganization and poverty (Kratzer & Hodgins, 1997; Moffitt, 1993, 2003; Moffitt et al., 2008). Youth with persistent conduct problems who have a childhood-onset are significantly more likely to show a family history of externalizing problems (i.e., CD, antisocial personality disorder, substance abuse disorders) than youth with an adolescent-onset to their conduct problems (Farrington, Jolliffe, Loeber, Stouthamer-Loeber, & Kalb, 2001; Farrington & Loeber, 2000; McCabe, Rodgers, Yeh, & Hough, 2004; Taylor, Iacono, & McGue, 2000). In addition to transmitting genetic risk for externalizing problems, antisocial parents are more likely to be of low socioeconomic status, engage in dysfunctional and sometimes abusive parenting practices, and often expose their children to chaotic and hostile home environments frequently marked by domestic violence (Jaffee, Belsky, Harrington, Caspi, & Moffitt, 2006; Kim-Cohen, Caspi, Rutter, Tomas, & Moffitt, 2006; McCabe et al., 2004).

Dysfunctional family environments also place the child at risk for developing cognitive deficits. For example, the experience of childhood physical abuse has been found to relate to a tendency to perceive innocuous experiences as hostile (i.e., hostile attribution bias), causing the child to react to perceived slights with anger and aggression (Dodge, Price, Bachorowski, & Newman, 1990). Also, children exposed to an inconsistent and noncontingent family environment may learn to become overly focused on the potential positive consequences of their behavior (i.e., obtaining a stereo) while ignoring the potential negative consequences (i.e., being arrested for stealing) (Barry et al., 2000; Pardini, Lochman, & Frick, 2003b). They also often display problems in the appropriate modulation of their behavior (i.e., delay gratification, conforming to parental and societal expectations) (Patterson, 1986). Importantly, these cognitive deficits can place the child at risk for rejection by conventional peers depriving him or her of important peer socializing experiences that foster the development of social and cognitive skills (Dodge, Bates, & Pettit, 1990; Price & Dodge, 1989). Further, peer rejection may cause the child to seek out associations with nonconventional and deviant peers, particularly when parents provide poor supervision (Coie, Terry, Zakriski, & Lochman, 1995; Dishion, Patterson, Stoolmiller, & Skinner, 1991; McCabe et al., 2004; Vitaro, Brendgen, Pagani, Tremblay, & McDuff, 1999).

With respect to course and prognosis, youth with childhood-onset CD show poorer outcomes in adulthood. For example, they show greater convictions and incarcerations, as well as greater social and occupational impairment (Frick & Loney, 1999; see Moffitt, 2003; Moffitt, 2006 for a review). In fact, research suggests that a third to a half of CD youth with childhood-onset will be diagnosed with antisocial personality disorder (APD) in adulthood (Loeber et al., 2002). In addition to showing poorer mental health outcomes, children in the childhood-onset group are also at great risk for physical health problems and show high mortality rates (Kratzer & Hodgins, 1997). They experience more physical injuries and illnesses, particularly chronic respiratory illness, contract more sexually transmitted diseases, and are more likely to suffer from periodontal disease (Farrington, 1995; Odgers et al., 2007; Piquero, Daigle, Gibson, Piquero, & Tibbetts, 2007). They are also at greater risk for school dropout and unwanted pregnancies (Bardone, Moffitt, Caspi, & Dickson, 1996; Capaldi & Stoolmiller, 1999). While research consistently demonstrates that youth with childhood-onset CD have poorer outcomes than youth with adolescent-onset CD, effects across gender are not uniform. The rate of antisocial outcomes is not as high for girls with CD as for boys with CD, although girls are at heightened risk for other adult adjustment problems, including somatization, emotional disorders, suicide attempts, and severe impairments in occupational and social adjustment (Robins, Tipp, & Pryzbeck, 1991; Silverthorn & Frick, 1999; Zoccolillo, 1993).

Assessment

The above review suggests that one of the most critical pieces of information that needs to be obtained in an assessment is the age at which various serious conduct problems began, as this provides some indication as to whether the child may be on the childhood-onset or adolescent-onset pathway and can be helpful in guiding intervention efforts. Age of onset has already been incorporated into several structured risk assessment measures (Augimeri et al., 2005; Borum et al., 2005). Although there is considerable support for the childhood- versus adolescent-onset distinction, there is some concern over the accuracy of age of onset information for differential diagnosis (see Moffitt et al., 2008). First, there is some suggestion that a childhood-limited subtype of CD may exist that is not included in the DSM-IV and is distinguished from the life-course-persistent type of childhood-onset CD by a pattern of desistance from conduct problems over development (see Moffitt, 2003; 2006 for a review). When identifying conduct problems in children younger than age 10, there is at present no empirically supported method for distinguishing between these two subtypes of childhood-onset CD. Second, when evaluating age of onset in adolescents, the accuracy of official records and informant judgments may be questionable given the research finding that the recall of this information tends to lag years later than the actual age of onset (Henry, Moffitt, Caspi, Langley, & Silva, 1994) and contact with law enforcement tends to occur 2–5 years after a youth's first criminal act (Moffitt et al., 2001). Also, by adolescence, youth with childhood-onset CD may be well on their way to a persistent pattern of CD and therefore assessing age of onset for conduct problems may be insufficient for assisting clinicians in treatment planning. That is, the DSM's disaggregation of CD into childhood- and adolescent-onset subtypes may not adequately capture the heterogeneity in causal pathways leading to severe antisocial and aggressive behavior in adolescence and adulthood.

SUBTYPES OF CHILDHOOD-ONSET CD

A primary purpose for distinguishing between childhood- and adolescent-onset patterns of conduct problems is to identify distinct developmental mechanisms underlying problem behaviors in more homogeneous subgroups of antisocial youth. This subtyping approach exemplifies the developmental psychopathology concept of *equifinality*, which proposes that the same developmental outcome (e.g., conduct problems) may result from divergent developmental pathways and processes (Cicchetti & Rogosch, 1996). The concept of equifinality has been applied to research on CD to explore the possibility that youth with a childhood-onset to their antisocial behaviors can be further disaggregated into subgroups with distinct etiological mechanisms underlying their problematic behaviors. Several attempts have been made to further distinguish subtypes of youth showing early conduct problems. For example, earlier editions of the DSM distinguished between aggressive and nonaggressive subtypes of CD (American

Psychiatric Association, 1980). This distinction was believed to be important in that children with aggressive CD show a more stable pattern of conduct problems that is particularly resistant to treatment efforts (Huesmann, Eron, Lefkowitz, & Walder, 1984).

Emotional Regulation

One subtyping approach distinguishes youth with childhood-onset CD based on distinct temperamental styles reflecting the level of emotional reactivity underlying their behaviors (Frick & Morris, 2004). One group experiences difficulty regulating their emotions and shows a tendency to react impulsively with strong angry and hostile emotions (i.e., emotionally dysregulated subtype), whereas a second group experiences low levels of emotional reactivity that may interfere with normal socialization (i.e., callous-unemotional subtype) (Christian, Frick, Hill, Tyler, & Frazer, 1997; Frick, Cornell, Bodin et al., 2003). Importantly, research suggests that different causal processes may underlie the conduct problems of both subtypes of youth with early conduct problems such that the former shows too high a level of emotional reactivity, and the latter shows too little affective response (see Frick & Morris, 2004).

The characteristic tendency of the emotionally dysregulated subtype toward angry reactivity can lead a child to engage in aggressive behaviors within contexts characterized by high emotional arousal and without thinking of the potential consequences of these acts (Hubbard et al., 2002; Kruh, Frick, & Clements, 2005; Loney, Frick, Clements, Ellis, & Kerlin, 2003). As a result, CD youth with emotion regulation problems are more likely to commit impulsive and unplanned antisocial acts for which they are typically remorseful afterwards (Frick & Morris, 2004; Pardini et al., 2003b). Consistent with this model, these children are more likely to engage in reactive types of aggression that are typically in response to real or perceived provocation by others (Frick, Cornell, Barry, Bodin, & Dane, 2003; Frick, Cornell, Bodin et al., 2003). They also show high rates of emotional distress (Frick, Cornell, Bodin et al., 2003; Frick et al., 1999), and are highly reactive to negative emotional stimuli, particularly the distress of others (Kimonis, Frick, Fazekas, & Loney, 2006; Loney et al., 2003; Pardini et al., 2003b). All of these findings support the contention that problems regulating emotion are critical for understanding the causes of their behavioral problems (Frick, 2006; Frick & Morris, 2004).

Biological risk factors. Unfortunately, few brain imaging studies have focused on specific subgroups of children with CD. However, a few studies have documented several neurological correlates that would be consistent with the problems in emotional regulation displayed by some children with childhood-onset CD. For example, one study documented reduced anterior cingulate responsivity to threatening emotional scenes under passive viewing in youth with conduct problems, which is believed to reflect deficits in emotional regulation (Stadler et al., 2007; Sterzer, Stadler, Krebs, Kleinschmidt, & Poustka, 2005). A more recent study using a passive viewing paradigm (i.e., serial presentation of slides with neutral, positive, and negative emotional valence) found increased amygdala activation when viewing negative slides (e.g., wounded children, violent scenes), partly related to co-morbid anxiety, in children with antisocial behavior (Herpertz et al., 2008). With regard to genetic risk, imaging studies suggest that the low-activity Monoamine Oxidase A genotype (MAOA-L) may relate specifically to children who show impulsive and reactive types of conduct problems (see Buckholtz & Meyer-Lindenberg, 2008 for a review).

Familial and environmental risk factors. Youth with CD who have problems with emotion regulation are also more likely to show deficits in verbal intelligence (Loney, Frick, Ellis, & McCoy, 1998) and come from families with high rates of dysfunctional parenting practices (Hipwell et al., 2007; Oxford, Cavell, & Hughes, 2003; Wootton, Frick, Shelton, & Silverthorn, 1997) and physical abuse (Dodge, Bates & Pettit, 1990; Strassberg, Dodge, Pettit, & Bates, 1994), compared to other youth with CD. Beyond the direct effect of problematic parenting, theory suggests that an emotionally dysregulated temperamental style may interfere with appropriate socialization by parents and peers (Frick & Morris, 2004). That is, the ability of these youths to interpret and use social cues within socialization experiences becomes detrimentally affected by their susceptibility to experiences of intense negative emotional arousal (Dodge & Pettit, 2003). As a result, within discipline encounters, they may not effectively process the parental message and internalize parental norms (Hoffman, 1994; Kochanska, 1993; 1997). Also, coercive cycles (i.e., a pattern of behavior occurring during the parent–child interaction in which a slight increase in aggression by the parent or child is reciprocated by equivalent or escalated aggression by the other person) may develop between the emotionally dysregulated youth and his or her parent, causing the child to learn to act in an aggressive and antisocial manner (Patterson, Reid, & Dishion, 1992b). With regard to peer relations, children showing intense, unregulated displays of negative emotion are more likely to be rejected by their classmates (Rubin, Bukowski, & Parker, 1998), putting them at greater risk for school truancy and association with delinquent peers who encourage future delinquent and aggressive behaviors (Keenan, Loeber, Zhang, Stouthamer-Loeber, & Van Kammen, 1995).

Callous-Unemotional Traits

Compared with the high levels of emotional arousal experienced by youth with CD who have problems with emotional regulation, a second subtype of youth with childhood-onset CD show the opposite pattern of too little emotional response – youth with callous-unemotional (CU) traits (e.g., absence of guilt and empathy, callous use of others for one's own gain). Research has consistently documented a subgroup of children with CD in school-based samples (Frick, Bodin, & Barry, 2000), outpatient mental health clinics (Christian et al., 1997; Frick, O'Brien, Wootton, & McBurnett, 1994), and juvenile forensic facilities (Caputo, Frick, & Brodsky, 1999; Silverthorn, Frick, & Reynolds, 2001) who show high levels of CU traits. Youth within the childhood-onset trajectory who also show CU traits are distinguished by higher levels of conduct problems that are more severe and stable (Frick, Stickle, Dandreaux, Farrell, & Kimonis, 2005;

Loeber et al., 2002). In their review of 24 published studies using child or adolescent samples, Frick and Dickens (2006) found that CU traits were associated with more severe conduct problems, delinquency, or violence and aggression. Eight additional studies published since this earlier review provide additional support for this finding (see Frick & White, 2008).

Compared to youth with CD and emotional regulation problems, those high on CU traits tend to be more aggressive and violent (Frick, Cornell, Barry et al., 2003). They also tend to engage in both instrumental (e.g., for gain) and reactive (e.g., in response to perceived provocation) forms of aggression (Enebrink, Andershed, & Langstrom, 2005; Fanti, Frick, & Georgiou, in press; Frick, Cornell, Barry et al., 2003; Frick & Marsee, 2006). In fact, many of the social–cognitive and affective differences that have been found between reactive and instrumental forms of aggression may be attributed to differences in their association with CU traits (Munoz, Frick, Kimonis, & Aucoin, 2008a; Pardini et al., 2003b; Waschbusch, Walsh, Andrade, King, & Carrey, 2007). Similar to findings with CD youth more generally, girls with CU traits are more likely to engage in relational forms of aggression than boys (Marsee & Frick, 2007; Odgers, Reppucci, & Moretti, 2005; Penney & Moretti, 2007).

With regard to course and prognosis, the presence of CU traits predicts greater rates of later delinquency, aggression and violent offending, as well as a shorter length of time to violent reoffending in antisocial adolescents (Brandt, Kennedy, Patrick, & Curtin, 1997; Forth, Hart, & Hare, 1990; Pardini, Obradovic, & Loeber, 2006; Ridenour, Marchant, & Dean, 2001). Further, youth with CU traits showed the highest rate of conduct problems, self-reported delinquency, and police contacts across a 4-year study period (Frick et al., 2005). They may also be at greater risk for developing antisocial personality disorders, such as psychopathy, in adulthood (Burke, Loeber, & Lahey, 2007; Loeber et al., 2002). In fact, the distinction between youth with CD who display a presence or absence of CU traits is similar to the distinction made within samples of antisocial adults using the construct of psychopathy. That is, the presence of psychopathic traits seems to designate an important subgroup of individuals with APD with distinct etiological mechanisms underlying their behaviors (Hare, 1996). Callous-unemotional traits are believed to tap the "deficient affective experience" (e.g., poverty of emotions, lack of empathy and guilt) of adult psychopathy (Cooke & Michie, 1997; Hare, 2003).

Biological risk factors. As noted previously, genetic influences seem to be particularly strong for youth with a childhood-onset to their CD. However, studies suggest that this may largely be due to the subgroup with CU traits. To date, two large twin studies have reported substantial genetic influences on measures of CU traits (Larsson, Andershed, & Lichtenstein, 2006; Taylor, Loney, Bobadilla, Lacono, & McGue, 2003), with both providing very similar estimates of the amount of variation in CU traits accounted for by genetic effects (i.e., 43% and 42%, respectively). However, Viding et al. (2005) more directly addressed the question of whether youth with and without CU traits show differences in the heritability of their conduct problems. Out of a total sample of 3,687 7-year-old twin pairs, they selected a sample of twins high on conduct problems and further divided them into those who were high and low on CU traits. When comparing the two groups, the group heritability (i.e., percentage of variance in conduct problems that could be accounted for by genetic factors) for the high conduct problem group was substantial (0.68) but the estimate was very different for those high on CU traits (0.81) and those low on CU traits (0.30). This finding was replicated in the same sample two years later at age 9 (Viding, Jones, Frick, Moffitt, & Plomin, 2008). Importantly, differences in heritability could not be attributed to differences in the severity of conduct problems or levels of hyperactivity. Interestingly, Viding et al. (2005) reported that in addition to the difference in genetic influences in the groups high and low on CU traits, the influence of shared environment was substantial for the group low on CU traits but negligible for the group high on these traits, which is consistent with studies finding that conduct problems are more strongly associated with dysfunctional parenting in children low on CU traits (e.g., Hipwell et al., 2007; Oxford et al., 2003; Wootton et al., 1997).

Genetic factors may underlie the distinct temperamental style found in youth with CU traits that is characterized by deficits in their emotional arousal to fear and distress in others and abnormalities in their response to cues of punishment and danger (Frick, 2006; Frick & Morris, 2004). Specifically, these youth have been described as displaying a temperamental style that has been variously labeled as low fearfulness (Rothbart & Bates, 1998) or low behavioral inhibition (Kagan & Snidman, 1991). Indeed, studies show that CU youth show deficits in response to stimuli that typically elicit a fear response. For example, youth with CU traits show a decreased sensitivity to punishment cues in laboratory and social settings (Blair, Peschardt, Budhani, Mitchell, & Pine, 2006; Dadds & Hawes, 2006; Fisher & Blair, 1998; Pardini et al., 2003b) and lower resting and stress-induced levels of cortisol (Loney, Butler, Lima, Counts, & Eckel, 2006; O'Leary, Loney, & Eckel, 2007). Importantly, fearless children may be at risk for impaired moral development as they are less likely to experience transgression-related arousal within socialization experiences in response to threats of punishment (Kochanska, 1993). A number of studies of normally developing children have documented both concurrent (e.g., Fowles & Kochanska, 2000; Kochanska, Gross, Lin, & Nichols, 2002) and predictive (Rothbart, Ahadi, & Hershey, 1994) associations between a fearless temperament and lower scores on measures of conscience development. Consistent with the hypothesized link to a fearless temperament, youth with CU traits show a preference for novel, exciting, and dangerous activities, are particularly prone to boredom, and show less trait anxiety than other youth with the same level of conduct problems (Andershed, Gustafson et al., 2002; Essau, Sasagawa, & Frick, 2006; Frick, Cornell, Bodin et al., 2003; Frick et al., 1999). That is, children with CU traits appear to be less distressed by the negative effects of their behavior problems on themselves and others compared to youth with comparable levels of conduct problems (Blair, Jones, Clark, & Smith, 1997; Pardini et al., 2003b).

In addition to showing deficits in their response to fear-inducing stimuli, antisocial youth with CU traits in clinical, community, and incarcerated settings also show abnormal processing of emotional stimuli (i.e., pictures, words, facial expressions, vocal tones) that typically evoke empathy (e.g., images of others crying). For example, antisocial youth with CU traits show less psychophysiological responsiveness to others' distress cues and sad facial expressions (Blair, 1999; Blair, Colledge, Murray, & Mitchell, 2001); impaired recognition of sad and fearful facial expressions and sad vocal tones (Blair & Coles, 2000; Blair et al., 2001; Stevens, Charman, & Blair, 2001); and reduced attention to images of others in distress (Kimonis et al., 2006). When studies have compared types of emotional stimuli, there is consistent evidence that youth with CU traits do not show abnormalities in how they process stimuli with positive emotional content, but specifically in the processing of negative and unpleasant emotional stimuli (Kimonis et al., 2006; Loney et al., 2003; Sharp, van Goozen, & Goodyer, 2006). Deficits in emotional reactivity that may tap underlying genetic or temperamental vulnerabilities make the child more difficult to socialize and place him or her at risk for problems in the normal development of guilt, empathy, and other aspects of conscience (Blair, 1995; Frick & Morris, 2004; Kagan, 1998; Kochanska, 1993).

The distinct temperamental characteristics and related cognitive and affective deficits displayed by youth high on CU traits may map onto potentially inherited predispositions toward distinct neurological functioning that may place these youth at greater risk for developing antisocial and aggressive behaviours (Viding & Jones, 2008). Specifically, Blair et al. (2005) and Viding (2004) have suggested that the unique constellation of deficits identified in youth with CU traits could implicate impaired functioning of the amygdala and related neural circuitry, including the orbitofrontal cortex, a pattern similar to that found in adults with psychopathy (Blair, Budhani, Colledge, & Scott, 2005; Kiehl et al., 2001). For example, in normal subjects, expressions of sadness and fear typically elicit activation of the amygdala (Blair, Morris, Frith, Perrett, & Dolan, 1999), which is also involved in several types of instrumental learning tasks involving the use of punishment information (Blair et al., 2005). Consistent with these hypothesized neural pathways, fMRI brain imaging studies have found that when performing an implicit emotion processing task (i.e., gender recognition), antisocial youth with CU traits show hypoactivation of the amygdala in response to fearful faces, compared with typically developing children and children with ADHD (Jones, Laurens, Herba, Barker, & Viding, 2009; Marsh et al., 2008). Abnormal ventromedial prefrontal cortex response to punishment has also been documented in youth with CU traits when performing a response modulation (i.e., "the relatively automatic shift of attention from the execution of a dominant response to relevant secondary and/or contextual cues that might be used to modify the ongoing response") task (Finger et al., 2008; Vitale et al., 2005, p. 462). This latter finding is consistent with studies demonstrating that youth with CU traits are less sensitive to punishment cues, especially when a reward-oriented response set is primed (Fisher & Blair, 1998; O'Brien & Frick, 1996; Pardini et al., 2003a).

Familial and environmental risk factors. Antisocial youth high on CU traits do not appear to show the same psychosocial risk factors reported for youth low on CU traits. For example, although dysfunctional parenting is consistently associated with CD, ineffective parenting is less strongly related to the presence of conduct problems in community samples (Hipwell et al., 2007; Oxford et al., 2003), clinic-referred youth (Wootton et al., 1997), and incarcerated juvenile offenders (Edens, Skopp, & Cahill, 2008) high on CU traits. Also, antisocial youth with CU traits are less likely to show deficits in verbal intelligence than other antisocial youth (Loney et al., 1998; Salekin, Neumann, Leistico, & Zalot, 2004). In fact, in one study of juvenile offenders, higher verbal abilities were linked to higher rates of violent offending in youth with CU traits (Munoz, Frick, Kimonis, & Aucoin, 2008b). Youth with CU traits, with and without conduct problems, are significantly more likely to affiliate with delinquent peers when compared with antisocial youth without CU traits (Kimonis, Frick, & Barry, 2004). Although exposure to a social context in which peers encourage deviant behaviors likely contributes to the maintenance and greater severity of antisocial behaviors, it is less likely to be a causal factor given that conduct problems in this subgroup of youth are more likely to emerge in childhood (i.e., Moffitt et al., 1996).

Assessment of CU traits. Given the importance of CU traits as a marker for a more severe and stable pattern of conduct problems across development, it is essential that clinicians assess for the presence of these traits in youth presenting with conduct problems. In fact, the inclusion of psychopathic/CU traits as a new specifier for conduct disorder is under consideration for the forthcoming DSM-V (see Moffitt et al., 2008). Several assessment tools have been developed for the measurement of CU traits in community and incarcerated youth. For children in community settings, the Antisocial Process Screening Device (APSD; Frick & Hare, 2001) and the Child Psychopathy Scale (CPS; Lynam, 1997) are behavior-rating scales that can be completed by parents, guardians, and teachers. Adjudicated youth are most often assessed with the Psychopathy Checklist: Youth Version (PCL:YV; Forth, Kosson, & Hare, 2003), which involves a lengthy clinical interview and review of the youth's institutional file. Self-report measures have also been developed for use with adolescent and pre-adolescent populations for a quicker assessment of CU traits, and are particularly useful for youth in the community for whom chart information is unavailable. These include the self-report APSD (Munoz & Frick, 2007) and the Youth Psychopathic Traits Inventory (Andershed, Kerr, Stattin, & Levander, 2002)

One issue that is important for assessing CU traits is that most measures that assess these traits typically were designed to assess multiple dimensions of psychopathy and include only a limited number of items specifically assessing CU traits, often with as few as four (Forth et al., 2003) or six (Frick & Hare, 2001) items. Further, and possibly due to this limited item pool, measures of CU traits often have had some significant psychometric limitations, such as displaying poor internal consistency in samples of adolescents (Poythress, Dembo, Wareham, & Greenbaum, 2006). One attempt to overcome these limitations is the development of the Inventory of Callous-Unemotional Traits (ICU; Frick, 2004), which is a self-report and informant-rated (i.e., parent, teacher) scale that provides a more extended assessment (e.g., 24 items) of the construct of CU traits.

The factor structure of this measure has been tested in community samples of adolescents in Germany (Essau, Sasagawa, & Frick, 2006) and Cyprus (Fanti et al., in press), and a sample of juvenile offenders in the United States (Kimonis et al., 2008). In all three samples, each using different translations of the scale, a similar bi-factor structure emerged with three factors (e.g., Uncaring, Callousness, Unemotional) loading on a higher-order CU dimension providing the best fit.

ADDITIVE, INTERACTIVE-EVOCATIVE, TRANSACTIONAL MODELS

The above review highlights the large number of risk factors associated with CD and the obvious inadequacy of etiological models that focus on any single risk factor to explain its development. Increasingly emerging research suggests that this large number of risk factors can act in additive, interactive, or transactional manners to contribute to the development of CD. The most basic method for integrating the influence of multiple risk factors is with a cumulative risk perspective. Rather than focusing on the type of risk factors, this approach emphasizes the additive effect of the total number of risk factors present. That is, the more risk factors that are present, the greater the child's risk for developing conduct problems (see Loeber & Farrington, 2000). A second perspective for integrating the effects of multiple risk factors is with an interactionist approach. From this perspective, a given risk factor (i.e., impulsivity) may constitute a moderate risk for conduct problems alone, but risk increases substantially in the presence of other risk factors (i.e., inadequate socializing experiences, poverty) (Lynam et al., 2000).

A third approach that incorporates the combined effect of multiple risk factors focuses on the reciprocal exchange between the child and his or her environment to explain the development of conduct problems. Similar to the interactionist perspective, normative developmental processes may become disrupted when particular combinations of risk factors co-occur. From the transactional perspective, a child with a given genetic predisposition to a particular temperamental style (i.e., emotional dysregulation) may elicit certain responses from others, which then feed back to the child to affect his or her own behavior. That is, ineffective reciprocal exchanges between the child and his or her parents in early childhood can function to reduce the effectiveness of socialization attempts and are likely to repeat later with teachers and peers when the child begins school. Support for the transactionist approach comes from an early study by Glueck and Glueck (1950) of 500 delinquents and 500 nondelinquents that reported that effective parenting strategies were undermined by delinquent children, resulting in erratic, threatening, and harsh discipline, poor supervision, and weak parent–child attachment. These ineffective parenting strategies further increased the risk for later delinquency (Sampson & Laub, 1994), demonstrating how a child's disposition can evoke dysfunctional responses in others and increase his or her risk for future conduct problems.

Gene-Environment Interactions

Given the transactional nature of risk factors, both biological and environmental, it is difficult to disentangle the effects of nature and nurture. The interaction of genes and environment suggest that individual genetic factors may moderate the relationship between environmental factors (e.g., childhood abuse) and the later development of conduct problems. For example, Caspi et al. (2002) found that the effect of childhood maltreatment on risk for conduct problems and aggressive behavior was moderated by a polymorphism in the Monoamine Oxidase A (MAOA) gene, which regulates serotonergic neurotransmission. That is, for individuals with the low-activity MAOA genotype (MAOA-L), the association between maltreatment and conduct problems was 0.30, whereas this association was significantly reduced (0.13) in individuals with the high-activity MAOA genotype. This suggests that for individuals with the genetic vulnerability conferred by MAOA-L, conduct problems may only manifest in the presence of an environmental trigger such as abuse.

Practical Implications: Assessment and Intervention

Research on the multiple developmental pathways to CD has a number of important implications for prevention and treatment (Frick, 2006). For clinicians, the first step in treatment planning should involve a comprehensive assessment of the youth that goes beyond simply documenting the presence of DSM-IV/TR CD criteria. That is, in order to adequately assess an individual child with conduct problems, clinicians must identify the unique constellation of risk factors that may be operating for him or her (Frick & McMahon, 2008; McMahon & Frick, 2005). This first step will assist the clinician in classifying the youth into a more homogenous subgroup to guide him or her in identifying the most critical targets of intervention and the most effective combination of services for that child (Frick, 2006; McMahon & Frick, 2005). To summarize, research suggests that there may be at least four subtypes of CD with distinct etiological processes underlying their antisocial behaviors, three of which are not currently included in the DSM-IV/TR: (a) a childhood-limited CD; (b) an adolescent-onset CD in which behavioral disturbance results from problems in identity formation; (c) a childhood-onset CD that may result from a temperamental style characterized by problems in emotion regulation (childhood-onset CD without CU traits); and (d) a childhood-onset CD that may result from a temperamental style characterized by low levels of emotional reactivity to cues of others' distress and threats of punishment that interferes with normal conscience development (childhood-onset CD with CU traits).

Research suggests that the most successful interventions for youth with severe antisocial and aggressive behaviors are both comprehensive and individualized. That is, they focus on treating a large number of risk factors that could lead to a child's behavioral problems and they are tailored to each child's unique constellation of needs (Conduct Problems Prevention Research Group., 2004; Henggeler, Schoenwald, Borduin, Rowland,

& Cunningham, 1998). For example, interventions that focus on anger control may be more effective for children within the childhood-onset pathway who do not exhibit CU traits but who often show problems with emotional regulation (Larson & Lochman, 2003). Importantly, a comprehensive and individualized approach to assessment and treatment can assist clinicians in (a) making judgments about a youth's long-term prognosis, (b) identifying youth in greatest need of intervention due to heightened risk for continued maladjustment, and (c) allocating greater resources to these targeted youth rather than squandering limited resources on lower-risk youth. For example, the above review suggests that children younger than age 10 who show an emotionally dysregulated or behaviorally uninhibited/ low fearful temperament may be a particularly important target group for violence prevention efforts.

Cornell and Frick (2007) found that behaviorally uninhibited preschool children who experienced strong, consistent, and obedience-oriented (i.e., authoritarian) parenting showed enhanced conscience development. This finding was interpreted to reflect the need for stronger methods of socialization in order to elicit an optimal level of arousal to allow for the internalization of parental norms for prosocial behavior in fearless children who suffer from reduced emotional arousal (see Kochanska, DeVet, Goldman, & Murray, 1994). However, this parenting approach may be less effective in youth prone to high levels of emotional arousal and may negatively affect the development of conscience for such youth (Kochanska, 1993), highlighting the importance of individualized interventions. Other researchers suggest that parenting practices that instead emphasize a warm and nurturing parent–child relationship may be more effective at buffering fearless children from developing later CU traits (Kochanska, 1997; Pardini, Lochman, & Powell, 2007). In another study of 4- to 9-year-old clinic-referred boys with conduct problems, Hawes and Dadds (2005) found that a punishment-oriented behavior modification program that taught parents more effective discipline strategies was not as effective in reducing disruptive behaviors in boys with CU traits, as they were with boys who were low on CU traits. However, in a different phase of treatment that focused on teaching parents methods for using positive reinforcement to encourage prosocial behaviors, children with CU traits were equally responsive to this parenting intervention as boys who were low on CU traits. This study appears consistent with the reward-oriented response style that has been identified in youth with CU traits that is outlined above. These studies further support the need for an individualized approach for providing more effective treatments to youth with conduct problems.

SUMMARY AND CONCLUSIONS

Youth with disruptive, antisocial, delinquent, and aggressive behaviors constitute a heterogeneous group. The common tendency to broadly study youth with conduct problems has resulted in the identification of a large number of risk factors. Importantly, there appear to be multiple developmental pathways to conduct problems, each with their own unique constellation of risk and protective factors. Various subtyping approaches have identified more homogeneous subgroups of youth with conduct problems that show distinct developmental trajectories, the most common of which distinguishes between conduct problems that onset in childhood versus adolescence. The childhood-onset subgroup begins to show oppositional behaviors early in life and this behavior worsens into more severe conduct problems over the course of development. There is significant research support for further distinguishing youth with a childhood-onset to their conduct problems into those with CU traits and those without (i.e., emotionally dysregulated type). Consistent with adult psychopathy, antisocial youth with CU traits show a number of distinct cognitive, emotional, and personality characteristics supporting the contention that the causal processes leading to their antisocial behavior is different from those operating for other antisocial youth. Further, CU traits are important for designating a group of antisocial youth who are at heightened risk for the development of early onset conduct problems, a more severe, stable, and aggressive pattern of antisocial behavior, and continued antisocial behavior and legal involvement into adulthood. Thus, when making important decisions about how to allocate limited therapeutic resources, this high-risk group may be particularly important to target. Importantly, interventions will be most effective when they are comprehensive and individualized and based on a thorough assessment of the child's unique constellation of risk factors.

REFERENCES

American Psychiatric Association. (1980). *Diagnostic and statistical manual of mental disorders* (3rd ed.). Washington, DC: American Psychiatric Association.

American Psychiatric Association. (1994). *Diagnostic and statistical manual of mental disorders* (4th ed.). Washington, DC: American Psychiatric Association.

American Psychiatric Association. (2000). *Diagnostic and statistical manual of mental disorders (4th edn. Text Revision)* (4th ed.). Washington, DC: American Psychiatric Association.

Abikoff, H., & Klein, R. G. (1992). Attention-deficit hyperactivity and conduct disorder: Comorbidity and implications for treatment. *Journal of Consulting and Clinical Psychology, 60*, 881–892.

Andershed, H. A., Gustafson, S. B., Kerr, M., & Stattin, H. (2002). The usefulness of self-reported psychopathy-like traits in the study of antisocial behaviour among non-referred adolescents. *European Journal of Personality, 16*(5), 383–402.

Andershed, H. A., Kerr, M., Stattin, H., & Levander, S. (2002). Psychopathic traits in non-referred youths: A new assessment tool. In E. Blauuw & L. Sheridan (Eds.), *Psychopaths: Current international perspectives* (pp. 131–158). The Hague: Elsevier.

Augimeri, L. K., Koegl, C. J., Levene, K. S., Webster, C. D., Grisso, T., Vincent, G. M., et al. (2005). *Early assessment risk lists for boys and girls: Mental health screening and assessment in juvenile justice* (pp. 295–310). New York, NY: Guilford Press.

Bardone, A. M., Moffitt, T., Caspi, A., & Dickson, N. (1996). Adult mental health and social outcomes of adolescent girls with depression and conduct disorder. *Development and Psychopathology, 8*(4), 811–829.

Barry, C. T., Frick, P. J., Grooms, T., McCoy, M. G., Ellis, M. L., & Loney, B. R. (2000). The importance of callous-unemotional traits for extending the concept of psychopathy to children. *Journal of Abnormal Psychology, 109*, 335–340.

Blair, R. J. R. (1995). A cognitive developmental approach to morality: Investigating the psychopath. *Cognition, 57*, 1–29.

Blair, R. J. R. (1999). Responsiveness to distress cues in the child with psychopathic tendencies. *Personality and Individual Differences, 27*, 135–145.

Blair, R. J. R., Budhani, S., Colledge, E., & Scott, S. (2005). Deafness to fear in boys with psychopathic tendencies. *Journal of Child Psychology and Psychiatry and Allied Disciplines, 46*(3), 327–336.

Blair, R. J. R., & Coles, M. (2000). Expression recognition and behavioral problems in early adolescence. *Cognitive Development, 15*, 421–434.

Blair, R. J. R., Colledge, E., Murray, L., & Mitchell, D. G. V. (2001). A selective impairment in the processing of sad and fearful expressions in children with psychopathic tendencies. *Journal of Abnormal Child Psychology, 29*(6), 491–498.

Blair, R. J. R., Jones, L., Clark, F., & Smith, M. (1997). The psychopathic individual: A lack of responsiveness to distress cues? *Psychophysiology, 34*, 192–198.

Blair, R. J. R., Morris, J. S., Frith, C. C., Perrett, D. I., & Dolan, R. J. (1999). Dissociable neural responses to facial expressions of sadness and anger. *Brain: A Journal of Neurology, 122*(5), 883–893.

Blair, R. J. R., Peschardt, K. S., Budhani, S., Mitchell, D. G. V., & Pine, D. S. (2006). The development of psychopathy. *Journal of Child Psychology and Psychiatry, 47*(3), 262–275.

Borum, R., Bartel, P. A., Forth, A. E., Grisso, T., Vincent, G. M., & Seagrave, D. (2005). *Structured assessment of violence risk in youth: Mental health screening and assessment in juvenile justice* (pp. 311–323). New York, NY: Guilford Press.

Boylan, K., Vaillancourt, T., Boyle, M., & Szatmari, P. (2007). Comorbidity of internalizing disorders in children with oppositional defiant disorder. *European Journal of Child Adolescent Psychiatry, 16*, 484–494.

Brandt, J. R., Kennedy, W. A., Patrick, C. J., & Curtin, J. J. (1997). Assessment of psychopathy in a population of incarcerated adolescent offenders. *Psychological Assessment, 9*, 429–435.

Brezina, T., & Piquero, A. R. (2007). Moral beliefs, isolation from peers, and abstention from delinquency. *Deviant Behavior, 28*(5), 433–465.

Brown, K., Atkins, M. S., Osborne, M. L., & Milnamow, M. (1996). A revised teacher rating scale for reactive and proactive aggression. *Journal of Abnormal Child Psychology, 24*(4), 473–480.

Buckholtz, J. W., & Meyer-Lindenberg, A. (2008). MAOA and the neurogenetic architecture of human aggression. *Trends in Neurosciences, 31*(3), 120–129.

Burke, J. D., Loeber, R., & Lahey, B. B. (2007). Adolescent conduct disorder and interpersonal callousness as predictors of psychopathy in young adults. *Journal of Clinical Child and Adolescent Psychology, 36*, 334–346.

Cantwell, D. P., & Baker, L. (1992). Attention deficit disorder with and without hyperactivity: A review and comparison of matched groups. *Journal of the American Academy of Child and Adolescent Psychiatry, 31*, 432–438.

Capaldi, D. (1992). The co-occurrence of conduct problems and depressive symptoms in early adolescent boys, II: A 2-year follow-up at grade 8. *Development and Psychopathology, 4*, 125–144.

Capaldi, D., & Stoolmiller, M. (1999). Co-occurrence of conduct problems and depressive symptoms in early adolescent boys: III. Prediction to young-adult adjustment. *Development and Psychopathology, 11*(1), 59–84.

Caputo, A. A., Frick, P. J., & Brodsky, S. L. (1999). Family violence and juvenile sex offending: Potential mediating roles of psychopathic traits and negative attitudes toward women. *Criminal Justice and Behavior, 26*, 338–356.

Caspi, A., McClay, J., Moffitt, T. E., Mill, J., Martin, J., Craig, I. W., et al. (2002). Role of genotype in the cycle of violence in maltreated children. *Science, 297*(5582), 851–854.

Christian, R. E., Frick, P. J., Hill, N. L., Tyler, L., & Frazer, D. R. (1997). Psychopathy and conduct problems in children: II. Implications for subtyping children with conduct problems. *Journal of the American Academy of Child and Adolescent Psychiatry, 36*, 233–241.

Cicchetti, D., & Rogosch, F. A. (1996). Equifinality and multifinality in developmental psychopathology. *Development and Psychopathology, 8*(4), 597–600.

Cohen, M. (1998). The monetary value of saving a high-risk youth. *Journal of Quantitative Criminology, 14*, 5–33.

Cohen, P., Cohen, J., Kasen, S., Velez, C. N., Hartmark, C., Johnson, J., et al. (1993). An epidemiological study of disorders in late childhood and adolescence, I: Age and gender-specific prevalence. *Journal of Child Psychology and Psychiatry, 34*, 851–867.

Coie, J. D., & Dodge, K. A. (1998). Aggression and antisocial behavior. In W. Damon & N. Eisenberg (Eds.), *Handbook of child psychology: Social, emotional, and personality development* (pp. 779–862). Toronto: Wiley.

Coie, J. D., Terry, R., Zakriski, A., & Lochman, J. (1995). Early adolescent social influences on delinquent behavior. In J. McCord (Ed.), *Coercion and punishment in long-term perspectives* (pp. 229–244). New York: Cambridge University Press.

Conduct-Problems-Prevention-Research-Group. (2004). The Effects of the Fast Track Program on Serious Problem Outcomes at the End of Elementary School. *Journal of Clinical Child and Adolescent Psychology, 33*(4), 650–661.

Cooke, D. J., & Michie, C. (1997). An item response theory analysis of the Hare Psychopathy Checklist – Revised. *Psychological Assessment, 9*(1), 3–14.

Cornell, A. H., & Frick, P. J. (2007). The moderating effects of parenting styles in the association between behavioral inhibition and parent-reported guilt and empathy in preschool children. *Journal of Clinical Child and Adolescent Psychology, 36*(3), 305–318.

Crick, N. R. (1996). The role of overt aggression, relational aggression, and prosocial behavior in the prediction of children's future social adjustment. *Child Development, 67*, 2317–2327.

Crick, N. R., Casas, J. F., & Mosher, M. (1997). Relational and overt aggression in preschool. *Developmental Psychology, 33*, 579–588.

Crick, N. R., & Dodge, K. A. (1996). Social information-processing mechanisms in reactive and proactive aggression. *Child Development, 67*, 993–1002.

Crick, N. R., & Grotpeter, J. K. (1995a). Relational aggression, gender, and social-aggression among children. *Developmental Psychology, 33*, 589–600.

Crick, N. R., & Grotpeter, J. K. (1995b). Relational aggression, gender, and social-psychological adjustment. *Child Development, 66*, 710–722.

Crick, N. R., Werner, N. E., Casas, J. F., O'Brien, K. M., Nelson, D. A., Grotpeter, J. K., et al. (1999). Childhood aggression and gender: A new look at an old problem. In D. Bernstein (Ed.), *The 45th Nebraska symposium on motivation: Gender and motivation* (pp. 75–141). Lincoln, NE: Nebraska University Press.

Dadds, M. R., & Hawes, D. J. (2006). *Integrated family intervention for child conduct problems: A behaviour-attachment-systems intervention for parents.* Bowen Hills: Australian Academic Press.

Dandreaux, D. M., & Frick, P. J. (in press). Developmental pathways to conduct problems: A further test of the childhood and adolescent-onset distinction. *Journal of Abnormal Child Psychology.*

Dishion, T. J., Patterson, G. R., Stoolmiller, M., & Skinner, M. L. (1991). Family, school, and behavioral antecedents to early adolescent involvement with antisocial peers. *Developmental Psychology, 27*, 172–180.

Dodge, K. A., Bates, J. E., & Pettit, G. S. (1990). Mechanisms in the cycle of violence. *Science, 250*, 1678–1683.

Dodge, K. A., Lochman, J. E., Harnish, J. D., Bates, J. E., & Pettit, G. S. (1997). Reactive and proactive aggression in school children and psychiatrically impaired chronically assaultive youth. *Journal of Abnormal Psychology, 106*(1), 37–51.

Dodge, K. A., & Pettit, G. S. (2003). A biopsychosocial model of the development of chronic conduct problems in adolescence. *Developmental Psychology, 39*, 349–371.

Dodge, K. A., Price, J. M., Bachorowski, J., & Newman, J. M. (1990). Hostile attributional biases in severely aggressive adolescents. *Journal of Abnormal Psychology, 99*, 385–392.

Eaves, L., Rutter, M., Silberg, J. L., Shillady, L., Maes, H., & Pickles, A. (2000). Genetic and environmental causes of covariation in interview assessments of disruptive behavior in child and adolescent twins. *Behavior Genetics, 30*(4), 321–334.

Edens, J. F., Skopp, N. A., & Cahill, M. A. (2008). Psychopathic features moderate the relationship between harsh and inconsistent parental discipline and adolescent antisocial behavior. *Journal of Clinical Child and Adolescent Psychology, 37*, 472–476.

Eley, T. C., Lichenstein, P., & Stevenson, J. (1999). Sex differences in the etiology of aggressive and nonaggressive antisocial behavior: Results from two twin studies. *Child Development, 70*(1), 155–168.

Enebrink, P., Andershed, H., & Langstrom, N. (2005). Callous-unemotional traits are associated with clinical severity in referred boys with conduct problems. *Nordic Journal of Psychiatry, 59*(6), 431–440.

Essau, C. A., Sasagawa, S., & Frick, P. J. (2006). Callous-unemotional traits in community sample of adolescents. *Assessment, 13*, 454–469.

Fabrega, J. H., Ulrich, R., & Mezzich, J. E. (1993). Do Caucasian and Black adolescents differ at psychiatric intake? *Journal of the American Academy of Child and Adolescent Psychiatry, 32*, 407–413.

Fanti, K. A., Frick, P. J., & Georgiou, S. (in press). Linking callous-unemotional traits to instrumental and non-instrumental forms of aggression. *Journal of Psychopathology and Behavioral Assessment.*

Farrington, D. P. (1995). Crime and physical health: Illnesses, injuries, accidents and offending in the Cambridge Study. *Criminal Behaviour and Mental Health, 5*(4), 261–278.

Farrington, D. P., Jolliffe, D., Loeber, R., Stouthamer-Loeber, M., & Kalb, L. M. (2001). The concentration of offenders in families, and family criminality in the prediction of boys' delinquency. *Journal of Adolescence, 24*(5), 579–596.

Farrington, D. P., & Loeber, R. (2000). Epidemiology of juvenile violence. *Child and Adolescent Psychiatric Clinics of North America, 9*(4), 733–748.

Fergusson, D. M., & Horwood, L. J. (2002). Male and female offending trajectories. *Development and Psychopathology, 14*, 159–177.

Finger, E. C., Marsh, A. A., Mitchell, D. G., Reid, M. E., Sims, C., Budhani, S., et al. (2008). Abnormal ventromedial prefrontal cortex function in children with psychopathic traits during reversal learning. *Archives of General Psychiatry, 65*, 586–594.

Fisher, L., & Blair, R. J. R. (1998). Cognitive impairment and its relationship to psychopathic tendencies in children with emotional and behavioral difficulties. *Journal of Abnormal Child Psychology, 26*, 511–519.

Forth, A. E., Hart, S. D., & Hare, R. D. (1990). Assessment of psychopathy in male young offenders. *Psychological Assessment, 2*, 342–344.

Forth, A. E., Kosson, D. S., & Hare, R. D. (2003). *The psychopathy checklist: Youth version manual.* Toronto: Multi-Health Systems.

Fowles, D. C., & Kochanska, G. (2000). Temperament as a moderator of pathways to conscience in children: The contribution of electrodermal activity. *Psychophysiology, 37*(6), 788–795.

Frick, P. J. (1998). *Conduct disorders and severe antisocial behavior.* New York: Plenum.

Frick, P. J. (2004). *The inventory of callous-unemotional traits.* New Orleans: The University of New Orleans.

Frick, P. J. (2006). Developmental pathways to conduct disorder. *Child Psychiatric Clinics of North America, 15*, 311–332.

Frick, P. J., Bodin, S. D., & Barry, C. T. (2000). Psychopathic traits and conduct problems in community and clinic-referred samples of children: Further development of the Psychopathy Screening Device. *Psychological Assessment, 12*, 382–393.

Frick, P. J., Cornell, A. H., Barry, C. T., Bodin, S. D., & Dane, H. A. (2003). Callous-unemotional traits and conduct problems in the prediction of conduct problem severity, aggression, and self-report of delinquency. *Journal of Abnormal Child Psychology, 31*, 457–470.

Frick, P. J., Cornell, A. H., Bodin, S. D., Dane, H. A., Barry, C. T., & Loney, B. R. (2003). Callous-unemotional traits and developmental pathways to severe conduct problems. *Developmental Psychology, 39*, 246–260.

Frick, P. J., & Dickens, C. (2006). Current Perspectives on Conduct Disorder. *Current Psychiatry Reports, 8*, 59–72.

Frick, P. J., & Hare, R. D. (2001). *The antisocial process screening device.* Toronto: Multi-Health Systems.

Frick, P. J., Lilienfeld, S. O., Ellis, M. L., Loney, B. R., & Silverthorn, P. (1999). The association between anxiety and psychopathy dimensions in children. *Journal of Abnormal Child Psychology, 27*(5), 383–392.

Frick, P. J., & Loney, B. R. (1999). Outcomes of children and adolescents with conduct disorder and oppositional defiant disorder. In H. C. Quay & A. Hogan (Eds.), *Handbook of disruptive behavior disorders* (pp. 507–524). New York: Plenum.

Frick, P. J., & Marsee, M. A. (2006). Psychopathy and developmental pathways to antisocial behavior in youth. In C. J. Patrick (Ed.), *Handbook of psychopathy* (pp. 355–374). New York: Guilford Press.

Frick, P. J., & McMahon, R. J. (2008). Child and adolescent conduct problems. *A guide to assessments that work*, 41–66.

Frick, P. J., & Morris, A. S. (2004). Temperament and developmental pathways to conduct problems. *Journal of Clinical Child and Adolescent Psychology, 33*, 54–68.

Frick, P. J., O'Brien, B. S., Wootton, J. M., & McBurnett, K. (1994). Psychopathy and conduct problems in children. *Journal of Abnormal Psychology, 103*, 700–707.

Frick, P. J., & Silverthorn, P. (2001). Psychopathology in children. In P. B. Sutker & H. E. Adams (Eds.), *Comprehensive handbook of psychopathology* (3rd ed., pp. 881–920). New York: Kluwer.

Frick, P. J., Stickle, T. R., Dandreaux, D. M., Farrell, J. M., & Kimonis, E. R. (2005). Callous-unemotional traits in predicting the severity and stability of conduct problems and delinquency. *Journal of Abnormal Child Psychology, 33*(4), 471–487.

Frick, P. J., & White, S. F. (2008). Research review: The importance of callous-unemotional traits for developmental models of aggressive and antisocial behavior. *Journal of Child Psychology and Psychiatry, 49*(4), 359–375.

Glueck, S., & Glueck, E. (1950). *Unraveling juvenile delinquency*. Oxford: Commonwealth Fund.

Hare, R. D. (1996). Psychopathy: A clinical construct whose time has come. *Criminal Justice and Behavior, 23*, 25–54.

Hare, R. D. (2003). *Hare psychopathy checklist-revised (PCL-R): 2nd edition, technical manual.* Canada: Multi-Health Systems.

Hawes, D. J., & Dadds, M. R. (2005). The treatment of conduct problems in children with callous-unemotional traits. *Journal of Consulting and Clinical Psychology, 73*(4), 737–741.

Henggeler, S. W., Schoenwald, S. K., Borduin, C. M., Rowland, M. D., & Cunningham, P. B. (1998). *Multisystemic treatment of antisocial behavior in children and adolescents.* New York: Guilford Press.

Henry, B., Moffitt, T. E., Caspi, A., Langley, J., & Silva, P. A. (1994). On the "remembrance of things past": A longitudinal evaluation of the retrospective method. *Psychological Assessment, 6*(2), 92–101.

Herpertz, S. C., Huebner, T., Marx, I., Vloet, T. D., Fink, G. R., Stoecker, T., et al. (2008). Emotional processing in male adolescents with childhood-onset conduct disorder. *Journal of Child Psychology and Psychiatry, 49*(7), 781–791.

Hinshaw, S. P., Lahey, B. B., & Hart, E. L. (1993). Issues of taxonomy and co-morbidity in the development of conduct disorder. *Development and Psychopathology, 5*, 31–50.

Hipwell, A. E., Pardini, D. A., Loeber, R., Sembower, M., Keenan, K., & Stouthamer-Loeber, M. (2007). Callous-unemotional behaviors in young girls: Shared and unique effects relative to conduct problems. *Journal of Clinical Child and Adolescent Psychology, 36*(3), 293–304.

Hoffman, M. L. (1994). Discipline and internalization. *Developmental Psychology, 30*, 26–28.

Hubbard, J. A., Smithmyer, C. M., Ramsden, S. R., Parker, E. H., Flanagan, K. D., Dearing, K. F., et al. (2002). Observational, physiological, and self-report measures of children's anger: Relations to reactive versus proactive aggression. *Child Development, 73*, 1101–1118.

Huesmann, L. R., Eron, L. D., Lefkowitz, M. M., & Walder, L. O. (1984). Stability of aggression over time and generations. *Developmental Psychology, 20*, 1120–1134.

Jaffee, S. R., Belsky, J., Harrington, H., Caspi, A., & Moffitt, T. E. (2006). When parents have a history of conduct disorder: How is the caregiving environment affected? *Journal of Abnormal Psychology, 115*(2), 309–319.

Jones, A. P., Laurens, K. L., Herba, C., Barker, G., & Viding, E. (2009). Amygdala hypoactivity to fearful faces in boys with conduct problems and callous-unemotional traits. *American Journal of Psychiatry, 166*, 95–102.

Kagan, J. (1998). Biology and the child. In N. Eisenberg (Ed.), *Handbook of child psychology: Vol. 3. Social, emotional, and personality development* (pp. 177–235). New York: Wiley.

Kagan, J., & Snidman, N. (1991). Infant predictors of inhibited and uninhibited profiles. *Psychological Science, 2*, 40–44.

Kazdin, A. E. (1995). *Conduct disorders in childhood and adolescence* (2nd ed.). Thousand Oaks, CA: Sage.

Keenan, K., Loeber, R., Zhang, Q., Stouthamer-Loeber, M., & Van Kammen, W. B. (1995). The influence of deviant peers on the development of boys' disruptive and delinquent behavior: A temporal analysis. *Development and Psychopathology, 7*, 715–726.

Keenan, K., & Shaw, D. S. (1997). Developmental and social influences on young girls' behavioral and emotional problems. *Psychological Bulletin, 121*, 95–113.

Kiehl, K. A., Smith, A. M., Hare, R. D., Mendrek, A., Forster, B. B., Brink, J., et al. (2001). Limbic abnormalities in affective processing by criminal psychopaths as revealed by functional magnetic resonance imaging. *Biological Psychiatry, 50*(9), 677–684.

Kim-Cohen, J., Caspi, A., Rutter, M., Tomas, M. P., & Moffitt, T. E. (2006). The caregiving environments provided to children by depressed mothers with or without an antisocial history. *American Journal of Psychiatry, 163*(6), 1009–1018.

Kimonis, E. R., Frick, P. J., & Barry, C. T. (2004). Callous-unemotional traits and delinquent peer affiliation. *Journal of Consulting and Clinical Psychology, 72*(6), 956–966.

Kimonis, E. R., Frick, P. J., Fazekas, H., & Loney, B. R. (2006). Psychopathy, aggression, and the processing of emotional stimuli in non-referred girls and boys. *Behavioral Sciences & the Law. Special Issue: Gender and Psychopathy Volume 2, 24*(1), 21–37.

Kimonis, E. R., Frick, P. J., Skeem, J., Marsee, M. A., Cruise, K., Munoz, L. C., et al. (2008). Assessing callous-unemotional traits in adolescent offenders: Validation of the Inventory of Callous-Unemotional Traits. *Journal of the International Association of Psychiatry and Law, 31*, 241–251.

Kochanska, G. (1993). Toward a synthesis of parental socialization and child temperament in early development of conscience. *Child Development, 64*, 325–347.

Kochanska, G. (1997). Multiple pathways to conscience for children with different temperaments: From toddlerhood to age 5. *Developmental Psychology, 33*, 228–240.

Kochanska, G., DeVet, K., Goldman, M., & Murray, K. (1994). Maternal reports of conscience development and temperament in young children. *Child Development, 65*(3), 852–868.

Kochanska, G., Gross, J. N., Lin, M. H., & Nichols, K. E. (2002). Guilt in young children: Development, determinants, and relations with a broader system of standards. *Child Development, 73*, 461–482.

Kratzer, L., & Hodgins, S. (1997). Adult outcomes of child conduct problems: A cohort study. *Journal of Abnormal Child Psychology, 25*, 65–81.

Kruh, I. P., Frick, P. J., & Clements, C. B. (2005). Historical and personality correlates to the violence patterns of juveniles tried as adults. *Criminal Justice and Behavior, 32*, 69–96.

Lahey, B. B., & Loeber, R. (1994). Framework for a developmental model of oppositional defiant disorder and conduct disorder. In D. K. Routh (Ed.), *Disruptive behavior disorders in childhood* (pp. 139–180). New York: Plenum.

Lahey, B. B., & Loeber, R. (1997). Attention-deficit/hyperactivity disorder, oppositional defiant disorder, conduct disorder, and adult antisocial behavior: A life span perspective. In D. M. Stoff, J. Breiling, & J. D. Maser (Eds.), *Handbook of antisocial behavior* (pp. 51–59). Hoboken, NJ: Wiley.

Lahey, B. B., Loeber, R., Hart, E., Frick, P. J., Applegate, B., Zhang, Q., et al. (1995). Four-year longitudinal study of conduct disorder in boys: Patterns and predictors of persistence. *Journal of Abnormal Psychology, 104*, 83–93.

Lahey, B. B., Miller, T. L., Gordon, R. A., & Riley, A. (1999). Developmental epidemiology of the disruptive behavior disorders. In H. Quay & A. Hogan (Eds.), *Handbook of the disruptive behavior disorders* (pp. 23–48). New York: Plenum.

Lahey, B. B., Van Hulle, C. A., Waldman, I. D., Rodgers, J. L., D'Onofrio, B. M., Pedlow, S., et al. (2006). Testing descriptive hypotheses regarding sex differences in the development of conduct problems and delinquency. *Journal of Abnormal Child Psychology, 34*(5), 737–755.

Larson, J., & Lochman, J. E. (2003). *Helping schoolchildren cope with anger*. New York: Guilford.

Larsson, H., Andershed, H., & Lichtenstein, P. (2006). A genetic factor explains most of the variation in the psychopathic personality. *Journal of Abnormal Psychology, 115*(2), 221–230.

Lilienfeld, S., & Waldman, I. D. (1990). The relation between childhood attention-deficit hyperactivity disorder and adult antisocial behavior reexamined: The problem of heterogeneity. *Clinical Psychology Review, 10*, 699–725.

Loeber, R., Burke, J. D., & Lahey, B. B. (2002). What are adolescent antecedents to antisocial personality disorder? *Criminal Behaviour and Mental Health, 12*(1), 24–36.

Loeber, R., Burke, J. D., Lahey, B. B., Winters, A., & Zera, M. (2000). Oppositional defiant and conduct disorder: A review of the past 10 years, part I. *Journal of the American Academy of Child and Adolescent Psychiatry, 39*(12), 1468–1482.

Loeber, R., & Farrington, D. P. (2000). Young children who commit crime: Epidemiology, developmental origins, risk factors, early interventions, and policy implications. *Development and Psychopathology, 12*, 737–762.

Loeber, R., Green, S. M., Keenan, K., & Lahey, B. B. (1995). Which boys will fare worse? Early predictors of the onset of conduct disorder in a six-year longitudinal study. *Journal of the American Academy of Child & Adolescent Psychiatry, 34*(4), 499–509.

Loney, B. R., Butler, M. A., Lima, E. N., Counts, C. A., & Eckel, L. A. (2006). The relation between salivary cortisol, callous-unemotional traits, and conduct problems in an adolescent non-referred sample. *Journal of Child Psychology and Psychiatry, 47*(1), 30–36.

Loney, B. R., Frick, P. J., Clements, C. B., Ellis, M. L., & Kerlin, K. (2003). Callous-unemotional traits, impulsivity, and emotional processing in antisocial adolescents. *Journal of Clinical Child and Adolescent Psychology, 32*, 139–152.

Loney, B. R., Frick, P. J., Ellis, M., & McCoy, M. G. (1998). Intelligence, psychopathy, and antisocial behavior. *Journal of Psychopathology and Behavioral Assessment, 20*, 231–247.

Lyman, R. D., & Campbell, N. R. (1996). *Treating children and adolescents in residential and inpatient settings*. Thousand Oaks, CA: Sage.

Lynam, D. R. (1996). The early identification of chronic offenders: Who is the fledgling psychopath? *Psychological Bulletin, 120*, 209–234.

Lynam, D. R. (1997). Pursuing the psychopath: Capturing the fledgling psychopath in a nomological net. *Journal of Abnormal Psychology, 106*, 425–438.

Lynam, D. R., Caspi, A., Moffitt, T. E., Wikstrom, P. O., Loeber, R., & Novak, S. P. (2000). The interaction between impulsivity and neighborhood context on offending: The effects of impulsivity are stronger in poorer neighborhood. *Journal of Abnormal Psychology, 109*, 563–574.

Marsee, M. A., & Frick, P. J. (2007). Exploring the cognitive and emotional correlates to proactive and reactive aggression in a sample of detained girls. *Journal of Abnormal Child Psychology, 35*(6), 969–981.

Marsh, A. A., Finger, E. C., Mitchell, D. G., Reid, M. E., Sims, C., Kosson, D. S., et al. (2008). Reduced amygdala response to fearful expressions in children and adolescents with callous-unemotional traits and disruptive behavior disorders. *American Journal of Psychiatry, 165*, 712–720.

McCabe, K. M., Rodgers, C., Yeh, M., & Hough, R. (2004). Gender differences in childhood onset conduct disorder. *Development & Psychopathology, 16*(1), 179–192.

McMahon, R. J., & Frick, P. J. (2005). Evidence-based assessment of conduct problems in children and adolescents. *Journal of Clinical Child and Adolescent Psychology, 34*(3), 477–505.

Moffitt, T. E. (1993). Adolescence-limited and life-course persistent antisocial behavior: A developmental taxonomy. *Psychological Review, 100*, 674–701.
Moffitt, T. E. (2003). Life-course persistent and adolescence-limited antisocial behavior: A 10-year research review and research agenda. In B. B. Lahey, T. E. Moffitt, & A. Caspi (Eds.), *Causes of conduct disorder and juvenile delinquency* (pp. 49–75). New York: Guilford.
Moffitt, T. E. (2005). The new look of behavioral genetics in developmental psychopathology: Gene-environment interplay in antisocial behaviors. *Psychological Bulletin, 131*(4), 533–554.
Moffitt, T. E. (2006). Life-course-persistent versus adolescence-limited antisocial behavior. In D. Cicchetti & D. J. Cohen (Eds.), *Developmental psychopathology, Vol 3: Risk, disorder, and adaptation* (2nd ed., pp. 570–598). Hoboken, NJ: Wiley.
Moffitt, T. E., Arseneault, L., Jaffee, S. R., Kim-Cohen, J., Koenen, K. C., Odgers, C. L., et al. (2008). Research review: DSM-V conduct disorder: Research needs for an evidence base. *Journal of Child Psychology and Psychiatry, 49*(1), 3–33.
Moffitt, T. E., & Caspi, A. (2001). Childhood predictors differentiate life-course persistent and adolescence-limited antisocial pathways among males and females. *Development and Psychopathology*, 355–375.
Moffitt, T. E., Caspi, A., Dickson, N., Silva, P., & Stanton, W. (1996). Childhood-onset versus adolescent-onset antisocial conduct problems in males: Natural history from ages 3 to 18 years. *Development and Psychopathology, 8*, 399–424.
Moffitt, T. E., Caspi, A., Harrington, H., & Milne, B. J. (2002). Males on the life-course persistent and adolescent-limited antisocial pathways: Follow-up at age 26 years. *Development and Psychopathology, 14*, 179–207.
Moffitt, T. E., Caspi, A., Rutter, M., & Silva, P. A. (2001). *Sex differences in antisocial behaviour: Conduct disorder, delinquency, and violence in the Dunedin Longitudinal Study*. New York: Cambridge University Press.
Munoz, L. C., & Frick, P. J. (2007). The reliability, stability, and predictive utility of the self-report version of the Antisocial Process Screening Device. *Scandinavian Journal of Psychology, 48*(4), 299–312.
Munoz, L. C., Frick, P. J., Kimonis, E. R., & Aucoin, K. J. (2008a). Types of aggression, responsiveness to provocation, and callous-unemotional traits in detained adolescents. *Journal of Abnormal Child Psychology, 36*(1), 15–28.
Munoz, L. C., Frick, P. J., Kimonis, E. R., & Aucoin, K. J. (2008b). Verbal ability and delinquency: Testing the moderating role of psychopathic traits. *Journal of Child Psychology and Psychiatry, 49*, 414–421.
O'Brien, B. S., & Frick, P. J. (1996). Reward dominance: Associations with anxiety, conduct problems and psychopathy in children. *Journal of Abnormal Child Psychology, 24*, 223–240.
O'Leary, M. M., Loney, B. R., & Eckel, L. A. (2007). Gender differences in the association between psychopathic personality traits and cortisol response to induced stress. *Psychoneuroendocrinology, 32*(2), 183–191.
Odgers, C. L., Caspi, A., Broadbent, J. M., Dickson, N., Hancox, R. J., Harrington, H., et al. (2007). Prediction of differential adult health burden by conduct problem subtypes in males. *Archives of General Psychiatry, 64*(4), 476–484.
Odgers, C. L., Reppucci, N. D., & Moretti, M. M. (2005). Nipping psychopathy in the bud: An examination of the convergent, predictive, and theoretical utility of the PCL-YV among adolescent girls. *Behavioral Sciences and the Law, 23*, 1–21.
Offord, D. R., Boyle, M. H., Szatmari, P., Rae-Grant, N. I., Links, P. S., Cadman, D. T., et al. (1987). Ontario Child Health Study: II. Six-month prevalence of disorder and rates of service utilization. *Archives of General Psychiatry, 44*, 832–836.
Ostrov, J. M., & Keating, C. F. (2004). Gender differences in preschool aggression during free play and structured interactions: An observational study. *Social Development, 13*(2), 255–277.
Oxford, M., Cavell, T. A., & Hughes, J. N. (2003). Callous-unemotional traits moderate the relation between ineffective parenting and child externalizing problems: A partial replication and extension. *Journal of Clinical Child and Adolescent Psychology, 32*, 577–585.

Pardini, D. A., Lochman, J. E., & Frick, P. J. (2003a). Callous/unemotional traits and social-cognitive processes in adjudicated youths. *Journal of the American Academy of Child & Adolescent Psychiatry, 42*(3), 364–371.

Pardini, D. A., Lochman, J. E., & Frick, P. J. (2003b). Callous/Unemotional traits and social cognitive processes in adjudicated youth. *Journal of the American Academy of Child and Adolescent Psychiatry, 42*, 364–371.

Pardini, D. A., Lochman, J. E., & Powell, N. (2007). The development of callous-unemotional traits and antisocial behavior in children: Are there shared and/or unique predictors? *Journal of Clinical Child and Adolescent Psychology, 36*, 319–333.

Pardini, D. A., Obradovic, J., & Loeber, R. (2006). Interpersonal callousness, hyperactivity/impulsivity, inattention, and conduct problems as precursors to delinquency persistence in boys: A comparison of three grade-based cohorts. *Journal of Clinical Child and Adolescent Psychology, 35*, 46–59.

Patterson, G. R. (1986). Performance models for antisocial boys. *American Psychologist, 41*, 432–444.

Patterson, G. R., Reid, J. B., & Dishion, T. J. (1992a). *Antisocial boys*. Eugene, OR: Castilia.

Patterson, G. R., Reid, J. B., & Dishion, T. J. (1992b). *A social learning approach: Vol. 4. Antisocial boys*. Eugene, OR: Castalia.

Peeples, F., & Loeber, R. (1994). Do individual factors and neighborhood context explain ethnic differences in juvenile delinquency? *Journal of Quantitative Criminology, 10*, 141–158.

Penney, S. R., & Moretti, M. M. (2007). The relation of psychopathy to concurrent aggression and antisocial behavior in high-risk adolescent girls and boys. *Behavioral Sciences & the Law, 25*(1), 21–41.

Piquero, A. R., Daigle, L. E., Gibson, C., Piquero, N. L., & Tibbetts, S. G. (2007). Are life-course-persistent offenders at risk for adverse health outcomes? *Journal of Research in Crime and Delinquency, 44*(2), 185–207.

Poulin, F., & Boivin, M. (2000). Reactive and proactive aggression: Evidence of a two-factor model. *Psychological Assessment, 12*, 115–122.

Poythress, N. G., Dembo, R., Wareham, J., & Greenbaum, P. E. (2006). Construct validity of the Youth Psychopathic Traits Inventory (YPI) and the Antisocial Process Screening Device (APSD) with justice involved adolescents. *Criminal Justice and Behavior, 33*, 26–55.

Price, J. M., & Dodge, K. A. (1989). Reactive and proactive aggression in childhood: Relations to peer status and social context dimensions. *Journal of Abnormal Child Psychology, 17*, 455–471.

Rhee, S. H., & Waldman, I. D. (2002). Genetic and environmental influences on antisocial behavior: A meta-analysis of twin and adoption studies. *Psychological Bulletin, 128*(3), 490–529.

Richters, J. E. (1997). The Hubble hypothesis and the developmentalist's dilemma. *Development and Psychopathology, 9*(2), 193–229.

Ridenour, T. A., Marchant, G. J., & Dean, R. S. (2001). Is the revised psychopathy checklist clinically useful for adolescents? *Journal of Psychoeducational Assessment, 19*(3), 227–238.

Robins, L. N., Tipp, J., & Pryzbeck, T. (1991). Antisocial personality. In L. N. Robins & D. A. Regier (Eds.), *Psychiatric disorders in America* (pp. 224–271). New York: Free Press.

Rothbart, M. K., Ahadi, S. A., & Hershey, K. (1994). Temperament and social behavior in childhood. *Merrill-Palmer Quarterly, 40*, 21–39.

Rothbart, M. K., & Bates, J. E. (1998). Temperament. In W. Damon (Ed.), *Handbook of child psychology: Vol. 3,Social, emotional, and personality development* (pp. 105–176). New York: Wiley.

Rubin, K. H., Bukowski, W., & Parker, J. G. (1998). Peer interactions, relationships, and groups. In W. Damon (Ed.), *Handbook of child psychology* (Social, emotional, and personality development, Vol. 3, pp. 619–700). New York: Wiley.

Russo, M. F., & Beidel, D. C. (1994). Comorbidity of childhood anxiety and externalizing disorders: Prevalence, associated characteristics, and validation issues. *Clinical Psychology Review, 14*, 199–221.

Salekin, R. T., Neumann, C. S., Leistico, A., & Zalot, A. A. (2004). Psychopathy in youth and intelligence: An investigation of Cleckley's hypothesis. *Journal of Clinical Child & Adolescent Psychology, 33*(4), 731–742.

Salmivalli, C., & Nieminen, E. (2002). Proactive and reactive aggression among school bullies, victims, and bully-victims. *Aggressive Behavior, 28*(1), 30–44.

Sampson, R. J., & Laub, J. H. (1994). Urban poverty and the family context of delinquency: A new look at structure and process in a classic study. *Child Development, 65*(2), 523–540.

Schwartz, D., Dodge, K. A., Coie, J. D., Hubbard, J. A., Cillessen, A. H. N., Lemerise, E. A., et al. (1998). Social-cognitive and behavioral correlates of aggression and victimization in boys' play groups. *Journal of Abnormal Child Psychology, 26*(6), 431–440.

Sharp, C., van Goozen, S., & Goodyer, I. (2006). Children's subjective emotional reactivity to affective pictures: Gender differences and their antisocial correlates in an unselected sample of 7-11-year-olds. *Journal of Child Psychology and Psychiatry, 47*(2), 143–150.

Silverthorn, P., & Frick, P. J. (1999). Developmental pathways to antisocial behavior: The delayed-onset pathway in girls. *Development and Psychopathology, 11*, 101–126.

Silverthorn, P., Frick, P. J., & Reynolds, R. (2001). Timing of onset and correlates of severe conduct problems in adjudicated girls and boys. *Journal of Psychopathology and Behavioral Assessment, 23*, 171–181.

Stadler, C., Sterzer, P., Schmeck, K., Krebs, A., Kleinschmidt, A., & Poustka, F. (2007). Reduced anterior cingulate activation in aggressive children and adolescents during affective stimulation: Association with temperament traits. *Journal of Psychiatric Research, 41*(5), 410–417.

Sterzer, P., Stadler, C., Krebs, A., Kleinschmidt, A., & Poustka, F. (2005). Abnormal neural responses to emotional visual stimuli in adolescents with conduct disorder. *Biological Psychiatry, 57*(1), 7–15.

Stevens, D., Charman, T., & Blair, R. J. R. (2001). Recognition of emotion in facial expressions and vocal tones in children with psychopathic tendencies. *Journal of Genetic Psychology, 16*, 201–211.

Strassberg, Z., Dodge, K. A., Pettit, G., & Bates, J. E. (1994). Spanking in the home and children's subsequent aggression toward kindergarten peers. *Development and Psychopathology, 6*, 445–461.

Taylor, J., Iacono, W. G., & McGue, M. (2000). Evidence for a genetic etiology of early-onset delinquency. *Journal of Abnormal Psychology, 109*(4), 634–643.

Taylor, J., Loney, B. R., Bobadilla, L., Iacono, W. G., & McGue, M. (2003). Genetic and environmental influences on psychopathy trait dimensions in a community sample of male twins. *Journal of Abnormal Child Psychology, 31*(6), 633–645.

Viding, E. (2004). On the nature and nurture of antisocial behavior and violence. In J. Devine, J. Gilligan, K. A. Miczek, R. Shaikh, & D. Pfaff (Eds.), *Youth violence: Scientific approaches to prevention* (pp. 267–277). New York: New York Academy of Sciences.

Viding, E., Blair, R. J. R., Moffitt, T. E., & Plomin, R. (2005). Evidence for a substantial genetic risk for psychopathic traits in 7-year-olds. *Journal of Child Psychology and Psychiatry, 46*(6), 592–597.

Viding, E., & Jones, A. P. (2008). Cognition to genes via the brain in the study of conduct disorder. *The Quarterly Journal of Experimental Psychology, 61*(1), 171–181.

Viding, E., Jones, A. P., Frick, P. J., Moffitt, T. E., & Plomin, R. (2008). Heritability of antisocial behaviour at 9: Do callous-unemotional traits matter? *Developmental Science, 11*(1), 17–22.

Vitale, J. E., Newman, J. P., Bates, J. E., Goodnight, J., Dodge, K. A., & Pettit, G. (2005). Deficient behavioral inhibition and anomalous selective attention in a community sample of adolescents with psychopathic traits and low-anxiety traits. *Journal of Abnormal Child Psychology, 33*(4), 461–470.

Vitaro, F., Brendgen, M., Pagani, L., Tremblay, R. E., & McDuff, P. (1999). Disruptive behavior, peer association, and conduct disorder: Testing the developmental links through early intervention. *Development and Psychopathology, 11*(2), 287–304.

Waschbusch, D. A. (2002). A meta-analytic examination of comorbid hyperactive-impulsive-attention problems and conduct problems. *Psychological Bulletin, 128*, 118–150.

Waschbusch, D. A., Walsh, T. M., Andrade, B. F., King, S., & Carrey, N. J. (2007). Social problem solving, conduct problems, and callous-unemotional traits in children. *Child Psychiatry & Human Development, 37*(4), 293–305.

Wiesner, M., Kim, H. K., & Capaldi, D. (2005). Developmental trajectories of offending: Validation and prediction to young adult alcohol use, drug use, and depressive symptoms. *Development and Psychopathology, 17*(1), 251–270.

Wootton, J. M., Frick, P. J., Shelton, K. K., & Silverthorn, P. (1997). Ineffective parenting and childhood conduct problems: The moderating role of callous-unemotional traits. *Journal of Consulting and Clinical Psychology, 65*, 301–308.

Zigler, E., Taussig, C., & Black, K. (1992). Early childhood intervention: A promising preventative for juvenile delinquency. *American Psychologist, 47*, 997–1006.

Zoccolillo, M. (1993). Gender and the development of conduct disorder. *Development and Psychopathology, 5*, 65–78.

4

Assessment of Conduct Problems Using an Integrated, Process-Oriented Approach

TRACY E. RHODES and MARK R. DADDS

This chapter presents a practical guide on how to assess conduct problems using an integrated process-oriented approach. We will present a model that builds on current evidence-based knowledge of child conduct problems and the family and school settings in which these problems flourish or fail to flourish, as well as our clinical experience with working with these children. Traditionally, terms such as "delinquent," "antisocial," "aggressive," "oppositional," and/or "impulsive" have been used in research and clinical settings to capture the core characteristics of disruptive behavior disorders. Here, however, we will use the term conduct problems (CPs) to refer to the broad range of behavioral difficulties that are characteristic of Oppositional Defiant Disorder (ODD) and Conduct Disorder (CD); non-compliance, defiance, aggression, and antisocial behaviors, such as lying, truancy, and theft.

Childhood CPs are a major burden and source of distress to the community, school and family and account for a large proportion of referrals to child and family mental health services. Children with CPs are not a homogenous group; CPs are multi-dimensional in nature and encompass a broad range of disruptive behaviors that exist on a continuum of severity. These behaviors range from context specific and minor acts of oppositional behavior or aggression to severe and pervasive acts of antisocial behavior within

TRACY E. RHODES • University of New South Wales
MARK R. DADDS • University of New South Wales

R.C. Murrihy et al. (eds.), *Clinical Handbook of Assessing and Treating Conduct Problems in Youth*, DOI 10.1007/978-1-4419-6297-3_4,

the community (Loeber, Burke, Lahey, Winters, & Zera, 2000). Depending on the constellation of risk factors and nature of the behaviors in question, CPs may be transitional or remain stable over the life course of the youth's development (Frick & Loney, 1999; Moffitt & Caspi, 2001). The negative consequences for these children may be minimal or pervasive – impacting on social, academic and familial domains (Moffitt & Caspi, 2001). CPs also feature in a range of childhood disorders, and in themselves represent a risk factor for other psychiatric, social and health problems at later stages of life (Loeber & Farrington, 2000). It is undoubtedly due to the ubiquity and far reaching impact of these problems that their prevention and treatment has been the subject of intense interest and research by clinicians and researchers involved in the care of these young people.

The simplistic matching of a child's diagnosis to a treatment is not a realistic goal of assessment. The last few decades have witnessed a significant expansion in the use of "diagnoses" such as those included in DSM-IV (APA, 1994), and the development of manual-based treatments designed for specific disorders. Thus, parents of a child with CPs might be referred to an evidence-based parent training programme which can lead to reductions in parent–child problems for a significant proportion of cases. However, CPs, and the contexts that facilitate their emergence, are notoriously heterogeneous and to maximise outcomes, assessment should be focused on elucidating individual child and family variables as much as is possible to "fine tune" a treatment approach.

Figure 4.1 outlines five elements of a state-of-the-art process-oriented assessment: (a) the application of evidence-based models of CPs as a guiding framework; (b) the application of multi-modal assessment tools to gain detailed information regarding the nature, developmental course, contextual factors and consequences of the specific conduct disturbance; (c) awareness of numerous therapeutic and family process issues that may impact on engagement, participation and therapeutic objectives; (d) the integration of relevant information, which at times will be discordant, to generate a clear functional analysis of the complex interacting, contributing, and maintaining factors; and finally, (e) using the functional analysis for treatment decision making regarding the "best fit" treatment intervention for a family.

This model emphasizes that assessment should be based on informed knowledge of the clinical science of CPs with regard to their causes, developmental stage, prognosis and treatment and should proceed using hypothesis testing strategies. Those areas most commonly implicated in the development of CPs include child characteristics (genetic vulnerability, temperament, social cognitive style), familial factors (parenting behaviors, family adjustment), and contextual social factors (school, deviant peers). The model also emphasizes that knowing "how to" collect the information required to generate hypotheses and operationalize problem behaviors is fundamental to conducting an accurate and useful assessment. This means that the clinician needs to be aware of the informants called upon and the most appropriate methods to employ with those informants. The selection of specific methods needs to be mindful of the psychometric

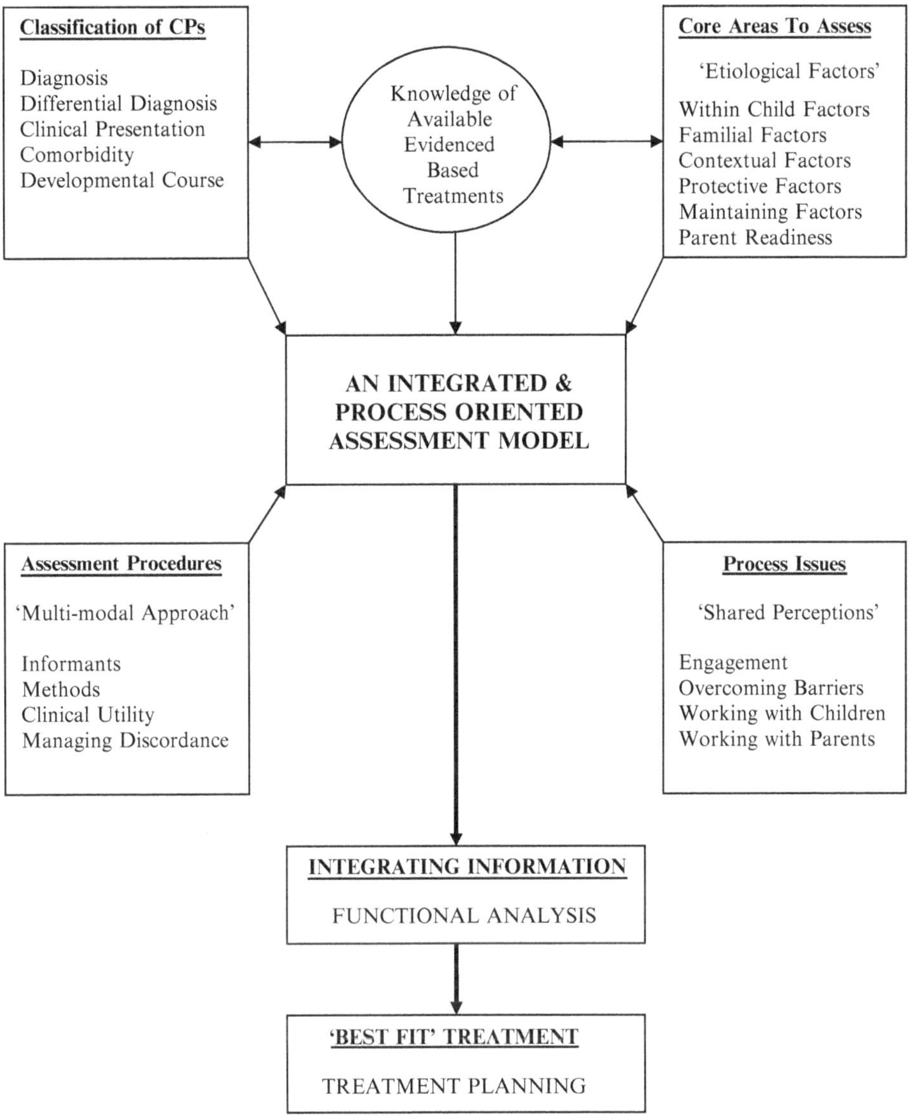

Fig. 4.1. An integrated process orientated model for assessing youth conduct problems.

properties and clinical utility of the chosen modes and instruments. Those methods most commonly employed include interviewing, behavioral rating scales, direct observations, and neuropsychological testing. Each mode of information provides unique "snapshots" of the child's functioning from different perspectives; when integrated, it should provide a detailed and complete picture of the nature, causes and prognosis of the youth's CPs and alternative more healthy pathways.

Throughout the assessment, a clinician should be guided by the main process issues that are relevant for the specific child and family. In our model, this includes both therapeutic processes that can be influenced by the clinician (e.g., engagement, overcoming therapeutic blocks) and familial processes that already exist within the child's immediate family system, such as the parental relationship and how it affects individual parenting. Recognition of process issues will facilitate an open dialogue with the family, increase engagement and identify potential barriers to participating in treatment. In adhering to each of these three interactive guiding principles within a process-oriented framework (i.e., application of knowledge, use of multi-modal methods and integration of information), what emerges is a multifaceted and fluid assessment process, involving the integration of both quantitative and qualitative procedures to construct a well-informed functional analysis. This chapter will address each of these core components in detail to provide a practical guide on how to conduct an integrated process-oriented assessment. This will lead into a discussion of how to integrate this information by generating a functional analysis. Finally, we highlight how to best provide assessment feedback and treatment recommendations that are driven by an integrated assessment and functional analysis.

DIAGNOSIS AND LEVEL OF IMPAIRMENT

A diagnosis is the outcome of matching the child's specific behavioral problems to scientifically based diagnostic criteria (see Chap. 1). Formal diagnostic systems, such as those outlined in the Diagnostic Manual of Mental Disorders (DSM-IV; APA, 1994) and the International Classification of Disorders (ICD-10; WHO, 1992), provide a universally recognized framework for classification, and are a good anchor point for clinicians and researchers to interpret a range of conduct-related problem behaviors. Some of the typical behaviors that attract the attention of educational and health professionals include aggression, non-compliance, impulsivity, lying and stealing. When a number of these behavioral problems cluster together and impact on a child's level of functioning, these specific constellations of "symptoms" are categorized according to one (or more) of the broadband externalizing disorders; ODD, CD and Attention Deficit Hyperactivity Disorder (ADHD).

Differential Diagnoses and Comorbidity

Diagnosis of CPs requires the clinician to adopt a scientific method of enquiry whereby specific hypotheses are generated and empirically tested throughout the assessment process. This means that prior to making a formal diagnosis, a number of potential differential, or alternative, diagnoses should be considered. This may be a challenging task as there are a range of childhood problems, such as neurological, mood and anxiety disorders, that have behavioral manifestations similar to the core characteristics of specific CPs (Jensen, Martin, & Cantwell, 1997). For instance, some children with a primary anxiety disorder, such as separation anxiety, often display intense levels of oppositional and aggressive behavior in anticipation of or on actual separation from a primary caregiver. This means that assessment requires an understanding of CPs generally and knowledge of multiple childhood disorders specifically.

High rates of co-occurrence of disorders in children with CPs further complicate the diagnostic picture. Research into childhood psychological disorders that commonly co-occur with CPs has received considerable attention (for comprehensive reviews see Boylan, Vaillancourt, Boyle, & Szatmari, 2007; Kazdin & Whitley, 2006; Ollendick, Jarrett, Grills-Taquechel, Seligman, & Wolff, 2008). When making a diagnosis, a clear distinction must be made between what constitutes a differential diagnosis and what constitutes a comorbid condition. This means that potential comorbid conditions must be evaluated, by investigating the developmental course of each disorder, and generating additional diagnoses that exist independent to the primary conduct disturbance. More often, children presenting with CPs will also have one or more co-occurring clinical disorders (Nock, Kazdin, Hiripi, & Kessler, 2006; Ollendick et al., 2008). Those most commonly associated with CPs across diagnostic categories include anxiety, depression and substance abuse disorders (Frick, Lilienfelt, Ellis, Loney, & Silverthorn, 1999). Comorbidity within externalising broadband categories is even higher, with ADHD being the most common comorbid condition (Bauermeister et al., 2007). Developmental trajectories of comorbid conditions are important to assess, as different disorders follow distinct developmental sequences of onset. For instance, in relation to CPs, the developmental trajectory is typically ADHD first; ODD, and then a transition to CD and substance abuse (Frick & Loney, 1999). This picture is slightly different for co-occurring internalizing problems, with anxiety and depression, especially in females, first emerging before CPs during puberty and adolescence (Boylan et al., 2007). Common comorbid and differential diagnoses within and without CPs include:

Oppositional Defiant Disorder and Conduct Disorder. Traditionally, ODD is regarded as a precursor to CD, and when criteria are met for CD, a sole diagnosis of CD is given. This can be difficult to differentiate at times, because like CD, severe levels of ODD are characterised by a pervasive level of defiance toward authority figures and aggressive outbursts. However, the key distinguishing feature between ODD and CD is that youths with ODD do not demonstrate a pervasive or persistent constellation of conduct-related behaviors that constitute a serious violation of rules and basic rights of others (Loeber & Farrington 2000). Furthermore, CD is typically associated with legal consequences that are unique to this constellation of behaviors (Connor, 2002).

Attention Deficit Hyperactivity Disorder. ADHD (inattentive, hyperactive, and combined types) is the leading comorbid problem and differential diagnosis in the area of CPs (Hinshaw, 2006). A meta-analysis by Waschbusch (2002) found that 36% boys and 57% of girls with CPs had comorbid ADHD. The core aspects that co-occur with CPs are inattention, impulsivity, and hyperactivity, and these influence the developmental course and severity of the child's problems (Moffitt, 1990). That is, research has found that a child with a co-occurring attentional-hyperactivity deficit has a more severe and chronic form of CPs that is both more stable and life persistent (Hinshaw, 2003). The challenge for the clinician is to disentangle the non-compliance, defiance, rule violation, and aggression that can and cannot be attributed to inattention, poor organization, and increased levels of motor activity (Bauermeister, et al., 2007).

Anxiety and Depression. Internalizing problems are frequently reported to co-occur with CPs, and CPs are associated with increased risk for the later development of problems with anxiety and depression (McMahon & Frick, 2005). For instance, of children who suffer from a primary anxiety disorder, 9–39% will experience a co-occurring externalising problem (Fergusson, Horwood, & Lynskey, 1993). Similarly, McConaughy and Skiba (1993) found that 51% of children in a community sample who had difficulties within the externalizing domain also had difficulties with internalizing symptoms (i.e., anxiety and depression). The challenge for the clinician is again to disentangle overlap and core problems; many behaviors arising from internalizing problems may be interpreted as CPs. Irritability is a characteristic of depression but may result in ODD type behavior. Research indicates that consideration of developmental course of the problems (which came first?) will often help disentangle these problems.

Adjustment Disorders. Stressful life events, such as death, parental divorce or trauma, during childhood are associated with an increase in all forms of physical and psychological difficulties (Willemen, Koot, Ferdinand, Goosens & Schuengel, 2008). Although environmental adversity is common in the development of CPs, they are not a specific and transient response to the event(s). A clear timeline of the stressor and onset of CPs should be ascertained. When considering an adjustment disorder, the key feature is that the problem behaviors need to have developed within 3 months of the psychosocial stressor and declined within a 6-month period (DSM-IV; APA, 1994). Careful consideration of the severity and range of behaviors are also important, so as not to preclude early identification of potentially more severe CPs developing.

CORE AREAS FOR A FUNCTIONAL ASSESSMENT

Figure 4.2 highlights the core assessment areas that feature in the developmental course of childhood CPs. The model presents the ecological approach to understanding a child's CPs that is based largely on the pioneering work of Bronfenbrenner (1977). This model highlights that children and families develop and function within many diverse ecological systems, such as the home, school, and wider community. A detailed investigation needs to consider the various contexts for the child's development, and how they interact. For example, how functional is the relationship between parents and the child's teachers?

Research consistently demonstrates that the emergence and continuance of CPs is influenced by the interaction of child, family, school, and broader ecological factors; and no one risk factor can be implicated as the sole causal mechanism for the onset of a conduct disturbance. Instead, what emerges from a strong body of theoretical and empirical work is that risk factors are multi-interactive and additive in contributing to both the expression of CPs and the level of impairment consequent to those problems. A broad enquiry that investigates each of these risk factors will include *within child factors*, such as neurobiological mechanisms, temperament and health issues; *familial factors* such as family adjustment,

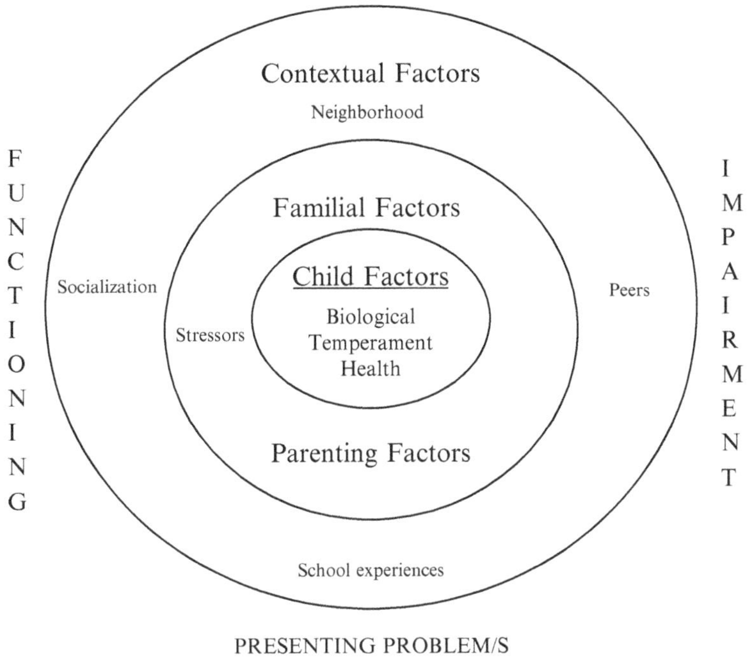

Fig. 4.2. An ecological-contextual model of core areas of assessment in CPs.

parenting behaviors and parent–child interactions; *external factors*, such as school functioning, community activities and peer groups; and *comorbid problems*, such as anxiety, depression or substance abuse. Throughout this process of investigation, specific exploration of the frequency, duration, severity, as well as antecedents, reinforcing agents and consequences that may lead to associated impairments in social, familial or academic functioning should be scrutinised.

THINKING ABOUT RISK FACTORS: TEMPERAMENT AND ENVIRONMENTAL ADVERSITY

Evaluating how child temperamental factors and environmental adversity interact to contribute to the nature and course of a child's CPs has important implications for prognosis and treatment decisions. Child factors such as genetic vulnerability, neuropsychological problems, and temperamental risk factors, such as early onset physical aggressive behavior, having high levels of negative affect versus "cold" or fearless traits, and poor social–emotional processing, have all been associated with the development of CPs and poorer treatment outcomes. Assessment questions that explore early developmental history and temperament are useful in gaining a clearer understanding of a child's temperamental risk to the emergence of later CPs. The child's temperament will interact with environmental variables to determine the specific protective and risk factors operating (Loeber et al., 2000). While there are exceptions to the rule, parenting behaviors of children with CPs are typically characterized by high punitive/low nurturing styles, low parental involvement and reinforcement of pro-social behavior, poor monitoring of the child's whereabouts and activities, and harsh and inconsistent discipline (Hoeve et al., 2008; Nelson & Coyne, 2009; Trentacosta & Shaw, 2008). These parenting behaviors are often related to various external stressors such as low parental education, psychopathology, poverty, social isolation and young single parent status (Dadds & McHugh, 1992; Webster-Stratton & Hammond, 1990). Other environmental factors of importance are school adjustment and peer factors. Table 4.1 summarizes the main areas of enquiry.

A MULTIMODAL ASSESSMENT PROCEDURE

Assessment should strive to be as objective and comprehensive as possible. This means that no one source of information should be solely relied upon to gain a clear picture of the child's problems. Rather, assessment should adopt a multi-modal approach. In essence, this encourages collection of information from multiple domains directly relating to the child's functioning, taken from multiple informants, using multiple methodologies. Monitoring changes over the course of treatment, as well as treatment outcome, also highlight the need to assess at multiple points in time. As previously outlined, assessment should be hypotheses driven and not simply a blind collection of information. Each method and procedure has its own unique function and the type of information gained during the assessment is dependent on the mode of assessment chosen. Established methods of assessment in the area of childhood CPs include clinical interviews, self report and behavioral rating scales, observation, and neuropsychological assessment. This section makes reference to the "how to" component of the model; that is, how to collect information needed for hypotheses testing and operationalization of the problem behavior/s, using a variety of established techniques and methods. It is not our intention to provide an exhaustive review of all the available modes of assessment, nor their psychometric properties or clinical utility.

Using a Multi-Informant Approach

An essential ingredient in conducting an inclusive assessment is to gain information from a range of sources. Informants include parents, teachers, child self reports, peers, and significant others (e.g., grandparents, professionals involved with the family). Each informant can provide unique insight into positive and negative aspects of the child's functioning, within different environments. Despite this, there are limitations embedded in the reliability and validity with each of these reports (see Bloomquist & Schnell, 2002 for a detailed discussion). Research shows that informants often disagree about the nature of the youth's problems and associated difficulties. Although, there is a higher rate of reliability between informants in relation to CPs compared to internalizing disorders, these concordance rates remain modest with reliability ranging from 0.5 to 0.6. (Hodges, 1993). Of significance to the clinician is that informants may provide infor-

Table 4.1. Application of research on etiological factors to clinical practice

Feature of CP	Specific areas of enquiry	Assessment mode	Informant
Child factors			
Genetic vulnerability (HPA axis, serotonin, MAOA)	Family history of males and CPs; including aggression, antisocial behavior, alcoholism, hyperactivity	Interview BRS (parent psychopathology)	Parents
Neurobiological deficits (ADHD, ASD, EF)	Emotional regulation, organization, attentional capacity, motor activity, VIQ, PIQ, speed of information processing	Interview, observation, neuropsychological assessment BRS (general and specific child dysfunction)	Parents, clinical observation, teacher, child
Temperamental risk			
Difficult temperament	Developmental history; restless, sleeping patterns, irritability	Interviews, resting heart rate, observation,	Parent, teacher, child, clinical observation
CU traits (hot versus cold)	Empathy, remorse, manipulation of others,	BRS (specific child dysfunction and parenting practices)	
Punishment insensitivity	Parenting strategies and child's responsiveness		
Aggression	Type of aggression (verbal, physical); reactive or proactive;		
Social cognitive style			
Information processing	Response to rewards versus punishment	Interviews	Parent, teacher, child, clinical observation
Thinking distortions (hostile attributions, threat perception)	Reactive to ambiguous stimuli; child's self talk and phrases when distressed/angry (e.g., Its not fair)	BRS (specific child dysfunction), observations	
Attachment representations	Childs internal representation of primary caregivers (secure versus insecure)	Story stem completion tasks	

(continued)

Table 4.1. (continued)

Feature of CP	Specific areas of enquiry	Assessment mode	Informant
Familial factors			
Parenting behavior			
Parent–child interactions	Parent–child coercive cycles; "dance steps" when in conflict	Interview, observation, BRS (parenting practices and styles)	Parents, child, clinical observation, Teacher
Parenting practices	Level of supervision and monitoring; modes of discipline (consistency, parenting team, harsh, authoritative)		
Parenting style	Level of warmth, nurturance and care		
Parenting expectations	Expectations of child's functioning and parenting (self, spouse)		
Parental adjustment			
Psychopathology	Level of stress; presence of psychological problems (depression, anxiety, substance abuse)	Interviews; observations BRS (family adjustment and parent psychopathology)	Parent, child, observations, health practitioners
Marital discord	Disagreements in parenting; cohesiveness as a couple		
Family stressors	Financial and health stressors		
Parent attributions	Perceptions regarding child's difficulties, significant areas of blame (self, child, spouse, relative)	Interviews, observations, BRS (parenting behaviors)	Parents, child, clinical observations
Family structure and systems	Physical family structure (hierarchical systems and power imbalances and dominance); family dynamics (chaotic, aggressive interpersonal relationships); Family subsystems (boundaries, teams); Family member roles	Interviews, observations	Parents, child, teachers, clinical observations

Contextual factors			
Demographics	SES[h], parent educational status. housing conditions (number of people in the home); number of children; parenting status (single, divorced, widowed, separated) and level of both parent involvement; history of child welfare involvement	Interviews, BRS (specific family adjustment); clinical rating of "quality of family environment" (e.g., DSM GAF; QFE questionnaire)	Parents, teachers, clinical observations Welfare reports
School	Cooperation and support from school, schools perceptions of child dysfunction, classroom versus playground behavior; academic failure (behavioral or specific learning deficit)	Interviews, BRS (teacher; general and specific child dysfunction); observations; neuropsychological assessment (academic & IQ)	Teachers, school personnel reports (counselor, principal) Observations
Peer groups	Social interaction functioning; number of peers; frequency of changed peer group; type of peers (deviant versus prosocial); level of exposure and/or participation regarding drugs, illegal activity and antisocial gangs	Interviews, BRS (general and specific child dysfunction)	Parents, teachers, peers, child
Protective	Intellectual functioning; temperament; competent social skills; stability of interpersonal relationships; secure attachment with parents; engagement in prosocial extracurricular activities	Interviews, BRS (teacher and child) Neuropsychological assessment Story stem completion tasks	Parents, teachers, child, peers, observation

Note. There is a strong body of literature in relation to each of these topics. For further information we have found that a literature search by combining key terms from the first two columns (+ assessment) will provide more detailed theoretical information, as well as advancements in relation to these areas of assessment and modes of assessment (e.g., aggression + reactive + assessment). Looking these terms up in an index of assessment and theory handbooks is also useful

ADHD Attention Deficit Hyperactivity Disorder. *ASD* Autistic Spectrum Disorder, *EF* Executive Functioning, *VIQ* Verbal Intelligence Quotation, *PIQ* Perceptual Intelligence Quotation, *BRS* stands for Behavioral Rating Scales, *CU* Callous-unemotional traits, *SES* Socio-economic status, *DSM* Diagnostic Statistical Manual, *QFE* Quality of Family Environment

mation that is influenced by a variety of factors, independent to the child's level of functioning and symptoms (Hinshaw & Zupan, 1997). For example, parent reports of youth's CPs tend to be exaggerated in the presence of parental stress or psychopathology, such as depression (Brennan, Le Brochque, & Hammen, 2003). Identifying limitations in the interview process and discordance in informant reports should not negate their clinical utility; rather, each person provides valuable "pieces" of information. When potential confounding factors are accounted for, parents are more reliable in terms of accuracy and validity in predicting future CPs (Loeber, Green, Lahey, & Stouthhamer-Loeber, 1990). Even discordance between sources can provide clinically meaningful information that informs case conceptualization and treatment planning (e.g., conflicting parent attributions about the severity of the child's problems).

Clinical Interviews

Interviewing is one of the most commonly used and oldest methods when assessing for CPs. It plays an important and valuable role; it enables a broad and in-depth collection of information and can be conducted with any individual who has significant contact with the youth, such as parents, teachers or welfare officers. The clinical interview serves a number of functions that guide the content of a comprehensive evaluation of the child's problems. Foremost, the interview is critical in establishing rapport with the parents and child (if present). This means that empathic listening and reflecting skills in conjunction with well-timed Socratic questioning will foster disclosure and development of a therapeutic alliance. Secondly, throughout the interview, the clinician should be considering hypotheses about the nature of the presenting problems within different contexts (e.g., home, school) in terms of the core areas for assessment discussed earlier.

Facilitating Discussion of Relevant Topics

Conducting a comprehensive assessment requires clinical skill and is not just a process of moving through a checklist of questions and content areas. Dadds and Hawes (2006) contend that when progressing through the components of the clinical interview, a consistent method should be used to facilitate the introduction and discussion of each new area for assessment. This method utilises a "funnelling" pattern in which new topics are approached first with broad, open-ended general inquiry questions (see Fig. 4.3). The specificity of questions should increase as the topic is addressed further, with an increasing movement from open to hypothesis-driven, closed-ended questions. Such a method allows parents to present their ideas and opinions freely, while also providing an account of relevant aspects of each topic in appropriate detail. At the end of each topic, key details are briefly summarised in the parents' own words, checked for accuracy with the parents, and then the clinician makes a smooth transition to the next area. Each summary includes a brief reiteration of the previous summary integrated with the new information; in this way, a clear picture of the child's problems is built steadily over the course of

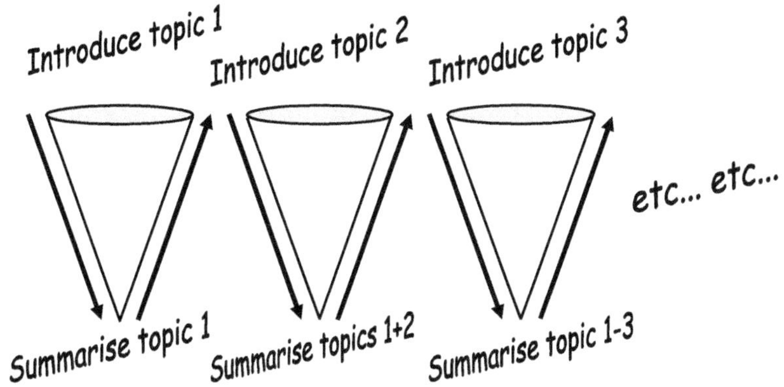

Fig. 4.3. An interviewing approach that maximizes the development of a shared perception with clients.

the interview, and the development of the picture is openly "owned" by both clinician and parents (and child). The goal of adopting a funnelling approach is the emergence of a *shared perception* of the child's difficulties and associated contextual factors.

Interviews with Parents

As children with CPs do not generally refer themselves or seek help on their own, parents (or caregivers) are often the first to be engaged in the assessment process. As a rule, parents should be interviewed first without the child present in order to allow them to privately vent about the child's problems and their own feelings and thoughts. Once this initial interview has been conducted and a shared perception developed with the parents, a similar opportunity can be provided to the child. An open dialogue between a clinician and parents relies heavily on establishing a good therapeutic relationship grounded in a shared spirit of scientific enquiry. Therefore, interviewing requires sensitivity to expectations, parental motivations and affective responses during the interview (Carr, 1999). From the outset, the primary goal of assessment is to develop a shared perception with all family members regarding the nature of the child's CPs. Therefore, irrespective of potential informant bias, parents should be regarded as "experts" when reporting on their child's functioning and family adjustment. Parents generally have the greatest amount of interpersonal involvement with their child under a variety of circumstances. Indeed, they are vital historians of their child's developmental status, both normal and deviant, as well as situations that may precipitate and reinforce specific conduct behaviors (McMahon & Frick, 2005).

It is common for mothers to be the primary, and at times sole source of information irrespective of their marital status. Even in two-parent family systems, the father's involvement in assessment and treatment is often lower in research, community, and clinical settings (Bagner & Eyberg, 2003) as mothers often have a greater proportion of day-to-day caretaking responsibilities of the child. When both parents are present, there are generally moderate levels of discordance, with mothers having a tendency to report a broader range and greater frequency of CPs compared to fathers (Bloomquist & Schnell, 2002). Research shows that parent agreement on the child's specific behaviors and level of impairment may be discrepant depending on (a) the level of involvement each parent has with the child; (b) the amount of time spent with the child in terms of parenting responsibilities; and (c) the way each parent historically manages the child and core parenting approaches. Regardless, each parent provides a unique perspective of the youth's difficulties, and gaining information from both parents' results in a comprehensive understanding of the youth's functioning from different viewpoints.

As indicated previously, there are multiple areas for assessment that are "core" to the development of CPs. Our experience is that a successful interview, both for clinicians and clients can be achieved by breaking these areas of enquiry down into a simple interview format. Table 4.2 outlines the core areas of an initial parent interview that a clinician should be familiar with prior to entering the interview. Additionally, we have outlined below some simple steps that can be incorporated into the interview procedure.

Table 4.2. Components of a comprehensive parent clinical interview (Adapted from Dadds and Hawes, 2006)

Broad areas of discussion	Specific content
Child and family details	Child details Parent details Structure of the family Genogram Individuals (non-family) in the home Childcare arrangements
The presenting problem (antecedents, maintaining factors, consequences)	Main concerns Operationalising behaviors (description) Frequency Duration Context (s) Impact
History of presenting problem	Onset Developmental progression Patterns of change (declines, escalations, significant events)
General functioning of the child	Home functioning Social functioning School Functioning
Parent and family functioning	Parents health and wellbeing Parent social support Childcare responsibilities Parents feelings and thoughts about their child Parent's childhood experiences History of mental illness Parents relationship (Family subsystems) Child's relationships with significant others Financial and environmental stressors Family system
Previous treatments and expectations for current treatment	What worked or did not work before A shared perception of processes and goals

These steps can help facilitate attendance, as well as foster parents in becoming active participants in the assessment and treatment process.

Facilitate Attendance. Several steps can be taken to ensure that parents attend the interview. Foremost, once an interview time has been scheduled, send out a confirmation letter that clearly states the date and time for the interview. This letter can also detail expectancies of the interview, such as duration and who should be in attendance (e.g., parents only on the first meeting). Sending a map with the clinic's location and details also reduces the risk of parents getting lost and choosing to not attend the interview. Research indicates that making small efforts, such as calling the day before to remind parents of the interview and confirm the appointment will also increase attendance rates (Watt, Holand, Best, & Dadds, 2007).

Foster the Attendance of Both Parents. Arrange for an appointment time that is suitable for both parents (where appropriate) to attend. The role of the father in the assessment process, and subsequent psychosocial intervention, is important if not fundamental. Each parent's observations, interpretations, and experiences of the child, within the familial system, inform the clinician of underlying interpersonal and systemic family processes. These processes, such as consistent parenting practices and variations in parenting belief systems often translate into current parent–child interactions. For these reasons alone, encouraging and motivating both parents to be engaged and active participants in the assessment process is vital. The likelihood of both parents participating in treatment is often diminished by parental disagreement regarding the extent to which professional help is felt necessary. For example, a mother may present with a child and the message conveyed may be that the father is not interested or is unwilling to be involved. In these cases, feeding back into the family system that each family member is considered an expert that has firsthand knowledge of the family's style and the child's problems is imperative. When resistance is encountered in relation to both parents attending, determine the reasons as to why and (if appropriate) offer to call the non-attending parent directly to outline the goal of the interview and reinforce the importance of his or her perspective regarding the child's difficulties. Nevertheless, disengagement from a parent in attending the assessment, or providing information, may be indicative of additional contributing and maintaining factors worth noting when constructing a functional analysis.

Address Parent Expectations. By clearly outlining expectations of the interview, the clinician commences the process of overcoming potential barriers to engagement in assessment and treatment. The clinician models from the outset what parents can expect by engaging in treatment. For instance, an initial interview should take 60 min, but may take up to 90 min. Therefore, tell the parents about how long the interview will take, so that they can make suitable child care arrangements and can allocate enough time to discuss their main concerns and complete an in-depth clinical interview. It is also useful at this stage to be upfront regarding what services are offered by the clinic, such as the focus being on child emotional and behavioral problems or length of treatment offered. This will establish clear boundaries regarding the clinician's role and what the focus of treatment will be.

It will also enable assessment of parents' readiness to engage based on parents' responses to what your service will offer.

Choose the Interview Format. There are three interview formats available: structured, semi-structured or unstructured interviews. Each format has its own unique set of strengths and limitations (see Bloomquist & Schnell, 2002). Specifically, choosing the structure of an interview is determined by the primary goal(s) of the interview, desired level of flexibility, level of expertise applying that format, the person/s being interviewed, developmental status of the child and the nature of their difficulties as outlined in the referral. The *semi-structured interview* is the most widely adopted interview method in the area of CPs. They can be used with all informants, and most formal semi-structured interviews have good psychometric properties offering parallel parent, teacher, and youth versions (Bloomquist & Schnell, 2002). When multiple behavioral problems are present, unstructured interviews are advantageous due to their flexibility and utility as a broad screening method (McMahon & Frick, 2005). However, unstructured formats rely heavily on clinical expertise of a range of childhood disorders and their etiological factors to critically drive the content of the interview. Semi-structured interviews offer a balance between a flexible enquiry of salient issues and a standardised set of questions and prompts that are based on diagnostic systems (e.g., DSM, ICD). An exhaustive description of the numerous empirically evaluated semi-structured interviews is outside the scope of this chapter. However, those that have received the most attention in the childhood psychopathology literature, due to their psychometric properties and clinical validity, include: The Child Assessment Schedule (CAS: Hodges & Fitch, 1979); the Child and Adolescent Psychiatric Assessment (CAPA: Angold, Cox, Prendergast, Rutter, & Simonoff, 1987); the Diagnostic Interview for Children and Adolescents (DICA: Herjanic, Herjanic, Brown, & Wheat, 1975); the Diagnostic Interview Schedule for Children (DISC: Costello, Edelbrocj, Dulcan, Kals, & Klaric, 1984), and its revisions (DISC-R: Shaffer et al., 1988; DISC-2: Fischer et al., 1993), and the Schedule for Affective Disorders and Schizophrenia for School-Aged Children (K-SADS-PL: Kaufman et al., 1997).

Interviews with Children and Adolescents

Traditionally, information provided by youth, especially below the age of 8 years, is often not called upon or relied on in the assessment phase. This is due to a child's self reports being regarded as unreliable and invalid because of their limited cognitive capacity and reduced self-awareness of their subjective internal experiences (Loney & Frick, 2003). However, despite apparent limitations in youth reports, increasing recognition is now afforded to the role a child plays as a valuable observer and informant of his or her own thoughts, feelings, and behaviors within various environments (Bloomquist & Schnell, 2002). Failure to consider these within child internal experiences has resulted in the under-recognition and detection of some of the core mediating processes, such as social cognitions and affective responses, in the development and persistence of CPs (see Crick & Dodge, 1994).

There are two important reasons why children are incorporated into the interview process; first to engage them as active participants in the assessment and treatment process which fosters a positive experience in disclosure and motivation to enter treatment; and second, to facilitate disclosure by the child of his or her perspectives and experiences of the CPs and associated difficulties to gain additional information to support or disconfirm hypotheses and consider appropriate treatment strategies. As a general rule, children are valuable informants of internalizing problems and covert CPs (Loeber & Schmaling, 1985; Ollendick & Hersen, 1984); however, younger children will typically underestimate overt CPs, such as aggressive behavior (David & Kistner, 2000). On the other end of the age spectrum, the older a youth is, especially as they move toward adolescence, the more reliable and informative their self reports of CPs (Loeber, 1990).

Suggestions for Interviewing Youths

Choosing to formally interview a youth, and determining how much of their self report is incorporated into the assessment process, will be dependent on a number of important factors. Predominantly, the main considerations revolve around the presenting problem, reliability of other informants, the youth's age, developmental level, and amount of motivation/resistance. In choosing to include the child's viewpoint, the following methods are available to facilitate generation of more reliable information.

Specific Interviewing Schedules. The development of youth interview schedules has enabled children to be brought into the interview stage in order to measure specific conduct-related behaviors from their perspective. For instance, the K-SADS Diagnostic Interview Schedule (K-SADS-PL, 1997; Kaufman et al., 1997) is appropriate for younger and older children and is useful as a broad diagnostic screening tool. It outlines child-friendly questions and uses prompts to facilitate an informative response. When used skilfully, content areas generate a behavioral diagnosis, level of impairment, and its parallel parent version enables identification of areas of discordance. Comparably, the Interview for Antisocial Behavior (IAB; Kazdin & Esveldt-Dawson, 1986) is a semi-structured interview appropriate for children aged 6–13 years designed to measure the presence/absence, severity and duration of a range of overt/covert CPs. In choosing to use a more structured interview format, it is imperative that interviewing questions are complemented with general interviewing techniques, especially on identification of more sensitive issues, such as suicidal ideation or illicit drug use. However, given reliability issues of interviewing youths, these schedules should always be supplemented with additional self report behavioral ratings scales.

Unstructured Questioning and Informal Observation. Interviewing children, especially those under 7 years, may be restricted to using more unstructured clinical skills that avoid technical jargon, such as open-ended questions that do not result in "yes" or "no" responses and declarative statements (e.g., you look angry versus are you angry?) (Ollendick & Hersen, 1984). During this time, important qualitative observations, including affect changes, attention capacity, or socialization skills can be noted, while simultaneously establishing rapport (Hinshaw & Zupan, 1997). It is also beneficial to conduct a formal Mental Status Examination of the child, which should be continually reviewed throughout treatment.

Encountering Hostility or Resistance in Children. Children typically do not present themselves to professionals in search of help for their CPs. Therefore, it should be anticipated that a child will display an initial resistance to engaging in the assessment process. This may be apparent through passive resistance to questions or explicit hostility toward parents, the clinician, and the whole process of attending a clinic. We have found the following aids useful in addressing this resistance and working with children. Firstly, we suggest that rapport building becomes the primary focus during initial contact. For younger children, playing a game or drawing a picture and asking about activities they enjoy are useful. For older children, discussing their hobbies and after school activities, normalizing their attendance and communicating that it is the family who is coming for treatment, not the youth per se. Secondly, it is important to minimize their distress and facilitate therapeutic rapport by clarifying the therapist's role as a stranger and normalizing their initial distrust. This distrust is then further counterbalanced by emphasizing that their perspective is important and this is a forum for them to provide opinions regarding their level of functioning at home and school. Thirdly, the clinician starts to develop a shared perception by providing empathy, normalization of feelings and validation of the child's experiences. Finally, the clinician outlines expectancies, as with parents, regarding the purpose and function of the assessment and what is expected of the child. This setting of boundaries helps to avoid the risk associated with the child attempting to collude with the clinician or the occurrence of "splitting" between significant others involved with the children, such as the clinician, parents or teacher.

RATING SCALES AND OBSERVATIONS

Once a clinical interview has been completed, more detailed assessment is conducted. The choice of conjunctive assessment methods is guided by the working hypotheses that have been formulated during the interview. For instance, in defining problem behaviors, you may want to determine the extent particular vulnerability traits (e.g., cold versus hot temperament) or social cognitive processes (e.g., hostile attribution bias) play in influencing the expression of these behaviors. The main modes of conjunctive assessment methods include behavioral rating scales (teacher, parent, and self report), observation methods and neuropsychological assessment.

Behavior rating scales are an evidence-based tool that are used to gain more detailed information in relation to a child's and family's level of functioning. More often, rating scales take a categorical approach with focus on the presence/absence of a specified symptom (Hinshaw & Zupan, 1997). However, some rating scales also measure severity and frequency of the conduct disturbance. Regardless of format, their clinical utility is widely recognized with most broad rating scales offering good psychometric properties and standardised parent, teacher and self-report versions. Therefore, they can be administered with relative ease within a variety of settings to capture different people's perspectives. The breadth and depth afforded by rating scales also enables identification of a range of difficulties; including specific antisocial behaviors and frequently co-occurring problems, such as internalizing disorders. On choosing to employ rating scales as a form of assessment, it should be noted that the informant's responses may be influenced by his or her personal level of distress, beliefs about CPs and motivations for participating in the assessment (Blader, 2006). This means that the interpretation of information provided should be guided by possible confounding factors, and where possible should always be supplemented with other modes of assessment, such as direct observations.

Overall, rating scales are separated into those that measure: (a) general child dysfunction; (b) specific areas of child dysfunction, such as temperamental traits; (c) general measures of parental dysfunction, including parenting behaviors or parent psychopathology; and (d) measures of marital and family functioning, such as quality of family environment. Table 4.3 outlines common rating scales used to measure different areas of child and family functioning. Care should be taken when selecting rating scales. A clinician should have a clear rationale for their choice of a particular rating scale, and preferably one that is compatible with therapeutic objectives. Often families who present to mental health services have family systems that are stressed, chaotic and disorganized (Sanders & Dadds, 1993). Therefore, overburdening family members with too many questionnaires, in a blind collection of information, places unnecessary burden on the system and may lead to treatment drop out.

Direct Observations

Behavioral observations are generally regarded as the "gold standard" of objective investigation into CPs as they occur in context. Structured observations of a child or youth in their natural setting (e.g., home, school) provide unique information that is not influenced by the perceptions, motivations and interpretations of any particular informant. There is broad consensus that the interpersonal dynamics occurring in parent–child dyads are critical to behavioral outcomes in children, both directly and in mediating the effects of other risk factors such as poverty (e.g.,Shaw, Bell, & Gilliom, 2000). The advent of Patterson's (1982) "coercion" model was associated with major conceptual and methodological advances in the application of social learning theory to explanations of antisocial development. To wit, Patterson (1982) suggested two main processes were operating in families of children with CPs, which could be explained using operant conditioning principles. The first of these is the parental modelling of antisocial or aggressive behavior. The second process involves "reinforcement traps," which can occur in a variety of ways (see Dadds & Hawes, 2006 for further discussion). In an effort to collect objective behavioral data concerning family processes, Patterson, Reid, and colleagues developed coding systems for recording moment-to-moment interactions between parents and children during innovative naturalistic-observational studies (see Reid, Patterson, & Snyder, 2002). Evidence in support of these processes has been reported over

Table 4.3. Broad and narrow based behavioral rating scales for child and parent dysfunction

Rating scale	Questionnaires	Informant
General areas of child dysfunction	Child Behavior Checklist (CBCL; Achenbach & Edlebrock, 1991)	Parent, teacher, youth (11–18 years)
	Revised Behavior Problem Checklist (Quay & Peterson, 1983)	Parents
	Connors Parent and Teacher Rating Scales (Conners, 1969).	Parents, teachers, youth (11–18 years)
Specific areas of child dysfunction	Child Depression Inventory (CDI; Kovacs, 1980); State-Trait Anxiety Scale for Children (Spielberger, 1973); Fear Survey Schedule (Wolpe & Lang, 1999).	Youth self report
	Eyberg Child Behavior Inventory (Eyberg & Pincus, 1999); The Parent Checklist and Teacher Checklist (Conduct Problems Prevention Research Group; Dodge & Coie, 1987); Aggressive Behavioral Rating Scale (Brown, Atkins, Osborne & Milnamow, 1996)	Youth, parent and teacher
	Antisocial Process Screening Device (APSD: Frick & Hare, 2001); Strengths & Difficulties Questionnaire (SDQ; Goodman, 2001)	
Parental dysfunction	Beck Depression Inventory (BDI; Beck, Ward, Mendelson, Mock & Erbaugh, 1961); General Health Questionnaire (Goldberg, 1972); Brief Symptom Inventory (Derogatis & Melisaraatos, 1983); The Perceived Social Supprt Scales (Procidano & Heller, 1983); Child Abuse Potential Inventory (Milner, 1980)	Parent self report
Marital and family functioning	Family Environment Scale (Moos, 1974); Dyadic Adjustment Scale (Spanier, 1976); Marital Adjustment Test (Locke & Wallace, 1959); The Parenting Problems Checklist (PPC; Dadds & Powell, 1991)	Parent self report

Note. This is not a comprehensive list of available behavioral rating scales and self report measures. For more detailed review see McMahon and Frick (2005)

decades of observational studies (see review by Snyder & Stoolmiller, 2002), and a range of efficacious behavioral interventions have directly flowed from this model (see McMahon & Forehand, 2003; Sanders & Dadds, 1993; Webster-Stratton & Hammond, 1998). While the goals of direct observation will vary, in general they are to: (a) assess the type, frequency, duration and intensity of problem behaviors; (b) identify how parents provide immediate antecedents and consequences for the problem behaviors; (c) assess the broader emotional tone of the parent–child relationship; and (d) observe how family structures provide a context for the behaviors.

Steps to Deciding an Observation Strategy

The next section outlines common steps that aid in making decisions regarding what observation strategy will be the most effective in meeting therapeutic objectives. It draws heavily from Sanders and Dadds (1993) and Dadds and Hawes (2006) methods of observation:

Generate Hypotheses for Testing. Given an assessment session with the parents has already been conducted, the therapist will have a number of hypotheses that can be tested during the observation. These hypotheses should be formulated in terms of observable behavior. These behaviors may vary greatly; however, in their amenability to direct observation. Thus, those behaviors selected should be compatible with using a direct observation procedure.

Select Target Behaviors. In selecting a target behavior that is amenable to observation in a natural or clinical setting, a number of questions need to be considered. Firstly, what are the overt behaviors that will be observed? Secondly, what are the circumstances under which these behaviors are generally expressed? Thirdly, who are the people that the target behavior is usually displayed with? On answering these questions, the clinician can start to select those behaviors that are most suitable for direct observation. Of significance in selecting target behaviors is that oppositional behavior in young children (e.g., crying, non compliance, and aggression) can be readily observed in the family home or clinic if the setting is selected appropriately. In the home, such behavior tends to escalate at times in which parents attempt to engage young children in routine activities such as bathing, bedtime, getting ready to leave on outings and meal times (Sanders, Dadds, & Bor, 1989). In clinic settings, oppositional behavior will similarly tend to occur when the parent tries to engage the child in structured teaching tasks or when compliance is enforced (e.g., cleaning up toys). Many problem behaviors are not readily observed. For example, stealing and fire setting are generally secretive and infrequent behaviors. Comparably, anxious or depressed behaviors may not occur in the presence of the clinician, and this should be factored into the chosen observational procedure.

Select Observational Procedure. Ideally, an observation procedure should be designed to elicit the problem behaviors and observe the family interaction patterns in which they are embedded (Patterson & Reid, 1984). Further, this needs to be done in a way that best approximates the natural occurrence of these patterns and yet provides sufficient procedural structure to prevent conflict or aggression escalating to a level that may be unusually distressing for participants. In our clinic, we incorporate a range of different tasks that tap into different aspects of spontaneous parenting behaviors (e.g., level of warmth; reinforcement of positive prosocial behaviors) and parent–child interactions (e.g., coercive cycles). These tasks generally include (a) a free play unstructured family task to assess normal interaction patterns in the absence of any direct induced stressors; (b) a structured play task that requires cooperation and family cohesion, alongside a range of parent–child interactions; and (c) explicit stress-inducing tasks, such as getting parents to give instructions to children (e.g., pack away the toys) or family problem-solving tasks.

We have found that each of these tasks will provide insight into parent–child interaction patterns, as well as parenting behaviors and target behaviors of the child under both nonstressful and highly stressful or emotive-based situations. When observing structured tasks, such as a family problem-solving discussion, the major points for observation include the extent to which family members actively listen to each other, the time taken to agree on a problem definition, and their ability to generate solutions and action strategies (Sanders & Dadds, 1993). What may become apparent are negative interaction patterns characterized by criticism, tangential discussion, failure to listen to one another, and poor problem solving, which is the result of vagueness, poor perseverance, or conflictual relations. These negative interaction patterns are of particular interest to the clinician who is trying to assess the quality of typical dyadic interactions and relationships within the family system.

As children approach middle childhood and adolescence, they become far more conscious of an observer's presence and are less likely to engage in open conflict with parents and siblings. With older children, it is more important to provide structured guidelines, or select settings, that prompt family interaction. Examples of such settings are family mealtimes and family meetings in which current problems are opened up for general discussion and potential problem solving. Similarly, where problems behaviors are secretive (stealing, truancy, sexual problems) or very low in frequency, direct observation of natural interactions are less likely to provide any useful data, and clinic-based family tasks or sole use of self report may need to be employed. Additional tasks that will target certain "high-risk" behaviors emerging can also be implemented within the bounds of ethical practice; using one's clinical judgment. For instance, the Issues Checklist (Robin, 1981) is a 5–10 min task that requires both parents and children to generate problems for discussion (Sanders & Dadds, 1993). Usually these problems result in heated discussions, and clinicians do need to be alert to the possibility of the discussion degenerating whereby the parent lectures or criticizes an overwhelmed child. Therefore, close monitoring of this task is required, with termination of the task taking place as quickly as is practical.

Select a Data Collection Method. There are a range of methods available for collecting and analyzing data that range from qualitative observations made by the clinician through to elaborate coding systems that specify the frequency, intensity and duration of a set of predetermined behaviors. Coding systems are dependent on a clinician's level of expertise, training with the coding system, and the target behaviors. However, many evidence-based observation coding systems are available and require only minimal levels of training and expertise. For instance, the Family Observation Schedule (FOS; Sanders, Dadds, & Bor, 1989) is a useful tool that has been shown to discriminate between distressed and non-distressed families (Sanders et al., 1989). This coding system measures a range of parent and child behavior, as well as specific parenting practices, such as level of warmth or hostility demonstrated during a nominated parent–child interaction.

Observation of a child in natural or clinical settings has been regarded as an additional assessment tool that provides further insight into family interpersonal dynamics. However, the choice of observation method must be driven by specific target behaviors and suitability of assessing behaviors via observation procedures. The greatest advantage of direct observation is that it provides objective information that can be used in conjunction with parent reports, and behavioral rating scales, to lend support to or disconfirm the clinicians working hypotheses.

NEUROPSYCHOLOGICAL ASSESSMENTS

Formal neuropsychological assessment of a child's intellectual ability, executive functioning and/or academic capacity identifies a child's neurocognitive strengths and weaknesses. This may have implications in the interpretation of the child's specific CPs and associated difficulties, prognosis and treatment planning. Used in conjunction with other assessment methods, a neuropsychological profile also provides information regarding the developmental course of the CPs and risk of developing additional problems, such as those associated with academic failure. As with all assessment tools, neuropsychological tests have a number of limitations that need to be taken into consideration (see Kaufman & Reynolds, 1984). The main consideration is that a range of within the child and external to the child factors, such as the child's motivation or experience of the examiner, may influence their performance on the day of testing. Therefore, observations of the child's thought processing, affective responses, and behavior need to be noted. These qualitative aspects of the child's functioning, such as attention or receptive language skills, also inform the examiner of additional risk factors that may have not been directly observed under comparable conditions (see Kaufman's research into these issues). One of the greatest advantages of neurocognitive assessment, however, is that comparisons between mental and chronological age are established (Kaufman & Reynolds, 1984). This baseline can be used to determine whether levels of cognitive, affective and behavioral functioning are developmentally appropriate, transitional or dysfunctional.

Intellectual Functioning

Tests of intellectual functioning identify a child's verbal and perceptual/organizational functioning. These abilities underpin the way a child comprehends, reasons, and responds to his or her environment. Typical abilities that are measured through an intellectual assessment include reasoning, planning, problem solving, speed of processing information, and attentional capacity (Bloomquist & Schnell, 2002). Past research has indicated an association between low intellectual functioning and severity of CPs (Moffitt, 1993). Specifically, compared to adjusted children, youths with a behavioral disturbance have a deficit in verbal intelligence (VIQ). However, recent research suggests that this link between low VIQ and CPs may only be true for children who are low on Callous Unemotional traits (Loney et al., 1999; Loney, Frick, Ellis, & McCoy, 1998). The most commonly used tests of intellectual functioning include the Weschler Intellectual Scale for Children (WISC-IV; Wechsler, 2003), its junior version the Weschler Preschool and Primary Scale of Intelligence (WPPSI-III; Weschler, 2002), and the Stanford–Binet IQ Test (SB5; Roid, 2003).

Executive Functioning

Executive functioning (EF) is an umbrella term that encapsulates an inter-related set of "sub-skills" that, as a whole, are primarily responsible for purposeful, goal-directed behavior, such as arousal of interest, intentional action and attainment of rewards (Kelly, Borrill, & Maddell, 1996). Contrary to popular belief, EF is not restricted to cognitive processes but is also related to emotional control and behavior (Gioia, Isquith, Guy, & Kenworthy, 2000). This means that EF serves an important role in relation to a child's cognitive, behavioral, emotional, and social functioning. There is an ever-increasing amount of research that indicates, even when developmental status is taken into account, that EF deficits are associated with aggression, delinquency, CPs, and attention-hyperactivity difficulties (Giancola, Mezzich, & Tarter, 1998; Sequin, Parent, Tremblay, & Zelazo, 2009). Findings also suggest that for children with stable and persistent physical aggression there may be a biological basis to their CPs (see Moffitt, 1993, and Chap. 3).

Academic Attainment

Formal assessment of a youth's academic functioning is generally not conducted unless some areas of academic difficulties have been indicated or identified. Learning difficulties and/or disorders have been associated with CPs (Powell, Lochman, & Bozmeyer, 2007), and may account for ongoing problems in the classroom and at home during tasks such as homework. When formally assessing a child with an academic impairment, it is important to distinguish between a learning difficulty and an actual learning disorder. Research consistently demonstrates that youths with CPs have negative learning experiences that are often associated with academic failure and school drop out (Loeber et al., 2000). However, the underlying reasons for this are varied and include; (a) an actual learning deficit, such as dyslexia; (b) poor performance due to non-compliance or classroom removal due to misbehavior; and (c) a neurobiological deficit, such as ADHD – inattentive or combined type, which impairs attention, working memory and organizational ability. Typically, academic evaluations will employ standardized tests of achievement, such as the Wechsler Individual Achievement Test (WIAT-III; Wechsler, 2008). The advantage of using the WIAT is that it can then be used to compare academic functioning against performance on intellectual tests (e.g., WISC-IV) to compute a discrepancy analysis score.

THE PROCESS OF ASSESSMENT

One of the most difficult issues in assessment and treatment of children revolves around treatment adherence and attrition rates. Families of children with CPs are well known for low readiness to engage with treatment services, high rates of treatment drop out, and poor adherence in implementing recommended treatment strategies (see Kazdin, Marciano, & Whitley et al., 2005, Kazdin, 2006 for comprehensive research into treatment barriers). While research typically focuses on treatment variables, Kazdin (1996) points out that important parent expectancies are established on first contact with clinics – at the time of assessment. That is, the treatment of CPs starts the moment the clinician comes into contact with the family. Reducing the occurrence of poor engagement and drop out is achieved through careful attention to the *process* of assessment as well as its content. Patterson and Chamberlain (1994) argued that parent engagement and cooperation is best enhanced through use of a stage model in which didactic input is suspended until client trust is built by giving parents adequate time to express their concerns in supportive client-centered sessions. Most evidence-based treatments now pay careful attention to explicating the therapist behaviors needed to maximize engagement and minimize drop out and poor engagement. For example, Sanders and Dadds (1993) similarly emphasise a stage model in which the therapist and parents form a team, jointly lead the assessment process, and then develop a shared perception of the problem and potential solutions prior to any treatment taking place. In our treatment, therapy process is modelled right from the first contact with the family through to termination in a way that emphasises teamwork, parent empowerment, and support.

There are numerous process issues involved in the assessment, and subsequent treatment, of families and children in the area of CPs. As outlined in the model, we conceptualise process issues in terms of therapeutic processes and familial processes. These two types of processes are distinct yet interactive; a skilled clinician who works within a process orientated approach will have a greater conceptualization of the nature of the family's difficulties and most appropriate treatment intervention. Specifically, sensitivity to these process issues will influence the family's level of engagement and disclosure; the degree of accuracy of the information gathered; cooperation with other agencies and professionals, such as teachers; and importantly development of a shared perception and motivation to enact change. Consequently, working with process issues should lead to a greater awareness and reduction of treatment barriers; participation in the recommended treatment plan; and more favourable outcomes for the child and their family. Throughout this chapter we have interwoven some of the more salient therapeutic process issues as they pertain to the various aspects of assessment, such as engagement/treatment barriers or encountering hostility from youths. This section discusses in more detail four of the most important familial processes that warrant attention, specific to assessment and treatment of CPs. We have drawn heavily from the work of Dadds and Hawes (2006), as they provide a useful summary of these core issues.

Facilitating the Involvement of Relevant Family Members

It is important to pay careful attention to making sure all members of the family feel heard and respected no matter how outrageous their perspectives, and to integrate their views into the larger conceptualization. The primary aim of assessment and treatment is to shape the behavior of those in most frequent contact with the referred child. In doing so, the clinician affects changes in the family system, as well as the environment in which the child lives and develops. Within such a model, parents function as agents of change, making their involvement and cooperation throughout assessment critical. In failing to allow both parents perspectives to be integrated into the assessment process, it becomes difficult to establish a trusting relationship with *both* parents (if there are two). The result is often that the parent whose thoughts have not been heard will disengage from the process, and may even drop out completely.

Another benefit of having both parents at the interview which is often neglected in assessment is to gain insight into the level they are functioning at as a "parenting team." There are robust findings in the literature that consistency in parenting practices has a direct influence on the nature, course, and developmental outcomes of a child with CPs. Assessment of the degree to which the child's parents (including step-parents) work together is important, for understanding both the current level of parent and family functioning and also for considering treatment goals. Further, it gives the clinician an indication of how well strategies are likely to be implemented in a consistent manner by both parents. When explored, these surface parenting practices can also reveal deeper underlying issues, such as marital functioning and discord, which is likely to have an impact on the development and maintenance of the youth's CPs.

Developing a Shared Perception with Different Family Members

Establishment of a facilitative relationship is a critical factor in enabling parents to explore the relationship of the child's problems to their management of the problem and to contextual factors such as marital distress. Viewing family problems in an interactional or systemic way can often inadvertently result in the clinician failing to form such a relationship with parents of behavior-disordered children. If parents commence treatment, as they often do, by complaining and blaming the child, and the clinician quickly focuses on the parents' management techniques, or worse, shifts focus onto other problems in the family, the parent may feel blamed and drop out. These social cognitive attributions about "who is to blame" should be recognised and addressed sensitively. As outlined, during initial interviews, it can be useful to build relationships with the parents and children separately, not proceeding to more formal assessments of parent–child patterns of interaction until open and trusting relationships with family members have been established.

Working with Parents Attributional Processes

A wealth of research has shown that parents of conduct problem children develop problematic attributions about the meaning of the child's behavior (e.g., Dadds, Mullins, McAllister, & Atkinson, 2003). Common examples include the parent feeling that the child's behavior is intentional and under the child's control, is designed to deliberately upset the parent, is a sign of serious mental problems, is inherited from other (disliked) family members (e.g., an abusive ex-spouse), or is in someway a punishment that the parent deserves. Further, parents may be horrified by the thought they sometimes have about the child, experiencing impulses of rejection and hatred. Finally, parents may have beliefs about models of discipline that are incompatible with the operant techniques typically taught in parent training programmes. All of these cognitions can make it very difficult to calmly parent a child and are risk factors for failure to implement traditional parent training programmes (e.g., Wahler & Dumas, 1989).

Integrating the Family Context with the Child's Problem

During the process of initial interviewing, it is important to explore and identify any issues that may be impacting adversely on the family system. Such issues may be sensitive, highly emotional, or frightening to clients. These "hot topics" should always be addressed in a way that maintains and maximises the client–therapist relationship, the dignity and self-esteem of the client, and the quality of the information obtained.

Problems with relating contextual aspects of family functioning (e.g., marital issues, financial stress, cultural differences) to a child's problems usually lie at two extremes. The first can happen when a clinician does not raise these issues for discussion, perhaps due to fear of confronting intimate family details or due to conceptual biases about the role of these variables. The other extreme occurs when these issues are raised in such a way that causes the parents to deny their importance, existence, or the right of the clinician to focus on them (suggestions for effectively raising questions about family functioning can be found in Dadds & Hawes, 2006).

When exploring such issues, the therapist should "funnel" questions in a similar way to the process used for progressing through the components of the broader intake interview. The therapist proceeds from the general (open-ended questions) to the specific (clarification, elaboration). This process should be conducted in a way that is client-centred, and again, develops a shared perception of these aspects of family functioning. During this discussion, it is also important to integrate parents' reports with other forms of assessment regarding family functioning. It is not unknown for parents to report absolutely no problem during this discussion, but to report problems such as marital distress on relevant inventories. Any discrepancies should be addressed with careful consideration of the individuals concerned. It may be that one parent is coerced by the other into not talking about any problems except those concerning the child.

THE PROCESS OF INTEGRATION

Functional Analysis: An Overview

A functional analysis is not a "method" of assessment but rather the product of a culmination of different assessment methods, such as interviews, behavioral rating scales, and self reports. Constructing a functional analysis should be a fluid process that is integrated into treatment; for this reason it serves a number of functions for the clinician and family (Sanders & Dadds 1993). Foremost, it enables the clinician to develop a clear conceptualization of the specific behaviors targeted for change and important causal factors that may be influencing the nature and course of the CPs. Second, it provides a concise framework to integrate all relevant information in a way that can be shared with the family to provide them with an understanding of targets for change. Lastly, it plays a critical role in treatment planning, establishing therapeutic objectives, and identifying clear treatment goals.

In adopting a scientific approach to treatment, a functional analysis is the apex upon which hypotheses testing and operationalization of problem behaviors occurs. Traditionally, functional analysis is concerned with specific testing and manipulation of the hypotheses generated (Cone, 1997; Ollendick & Hersen, 1984). However, this term is now broadened to incorporate other important factors, such as distal, contextual, and immediate antecedents of target behaviors. These possible maintaining factors are generally causally interrelated, meaning that behavior is seen as reciprocally determined rather than unidirectional (Sanders & Dadds, 1993). Thus, a behavioral analysis adds important dimensional information, such as a "snap shot" of reciprocal parent–child interactions frozen in time, to understand the function of particular behaviors. Once generated, underlying functional variables that play a role in influencing a child's problematic behavior can be manipulated through selection of appropriate treatment strategies (Sturmey, 1994).

Steps in Developing a Functional Analysis

The clinical purpose of a functional assessment is to gather information to confirm hypotheses, further operationalise presenting problems, and drive the implementation of appropriate treatment strategies (Ollendick & Hersen, 1984). Most importantly, a functional analysis is an interpretive framework to understand a child within context and is ultimately going to be shared with relevant family members, and significant others (e.g., teachers), who will be involved in treatment. Thus, four important questions that aid in developing a functional analysis include:

1. What is the larger diagnostic framework most applicable to the behavioral expression of this child's problem behaviors?
2. What are the target behaviors and the child's internal experience when they occur (e.g., thoughts, beliefs, emotions, physiological responses)?
3. How did these problems develop?
4. How are these problems maintained (who, when, where, and how)?

These questions tap into the core components of a functional analysis that should be identified and integrated; these include (a) identification and definition of target behaviors; (b) antecedents, including within child factors and wider social contextual factors; (c) reinforcing agents, such as coercive parent–child interactions; and (d) consequences and related skills deficits, as they occur in diverse contexts.

Identify and Define Target Behaviors. By the time a clinician is ready to develop a functional analysis, they should start to have some idea of the core presenting problem/s. The most fundamental and necessary step in conducting a detailed functional analysis is to identify and clearly define target behaviors. To begin, specific behaviors should be listed and clearly defined in terms of their observable behaviors. This means that broad terms such as "aggressive" or "oppositional" should be clearly defined in terms of identifiable discrete behaviors such as "slams doors, verbal insults to parents" or "refuses to get dressed, argues at bedtime" (Sanders & Dadds, 1993). Listing observable behaviors should not be restricted to the child, but also other relevant individuals. For instance, a mother's behavior when responding to her child should be noted, such as "ignores verbal insults" or "screaming when instructions not followed." The methods that were used to define these behaviors should also be noted down, such as "child's hits when told no" was based on observations and parent reports.

On completion of this list a range of behaviors will be detailed, therefore a selection process of which behaviors to target should be implemented. Sanders and Dadds (1993) recommend following a specified criteria for determining which target behaviors to choose taking into account: (a) the expressed concerns of the family; (b) the importance of the behavior in terms of its adverse consequences for the child and family; (c) the likelihood of success in changing the behavior; (d) the inter-relationships between the target behaviors, that is, particular behaviors dependent upon other behaviors that are expected to decrease if the behaviors they are dependent on are targeted. For example, it may be unnecessary to target swearing if it only occurs during tantrums that result from the ineffective management of noncompliance; and (e) the ability of the parents to implement strategies for a particular behavior. Once the target behaviors are chosen and defined, these should be fedback to the family, and agreement between the clinician, parents, and child (if appropriate) reached before proceeding to examine these targets in greater detail.

Identify Important Child Characteristics. Within child characteristics, such as cognitive, emotional, and physical factors all play a role in influencing the expression and maintenance of target behaviors. These characteristics may be inherent within the child's biological make up (temperament style) or those internal experiences that occur in the actual moment of problematic behavior.

Identify Distal, Contextual and Immediate Antecedents of Target Behaviors. Immediate antecedents to the behavior are listed. These triggers occur immediately prior to the target behavior (i.e., precipitants that occur within a few minutes or less). Again, these events should be listed in clearly observable terms. Distal and contextual events that are associated with the occurrence of the target behavior should also be listed. These events do not directly elicit the occurrence of the target behavior, but exert their influence by either increasing the probability that an antecedent will occur, or by increasing the probability that the target behavior will follow the relevant antecedent stimuli.

Identify Consequences of Target Behaviors. The consequences of target behaviors are divided into (a) stimuli that occur immediately following the problem behavior; these reinforcing or punishing stimuli are often hypothesised to be associated with maintenance of the problem behavior and; (b) delayed consequences of the problem behavior. The latter are often not directly related to the performance, but operate indirectly by feeding back into antecedent conditions and organismic states.

Identify Maintaining Coercive and Vicious Cycles. Identification of maintaining cycles is achieved by examining all of the core components of the functional analysis and making functional links between the antecedents, target behavior, reinforcers, and consequences. Each functional link can be highlighted as a typical interaction pattern that serves to maintain a coercive cycle that reinforces problem behaviors in the long term.

Share the Analysis with Family Members. The final step is to share the functional analysis with family members in order to facilitate a common agreement of those behaviors and maintaining factors that should be targeted in treatment. This can be presented in a diagrammatic form that highlights all of the components of the functional analysis in a simplistic model that shows clear patterns in relation to antecedents, reinforcers, and consequences of the target behavior. Presenting more distal and historical factors is a helpful way to illustrate to the family the potential origins of the presenting problems.

CASE STUDY: JACK

Jack, 5 years, was referred by his mother, Mrs. Cooper, due to her inability to manage his behavior and concerns raised by his kindergarten teacher regarding disruptive behavior at school. Mrs. Cooper reported that Jack had problems at home and school that were characterized by numerous, frequent and intense temper outbursts, physical/verbal aggression toward adults and peers, non-compliance, argumentativeness, and more recently malicious acts toward others. She stated that "at the rate his behavior is worsening he will be expelled from school and will lead to me having a nervous breakdown." Jack was assessed using interviews with both parents, a clinic based observation of structured and unstructured tasks, a telephone conference with his school teacher, and completion of behavioral rating scales (general and specific to child dysfunction and specific to parental psychopathology and family adjustment). On the basis of the available assessment information, Jack was diagnosed with having ODD (DSM-IV) with a moderate level of impairment because his CPs were evident across all settings. Jack's quality of family environment was rated as poor due to moderate levels of marital discord, current maternal depression, and a longstanding history of paternal substance abuse. Furthermore, numerous additional stressors, such as financial instability and low levels of social support indicated poor family adjustment.

Mrs. Cooper's parenting responses to Jack's oppositional behavior centered around the use of vague instructions, the most common form being to simply repeat her son's name over and over in increasingly aggressive tones. Her exhaustion with Jack was leading her to no longer notice any of his positive behaviors and thus there was a clear lack of attention to appropriate behavior. For Mr. Cooper, parenting behaviors were observed to be similar to Mrs. Cooper except that he had no praise skills in his repertoire, and offered little contribution to the management of Jack or day to day chores around the home. He would often criticize his wife for Jack's behavior and her inability to handle him, rather than offering to help. Thus, Jack's behavior had become a major source of tension in the marital relationship causing Mrs. Cooper to become increasingly burdened with the care of Jack, and Mr. Cooper to withdraw more and more into work and other activities outside the home. There was little positive engagement between Mr. and Mrs. Cooper except for aversive discussions about Jack's problems.

The next step is to decide upon priorities and goals for treatment and to conduct a functional analysis of the selected target behaviors. In this case, Mr. and Mrs. Cooper's priorities for change focused on Jack's excesses viz. noncompliance, hitting, kicking, swearing, and tantrums. These behaviors were interrelated in that they occurred in a cluster. Attempts by Mr. and Mrs. Cooper to direct Jack's behavior would result in noncompliance and the ensuing battle would escalate to include hitting, kicking, swearing, and tantrums. Thus, these behaviors could be targeted with a behavior management routine that was well within the capacity of Mr. and Mrs. Cooper to implement. The maintenance of these problems was functionally related to Mr. and Mrs. Cooper's ability to work as an effective team, to avoid criticizing each other, and to encourage and support each other's role in the family. These problems were openly discussed with Mr. and Mrs. Cooper and agreement was achieved to target this area for change. Given the above rationale, we conducted a functional analysis, for the problem clusters listed above. On reviewing all of the available information the following functional analysis was conducted for Jack's main oppositional behaviors (see Fig. 4.4).

ASSESSMENT FEEDBACK AND TREATMENT RECOMMENDATIONS

Clinical skills are required to successfully communicate assessment findings in open dialogue with the family (Dadds & Hawes, 2006; Sanders et al., 1993). These involve developing a shared perception with clients by presenting a summary of the assessment findings, with feedback of available diagnostic and prognostic information, and a discussion of treatment options, including strategies, therapy duration, and contact frequency. Just as important as the content of this feedback is the process of encouraging a positive attitude in parents toward actively confronting the identified problems. This is best achieved by ensuring the following processes have been incorporated; (a) the informants felt listened to and an empathetic therapeutic alliance is established; (b) informants have confidence in the therapist's clinical skills, as well as the therapist's conceptualization and feedback of the more salient issues raised by them; and (c) that the informant has gained insight into the youth's patterns of behaviors, including their own potential role in fostering unhelpful patterns.

The task that follows assessment consists of the scheduling, sequencing, and integrating of interventions. At this point, it is assumed that the

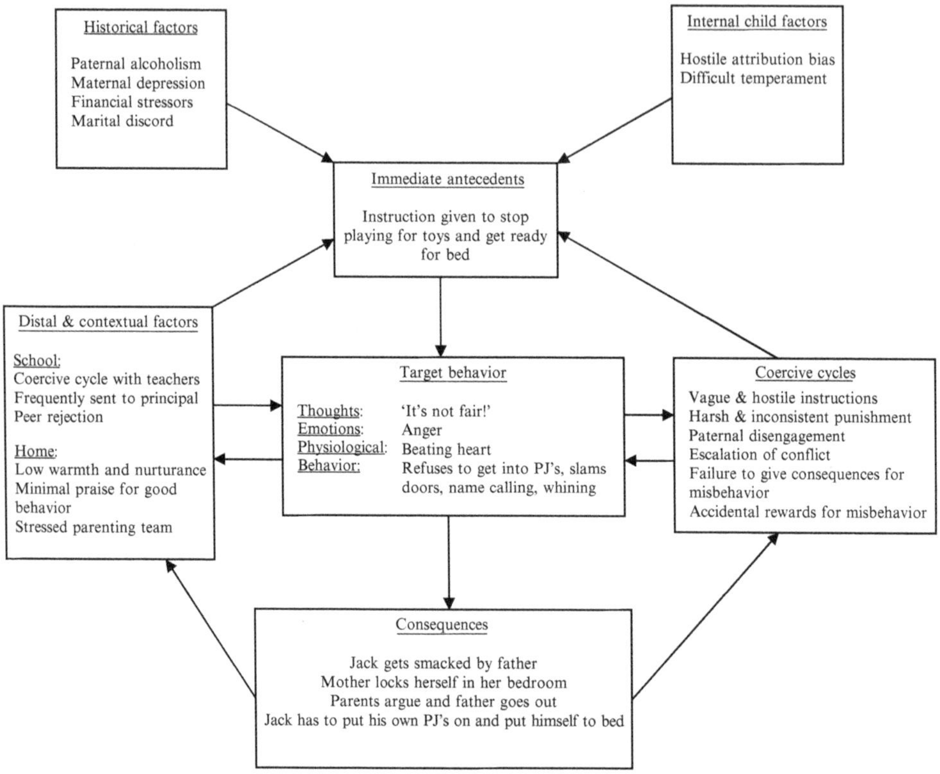

Fig. 4.4. Functional analysis of Jack's target behavior.

family has established an open trusting relationship with the clinician, and the child has been assessed as exhibiting behavior problems warranting a family intervention (Dadds & Hawes, 2006). When making treatment decisions, it is important to be mindful that manualised and popular treatment approaches are only as effective as the information gained in relation to the youth's difficulties. Therefore, treatment decisions are based on the functional analysis and a shared perception of the child's difficulties. Associated factors, such as familial adjustment, are also considered when considering a "best fit" treatment intervention. The remaining chapters in this handbook detail the various treatment approaches that have been developed in the area of youth CPs.

CONCLUDING COMMENTS: STAYING POSITIVE!

Throughout the assessment process the clinician needs to remember they are assessing and treating people, not just diagnostic categories or constellations of "symptoms." Therefore, adopting a process oriented approach to assessment that empowers people and fosters positive growth through empathic and open enquiry is the goal. Because the present topic of assessment is a psychological or behavioral disorder, this chapter has been largely focussed on the discernment and characterization of "pathology." As a balance to this, it is very useful to think about positive pathways that the child's life could take. Of course, a common pathway for children with CPs is into chronic problems. On the other hand, children do desist from negative pathways and evidence-based treatments show good results in ameliorating problems. Thus, it is advisable to think about the child in terms of positive pathways as well. What strengths does this child and his or her family have that can be built on? What would a healthy road look like for this child? What changes will promote health and well being? What positive potentials can be identified for this child?

REFERENCES

Achenbach, T. M., & Edelbrock, C. S. (1991). *Manual for the child behavior checklist and the revised child behavior profile*. Burlington, VT: University Associates in Psychiatry.

American Psychiatric Association. (1994). *Diagnostic and statistical manual of mental disorders* (4th ed.). Washington, DC: American Psychiatric Association.

Angold, A., Cox, A., Prendergast, M., Rutter, M., & Simonoff, E. (1987, 1989). *Child and adolescent psychiatric assessment*. Durham, NC: Developmental Epidemiology Program, Department of Psychiatry, Duke University.

Bagner, D. M., & Eyberg, S. (2003). Father involvement in parent training does it matter? *Journal of Clinical Child and Adolescent Psychology, 32*, 599–605.

Bauermeister, J. J., Shrout, P. E., Ramírez, R., Bravo, M., Alegría, M., Martínez-Taboas, A., et al. (2007). ADHD correlates, comorbidity, and impairment in community and treated samples of children and adolescents. *Journal of Abnormal Child Psychology, 35*(6), 1573–2835.

Beck, A. T., Ward, C. H., Mendelson, M., Mock, J., & Erbaugh, J. (1961). An inventory for measuring depression. *Archives of General Psychiatry, 4*, 53–63.

Blader, J. C. (2006). Which family factors predict children's externalizing behaviors following discharge from psychiatric inpatient treatment? *Journal of Child Psychology and Psychiatry, 47*(11), 1133–1142.

Blazei, R. W., Iacono, W. G., & McGue, M. (2008). Father–child transmission of antisocial behavior: The moderating role of father's presence in the home. *Journal of the American Academy of Child and Adolescent Psychiatry, 47*(4), 406–415.

Bloomquist, M. L., & Schnell, S. V. (2002). *Helping children with aggression and conduct problems: Best practices for intervention*. New York: Guildford Press.

Brennan, P. A., Le Brocque, R., Hammen, C. (2003). Maternal depression, parent-child relationships, and resilient outcomes in adolescence. *Journal of the American Academy of Child & Adolescent Psychiatry, 42* (12), 1469–1477.

Brown, K., Atkins, M. S., Osborne, M. L., & Milnamow, M. (1996). A revised teacher rating scale for reactive and proactive aggression. *Journal of Abnormal Child Psychology, 24*, 473–480.

Bronfenbrenner, U. (1977). Toward an experimental ecology of human development. *American Psychologist, 32* (7), 513–531.

Boylan, K., Vaillancourt, T., Boyle, M., & Szatmari, P. (2007). Comorbidity of internalizing disorders in children with oppositional defiant disorder. *European Journal of Child and Adolescent Psychiatry, 16*(8), 484–494.

Carr, A. (1999). *The handbook of child and adolescent clinical psychology*. London: Routledge.

Cone, J. D. (1997). Issues in functional analysis in behavioral assessment. *Behavior Research and Therapy, 35*, 259–275.

Conners, C. K. (1997). *Conners rating scales – revised manual*. New York: Multi-Health Systems.

Connor, D. F. (2002). *Aggression & antisocial behavior in children and adolescents. Research and treatment.* New York: Guilford Press.

Costello, A., Edelbrock, L., Dulcan, M., Kalas, R., & Klaric, S. (1984). *Report on the NIMH diagnostic interview schedule for children (DISC).* Washington, DC: National Institute of Mental Health.

Crick, N. R., & Dodge, K. A. (1994). A review and reformulation of social information-processing mechanisms in children's social adjustment. *Psychological Bulletin, 115* (1), 74–101.

Conners, C. K. (1969). A teacher rating scale for use in drug studies with children. *American Journal of Psychiatry, 126,* 884–888.

Dadds, M. R., & Hawes, D. (2006). *Integrated family intervention for child conduct problems: A behavior-attachment-systems intervention for parents.* Brisbane: Australian Academic Press.

Dadds, M. R., & McHugh, T. A. (1992). Social support and treatment outcome in behavioral family therapy for child conduct problems. *Journal of Consulting and Clinical Psychology, 60* (2), 252–259.

Dadds, M. R., Mullins, M. J., McAllister, R. A., & Atkinson, E. (2003). Attributions, affect, and behavior in abuse-risk mothers: A laboratory study. *Child Abuse and Neglect, 27*(1), 21–45.

Dadds, M., & Powell, M. B. (1991). The relationship of interparental conflict and global marital adjustment to aggression, anxiety, and immaturity in aggressive and non-clinic children. *Journal of Abnormal Child Psychology, 19,* 553–567.

David, C., & Kistner, J. (2000). Do positive self-perceptions have a "dark side"? Examination of the link between perceptual bias and aggression. *Journal of Abnormal Child Psychology, 28*(4), 327–337.

Derogatis, L. R., & Melisaraatos, N. (1983). The brief symptom inventory (BSI): An introductory report. *Psychological Medicine, 13,* 595.

Dodge, K. A., & Coie, J. D. (1987). Social-information-processing factors in reactive and proactive aggression in children's peer groups. *Journal of Personality and Social Psychology, 53,* 1146–1158.

Eyberg, S. M., & Pincus, D. (1999). *The Eyberg child behvior inventory and Sutter–Eyberg student behavior inventory: Professional manual.* Lutz, FL: Psychological Assessment Resources.

Fergusson, D. M., Horwood, L. J., & Lynskey, M. T. (1993). Prevalence and comorbidity of DSM-III-R diagnoses in a birth cohort of 15 year olds. *Journal of the American Academy of Child and Adolescent Psychiatry, 33,* 1127–1134.

Fisher, P. W., Shaffer, D., Piacentini, J., Lapkin, J., Kafantaris, V., et al (1993). Sensitivity of the diagnostic interview schedule for children, 2nd Edition (DISC-2.1) for specific diagnoses of children and adolescents. *The American Academy of Child and Adolescent Psychiatry, 32* (3), 666–673.

Frick, P. J., & Hare, R. D. (2001). *The antisocial process screening device.* Toronto: Multi-Health Systems.

Frick, P. J., & Loney, B. R. (1999). Outcomes of children and adolescents with conduct disorder and oppositional defiant disorder. In H. C. Quay & A. Hogan (Eds.), *Handbook of disruptive behavior disorders* (pp. 507–524). New York: Plenum Press.

Frick, P. J., Lilienfeld, S. O., Ellis, M., Loney, B., & Silverthorn, P. (1999). The association between anxiety and psychopathy dimensions in children. *Journal of Abnormal Child Psychology, 27,* 383–392.

Goldberg, D. (1972). *Detecting psychiatric illness by questionnaire.* Oxford: Oxford University Press.

Giancola, P. R., Mezzich, A. C., Tarter, R. E. (1998). Executive cognitive functioning, temperament, and antisocial behaviour in conduct-disordered adolescent females. *Journal of Abnormal Psychology, 107,* 629–641.

Gioia, G. A., Isquith, P. K., Guy, S. C., & Kenworthy, L. (2000). Behavior rating inventory of executive function. *Child Neuropsychology: A Journal on Normal and Abnormal Development in Childhood and Adolescence, 6*(3), 235–8.

Goodman, R. (2001). Psychometric properties of the strengths and difficulties questionnaire. *Journal of the American Academy of Child & Adolescent Psychiatry, 40* (11), 1337–1345.

Herjanic, B., Herjanic, M., Brown, F., & Wheatt, T. (1975). Are children reliable reporters? *Journal of Abnormal Child Psychology, 3*, 41–48.

Hinshaw, S. P. (2003). Impulsivity, emotion regulation, and developmental psychopathology: Specificity vs. generality of linkages. *Annals of the New York Academy of Sciences, 1008*, 149–159.

Hinshaw, S. P. (2006). Attention-deficit hyperactivity disorder. In P. C. Kendall (Ed.), *Child and adolescent therapy: Cognitive-behavioral procedures* (Vol. 3, pp. 46–68). New York: Guildford Press.

Hinshaw, S. P., & Zupan, B. A. (1997). Assessment of antisocial behavior in children and adolescents. In D. M. Stoff, J. Breiling, & J. D. Maser (Eds.), *Handbook of antisocial behavior* (pp. 36–50). New York: Wiley.

Hodges, K., & Fitch, P. (1979). *Development of a mental status examination interview for children*. Kansas City, MO: Paper presented at the Missouri Psychological Association meeting.

Hodges, K. (1993). Structured interviews for assessing children. *Journal of Child Psychology and Psychiatry, 34*, 49–68.

Hoeve, M., Blokland, A., Dubas, J. S., Loeber, R., Gerris, J. R., & van der Laan, P. H. (2008). Trajectories of delinquency and parenting styles. *Journal of Abnormal Child Psychology, 36*(2), 223–235.

Jensen, P., Martin, D., & Cantwell, D. (1997). Hyperactive/impulsive/inattention problems and conduct problems. *Journal of the American Academy of Child & Adolescent Psychiatry, 36*(2), 1065–1079.

Kazdin, A. E. (2006). Premature termination from treatment among children referred for antisocial behavior. *Journal of Child Psychology and Psychiatry, 31* (3), 415–425.

Kazdin, A. E. (1996). Dropping out of child psychotherapy: Issues for research and implications for practice. *Clinical Child Psychology and Psychiatry, 1*, 133–156.

Kazdin, A. E., & Whitley, M. K. (2006). Pretreatment social, relations, therapeutic alliance and improvements in parenting practices in parent management training. *Journal of Consulting and Clinical Psychology, 74*(2), 346–355.

Kazdin, A. E., Marciano, P. L., & Whitley, M. K. (2005). The therapeutic alliance in cognitive behavioral treatment of children referred for oppositional, aggressive, and antisocial Behavior. *Journal of Consulting and Clinical Psychology, 73*(4), 726–730.

Kaufman, J., Birmaher, B., Brent, D., Rao, U., Flynn, C., et al. (1997). Schedule for affective disorders & lifetime version: Initial reliability and validity data. *Journal of the American Academy of Child & Adolescent Psychiatry, 36*, 980–989.

Kaufman, A. S., & Reynolds, C. R. (1984). Intellectual and academic achievement tests. In T. H. Ollendick & M. Hersen (Eds.), Child Behavioral Assessment: Principals and Procedures. New York: Pergamon Press.

Kelly, T. P., Borrill, H. S., & Maddell, D. L. (1996). Development and assessment of executive function in children. *Child Psychology and Psychiatry Review, 1*, 46–51.

Kazdin, A. E., & Esveldt-Dawson, K. (1986). The interview for antisocial behavior: Psychometric characteristics and concurrent validity with child psychiatric inpatients. *Journal of Psychopathology and Behavioral Assessment, 8*, 289–303.

Kovacs, M. (1980–1981). Rating scales to assess depression in school aged children. *Acta Paedopsychiatrica, 46*, 305–315.

Loney, B. R., & Frick, P. J. (2003). Structured diagnostic interviewing. In C. R. Reynolds & R. W. Kamphaus (Eds.), *Handbook of educational assessment of children, 2nd ed* (pp. 235–247). New York: Guilford.

Locke, H. J., & Wallace, K. M. (1959). Short marital-adjustment and prediction tests: Their reliability and validity. *Marriage & Family Living, 21*, 251–255.

Loeber, R., & Farrington, D. P. (2000). Young children who commit crime: Epidemiology, developmental origins, risk factors, early interventions, and policy implications. *Development and Psychopathology, 12*, 737–762.

Loeber, R. (1990). Development and risk factors of juvenile antisocial behavior and delinquency. *Clinical Psychology Review, 10*, 1–41.

Loeber, R., Burke, J. D., Lahey, B. B., Winters, Q., & Zera, M. (2000). Oppositional defiant and conduct disorder: A review of the past 10 years, part 1. *Journal of the American Academy of Child and Adolescent Psychiatry, 39*(12), 1468–1484.

Loeber, R., & Farrington, D. P. (2000). Young children who commit crime: Epidemiology, developmental origins, risk factors, early interventions, and policy implications. *Development and Psychopathology, 12*, 737–762.

Loeber, R., Green, S., Lahey, B., & Stouthamer-Loeber, M. (1990). Optimal informants on childhood disruptive behaviors. *Development and Psychopathology, 1*, 317–337.

Loeber, R., & Schmaling, K. (1985). Empirical evidence for overt and covert patterns of antisocial conduct problems. *Journal of Abnormal Child Psychology, 13*, 337–352.

Loney, B. R., Frick, P. J., Ellis, M., & McCoy, M. G. (1998). Intelligence, psychopathy, and antisocial behavior. *Journal of Psychopathology and Behavioral Assessment, 20*, 231–247.

McConaughy, S. H., & Skiba, R. J. (1993). Comorbidity of externalizing and internalizing problems. *Journal of School Psychology Review, 22*, 421–436.

McMahon, R. J., & Forehand, R. (2003). *Helping the noncompliant child: Family-based treatment for oppositional behavior* (2nd ed.). New York: Guilford Press.

McMahon, R. J., & Frick, P. J. (2005). Evidence-based assessment of conduct problems in children and adolescents. *Journal of Clinical Child and Adolescent Psychology, 34*, 477–505.

Milner, J. S. (1980). *The child abuse potential inventory: Manual.* Webster, NC: Psytec.

Moffitt, T. E. (1990). Juvenile delinquency and attention-deficit disorder: Developmental trajectories from age 3 to 15. *Child Development, 61*, 893–910.

Moffitt, T. E., & Caspi, A. (2001). Childhood predictors differentiate life-course persistent and adolescence limited pathways, among males and females. *Development and Psychopathology, 13*, 355–375.

Moffitt, T. E. (1993). Adolescence-limited and life-course-persistent antisocial behavior: A developmental taxonomy. *Psychological Review, 100*, 674–701.

Moos, R. (1974). *Family environment scale and preliminary manual.* Palo Alto, CA: Consulting Psychologists Press.

Nelson, D. A., & Coyne, S. M. (2009). Children's intent attributions and feelings of distress: Associations with maternal and paternal parenting practices. *Journal of Abnormal Child Psychology.*

Nock, M. K., Kazdin, A. E., Hiripi, E., & Kessler, R. C. (2006). Prevalence, subtypes, and correlates of DSM-IV conduct disorder in the National Comorbidity Survey Replication. *Psychological Medicine, 36*, 699–710.

Ollendick, T. H., & Hersen, M. (1984). *Child behavioral assessment, principles and procedures* (pp. 3–19). New York: Pergamon Press.

Ollendick, T. H., Jarrett, M. A., Grills-Taquechel, A. E., Seligman, L. D., & Wolff, J. C. (2008). Moving beyond treatment efficacy: Comorbidity as a predictor and moderator of treatment outcome in youth with anxiety, affective, attentional and oppositional/conduct disorders. *Clinical Psychology Review, 28*, 1447–1471.

Patterson, G. R. (1982). *A social learning approach: 3. Coercive family process.* Eugene, OR: Castalia.

Patterson, G. R., & Chamberlain, P. (1994). A functional analysis of resistance during parent training therapy. *Journal of Clinical Psychology: Science and Practice, 1*(1), 53–70.

Patterson, G. R., & Reid, J. B. (1984). Social interactional processes within the family: The study of moment-by-moment family transactions in which human social development is embedded. *Journal of Applied Developmental Psychology, 5*, 237–262.

Powell, N. R., Lochman, J. E., & Boxmeyer, C. L. (2007). The prevention of conduct problems. *International Review of Psychiatry, 19*(6), 597–605.

Procidano, M. E., & Heller, K. (1983). Measures of perceived social support from friends and from family: Three validation studies. *American Journal of Community Psychology, 11*, 1–24.

Quay, H. C., & Peterson, D. R. (1983). *Interim manual for the revised behavior problem checklist.* Coral Gables, Florida: University.

Reid, J. B., Patterson, G. R., & Snyder, J. J. (Eds.) (2002). *Antisocial behavior in children and adolescents: A developmental analysis and a model for intervention.* Washington DC: American Psychological Association.

Robin, A. L. (1981). A controlled evaluation of problem-solving communication training with parent-adolescent conflict. *Behavior Therapy, 12*, 593–609.

Roid, G. H. (2003). *Stanford-Binet intelligence scales* (5th ed.). Riverside: Examiner's Manual.

Sanders, M. R., Dadds, M. R., & Bor, W. (1989). Contextual analysis of child oppositional and maternal aversive behaviors in families of conduct-disordered and problem children. *Journal of Clinical Child Psychology, 18*(1), 72–83.

Sanders, M. R., & Dadds, M. R. (1993). *Behavioral family intervention.* Needham Heights, MA: Allyn and Bacon.

Séguin, J. R., Parent, S., Tremblay, R. E., & Zelazo, P. D. (2009). Different neurocognitive functions regulating physical aggression and hyperactivity in early childhood. *Journal of Child Psychology and Psychiatry*, 50 (6), 679-687.

Shaffer, D., Schwab-Stone, M., Fisher, P., Davies, M., Piacentini, J., Gioia, P. (1988). A revised version of the Diagnostic Interview Schedule for children (DISC-R): results of a field trial and proposals for a new instrument (DISC-2). Report submitted to the National Institute of Mental Health.

Shaw, D. S., Bell, R. Q., Gilliom, M. (2000). A truly early starter model of antisocial behavior revisited. Clinical Child and Family Psychology Review, 3 (3), 155-172.

Snyder, J., & Stoolmiller, M. (2002). Reinforcement and coercion mechanisms in the development of antisocial behavior: The family. In J. B. Reid, G. R. Patterson, & J. Snyder (Eds.), *Antisocial behavior in children and adolescents: A developmental analysis and model for intervention* (pp. 65–100). Washington, DC: American Psychological Association.

Spanier, G. B. (1976). Measuring dyadic adjustment: New scales for assessing the quality of marriage and similar dyads. *Journal of Marriage and the Family, 38*, 15–28.

Spielberger, C. D. (1973). *Preliminary manual for the state-trait anxiety inventory for children ("How I Feel Questionnaire").* Palo Alto, CA: Consulting Psychologist Press.

Sturmey, P. (1994). Assessing the functions of aberrant behaviors: A review of psychometric instruments. *Journal of Autism and Developmental Disorders, 24*, 293–304.

Trentacosta, C. J., & Shaw, D. S. (2008). Maternal predictors of rejecting parenting and early adolescent antisocial behavior. *Journal of Abnormal Child Psychology, 36*, 247–259.

Waschbusch, D. A. (2002). A meta-analytic examination of comorbid hyperactive- impulsive-attention problems and conduct problems. *Psychological Bulletin, 128*, 118–150.

Wahler, R. G., & Dumas, J. E. (1989). Attentional problems in dysfunctional mother- child interactions: An interbehavioral model. *Psychological Bulletin, 105* (1), 116–130.

Watt, B. D., Hoyland, M., Best, D., & Dadds, M. D. (2007). Treatment participation among children with conduct problems and the role of telephone reminders. *Journal of Child Family Studies, 16*, 522–530.

Webster-Stratton, C., & Hammond, M. (1990). Predictors of treatment outcome in parent training for families with conduct problem children. *Behavior Therapy, 21* (3), 319–337

Webster-Stratton, C., & Hammond, M. (1998). Conduct problems and level of social competence in Head Start children: Prevalence, pervasiveness, and associated risk factors. *Clinical Child and Family Psychology Review, 1*(2), 101–124.

Wechsler, D. (2002). *Wechsler preschool and primary scale of intelligence – third edition.* San Antonio, TX: The Psychological Corporation.

Wechsler, D. (2003). *Wechsler intelligence scale for children – fourth edition.* San Antonio, TX: The Psychological Corporation.

Wechsler, D. (2008). *Wechsler individual achievement test – third edition.* San Antonio, TX: The Psychological Corporation.

Willemen, A. M., Koot, H. M., Ferdinand, R. F., Goossens, F. A., & Schuengel, C. (2008). Change in psychopathology in referred children: the role of life events and perceived stress. *Journal of Child Psychology and Psychiatry, 49* (11), 1175–1183.

Wolpe, J., & Lang, P. J. (1964). A fear survey schedule for use in behavior therapy. *Behavior Research and Therapy, 2*, 27–30.

Section II

Evidence-Based Treatments of Conduct Problems: An Applied Approach for Practitioners

5

The Incredible Years Program for Children from Infancy to Pre-adolescence: Prevention and Treatment of Behavior Problems

CAROLYN H. WEBSTER-STRATTON and M. JAMILA REID

OVERVIEW

The incidence of Oppositional Defiant Disorder (ODD) and Conduct Disorder (CD) in children is alarmingly high, with reported cases of early-onset conduct problems occurring in 4–6% of young children (Egger & Angold, 2006), and as high as 35% of young children in low-income families (Webster-Stratton & Hammond, 1998). Developmental theorists have suggested that "early starter" delinquents who first exhibit ODD symptoms in the preschool years have a twofold to threefold risk of becoming chronic juvenile offenders (Loeber et al., 1993; Patterson, Capaldi, & Bank, 1991) compared to typically developing children (Snyder, 2001). Children with early-onset CD also account for a disproportionate share of delinquent acts in adolescence and adulthood, including interpersonal violence, substance abuse, and property crimes. In fact, the primary developmental pathway for serious CDs in adolescence and adulthood appears to be established during the preschool period. Early onset conduct problems represent one of the most costly mental disorders to society because such a large proportion of

CAROLYN H. WEBSTER-STRATTON • University of Washington
M. JAMILA REID • University of Washington

R.C. Murrihy et al. (eds.), *Clinical Handbook of Assessing and Treating Conduct Problems in Youth*, DOI 10.1007/978-1-4419-6297-3_5,

antisocial children remain involved with mental health agencies or criminal justice systems throughout the course of their lives.

Risk factors from a number of different areas contribute to child conduct problems including ineffective parenting (e.g., harsh discipline, low parent involvement in school, and low monitoring) (Jaffee, Caspi, Moffitt, & Taylor, 2004); family risk factors (e.g., marital conflict and parental drug abuse, mental illness, and criminal behavior) (Knutson, DeGarmo, Koeppl, & Reid, 2005); child biological and developmental risk factors (e.g., attention deficit hyperactivity disorders [ADHD], learning disabilities, and language delays); school risk factors (e.g., poor teacher classroom management, high levels of classroom aggression, large class sizes, and poor school–home communication); and peer and community risk factors (e.g., poverty and gangs) (Collins, Maccoby, Steinberg, Hetherington, & Bornstein, 2000). Effective interventions for children with conduct problems ideally target multiple risk factors and are best offered as early as possible. Conduct disorder becomes increasingly resistant to change over time, so early intervention is a crucial strategy for the prevention or reduction of conduct problems, violence, substance abuse, and delinquency. Children with ODD and CD are clearly identifiable as early as 3–4 years of age, and there is evidence that the younger the child is at the time of intervention, the more positive the behavioral adjustment at home and at school following treatment. Intervention that is delivered prior to school entry and during the early school years can strategically target risk factors across multiple domains; home and school, and through multiple change agents; parent, teacher, and child. Unfortunately, less than 20% of young children meeting DSM-IV criteria for ODD are referred for mental health services (Horwitz, Leaf, Jeventhal, Forsyth, & Speechley, 1992). Even fewer of those referred obtain evidence-based interventions.

THE INCREDIBLE YEARS TREATMENT PROGRAMS

To address the parenting, family, child, and school risk factors for children or adolescents with conduct problems, we have developed three complementary training curricula, known as the Incredible Years (IY) Training Series, targeted at parents, teachers, and children (from birth to 12 years). This chapter reviews these training programs and their associated research findings.

Incredible Years Parent Interventions

Goals of the parent programs. Goals of the parent programs are: (a) to promote parent competencies and strengthen families by increasing positive parenting, parent–child bonding and attachment, and self-confidence about parenting; (b) to increase parents' ability to use play interactions to coach children's social–emotional, academic, verbal, and persistence skills; (c) to reduce critical and physically violent discipline and increase positive discipline strategies such as ignoring and redirecting, logical consequences, time-out, and problem solving; (d) to improve parental self-control, depression, anger management, communication skills, and problem solving; (e) to increase family support networks; and (f) to improve home–school bonding and increase parents' involvement in school-related activities so as to support their children's academic competence.

After more than 28 years of program development and evaluation, the IY parent treatment consists of a variety of comprehensive, empirically validated programs. Below we describe each of the well-researched parent programs and their targeted populations.

BASIC parent training treatment program. In 1980, we developed an interactive, video-based parent intervention program (BASIC) for parents of children ages 2–7 years. In subsequent years, we revised and updated this program to include three separate age range BASIC programs: the baby/toddler age (0–3 years), preschool (3–5 years), and school-age (6–13 years). Each of these revised programs include age appropriate examples of culturally diverse families, children with varying temperaments, and added emphases on social and emotional coaching, problem solving, how to set up predictable routines, and support children's academic success. The BASIC toddler parent training programs are completed in 12 weekly, 2 hour sessions while the preschool and school-age programs are 18–20 weekly, 2 hour sessions. The foundation of the program is brief video vignettes of modeled parenting skills (each program has over 300 vignettes) shown by a therapist to groups of 8–12 parents. The videos demonstrate social learning and child development principles and serve as the stimulus for focused discussions, problem solving, and collaborative learning. The program is also designed to help parents understand normal variations in children's development, emotional reactions, and temperaments.

The BASIC program begins with a focus on enhancing positive relationships between parents and children by teaching parents to use child-directed interactive play, academic and persistence coaching, social and emotional coaching, praise, and incentive programs. Next, parents learn how to set up predicable home routines and rules, followed by learning a specific set of nonviolent discipline techniques including monitoring, ignoring, commands, natural and logical consequences, and ways to use time-out to teach children to calm down. Finally, parents are taught how they can teach their children problem-solving and self-regulation skills.

ADVANCE parent training treatment program. In 1989, we expanded our theoretical and causal model concerning conduct problems and developed the ADVANCE treatment program (updated in 2008). This program was designed to be offered after parents complete the BASIC parenting program and focuses on helping parents with adult intra- and interpersonal skills. The content of this 10–12-session video program (over 90 vignettes) consists of five components: (a) personal self-control, anger management, positive self-talk, and other coping strategies; (b) communication skills for talking effectively with partners, teachers, and other adults; (c) problem-solving conflict situations with partners, extended family members, teachers, and employers; (d) problem solving with children and conducting family meetings; and (e) strengthening social support and self care. We theorized that a broader-based training model would help mediate the negative influences of these personal and interpersonal factors on parenting skills and promote increased maintenance and generalizability of treatment effects.

The content of both the BASIC and ADVANCE programs is also provided in the recently revised text that parents use for the program, titled *The Incredible Years: A Troubleshooting Guide for Parents* (Webster-Stratton, 2006)

SCHOOL parent training treatment. More than 50% of parents who completed our parent training programs requested guidance on issues surrounding homework, communication with teachers, behavior problems at school, and promoting their children's academic and social skills. In addition, 40% of teachers reported problems with children's compliance and aggression in the classroom and requested advice on how to manage these problems. Clearly, integrating interventions across settings (home and school) and agents (teachers and parents) to target school and family risk factors fosters greater between-environment consistency and offers the best chance for long-term reduction of antisocial behavior.

In 1990, we developed an academic skills training intervention (SCHOOL) as an adjunct to our school-age BASIC program, and in 2003, a school readiness intervention as an adjunct to our preschool BASIC program. These two interventions each consist of four to six additional sessions usually offered to parents after the BASIC program is completed. For parents of school-age children, these sessions focus on collaboration with teachers, ways to foster children's academic readiness and school success through parental involvement in school activities and homework, and the importance of after-school and peer monitoring. For the parents of preschool children, the sessions focus on interactive reading skills and ways to promote children's social, emotional, self-regulation, and cognitive skills. Program components include teaching parents to: (a) help children feel confident in their own ideas and ability to learn; (b) prepare children for school by facilitating pre-reading skills (pre-school) and supporting/encouraging older children with homework routines and limits on "screen time"; (c) support children's discouragement and learning difficulties by setting realistic goals, encouraging their persistence with difficult tasks, and using academic coaching to motivate and reinforce learning progress at home; and (d) collaborate with teachers to jointly develop plans that address behavioral issues at school.

Incredible Years Teacher Training Intervention

When children with behavior problems enter school, negative academic and social experiences escalate the development of conduct problems. Aggressive, disruptive children quickly become socially excluded, and peers begin to respond to aggressive children in ways that increase the likelihood of reactive aggression. This peer rejection leads to association with deviant peers, which increases the risk for higher levels of antisocial behavior. In addition, teacher behaviors (low rates of praise, high rates of critical/harsh discipline, ineffective management strategies, low emphasis on teaching social–emotional competence) and classroom/school characteristics (high student–teacher ratio, no tolerance school discipline policies, high classroom levels of children with special needs) are associated with increased aggression, delinquency, and poor academic performance. Rejecting and non-supportive responses from teachers further exacerbate the problems of aggressive children.

In 1995 (revised 2003), we developed a 6-day (42 h) teacher-training program with the goal of promoting teacher competencies and strengthening home–school connections by doing the following: (a) improving teachers' classroom management skills, including proactive teaching approaches and effective discipline; (b) increasing teachers' use of academic, persistence, social, and emotional coaching with students; (c) strengthening teacher–student bonding; (d) improving home–school collaboration and parent–teacher bonding; and (e) increasing teachers' ability to teach social skills, anger management, and problem-solving skills in the classroom. A complete description of the content included in this curriculum is described in the book that teachers use for the course, titled *How to Promote Social and Emotional Competence* (Webster-Stratton, 2000).

Incredible Years Child Training Intervention (Dinosaur School)

Research has indicated that children with conduct problems are more likely to have certain temperamental characteristics such as inattentiveness, distractibility, impulsivity, and ADHD. Other child factors have also been implicated in early-onset CD. For example, deficits in social–cognitive skills and negative attributions contribute to poor emotional regulation and aggressive peer interactions. In addition, studies indicate that children with conduct problems have significant delays in their peer-play skills – in particular, difficulty with reciprocal play, cooperative skills, taking turns, waiting, and giving suggestions (Gottman, 1983; Webster-Stratton & Lindsay, 1999). Finally, reading, learning, and language delays are also associated with conduct problems, particularly for "early life course persisters" (Moffitt & Lynam, 1994). Academic difficulties and behavior problems exacerbate one another in a bidirectional spiral whereby academic problems lead to disengagement, increased frustration, and lower self-esteem, which contribute to the child's behavior problems. At the same time, negative classroom behavior limits a child's ability to be engaged in learning, to follow teacher's instructions, and to achieve academically. Thus, a cycle is created in which one problem exacerbates the other. This combination of academic delays and conduct problems contributes to the development of more severe CD and school failure.

In 1990, we developed a child treatment program to directly focus on the social learning and academic deficits of children diagnosed with ODD or conduct problems (ages 4–8). This 22-week program (revised 2006) consists of a series of DVD programs (over 180 vignettes) that teach children problem solving and social skills. Organized to dovetail with the content of the parent-training program, the program consists of seven main topic areas: Introduction and Rules; Empathy and Emotion; Problem Solving; Anger Control; Friendship Skills; Communication Skills; and School Skills.

The children meet weekly in groups of six children for 2 h. To enhance generalization, the video vignettes involve real-life conflict situations at home and at school (playground and classroom), such as teasing, being rejected, and destructive behavior. The goals of this program are to promote children's competencies and reduce aggressive and noncompliant behaviors by doing the following: (a) strengthening social skills (turn taking, waiting, asking, sharing, helping, and complimenting); (b) promoting use of self-control and self-regulation strategies; (c) increasing emotional awareness by labeling feelings, recognizing the differing views of oneself and others, and enhancing perspective taking; (d) promoting children's ability to persist with difficult tasks; (e) improving academic success, reading, and school readiness; (f) reducing defiance, aggression, peer rejection, bullying, stealing, lying, and promoting compliance with teachers and peers; (g) decreasing negative cognitive attributions and conflict management approaches; and (h) increasing self-esteem and self-confidence.

Group Process and Methods Used in Parent, Teacher, and Child Training Programs

All three treatment approaches rely on performance training methods and group support training including video modeling, role play, practice activities, and live feedback from the therapist and other group members. In accordance with modeling and self-efficacy theories of learning, parents, teachers, and children participating in the program develop their skills by watching video examples of key skills, discussing and sharing their reactions to the videos, and then modeling or role playing skills themselves. Video examples provide a more flexible method of group training than didactic verbal instruction or sole reliance on role play because a wide variety of models, settings, and situations can be used as examples. The goals of this approach are to provide better generalization of the content and, therefore, better long-term maintenance; to provide a variety of learning methods – visual, verbal, and performance; to be low-cost because of the group format; and easily disseminated because of the extensive videos and manuals.

The video vignettes show parents, teachers, and children of differing ages, cultures, socioeconomic backgrounds, temperaments and developmental abilities, so that participants will perceive at least some of the models as similar to themselves and will therefore accept the vignettes as relevant. Vignettes show models (unrehearsed) in natural situations responding effectively as well as times when they are responding less effectively in order to demystify the notion that there is "perfect parenting or teaching" and to illustrate how one can learn from one's mistakes. This approach also emphasizes our belief in a coping and collaborative interactive model of learning (Webster-Stratton & Herbert, 1994); that is, participants' view a video vignette of a situation and then discuss and role play how the individual might have handled the interaction more effectively. Thus participants improve upon the interactions they see in the vignettes. This approach enhances participants' confidence and develops their ability to analyze interpersonal situations and select an appropriate response. In this respect, our training differs from some training programs where the therapist provides the analysis and recommends a particular strategy.

The video vignettes demonstrate behavioral principles and serve as the stimulus for focused discussions, problem solving, and collaborative learning. After each vignette, the therapist solicits ideas from group members and involves them in the process of problem solving, sharing, and discussing ideas and reactions. The therapists' role is to support and empower group members by teaching, leading, reframing, predicting, identifying key developmental or teaching principles, and role playing (Webster-Stratton & Hancock, 1998). The collaborative context is designed to ensure that the intervention is sensitive to individual cultural differences and personal values. The program is "tailored" to each teacher, parent, or child's individual needs and personal goals as well as to each child's personality and behavior problems.

This program also emphasizes a commitment to group members' self-management. We believe that this approach empowers participants in that it gives back dignity, respect, and self-control to parents, teachers, and children who are often seeking help at time of low self-confidence and intense feelings of guilt and self-blame (Webster-Stratton, 1996). By using group process, the program not only is more cost-effective but also addresses an important risk factor for children with conduct problems; the family's isolation and stigmatization. Parent groups provide that support and become a model for parent support networks (see Webster-Stratton & Herbert, 1994.) The child groups provide children with conduct problems some of their first positive social experiences with other children. Moreover, it was theorized that the group approach would provide more social and emotional support and decrease feelings of isolation for teachers as well as parents and children.

As with the teacher and parent programs, the child treatment program uses video modeling examples in every session to foster discussion, problem solving, and modeling of prosocial behaviors. The scenes selected for each of the units involve real-life conflict situations at home and at school (playground and classroom). The videotapes show children of differing ages, sexes, and cultures interacting with adults or with other children. After viewing, the vignettes, children discuss feelings, generate ideas for more effective responses, and role play alternative scenarios. In addition to the interactive video vignettes, the therapists use life-size puppets to model appropriate behavior and thinking processes for the children. The use of puppets appeals to children on the fantasy level so predominant in this preoperational age group. Because young children are more vulnerable to distraction, are less able to organize their thoughts, and have poorer memories, we use a number of strategies for reviewing and organizing the material, such as: (a) playing "copy cat" to review skills learned; (b) using many video examples of the same concept in different situations and settings; (c) using cartoon pictures and specially designed stickers as "cues" to remind children of key concepts; (d) role playing with puppets and other children to provide practice opportunities and experience with different perspectives; (e) reenacting video scenes; (f) rehearsing skills with play, art, and game activities; (g) homework, so children can practice key skills with parents; and (h) letters to parents and teachers that explain the program's key concepts and asking them to reinforce these behaviors.

EVIDENCE FOR THE EFFECTS OF TREATMENT

Effects of Parent Training Program

The efficacy of the IY BASIC parent treatment program for children (ages 3–8 years) diagnosed with ODD/CD has been demonstrated in six published randomized control group trials by the program developer and colleagues at the University of Washington Parenting Clinic (Reid, Webster-Stratton, & Hammond, 2007; Webster-Stratton, 1981; Webster-Stratton, 1982, 1984, 1990a, 1992, 1994, 1998; Webster-Stratton & Hammond, 1997; Webster-Stratton, Hollinsworth, & Kolpacoff, 1989; Webster-Stratton, Kolpacoff, & Hollinsworth, 1988; Webster-Stratton, Reid, & Hammond, 2004). In all of these studies, the BASIC program has been shown to significantly improve parental attitudes and parent–child interactions, and significantly reduce harsh discipline, and child conduct problems compared to wait-list control groups and other treatment approaches. In the third of these studies, treatment component analyses indicated that the combination of group discussion, a trained therapist, and video modeling produced the most lasting results in comparison to treatment that involved only one training component (see Webster-Stratton, Hollinsworth, & Kolpacoff, 1989, and Webster-Stratton, Kolpacoff, & Hollinsworth, 1988).

In addition, the BASIC program has been replicated in five projects by independent investigators in mental health clinics with families of children diagnosed with conduct problems (Drugli & Larsson, 2006; Larsson et al., 2008; Lavigne et al., 2008; Scott, Spender, Doolan, Jacobs, & Aspland, 2001; Spaccarelli, Cotler, & Penman, 1992; Taylor, Schmidt, Pepler, & Hodgins, 1998). These replications were "effectiveness" trials; that is, they were done in applied mental health settings, not a university research clinic, and the therapists were typical therapists at the centers not research therapists. Three of the above replications were conducted in the United States, two in United Kingdom, and one in Norway. This illustrates the transportability of the BASIC parenting program to other cultures.

In our fourth study, we examined the effects of adding the ADVANCE intervention (parent intra- and interpersonal skills) component to the BASIC intervention (Webster-Stratton, 1994) by randomly assigning families to either BASIC parent training or BASIC + ADVANCE training. Both treatment groups showed significant improvements in child adjustment and parent–child interactions and a decrease in parent distress and child behavior problems. These changes were maintained at follow-up. ADVANCE children showed significant increases in the number of prosocial solutions generated during problem solving, in comparison to children whose parents received only the BASIC program. Observations of parents' marital interactions indicated significant improvements in ADVANCE parents' communication, problem-solving, and collaboration skills when compared with parents who did not receive ADVANCE. Moreover, ADVANCE parents reported significantly greater consumer satisfaction than parents who did not receive ADVANCE. These results suggest that focusing on helping parents to manage personal distress and interpersonal issues through a video modeling group discussion treatment (ADVANCE) added significantly to treatment outcomes for our BASIC program. Consequently, a 20–24-week program that combines BASIC with ADVANCE has become our core treatment for parents with children with conduct problems.

In our sixth and seventh studies respectively, we examined the additive effects of combining the child training intervention (Dinosaur School) and teacher training with the parent training program (BASIC + ADVANCE). Both studies replicated positive results from the ADVANCE study and provided data on the advantages of training children and teachers as well as parents. (Study results are presented below, see section on Effects of Teacher- and Child-Training Treatment and Prevention Programs.)

Parent training treatment: Who benefits and who does not? We have followed families longitudinally (1, 2, and 3 years post treatment), and have completed a 10–15-year follow-up of the children and their families. We assessed both the statistical and clinical significance of treatment effects. In assessing clinical significance, we looked at the extent to which parent or teacher reports indicated that the children were within the nonclinical range of functioning or showed a 30% improvement if there were no established normative data, and whether families requested further therapy for their children's behavior problems at the follow-up assessments. These outcome criteria were chosen to avoid reliance on a single informant or criterion measure, thereby providing greater validity to the findings. In our 3-year follow-up of 83 families treated with the BASIC program, we found that while approximately two-thirds of children showed clinically significant behavior improvements, 25–26% of parents and 26% of teachers still reported clinically significant child behavior problems (Webster-Stratton, 1990b). We also found that the families whose children had continuing externalizing problems (according to teacher and parent reports) at our 3-year follow-up assessments were more likely to be characterized by marital distress or single-parent status, maternal depression, lower social class, high levels of negative life stressors, and family histories of alcoholism, drug abuse, and spouse abuse (Webster-Stratton, 1990b; Webster-Stratton & Hammond, 1990).

Hartman (Hartman, Stage, & Webster-Stratton, 2003) examined whether child ADHD symptoms (i.e., inattention, impulsivity, and hyperactivity) predicted poorer treatment results from the parent-training intervention. Contrary to Hartman's hypothesis, analyses suggested that the children with ODD/CD who had higher levels of attention problems showed *greater* reductions in conduct problems than children without attention problems. Similar findings for children with ADHD were reported in the UK study (Scott et al., 2001). An ongoing study is evaluating the parent and child treatments with young children whose primary diagnosis is ADHD.

Webster-Stratton et al. (in press) conducted an 8- to 12-year follow-up of families who were in the ADVANCE study previously discussed. She interviewed 83.5% of the parents and adolescents from the original study (now 12–19 years of age). Results indicated that over 75% of the teenagers were typically adjusted with minimal behavioral and emotional problems. Furthermore, parenting skills taught in the intervention had lasting effects. Important predictors of long-term outcome were mothers' post-treatment level of critical statements and fathers' use of praise. In addition, the level of mother–child coercion immediately post treatment was a significant predictor of teen adjustment.

Evidence for Effects of Parent Programs as Prevention

In the past decade, we have also evaluated the parent programs as a selective prevention program with multiethnic, socioeconomically disadvantaged families in two randomized studies; one with low income Head Start families and another with unselected primary school children. Results of all these studies suggest the program's effectiveness as a method of preventing the development of conduct problems and strengthening social competence in preschool children (Reid, Webster-Stratton, & Hammond, 2007; Webster-Stratton, 1998; Webster-Stratton, Reid, & Hammond, 2001). These studies also showed that programs were equally effective for families from diverse cultural and ethnic backgrounds including Latino, Asian, and African American families. (Reid, Webster-Stratton, & Beauchaine, 2001). The study with primary school children evaluated the effects of the parent intervention with an indicated, culturally diverse population. Children who received the intervention showed fewer externalizing problems, better emotion regulation, and stronger parent–child bonding than control children. Mothers in the intervention group showed more supportive and less coercive parenting than control mothers (Reid, Webster-Stratton, & Hammond, 2007). Similar results were reported by independent investigators with selective and indicated prevention populations including a study conducted in the United Kingdom (Gardner, Burton, & Klimes, 2006; Gross et al., 2003; Hutchings & Gardner, 2006; Miller Brotman et al., 2003). One study reported the effectiveness of the IY parent program with foster parents (Linares, Montalto, MinMin, & Oza, 2006).

Summary and significance. Over the past 28 years, studies have shown that parent training is a highly effective therapeutic method for producing significant behavior change in children with conduct problems and with high-risk populations (i.e., socioeconomically disadvantaged). These findings provide support for the notion that parenting practices play a key role in children's social and emotional development.

Effects of Teacher- and Child-Training Treatment and Prevention Programs

To date, there have been two randomized studies by the developer and one by an independent evaluator evaluating the effectiveness of the child-training program for reducing conduct problems and promoting social competence in children diagnosed with ODD/CD. In the first two studies (Drugli & Larsson, 2006; Webster-Stratton & Hammond, 1997), clinic-referred children (with ODD) and their parents were randomly assigned to one of four groups: a parent-training treatment group (PT), a child-training group (CT), a child- and parent-training group (CT + PT), or a waiting-list control group (CON). Post-treatment assessments indicated that all three treatment conditions resulted in significant improvements in parent and child behaviors in comparison to controls. Comparisons of the three treatment conditions indicated that CT and CT + PT children showed significant improvements in problem solving as well as conflict management skills, as measured by observations of child interactions with a best friend; differences among treatment conditions on these measures consistently favored the CT conditions over the PT only condition. On measures of parent and child behavior at home, PT and CT+ PT parents and children had significantly more positive interactions in comparison to CT parents and children.

One-year follow-up assessments indicated that all the significant changes noted immediately post treatment were maintained over time. Moreover, child conduct problems at home significantly decreased over time. Analyses of the clinical significance of the results suggested that the combined CT + PT condition produced the most significant improvements in child behavior at 1-year follow-up. However, children from all three treatment conditions showed increases in behavior problems at school 1 year later, as measured by teacher reports (Webster-Stratton & Hammond, 1997).

Another study (Webster-Stratton, Reid, & Hammond, 2004) tested the effects of different combinations of parent, child, and teacher training. Families with a child diagnosed with ODD were randomly assigned to one of six groups: (a) Parent training only; (b) Child training only; (c) Parent training and teacher training; (d) Parent training, teacher training, and child training; (e) Child training and teacher training; or (f) Waitlist control.

As expected, results for the parent training component replicated earlier studies with parents in all three conditions that received parent training showing significantly less negative and more positive parenting than parents in conditions that did not receive training (Webster-Stratton & Reid, 1999). Children in all five treatment conditions showed reductions in aggressive behaviors with mothers at home, and at school with peers and teachers, compared with controls. Treatment effects for children's positive social skills with peers were found only in the three conditions with child training compared with controls. Trained teachers were rated as less critical, harsh, and inconsistent, and more nurturing than control teachers. Most treatment effects were maintained at 1-year follow-up. In summary, this study replicated our previous findings on the effectiveness of the parent- and child-training programs and indicated that teacher training significantly improves teachers' classroom management skills and improves children's classroom aggressive behavior. In addition, treatment combinations that added either child training or teacher training to the parent training were most effective.

Three other randomized control group studies (Raver et al., 2007; Webster-Stratton, Reid, & Hammond, 2001; Williford & Shelton, 2008) have evaluated the teacher-training curriculum in a prevention setting with Head Start teachers. In the study by the developer, parent–teacher bonding was reported to be significantly higher for experimental than for control mothers. Experimental children showed significantly fewer conduct problems at school than control children, and trained teachers showed significantly better classroom management skills than control teachers. In the second study by an independent investigator (Raver et al., 2007) 5 days of the IY Teacher Program were delivered to teachers in combination with weekly visits by mental health consultants who "coached" teachers as they implemented management strategies. Results showed that Head Start classrooms in the treatment condition had significantly higher levels of positive classroom climate, teacher sensitivity and behavior management than classrooms in the control condition with medium to high effect sizes.

Lastly, a recent study (Webster-Stratton, Reid, & Stoolmiller, 2008) was completed using the teacher training and classroom Dinosaur curriculum in Head Start and with primary schools that serve high numbers of economically disadvantaged children. Results showed significant improvements in conduct problems, self-regulation, and social competence compared with control students. Effect size was particularly high for children with high baseline levels of conduct problems. Another prevention study using the curriculum in schools reported reductions in playground aggressive behavior compared to control schools (Barrera et al., 2002).

Who benefits from Dinosaur child training? Analyses on 99 children diagnosed with ODD who received child treatment were conducted to examine the effects of child hyperactivity, parenting style, and family stress on treatment outcome. The hyperactivity or family stress risk factors did not have an impact on children's treatment response. Negative parenting, on the other hand, did negatively impact children's treatment outcome. Fewer children who had parents with one of the negative parenting risk factors (high levels of criticism or physical spanking) showed clinically significant improvements compared to children who did not have one of the negative parenting risk factors. This finding suggests that for children whose parents exhibit harsh and coercive parenting styles, it is important to offer a parenting intervention in addition to a child intervention (Webster-Stratton, Reid, & Hammond, 2001). Our studies also suggest that child training significantly enhances the effectiveness of parent training treatment for children with pervasive conduct problems (home and school settings) because of its added benefits for children's classroom peer interactions and social competence.

CASE EXAMPLE: STEWART

The following section presents a case in which the IY Parent, Teacher, and Child Training Programs were used to treat a young boy, Stewart. Stewart is a 6-year-old who presented with ODD and ADHD. His problems occurred at home, at school, and with peers. This case study outlines how the three different IY Programs (parent, teacher, and child) can be applied flexibly and synergistically to attend to individual family needs and address issues of comorbidity.

INTAKE INFORMATION

Susan and Tim Jones were referred to the Parenting Clinic by their school psychologist because of difficulties at home and at school with their 6-year-old son, Stewart. Stewart had a substantial reputation at the school for his aggressive and oppositional behavior. At the time that the Joneses came to the clinic, his teacher had told his parents that she did not believe her classroom was an appropriate place for Stewart. In addition to these problems at school, Stewart's behavior at home was extremely volatile. He would frequently "lose control of his behavior" and engage in extended temper tantrums during which he would call his parents names, refuse to comply with any requests, and become aggressive or destructive. Both parents described feeling helpless to change Stewart's behavior once it reached these proportions. Their usual parenting style was to talk and reason with Stewart, but they felt that this merely escalated his behavior. They also had tried a number of different discipline strategies (e.g., time-out, loss of privileges), that did not seem to work to change Stewart's behavior. Susan and Tim were also concerned about the effect that his difficulties were having on his self-esteem. Stewart had begun talking about the fact that no one liked him at school, that he had no friends, and that he was the dumbest kid in his class. Lastly, Susan and Tim reported that Stewart's behaviors were putting a significant strain on the family's functioning. Both felt his problems were their main focus, to the exclusion of other activities and interests. They felt that they no longer had control over their family and were worried that Stewart's behavior was on an irreversible trajectory.

TREATMENT

Treatment began in October, following the assessment period. Stewart and his parents came to the University of Washington Parenting Clinic each week for a 2 h group that lasted 24 weeks. During that time, Stewart attended the child group with five other children (three boys and two girls, ages 4–7), and his parents attended the parenting group.

Parent group. During the initial group, parents described their children and their reasons for coming to the clinic. Many of the parents, and Susan, in particular, described how isolated she felt as a parent of a "problem child." She felt that they could no longer socialize with their friends because Stewart was not able to behave appropriately. She felt judged by other parents and felt that she was a bad parent because nothing she did worked with Stewart. Tim expressed a sense of relief at being in a group where he was free to talk about his son's issues without judgment from other parents. Susan and Tim expressed goals for Stewart primarily in terms of his happiness and self-esteem, although they believed that to achieve these goals, they would need to find ways to reduce his oppositional behavior, improve his social skills, and increase his cooperation with authority.

The first four to five sessions of the group were focused on child-directed play interactions. Since almost all adult–child interactions with Stewart involved a power struggle, and since his negative behaviors had placed such great strain on the parent–child relationship, the first goal of therapy was to use child-directed play to begin to change the dynamic of this relationship. Tim and Susan were encouraged to play with Stewart on a daily basis where their job was to follow Stewart's lead, be an "appreciative audience," and not to make demands, give instructions or even ask questions as long as he was appropriate in his behavior. These play sessions were designed to give Stewart some power in the relationship in an appropriate setting, to show him that his parents valued him, and to give his parents a time when they could just enjoy his creativity and playfulness without feeling as if they had to make him behave in a certain way. At first, Tim and Susan reported that he rejected their attempts to play with him. They were encouraged to be persistent and to make regular attempts each day to engage with him in this positive way. Gradually Stewart began to look forward to this time playing with his parents and seemed excited that they were willing to play on his terms. Although much of Stewart's behavior outside of the play sessions continued to be negative and challenging, Stewart's parents reported that he seemed calmer after play sessions, and that they had moments of feeling connected and appreciative of his strengths. They gradually also began to address some of Stewart's ADHD behaviors during these play sessions by using focused persistence coaching to comment when they saw Stewart being persistent, calm, or patient with an activity. For example, they learned to say such things as, "You are really concentrating and working hard on that puzzle, you just keep trying and are going to figure it out."

As these play sessions became more enjoyable, parents were taught to use social and emotion coaching with him one-on-one. This coaching helped him to develop emotional literacy, to express his feelings rather than to strike out at someone when frustrated. He also was helped to use social skills by coaching him when he was sharing, waiting, helping, and taking turns.

The ignoring and limit setting units were challenging for Tim and Susan. Both were used to reasoning with Stewart when he was misbehaving. They understood the principle of ignoring when Stewart was annoying or verbally abusive; however, they had difficultly following through. Stewart was very persistent with his whining and tantrums, and both parents needed support and encouragement to stick to their discipline plans. Stewart frequently swore and called his parents names, which they found difficult to ignore. When they did ignore, he would also cry and yell that they didn't love him and would then become very destructive. Strategies to help Tim and Susan involved teaching them to use calming self-talk (e.g., " I can stay calm, I can handle this") and reframing strategies (e.g., "He will feel safer when he learns there are predictable limits"). They had tried using time-out but had always given up part way through the process because of Stewart's aggressive and destructive behavior. Group problem solving helped them to plan ways to keep Stewart and the house safe during a destructive time-out. All of these solutions were role played with the group so that Tim and Susan felt equipped to try them out at home and prepared for his oppositional responses. With this support, they managed to successfully complete several lengthy time-out sequences with Stewart. There was a marked shift in their self-confidence after this point. Although Stewart continued to have very difficult days, they felt more equipped to handle his behavior at home. They also noticed that the frequency of these very intense tantrums decreased markedly.

The adult communication and problem-solving material was also useful to Tim and Susan. They had a strong relationship; however, their focus on Stewart was so all-consuming and so reactive that they rarely spent time communicating about their plan for working together to manage his behavior. Consequently, they sometimes had difficulty backing each other up because they hadn't agreed in advance about how to handle a problem. The communication and problem-solving sections of the curriculum helped them to set aside time to make proactive plans for managing family issues, as well as helping them realize that they also needed some time for themselves to reconnect on adult issues.

Working with the school and teacher training. Although Susan and Tim grasped the concepts in the parenting group and worked hard to implement new strategies at home, they were experiencing significant conflict with the school. Even after Stewart's behavior began to improve at home, it continued to worsen at school. His teacher repeatedly requested that he be removed from her classroom, and Stewart was so unhappy at school that it became a battle to get him to school in the mornings. Susan and Tim received daily negative reports about Tim's behavior. Tim, Susan, and Stewart's teacher and principal were all frustrated, and the parent–school relationship had become quite adversarial. Tim and Susan reported that whenever they met with the principal and the teachers, they felt personally attacked, and felt responsible for defending Stewart, even though they agreed that his behavior had been unacceptable.

Although Stewart's teacher was not happy about having him in her class, she did agree to attend 4 days of teacher training at the clinic. This training gave her a chance to express her frustration with the classroom situation and to share ideas with other teachers who also had challenging students. She reported that she had a class of 25 children, five of whom had special needs. Stewart's behavior was the most severe, and, in her opinion, he frequently set off her other challenging children so that she felt unable to manage the situation. Through a series of parent–teacher conferences, a meeting with the principal, and support from other teachers during the teacher training as well as help from the therapists, things slowly began to improve. Stewart's parents, teacher, and the IY therapists worked collaboratively to set up a simple behavior plan for Stewart in the classroom. This plan focused on a few positive behavioral goals with frequent reinforcement, a wiggle space for times when Stewart was having difficulty sitting still, and a back-up time-out plan for severe negative behavior. Stewart was able to earn breaks for successfully completing manageable parts of his school work. He was also given sanctioned reasons to move around the classroom since it was difficult for him to sit still for long periods of time. Peer issues were also addressed. His teacher made a concerted effort to highlight Stewart's strengths to the class. As part of his behavior plan, he was able to earn chances to assist other children (an activity that had proven to be very reinforcing to him in our child Dinosaur group at the clinic). On the playground, Stewart was initially limited to activities in a smaller, well-supervised area, and through appropriate behavior was able to earn the privilege of expanded recess. Lastly, Stewart was also referred for a special education evaluation, which eventually led to a part-time classroom assistant who was able to relieve some of the pressure on his teacher.

Child dinosaur social skills and problem solving group. Stewart was initially resistant to the idea of coming to the child groups. His negative experience with school made him extremely reluctant to participate in any activity that seemed remotely like school. During the first few sessions, the therapists had the puppets model that they, too, had been scared or mad when they first came to Dinosaur school, but that they soon started to like the group and had made good friends. After this initial processing, the therapists ignored Stewart's complaints about being in the group and instead focused on praising and giving tokens for any appropriate behavior that he exhibited. They noticed that while he was reluctant to volunteer answers or participate on his own, if he was asked to help another child with an answer or a project, he quickly became involved. Initially Stewart sought attention from the other children in the group by being disruptive and inappropriate. The other children were taught to ignore this inappropriate behavior. Stewart was also put in charge of helping to monitor other children's friendly and positive behavior. This provided him with an opportunity to receive attention and positive approval from others. After four sessions, Stewart began to report to his parents that he liked Dinosaur school. Two of the other boys in the group became friends with Stewart, and they began to have some play dates after school. From this point on, Stewart was consistently positive about coming to the group, and his parents reported that he seemed happy about a group peer activity for the first time in his life.

A second issue for Stewart during the child groups was difficulty sitting and attending for more than a few minutes at a time. The therapists arranged the format of the group such that children had frequent opportunities to change activities and move around. After showing the children a video vignette, therapists would lead a brief discussion with the puppet and then have children role play the situation. They continually interspersed sedentary activities with more active rehearsal and "hands-on" learning. Stewart was reinforced for attentive behavior, but the therapist also ignored considerable wiggling and movements, if he was engaged in the lesson. Stewart was also allowed to leave the group and go to a "wiggle space" if he was unable to sit still. As long as the activities changed frequently and the therapists monitored Stewart's attention level and need to move around, they were able to keep him engaged and on-task.

Social, persistence, and emotion coaching were also an important part of Stewart's treatment plan. In order to gradually increase Stewart's ability to focus and concentrate on a given activity, therapists worked hard to identify times when Stewart was focused, calm, working hard, working carefully, and sticking with an activity. They noticed that Stewart's attention span was immediately longer whenever descriptive commenting was used, most likely because he enjoyed the attention and wanted it to continue. This provided many opportunities to comment on his persistence. Since Stewart was also easily dysregulated and quick to get angry, attention was given to times when he was calm, regulated, and content. When Stewart started to become angry, his feelings were labeled, and then the therapist predicted that he would be able to stay calm and try again (if he tantrumed, he was ignored.) Stewart's social behaviors were also encouraged through a combination of descriptive commenting, modeling, and coaching. If Stewart spontaneously engaged in a friendly behavior, the therapists' labeled that behavior: e.g., "Wow, Stewart, you just asked for that block in a friendly voice." At times, they also modeled a behavior themselves (or used a puppet to model the behavior). "Stewart, I've got an extra train car. I would like to share it with you." They also provided direct coaching to Stewart when they saw he wanted something but was not expressing himself. "Stewart, it looks like you're frustrated that you don't have more train track. Can you ask Dylan if he will let you use some more pieces?"

Summary of treatment. Stewart's behavior improved at home as Susan and Tim begin to use more effective limit setting, combined with frequent positive interactions and coaching his social behaviors. There continued to be explosive incidents throughout the treatment period, but they became less frequent, and Susan and Tim became confident in their ability to handle the problems. The Dinosaur child group quickly became a reinforcing activity for Stewart, and he made some of his first friends in the group and was proud of these interactions. This was in sharp contrast to his negative feelings about peers and school. He also learned specific social and problem-solving skills that he began to use with peers in social situations. School changes were most difficult, but parents, teachers, and therapists all worked hard to continue to implement new strategies there. Stewart's difficult behavior and explosive episodes at school continued, but were reported to be less frequent and less intense. In addition, the school and the teacher began to feel equipped to handle the behaviors and they worked collaboratively with Stewart's parents to set goals and modify his behavior plan as needed.

NEW PROGRAMS

In recent years, the IY parent programs (BASIC) have been extended to include new programs for older children (8–13 years) as well as infants (0–12 months) and toddlers (1–3 years). Current studies are in progress to evaluate the effectiveness of these programs. The intervention model for these two programs is similar to all of our other programs and includes video vignettes of families and their young children. Below is a summary of the content for each program.

BABY-TODDLER program. The new BABY-TODDLER curriculum is split into two programs. The first program covers the baby 0–12 months of age and can be completed in 8–10 sessions (the toddler program is delivered in 18 sessions and is described above). The content of the Baby Program includes: (a) getting to know your baby; (b) parents as responsive communicators and babies as intelligent language learners; (c) providing physical and visual stimulation for your baby; (d) learning to read babies' minds; (e) gaining support; and (f) the emerging sense of self. Parents attend these groups with their babies and participate in hands-on role plays and exercises with their own babies. Pilot groups are currently being run in Seattle with parents referred by the child welfare system and in Wales with low-income families. Preliminary clinical reports show that these groups are well evaluated by parents; attendance and satisfaction ratings have been very high in both pilot programs.

SCHOOL-AGED program. The new SCHOOL-AGED curriculum for 8–13 year olds consists of 16–18 sessions. New vignettes for this age group include: (a) special time and projects; (b) social, emotional and persistence coaching; (c) encouraging home responsibilities; (d) rules and discussions regarding computer and TV use, and drugs and alcohol; (e) following through with rules; (f) selective ignoring and avoiding arguments; and (g) imposing consequences. The first 12 weeks focus on social and emotional skills and home behavior followed by four sessions in which parents learn how to encourage and support their child's academic competence. This includes promoting reading habits, helping children with homework assignments, fostering good learning habits and routines, and working with schools. It is highly recommended that the ADVANCE program with its focus on problem solving and family meetings is also delivered in conjunction with the BASIC program, especially when working with parents of antisocial children. Over the past year, this program has been evaluated in England with severely antisocial children ages 9–13 years. Preliminary results show high parent evaluations by parents as well as high program attendance.

DIRECTIONS FOR FUTURE RESEARCH

Although our programs were first designed and evaluated to be used as clinic-based treatments for diagnosed children and their parents and teachers, our more recent evaluations have shown the programs to be equally effective in preventive settings with high-risk families and children. This prevention model has allowed us to research our intervention with families who might not seek or receive mental health services in traditional clinic settings, and also with at-risk children before their behaviors have reached clinical levels.

As more is known about the type, timing, and dosage of interventions needed to prevent and treat children's conduct problems, we can further target children and families to offer treatment and support at strategic points. By providing a continuum of services we believe we will be able to prevent the further development of CDs, delinquency, and violence. For example, the prevention versions of the classroom social skills intervention, parent training, and/or teacher training might be offered as universal prevention to all children in a school. Children who continue to exhibit significant behavior problems might be offered the treatment versions of the programs. For those children requiring additional treatment, more research is needed to understand what constellation of treatments (parent, teacher, child) would best fit their particular needs.

Ongoing research is evaluating the IY programs with new populations including neglectful and abusive families referred by Child Protective Services, children with ADHD, and families from many different countries around the world including Russia, Turkey, Australia, Holland, and Scandinavia.

SUMMARY AND CONCLUSIONS

In summary, a review of our research suggests that interactive video training methods are effective treatments for early-onset ODD/CD. Our most effective parent intervention includes both parenting skills and training in marital communication, problem solving and conflict resolution, and ways to foster children's academic and social emotional competence. These findings document the need for interventions that strengthen families' protective factors (specifically, parents' interpersonal skills and coping skills) so that they can cope more effectively with the added stress of having a child with conduct problems. Our research has also suggested that child and teacher training are highly effective strategies for addressing children's social deficits and improving social skills, problem-solving strategies, and peer relationships. The addition of child or teacher training seems to be particularly helpful for children with pervasive conduct problems (school and home) and with peer relationship difficulties.

Our intervention studies, which target different combinations of risk factors, can be seen as an indirect test of the different theoretical models regarding the development of CDs. We started with a simple parenting skills deficit model and have evolved to a more complex interactional model. In our current model, we hypothesize that the child's eventual outcome will be dependent on the interrelationship between child, parent, teacher, and peer risk factors. Therefore, the most effective interventions should be those that involve schools, teachers, and the child's peer group as well as parents.

ACKNOWLEDGEMENTS

This research was supported by the NIMH Research Scientist Development Award MH00988, NIMH 5 R01 MH067192, and 5 R01 MH074497. Correspondence concerning this chapter should be addressed to Carolyn Webster-Stratton, University of Washington, School of Nursing, Parenting Clinic, 1141 8th Avenue West, Seattle, WA 98119. The senior author of this paper has disclosed a potential financial conflict of intererst because she disseminates these interventions and stands to gain from a favorable report. Because of this, she has voluntarily agreed to distance herself from certain critical research activities (i.e., recruiting, consenting, primary data handling, and analysis), and the University of Washington has approved these arrangements.

REFERENCES

Barrera, M., Biglan, A., Taylor, T. K., Gunn, B., Smolkowski, K., Black, C., et al. (2002). Early elementary school intervention to reduce conduct problems: A randomized trial with Hispanic and non-Hispanic children. *Prevention Science, 3*(2), 83–94.

Collins, W. A., Maccoby, E. E., Steinberg, L., Hetherington, E. M., & Bornstein, M. H. (2000). Contemporary research on parenting: The case for nurture and nature. *American Psychologist, 55*, 218–232.

Drugli, M. B., & Larsson, B. (2006). Children aged 4–8 years treated with parent training and child therapy because of conduct problems: Generalisation effects to day-care and school settings. *European Child and Adolescent Psychiatry, 15*, 392–399.

Egger, H. L., & Angold, A. (2006). Common emotional and behavioral disorders in preschool children: Presentation, nosology, and epidemiology. *Journal of Child Psychology and Psychiatry, 47*, 313–337.

Gardner, F., Burton, J., & Klimes, I. (2006). Randomized controlled trial of a parenting intervention in the voluntary sector for reducing conduct problems in children: Outcomes and mechanisms of change. *Journal of Child Psychology and Psychiatry, 47*, 1123–1132.

Gottman, J. M. (1983). How children become friends. *Monographs of the Society for Research in Child Development, 48 (2, Serial No. 201).*

Gross, D., Fogg, L., Webster-Stratton, C., Garvey, C. W. J., & Grady, J. (2003). Parent training with families of toddlers in day care in low-income urban communities. *Journal of Consulting and Clinical Psychology, 71* (2), 261–278.

Hartman, R. R., Stage, S., & Webster-Stratton, C. (2003). A growth curve analysis of parent training outcomes: Examining the influence of child factors (inattention, impulsivity, and hyperactivity problems), parental and family risk factors. *The Child Psychology and Psychiatry Journal, 44*(3), 388–398.

Horwitz, S. M., Leaf, P. J., Jeventhal, J. M., Forsyth, B., & Speechley, K. N. (1992). Identification and management of psychosocial and developmental problems in community-based, primary care pediatric practices. *Pediatrics, 89*, 480–485.

Hutchings, J., & Gardner, F. (2006). Evaluation of Incredible Years Parenting Program with Sure Start Parents

Jaffee, S. R., Caspi, A., Moffitt, T. E., & Taylor, A. (2004). Physical maltreatment victim to antisocial child: Evidence of environmentally mediated process. *Journal of Abnormal Psychology, 113*, 44–55.

Knutson, J. F., DeGarmo, D., Koeppl, G., & Reid, J. B. (2005). Can neglect, supervisory neglect and harsh parenting in the development of children's aggression: A replication and extension. *Child Maltreatment, 10*, 92–107.

Larsson, B., Fossum, B., Clifford, G., Drugli, M., Handegard, B., & Morch, W. (2009). Treatment of oppositional defiant and conduct problems in young Norwegian children: Results of a randomized trial. *European Child Adolescent Psychiatry 18*(1), 42–52.

Lavigne, J. V., LeBailly, S. A., Gouze, K. R., Cicchetti, C., Pochyly, J., Arend, R., et al. (2008). Treating Oppositional Defiant Disorder in primary care: A comparison of three models. *Journal of Pediatric Psychology, 33*(5), 449–461.

Linares, L. O., Montalto, D., MinMin, L., & Oza, S. V. (2006). A Promising Parent Intervention in Foster Care. *Journal of Consulting and Clinical Psychology, 74*(1), 32–41.

Loeber, R., Wung, P., Keenan, K., Giroux, B., Stouthamer-Loeber, M., Van Kammen, W. B., et al. (1993). Developmental pathways in disruptive child behavior. *Development Psychopathology, 5*, 103–133.

Miller Brotman, L., Klein, R. G., Kamboukos, D., Brown, E. J., Coard, S., & Sosinsky, L. S. (2003). Preventive intervention for urban, low-income preschoolers at familial risk for conduct problems: A randomized pilot study. *Journal of Child Psychology and Psychiatry, 32*(2), 246–257.

Moffitt, T. E., & Lynam, D. (1994). The neuropsychology of conduct disorder and delinquency: Implications for understanding antisocial behavior. In D. C. Fowles, P. Sutker, & S. H. Goodman (Eds.), *Progress in experimental personality and psychopathology research* (pp. 233–262). New York: Springer.

Patterson, G. R., Capaldi, D., & Bank, L. (1991). An early starter model for predicting delinquency. In D. J. Pepler & K. H. Rubin (Eds.), *The development and treatment of childhood aggression* (pp. 139–168). Hillsdale, NJ: Erlbaum.

Raver, C. C., Jones, S., Li-Grining, C., Metzger, M., Smallwood, K., & Sardin-Adjei, L. (2007). *Improving preschool classroom processes: Preliminary findings from a randomized trial implemented in Head Start. Early Childhood Research Quar.* terly, Chicago: University of Chicago.

Reid, M. J., Webster-Stratton, C., & Beauchaine, T. P. (2001). Parent training in Head Start: A comparison of program response among African American, Asian American, Caucasian, and Hispanic mothers. *Prevention Science, 2*(4), 209–227.

Reid, M. J., Webster-Stratton, C., & Hammond, M. (2007). Enhancing a classroom social competence and problem-solving curriculum by offering parent training to families of moderate-to-high-risk elementary school children. *Journal of Clinical Child and Adolescent Psychology, 36*(5), 605–620.

Scott, S., Spender, Q., Doolan, M., Jacobs, B., & Aspland, H. (2001). Multicentre controlled trial of parenting groups for child antisocial behaviour in clinical practice. *British Medical Journal, 323*(28), 1–5.

Snyder, H. (2001). Child delinquents. In R. Loeber & D. P. Farrington (Eds.), *Risk factors and successful interventions*. Thousand Oaks, CA: Sage.

Spaccarelli, S., Cotler, S., & Penman, D. (1992). Problem-solving skills training as a supplement to behavioral parent training. *Cognitive Therapy and Research, 16*, 1–18.

Taylor, T. K., Schmidt, F., Pepler, D., & Hodgins, H. (1998). A comparison of eclectic treatment with Webster-Stratton's Parents and Children Series in a children's mental health center: A randomized controlled trial. *Behavior Therapy, 29*, 221–240.

Webster-Stratton, C. (1981). Modification of mothers' behaviors and attitudes through videotape modeling group discussion program. *Behavior Therapy, 12*, 634–642.

Webster-Stratton, C. (1982). Teaching mothers through videotape modeling to change their children's behaviors. *Journal of Pediatric Psychology, 7*(3), 279–294.

Webster-Stratton, C. (1984). Randomized trial of two parent-training programs for families with conduct-disordered children. *Journal of Consulting and Clinical Psychology, 52*(4), 666–678.

Webster-Stratton, C. (1990a). Enhancing the effectiveness of self-administered videotape parent training for families with conduct-problem children. *Journal of Abnormal Child Psychology, 18*, 479–492.

Webster-Stratton, C. (1990b). Long-term follow-up of families with young conduct problem children: From preschool to grade school. *Journal of Clinical Child Psychology, 19*(2), 144–149.

Webster-Stratton, C. (1992). Individually administered videotape parent training: "Who benefits?". *Cognitive Therapy and Research, 16*(1), 31–35.

Webster-Stratton, C. (1994). Advancing videotape parent training: A comparison study. *Journal of Consulting and Clinical Psychology, 62*(3), 583 593.

Webster-Stratton, C. (1996). Parenting a young child with conduct problems: New insights using grounded theory methods. In T. H. Ollendick & R. S. Prinz (Eds.), *Advances in clinical child psychology* (pp. 333–355). Hillsdale, NJ: Lawrence Erlbaum Associates.

Webster-Stratton, C. (1998). Preventing conduct problems in Head Start children: Strengthening parenting competencies. *Journal of Consulting and Clinical Psychology, 66*(5), 715–730.

Webster-Stratton, C. (2000). *How to promote social and academic competence in young children*. London: Sage.

Webster-Stratton, C. (2006). *The Incredible Years: A trouble-shooting guide for parents of children ages 3–8 years.* Seattle, WA: Incredible Years Press.

Webster-Stratton, C., & Hammond, M. (1990). Predictors of treatment outcome in parent training for families with conduct problem children. *Behavior Therapy, 21*, 319–337.

Webster-Stratton, C., & Hammond, M. (1997). Treating children with early-onset conduct problems: A comparison of child and parent training interventions. *Journal of Consulting and Clinical Psychology, 65*(1), 93–109.

Webster-Stratton, C., & Hammond, M. (1998). Conduct problems and level of social competence in Head Start children: Prevalence, pervasiveness and associated risk factors. *Clinical Child Psychology and Family Psychology Review, 1*(2), 101–124.

Webster-Stratton, C., & Hancock, L. (1998). Parent training: Content, methods and processes. In E. Schaefer (Ed.), *Handbook of parent training* (2nd ed., pp. 98–152). New York: Wiley.

Webster-Stratton, C., & Herbert, M. (1994). *Troubled families – problem children: Working with parents: A collaborative process.* Chichester: Wiley.

Webster-Stratton, C., Hollinsworth, T., & Kolpacoff, M. (1989). The long-term effectiveness and clinical significance of three cost-effective training programs for families with conduct-problem children. *Journal of Consulting and Clinical Psychology, 57*(4), 550–553.

Webster-Stratton, C., Kolpacoff, M., & Hollinsworth, T. (1988). Self-administered videotape therapy for families with conduct-problem children: Comparison with two cost-effective treatments and a control group. *Journal of Consulting and Clinical Psychology, 56*(4), 558–566.

Webster-Stratton, C., & Lindsay, D. W. (1999). Social competence and early-onset conduct problems: Issues in assessment. *Journal of Child Clinical Psychology, 28*, 25–93.

Webster-Stratton, C., & Reid, M. J. (1999, November, 1999). *Treating children with early-onset conduct problems. The importance of teacher training.* Toronto: Paper presented at the association for the advancement of behavior therapy.

Webster-Stratton, C., Reid, M. J., & Hammond, M. (2001). Preventing conduct problems, promoting social competence: A parent and teacher training partnership in Head Start. *Journal of Clinical Child Psychology, 30*(3), 283–302.

Webster-Stratton, C., Reid, M. J., & Hammond, M. (2004). Treating children with early-onset conduct problems: Intervention outcomes for parent, child, and teacher training. *Journal of Clinical Child and Adolescent Psychology, 33*(1), 105–124.

Webster-Stratton, C., Reid, M. J., & Stoolmiller, M. (2008). Preventing conduct problems and improving school readiness: Evaluation of the Incredible Years Teacher and Child Training Programs in high-risk schools. *Journal of Child Psychology and Psychiatry, 49*(5), 471–488.

Webster-Stratton, C., Rinaldi, J., & Reid, M. J. (in press). Long-term outcomes of Incredible Years Parenting Program: predictors of adolescent adjustment. *Journal of Child Psychology and Psychiatry.*

Williford, A. P., & Shelton, T. L. (2008). Using mental health consultation to decrease disruptive behaviors in preschoolers: Adapting an empirically-supported intervention. *Journal of Child Psychology and Psychiatry, 49*(2), 191–200.

6

Parent–Child Interaction Therapy for Preschool Children with Conduct Problems

SHEILA M. EYBERG and REGINA BUSSING

This chapter describes Parent Child Interaction Therapy (PCIT), an evidence-based treatment for preschool children with conduct-disordered behavior and their parents (Eyberg, Nelson, & Boggs, 2008). Originally developed for children with severely disruptive behavior, PCIT has also been used for the treatment of behavior problems associated with children's medical, developmental, and neurological disorders and internalizing disorders such as separation anxiety as well as the treatment of parental physical abuse and neglect (Bagner & Eyberg, 2007; Chaffin et al., 2004, Choate, Pincus, Eyberg, & Barlow, 2005). Although parent training for young children with conduct disorders has historically focused on either relationship enhancement (e.g., Guerney, 1964) or behavior change (e.g., Patterson, 1974), PCIT integrates these approaches by teaching parents to establish a nurturing relationship while increasing their child's prosocial behavior and decreasing conduct-disordered behaviors. PCIT seeks to effect behavior change in both participants in the parent–child relationship, and it does so through assessment-based teaching and live coaching techniques, supplemented by targeted homework assignments and systematic skill generalization. Treatment completion is dependent on parenting skill mastery and normalization of child behavior. Parents progress

---

SHEILA M. EYBERG • University of Florida
REGINA BUSSING • University of Florida

R.C. Murrihy et al. (eds.), *Clinical Handbook of Assessing and Treating Conduct Problems in Youth*, DOI 10.1007/978-1-4419-6297-3_6,

through two phases of treatment, first learning a child-directed interaction (CDI) and then incorporating a parent-directed interaction (PDI). The CDI focuses on parent–child bonding, positive parenting skills, and child social skills enhancement, whereas the PDI focuses on parental discipline skills and reduction of child conduct problems.

Conduct-disordered behavior in preschoolers refers to a constellation of "acting out" behaviors, such as noncompliant, stubborn, aggressive, and destructive behaviors. Although there remains controversy as to whether a diagnosis of conduct disorder should be applied to children at such a young age, telltale symptoms such as lying, bullying or threatening, initiating physical fights, being physically cruel to animals, and deliberately destroying property are not uncommon in clinical preschool samples (Brinkmeyer, 2006), and conduct-disordered behavior is the most common reason for referral of young children to mental health services (Loeber, Burke, Lahey, Winters, & Zera, 2000).

Early intervention in families of young children with conduct-disordered behavior may be critical. Conduct-disordered behavior represents the single most important behavioral risk factor for later antisocial behavior (Loeber & Dishion, 1983; White, Moffit, Earls, Robins, & Silva, 1990) and can be reliably identified in children as young as 3 (Olweus, 1979). Families of young children are more apt to complete treatment than families of older children (Dishion & Patterson, 1992), and positive treatment-related behavior changes in young children with conduct-disordered behavior tend to last over long periods of time (Eyberg, Edwards, Boggs, & Foote, 1998; Reid, Webster-Stratton, & Hammond, 2003). Effective intervention prior to school entry may prevent the associated problems with academic performance and peer relationships that require multiple interventions only a few years later (Campbell, 1997; Webster-Stratton & Herbert, 1994).

PARENT–CHILD INTERACTION THERAPY MODEL

Theoretical Foundations of PCIT

On the basis of Baumrind's (1966) developmental theory of parenting, PCIT draws from both attachment and social learning principles to teach authoritative parenting – a combination of nurturance, good communication, and firm control. Baumrind transformed her original authoritative-authoritarian-permissive parenting model to one based on two orthogonal constructs, parent responsiveness and parent demandingness (Baumrind, 1991). Her research demonstrated that parents who do not meet young children's needs for both nurturance and limit-setting are less likely to raise healthy adolescents. The authoritative parenting style has been associated with fewer child behavior problems than other styles across a diverse range of clinical populations (e.g., Azar & Wolfe, 1989; Querido, Warner, & Eyberg, 2002), and consistent with this literature, PCIT seeks to promote an authoritative parenting style, drawing from both attachment and social learning theories to achieve optimal child outcomes.

According to attachment theory, parental warmth and responsiveness to the emotional needs of young children contribute to the development of a secure working model of relationships, which in turn leads to greater emotional regulation and enhances the child's desire to please and willingness to comply. Conversely, parents who are unresponsive to their children's emotional expression and needs foster an insecure attachment. Maladaptive parent–child attachment has been consistently linked to children's aggressive behavior, low social competence, poor coping skills, low self-esteem, and poor peer relationships. Moreover, an insecure parent–child attachment is related to increased maternal stress as well as child abuse and neglect (Coie et al., 1993; Earls, 1980).

The specific behavior management techniques taught in PCIT are based on social learning theory, which emphasizes the contingencies that shape dysfunctional interactions between disruptive children and their parents. Patterson's (1982) coercion hypothesis provides a social learning account in which the development and maintenance of disruptive behaviors occur via maladaptive parent–child interactions. These interactions are characterized by mutual and escalating aversive behaviors resulting from the attempts of both the parent and child to control the actions (e.g., arguing, criticizing, whining, aggression) of the other. To interrupt this cycle, parents must change their behavior to incorporate clear limit setting in the context of an authoritative relationship. Thus, the goals of PCIT are both to improve the parent–child relationship and to improve parental behavior management skills.

Goals of PCIT

PCIT theory posits that a warm, nurturing relationship is a necessary foundation for establishing effective limit setting and consistency in discipline that will lead to lasting change in the behaviors of both parent and child. Therefore, in the first phase of PCIT, the CDI, parents learn to follow the child's lead in play. The specific goals of CDI are to increase parental responsiveness and establish a secure and nurturing relationship between parent and child. Once parents have mastered the CDI skills (detailed below), the second phase of treatment adds the PDI, in which parents learn to lead the child's behavior when needed. The goal of PDI is to improve parental limit setting and consistency in discipline to reduce the child's noncompliance, aggression, and other negative behaviors. Therapists teach parents problem-solving skills to assist them in applying the principles and skills taught in CDI and PDI to new situations and new problems as they arise.

Characteristics of the Treatment Program

Assessment Driven. The initial assessment for PCIT uses multiple informants and methods to arrive at an accurate conceptualization of the child's behavior problems, including parent and teacher behavior rating scales and coding of behavioral observations of the parent–child interaction and the child's behavior at school. This assessment information is integral to PCIT to define treatment needs, guide the course of therapy, assess progress through treatment, and evaluate outcomes.

During the pretreatment assessment, and weekly throughout treatment, parents complete the 36-item *Eyberg Child Behavior Inventory* (ECBI, Eyberg & Pincus, 1999) *Intensity Scale* to quantify the frequency of the child's behavior problems relative to norms. If the child also exhibits problems in the school setting, the child's teacher is asked to complete the *Sutter-Eyberg Student Behavior Inventory-Revised* (SESBI-R; Eyberg & Pincus, 1999), which is similar in format to the ECBI and assesses disruptive behavior at school.

The final component of the assessment involves direct observation of parent–child interactions conducted in the clinic and, if needed, observations of the child's behavior at school. The *Dyadic Parent–Child Interaction Coding System* (DPICS; Eyberg, Nelson, Duke, & Boggs, 2004) is used to assess the quality of parent–child social interactions during three 5 min standard situations that vary in the degree of parental control required (i.e., child-led play, parent-led play, and clean-up). It permits coding of important parental antecedents (e.g., direct or indirect commands) and consequences (e.g., praise, criticism) of child behavior. The *Revised Edition of the School Observation Coding System* (REDSOCS; Jacobs et al., 2000) is an easy-to-use interval coding system designed to measure inappropriate, noncompliant, and off-task behaviors during a brief period of structured classroom activities on three consecutive days.

The pretreatment assessment information serves as baseline data for monitoring treatment progress. Parent skill acquisition is monitored at each session through DPICS-III coding, and improvement in child behavior outside the clinic is assessed through weekly ECBI Intensity Scale ratings at the beginning of each session. Treatment is effectively completed when (a) ongoing DPICS-III assessment indicates that the parents have met mastery criteria for the CDI and PDI interaction skills; (b) the behavior problems have declined to a *T* score of 55 or lower on the ECBI; and (c) the parents express confidence in their ability to manage future child behavior problems independently and feel ready for treatment to end.

Family Characteristics. Children and their parents are seen together in PCIT. Treatment includes both parents and other significant caregivers in the child's life, if possible, such as a grandparent. Although originally designed for individual family treatment, several research teams are examining the efficacy of group PCIT (e.g., Niec, Hemme, Yopp, & Brestan, 2005). In group PCIT, the dyadic parent–child coaching component is retained, and group size is typically three to six families per group.

Therapy Structure

Each phase of treatment begins with a teaching session in which the therapist explains, models, and role-plays the CDI or PDI skills with the parents, followed by coaching sessions in which parents practice the skills with their child while the therapist coaches them on the new behaviors. Parents complete the ECBI Intensity Scale before each session to monitor child behavior problems at home. The coaching sessions begin with a brief review of the previous week followed by a 5 min observation of the parent–child interaction to determine which skills parents have mastered and which will be important targets for in-session coaching.

Coaching constitutes the majority of session time. Therapists typically coach from an observation room with a one-way mirror into the playroom, using a "bug-in-the-ear" system for communicating to the parent playing with the child. Coaching consists of frequent, brief statements that give parents immediate feedback on their CDI or PDI skills (e.g., "Nice labeled praise," "Good direct command"), their manner (e.g., "Great enthusiasm," "Good job staying calm"), or their effect (e.g., "He stays on task longer when you describe what he is doing"). The therapist also offers suggestions (e.g., "Give her as many praises as you can when she's playing so quietly and gently with the toys").

At the end of each session, therapists review with parents a summary sheet showing how often they used each CDI or PDI skill during the initial 5 min observation period. The parents can track their weekly skills progress on the summary sheet and decide which skill to emphasize during their daily practice sessions the following week. The therapist and parents also review a graph of the child's progress based on the parents' weekly behavior ratings on the ECBI.

Content of the Treatment Sessions

Child-Directed Interaction. The primary rule for parents during CDI is to follow their child's lead. Parents learn three important communication skills – behavioral descriptions, reflections, and labeled praises – to give positive attention to their child's positive behaviors as they play together. Parents also learn not to use commands, questions, or criticisms, which can be intrusive in child-led play (see Table 6.1 for CDI skill descriptions with examples). Parents learn to ignore mild negative behaviors that occur. By giving attention only to positive child behaviors, parents learn to use the technique of *differential social attention* to shape their child's behavior in this initial phase of treatment. At the end of the CDI Teach session, therapists provide parents with a handout summarizing the skills and ask parents to practice the interaction for 5 min each day. They give parents a separate handout to record their daily home practice and any problems that arise during home sessions.

In the first CDI coaching session, therapists focus exclusively on reinforcing parents' use of any CDI skill. In subsequent sessions, the focus remains on praising the positive parenting skills although therapists may also give suggestions or directions during coaching as the parents become more comfortable and trusting of their therapist. For example, a therapist might focus on increasing labeled praise, and whenever the parent gives an unlabeled praise (e.g., "Good job"), the therapist might cue the parent to label it by saying "Good job of what?" or just "Of what?" The therapist would also reinforce the parent specifically for each use of labeled praise (e.g., "Great labeling that praise!").

If the child becomes disruptive during a CDI session, parents are coached to ignore the child by looking away and not talking or gesturing to the child. Parents are advised that the ignored behavior is likely to get

Table 6.1. CDI skills

Skills	Reasons	Examples
"Do" skills		
Labeled praises	• Increases behavior that is praised	• Good job of cleaning up!
	• Shows approval	• I like how you're building so quietly
	• Increases self-esteem	• Great idea to make a house
	• Creates positive feelings	• Thank you for sharing with me
Reflections	• Lets child lead the conversation	• Child: I drew a tree Parent: Yes, a big tree by the house
	• Shows that you are listening	
	• Show that you understand	• Child: This isn't very easy Parent: It's pretty hard to balance that
	• Improves speech	• Child: I made a choo choo Parent: You did make a train
	• Clarify ideas	• Child: It's gone all over Parent: It melted all over the table
Behavior descriptions	• Lets child lead activity	• You are building a fort
	• Shows you are interested	• You're putting the monkeys where they can watch all the other animals
	• Teaches concepts and builds vocabulary	• You drew six petals on your flower
	• Holds child's attention on the task	• Now you're searching for the letters for the next word
"Don't" skills		
Commands	• Takes lead away from child	Indirect Commands: • Let's play with the cars
	• Risks negative interaction	Direct Commands: • Give me the red car
Questions	• May be hidden commands	• Can you tell me what color this is? • We're building a big house, aren't we?
	• Suggests you are not listening	• Child: I want to play with the animals Parent: The animals?
	• Suggests you disapprove	• You're putting round blocks on the tower?
Critical statements	• Lowers self-esteem	• You still have it wrong
	• Creates unpleasant interaction	• Your tower is crooked
	• Increases the criticized behavior	• That's not a good idea • Stop fidgeting

worse before it gets better and that they must follow-through with ignoring until the child's behavior improves. Parents are then coached to return to the positive CDI skills when their child is again behaving appropriately. Parents are also taught to stop the interaction for negative behaviors that cannot be ignored such as aggressive or destructive behaviors like hitting, biting, or breaking toys. Therapists coach the parent to state that special time is over because of the destructive or aggressive behavior, and parents are encouraged to reengage in the CDI after the child has calmed down.

Therapists continue to coach parents in using the CDI skills until parents meet the minimum criteria for mastery during the initial 5 min observation: (a) 10 behavioral descriptions; (b) 10 reflective statements; (c) 10 labeled praises; and (d) no more than three total questions, commands, and criticisms. Once parents have met these criteria, they move into the second phase of treatment, the PDI. Because the CDI skills form an important foundation for establishing and maintaining effective discipline, however, the therapist continues to code 5 min of CDI at the beginning of subsequent therapy sessions. If a parent falls below criterion on any of the CDI skills, the therapist will coach these skills before beginning the PDI. The 5 min CDI home practice sessions also continue.

Parent-Directed Interaction. Primary goals of PDI include decreasing noncompliance and other negative behaviors that are not extinguished by active ignoring. Parents continue to give positive attention to appropriate behaviors in PDI, but rather than exclusively following the child's lead, parents learn to give effective directions and to follow through consistently with calm, predictable responses to their child's behavior. Both parents and children know what consequences will follow the child's obedience or disobedience, which reduces parental anxiety and helps parents to feel more in control of their child's behavior.

Therapists teach parents to give their children clear, positively stated, direct commands rather than criticisms (e.g., "Ask me quietly" rather than "Stop yelling") or indirect commands that suggest optional compliance (e.g., "Please give me the hammer" rather than "Will you give me the hammer?"). Parents also learn correct timing for reasoning; they learn to give reasons for their commands either before they are given ("It is time for us to go. The room has to be clean before we can leave. Please put the blocks in the container.") or after they are obeyed ("Good job of cleaning up! The room is nice and clean for others now.") rather than after they are given and before they are obeyed, which can lead to arguing and can reinforce children's delay tactics. In addition to practicing commands during the teaching session, parents receive a handout summarizing the rules to review at home (see Table 6.2).

Next, therapists teach parents specific steps to follow once a command has been given. If the child obeys, the parent gives a labeled praise for compliance (e.g., "Thank you for listening!") and then returns to the CDI skills until the next command is needed. If the child disobeys, the parent initiates the timeout sequence. Parents are taught never to ignore noncompliance, because noncompliant behavior is reinforced if children are permitted to disobey. The timeout procedure provides concrete steps to follow after disobedience, with three levels: warning, chair, and room. At each level, the child may choose to obey the parent and end the timeout. The procedure does not end until the child obeys the original command.

The Warning. The warning is given after the child first disobeys a direct command. Before giving the warning, parents may give the child up to 5 s to begin obeying the command when it is unclear if the child intends to obey. This "5-second rule" is not used when the child clearly disobeys (e.g., after a command to hand the parent the block, the child throws the block on the floor). The warning is the statement: "If you don't [original command], then

Table 6.2. Rules for effective commands

Rule	Reasons	Examples
Make commands direct rather than indirect	• Leaves no question that the child is being instructed to do something • Does not imply a choice, nor suggest that the parent might do the task for the child • Reduces confusion for the child	• Please hand me the car • Put the block in the box • Draw a circle *Instead of* Will you draw a circle? Let's draw a circle
State commands positively	• Tells child what to do ratherthan what not to do • Avoids criticism of the child's actions • Provides a clear statement of what the child should do	• Come sit beside me *Instead of* Stop running around the room! • Put your hands in your pockets *Instead of* Don't touch the glass
Give commands one at a time	• Helps child remember the whole command • Enables parent to determine if child completed entire command	• Put the crayons in the box *Instead of* Put the crayons in the box, and put the box in the cupboard, and close the cupboard door • Put all your shoes in the closet *Instead of* Clean your room
Make commands specific rather than vague	• Tells child exactly what is supposed to be done	• Get down off the table *Instead of* Be careful. • Please sit quietly. *Instead of* Behave!
Make commands age-appropriate	• Assures that child can understand what is expected	• Put these blue Legos (pointing) back in their box. *Instead of* Put the navy pieces in the proper container • Draw a square. *Instead of* Draw a cube

Give commands politely and respectfully	• Prevents child from learning to obey only if yelled at • Teaches children to obey polite and respectful commands • Prepares child for school	• Child: (banging block) Parent: (in normal voice) Please give me the block. *Instead of* Parent: (loudly) Stop banging and give me that block now!
Explain commands only before they are given or after they are obeyed	• Explanations before commands help orient the child to the task • Explanations after commands are obeyed are "heard" and meaningful • Explanations after the command is given but before it is obeyed reinforce dawdling and often are not "heard"	• Parent: It is just about time for dinner. Please wash your hands Child: Why? Parent: (ignores) Child: (obeys) Parent: Thank you for washing your hands before dinner. Clean hands keep germs away from your food so you won't get sick
Use direct (effective) commands only when they are really necessary	• If a task is optional, better to use an indirect (optional) command – or none at all • If commands are reserved for important tasks, children will be less likely to "test" them	• (Child is running around room) Parent: Please sit in this chair. (Good time to use this command) *Instead of* Please get me a tissue. (Not a good time to give this command, and important to consider if this command is necessary)

you have to go to the timeout chair." If the child obeys the warning, the parent gives the child a labeled praise and the play continues.

The Chair. After the warning, the parent again uses the 5 s rule. If the child has not started to obey the warning within 5 s, the parent calmly and quickly takes the child to the timeout chair while saying, "You didn't do what I told you to do, so you have to sit on the timeout chair." This statement reminds the child of the reason for the timeout and reiterates the connection between noncompliance to a direct command and a negative consequence. The parent may lead the child to the chair with just a touch, or may carry the child from behind, if necessary, with arms under the child's arms and crossed over the child's chest. After placing the child on the chair, the parent says only, "Stay here until I say you can get off." This statement has a very different meaning than a statement such as "Stay here until you are ready to behave." It is important for the parent to establish control of the time the child spends on the chair. If a child could get off the chair whenever he or she wished, timeout would be much less effective.

Therapists teach parents to ignore all negative behavior as long as the child stays on the chair. This skill may be difficult for parents, because children often resort to various forms of emotional manipulation (e.g., "I don't love you anymore," "I'm really really sorry") or, more rarely, negative physical behavior (e.g., taking off their clothes). The child must stay on the chair for 3 min, plus 5 s of quiet at the end of 3 min. These 5 s of quiet ensure that the child does not leave the chair with the impression that whatever he or she said or did on the chair immediately before the end of timeout caused the parent to end timeout.

Once the child's time on the chair is up, the parent is instructed to walk over to the child and say, "You are sitting quietly on the chair. Are you ready to [original command]?" If the child says "No," begins to argue, or ignores the parent, the parent says, "Then stay on the chair until I say you can get off." The parent then walks away and begins the 3 min time period again. If the child indicates that he or she is ready, either by saying, "Yes" or by getting off of the chair in a compliant manner, the parent walks the child back to the task. The parent then indicates that the child should obey the original command (e.g., pointing to the block that the child was originally instructed to hand to the parent). A child rarely refuses to obey at this point, but if the child did disobey, the parent would say again, "You didn't do what I told you to do, so you have to sit on the chair," and then follow through as before.

When the child does obey the original command, the parent gives only a brief acknowledgement, such as "Fine." The parent does not give the child extensive labeled praise at this point because the child did not comply until he or she was sent to timeout. Instead the parent immediately gives the child another similar but very simple command. The child will very likely obey this command, and at this point the parent gives the child highly enthusiastic labeled praise for minding and returns to CDI. This way, the child begins to distinguish between the positive responses that follow immediate compliance and the less-reinforcing responses that follow compliance that required timeout.

The Room. When timeout is necessary, the timeout chair alone may not be sufficient in the beginning of treatment if the child gets off the chair without permission. For this reason, parents are taught to use a timeout room as a backup to teach their child to stay on the chair. Parents rarely need to use the timeout room after the first 2 or 3 weeks of PDI because children learn quickly to stay seated once they realize they will have to go to the timeout room if they get off of the chair without permission.

The first time a child gets off the timeout chair without permission, the parent gives a timeout room warning, places the child back on the chair, and starts the 3 min timing again. After that one warning, whenever a child gets off the timeout chair without permission in the future, the parent leads or carries the child to the timeout room while saying, "You got off the chair before I said you could, so you have to go to the timeout room." Once the child is in the timeout room, the parent stays just outside the door and keeps close track of the time. The child stays in the room for 1 min plus 5 s of quiet. The parent then leads the child back to the timeout chair and says, "Stay on the chair until I say you can get off." The child's 3-min timeout on the chair then starts over. This process may need to be repeated several times during the first timeout, so it is essential that parents and therapists allow adequate time to follow through until the child learns to stay on the chair.

The timeout room used in PCIT sessions should be easily accessible from the playroom and should be empty or contain only heavy furniture that the child cannot move. Ideally, this room is constructed with a "Dutch door," – a half-door just high enough to prevent a child from climbing over it. The room should also have an observation window or camera through which the therapist can monitor the child's behavior. The timeout room selected for use in the child's home must be at least 5×5 ft^2 in size and well lit. Although the timeout room will need to be used for only a short time, it is important to prepare well so that it is both safe and effective. Some families have large laundry rooms that can be emptied for a few weeks. Use of a bathroom as a timeout room requires careful discussion of safety requirements, such as removing all cleaning solutions and medicines from cabinets and turning down the water temperature or disconnecting the water supply to a spare bathroom. Some families clear the child's bedroom of all but basic furniture for use as a timeout room during the first few weeks of PDI.

Children often escalate their negative reactions (crying, yelling, kicking) when their parents do not give in to them during the timeout procedure. Coaching timeout during the first and second PDI sessions allows therapists to support parents during the emotionally difficult process of learning consistency so that they do not give up, and it gives therapists many opportunities to teach parents about their own and their child's behavior. Therapists can convey accurate attributions about the reasons for the child's behavior and can provide behavioral interpretations of the change as it is occurring. They can coach parents in relaxation or anger-control techniques in vivo, if indicated, and if the child makes many journeys between the timeout chair and timeout room, they can assure parents that their child does understand the process, is choosing timeout over obeying, but will complete the procedure and obey the original command within the session. Further information on the treatment protocol may be found in the PCIT treatment manual, accessible at www.pcit.org.

As PDI progresses, generalization of PDI skills from practice sessions to real life is emphasized. Parents learn to use commands for behaviors that are incompatible with problem behaviors (called "positive opposites"), such as, "Use your indoor voice" and "Pet the cat gently." Parents are coached to use direct commands with correct follow-through at the clinic at all times, including time in the waiting room and during the parent–therapist wrap-up at the conclusion of sessions if indicated by child disruptive behavior. After children learn to respond to the running commands of PDI, parents learn to develop "House Rules," a standing command variation of the PDI algorithm to address aggressive or destructive behaviors that have not changed despite focused praise for positive opposite behavior. Before setting up a house rule (e.g., no jumping on furniture), parents will spend a day or two labeling the specific undesirable behavior explicitly for the child when it occurs, to avoid any confusion and reduce debating once the rule is in place. The parent then explains to the child that he or she will be taken to the timeout chair immediately any time the rule is broken.

In the latter treatment sessions, parents learn and practice variations of PCIT as needed to achieve treatment completion criteria such as managing their child's behavior in public situations' or with siblings. For example, if sibling conflict remains a problem after the parents and child have mastered the PDI procedure, the therapist would schedule a sibling-attended session and coach the parents in how to alternate their CDI skills between children, with emphasis on the siblings' positive interactions with one another, and how to insert targeted commands to each child for specific cooperative behaviors, particularly those that resolve a conflict, followed by targeted labeled praises.

Throughout PDI, therapists teach and coach parents toward mastery level for PDI skills, defined as (a) making at least 75% of their commands "effective" during the DPICS-III observation of PDI at the beginning of the session (i.e., direct, positively stated, single commands that provide opportunity for compliance); (b) at least 75% correct follow-through (labeled praise after obey; warning after disobey; and (c) if the child requires a timeout during the PDI coding, successful follow-through, so that the interaction ends with a labeled praise for compliance to the follow-up command). Some parents achieve mastery of PDI skills within four PDI sessions; however, for children with significant conduct disorder, parents usually require the detailed teaching and coaching offered in the later PDI sessions to achieve a normalization of child behavior.

Maintenance Strategies

To ensure optimal maintenance of learned skills and problem-solving techniques, therapists encourage increasing parental responsibility for problem solving as treatment progresses. Throughout treatment, emphasis is placed on teaching parents how to generate and evaluate applications of PCIT principles and skills to new problems they encounter with their child. In addition, the last session specifically addresses ways in which parents can use problem solving to deal with new issues that may arise after treatment has ended.

Measuring Therapy Progress

Therapists assess the families' progress through PCIT in several ways. First, the observation and DPICS-III coding of parent–child interactions at the start of each session are used both to select the skills to target during the session and to determine when parents have met the mastery criteria for moving from one phase of treatment to the next and for completing treatment. Before each session, parents also fill out the ECBI Intensity Scale, which measures the child's current frequency of disruptive behavior at home. The therapist graphs the parents' scores each week to monitor the child's progress toward the treatment completion goal of scoring within ½ standard deviation of the normal mean (114 or lower), and at various points in treatment shares this graph with the parents. PCIT is performance-based rather than time-limited, and the number of treatment sessions varies widely. The average length of treatment is 15 sessions, although completion in the range of 10–20 sessions is not uncommon.

THE EVIDENCE BASE FOR PCIT

Treatment Efficacy

In the first randomized controlled trial of PCIT, Schuhmann et al. (1998) compared families receiving PCIT to wait-list controls. Following an initial assessment, 64 clinic-referred families were randomly assigned to an immediate treatment (IT) or wait-list control (WL) group. After treatment, parents in the IT group interacted more positively with their child and reported clinically and statistically significant improvements in their child's behavior. These parents also reported less parenting stress and a more internal locus of control than WL parents.

In a second randomized controlled trial, investigating the efficacy of PCIT for treating disruptive behaviors of young children with mental retardation and comorbid ODD, Bagner and Eyberg (2007) found that, after treatment, mothers interacted more positively with their children, and their children were more compliant and less disruptive than WL children.

PCIT outcomes for children with ODD and other diagnostic comorbidities have been studied as well (Chase & Eyberg, 2008; Floyd, 2005). A recent study comparing clinical characteristics and treatment outcomes of preschoolers with CD versus ODD-only found that preschoolers with CD took longer to reach PCIT completion criteria but did not have higher attrition or relapse rates than preschoolers with ODD only (Brinkmeyer, 2006).

Longitudinal Outcomes

Several follow-up studies have demonstrated maintenance of treatment effects after PCIT. At a 2-year follow-up of 13 families that completed treatment, parent ratings of child behavior problems, child activity level, and parenting stress remained similar to post-treatment levels, and most of the children remained free of disruptive behavior diagnoses. Further, these parents continued to report high satisfaction with the process and outcome of PCIT (Eyberg et al., 2001).

In a study comparing longitudinal outcomes of 23 treatment completers and 23 treatment dropouts, Boggs et al. (2004) found that after 1–3 years, families that completed treatment continued to show significant positive change in ratings of their child's disruptive behavior and their own parenting stress, whereas families that dropped out of treatment reported little change in their children's behavior or their level of parenting stress from pretreatment levels. Results clearly indicated consistently better long-term outcomes for the treatment completers than the dropouts. Hood and Eyberg (2003) found that 3–6 years following treatment completion, 23 treatment completers not only maintained their treatment gains but also showed continuing behavioral gains with time. Maternal confidence in their ability to control their children's behavior was also maintained over the 3–6 year follow-up period.

Although research examining maintenance of treatment effects has been encouraging, with group-level analyses demonstrating that treatment gains are maintained, further research is necessary to evaluate individual differences that affect maintenance. Hood and Eyberg (2003) found that 75% of children showed clinically significant change 3–6 years following treatment. However, 25% did not maintain their post-treatment gains. It is important to understand factors that place some families at risk for relapse. It is possible that "at risk" families may require a period of consolidation (i.e., a few additional sessions after treatment goals have been met) to achieve durable effects from treatment. Alternatively, disruptive behavior disorders or maladaptive parenting styles may be chronic conditions within some families that require ongoing monitoring and treatment. Families that have previously demonstrated the commitment to succeed in treatment may rally quickly with timely booster treatment.

Treatment Attrition

PCIT attrition rates for conduct-disordered children have ranged from 33% to 36% (e.g., 35% in Eisenstadt, Eyberg, McNeil, Newcomb, & Funderburk, 1993; 33% in Werba et al., 2006; 36% in Fernandez & Eyberg, 2009), which compares favorably to attrition statistics for parent training ranging from 40% to 65% (Wierzbicki & Pekarik, 1993). The most common reasons for dropout from PCIT have been disagreement with the treatment approach, followed by being too busy to participate in treatment, having additional stressors that interfered with treatment participation, or having logistical problems that interfered (Fernandez & Eyberg, 2009). Because treatment is performance-based and continues until the treatment goals are met, the only way a family cannot succeed, theoretically, is by dropping out. In reality, most families complete PCIT in 16 or fewer sessions (Werba, Eyberg, Boggs, & Algina, 2006), and families that drop out after 20 sessions may not have succeeded with further sessions. Preventing treatment dropout continues to be a challenge in PCIT research and treatment.

Moderators and Mediators of Outcome

Most PCIT outcome studies have been conducted in psychology clinics at major metropolitan medical centers using culturally heterogeneous samples of referred boys and girls with disruptive behavior. Despite this demographic diversity, no PCIT moderator studies have yet been reported. Research in this area may reveal ways to refine treatment to improve long-term outcomes. However, the principles of parenting that derive from attachment and social learning theories and form the basis of PCIT have broad application. For example, Querido et al. (2002) found that the authoritative parenting style predicted optimal child outcomes among African–American families. Studies assessing mediators of PCIT outcome have shown that increases in the CDI "Do" skills and decreases in the CDI "Don't" skills mediated change in child disruptive behaviors during PCIT (e.g., Bagner & Eyberg, 2007).

Application to New Populations

PCIT has been implemented in treatment with abusive families, where the identified patient is typically the parent. Coercive parent–child relationships that characterize families of disruptive children are central to physically abusive families. Further, because abusive families tend to experience few positive interactions, they seem to benefit greatly from coaching in positive parenting skills that facilitate warm, enjoyable family experiences. A randomized controlled trial conducted by Chaffin et al. (2004) found that physically abusive parents who underwent PCIT were significantly less likely to be reported again for child abuse than parents assigned to a standard community treatment condition. The reduction of coercive parent–child interactions in the PCIT condition was shown to mediate the re-abuse outcome.

Even though originally developed as an intervention for child disruptive behaviors, PCIT has been shown to have beneficial effects on child internalizing behaviors as well. In addition to general reductions in internalizing behavior, Chase and Eyberg (2008) found that PCIT reduced the symptoms of separation anxiety disorder (SAD) to non-diagnostic levels among children with comorbid ODD and SAD. Furthermore, an adaptation of PCIT has been developed and pilot tested for children with primary SAD that includes the addition of an anxiety-specific treatment phase, Bravery Directed Interaction, to facilitate exposure to previously avoided situations (Pincus, Santucci, Ehrenreich, & Eyberg, 2008).

The efficacy of PCIT has been documented across cultural groups including Mexican American families (McCabe & Yeh, 2009); Puerto Rican families (Matos, Bauermeister, & Bernal, 2009); African–American families (Fernandez, Butler, & Eyberg, in press); Chinese families (Leung, Tsang, Heung, & Yiu (2009); and Australian families (Nixon, Sweeny, Erickson, & Touyz, 2003). In addition, Phillips and colleagues successfully implemented PCIT by Australian nurse clinicians in a community health clinic (Phillips, Morgan, Cawthorne, & Barnett, 2008).

Successful implementation of PCIT in diverse populations necessitates careful consideration of the cultural factors related to mental health utilization, family structure, discipline norms, and language. As PCIT has been investigated in different populations, the protocol has been adapted to strengthen treatment acceptance and success. For example, McCabe & Yeh (2009) presented PCIT as an educational/skill-building intervention to reduce the stigma associated with seeking mental health services among the Mexican–American community. The Mexican–American adaptation also extended the length of treatment sessions to permit more time for social exchanges deemed important to rapport in that culture.

CASE STUDY

Mickey is a 5-year-old boy referred by his school guidance counselor for assessment and treatment of his longstanding oppositional and aggressive behavior, which includes hitting, kicking and biting other students, and defying teachers' instructions. His mother, Ms. A, reports similar problems at home and with neighborhood children. She is particularly concerned about his violent behavior towards his sister, whom he hits in response to the slightest provocation. To avoid getting into trouble for aggressive behavior, Mickey has begun lying to his mother. Ms. A is concerned that these problem behaviors indicate her son is a budding criminal.

Mickey lives with his mother and 3-year-old sister, Sascha. His parents separated 2 years ago, after a period of marital problems that escalated to domestic violence. Ms. A is a part-time student at the community college and works part-time; she appeared both anxious and tired during the interview. Mickey's father has unstable employment, does not pay child support, and cannot be relied on to follow through with planned visits or phone calls with the children. Although Mickey has witnessed domestic violence, his mother indicated that he has not been physically or sexually abused himself.

Mickey's response to his mother's discipline has left her frustrated and feeling helpless. Ms. A tries to reason with him, and uses restriction and timeout, but has found nothing effective. Mickey refuses to listen, will not stay in timeout, and argues and tantrums at home and in public places when he does not get his way. Ms. A does not believe in physical punishment, but occasionally will spank him out of frustration when he gets very defiant or threatening.

Results of the pretreatment assessment were consistent with a diagnosis of CD. Ms. A's responses on the ECBI indicated significantly disruptive behavior, with an Intensity score of 182. Teacher ratings on the SESBI-R indicated significant problems at school as well. During the first DPICS situation, child-led play, Mickey played with many different toys, each only briefly. His mother tried to follow his lead and asked many questions about his play activities, which Mickey tended to ignore, and she repeatedly criticized him for playing roughly with toys. She praised him twice in the 5 min period, saying "thank you" when he offered toys to her. During the parent-led play situation, Mickey initially engaged with his mother's choice of coloring, but after a minute left the table and began playing with Legos. When Ms. A instructed him to return to the table, he began whining that her game was boring and that he wanted to play with the Legos instead. He continued to play with the Legos, and his mother then joined him. In the third DPICS situation, clean-up, Ms. A was instructed to get Mickey to clean up the toys by himself. She asked him to "put all the toys away," but he continued playing. She asked him again, explaining that the doctors needed him to pick up the toys so the playroom would be clean for other children. Mickey started putting Legos into the toy box while his mother watched silently, but after 20 s he crawled under a chair with some of the Legos and started building. When his mother reminded him to continue cleaning up, he threw a few of the Legos at her and laughed. She told him sternly to stop and finish cleaning up the toys. After he threw a few more Legos at her, she tried to pull him out from under the chair, but he started kicking at her. Following this observation, Ms. A confirmed that Mickey's behavior in the session was quite typical of his behavior at home and school. The therapist informed her that PCIT was an appropriate treatment for the kinds of behavior problems he was showing, and they scheduled the first session.

During the didactic CDI Teach session, Ms. A was attentive and seemed eager to learn ways to provide positive attention to Mickey. She was able to understand and recall the "do" skills (labeled praise, reflections, and behavioral descriptions) and the "don't" skills (commands, questions, and criticism) easily, and role-played the "do" skills well. She was less enthusiastic about the practice of ignoring unwanted behavior. She acknowledged that the bond between herself and Mickey needed strengthening, but expressed her fear that Mickey would turn out like his father if she were to ignore his misbehavior. The therapist reassured her that the CDI would enable her to give Mickey much more attention for his positive behaviors and that the need for ignoring would decrease as Mickey learned how to gain attention in a new way. The therapist further reassured her that this new interaction was a way for her to strengthen the parent–child bond without leading to overly permissive parenting.

Ms. A attended subsequent CDI Coach sessions with her son regularly over the next 7 weeks. In the first 2 weeks of treatment, her homework completion was inconsistent, slowing her progress in learning the skills. Although committed to Mickey's treatment, she frequently felt overwhelmed by the time demands of single parenting along with her college course work and part-time job, and tended to drop "special time," the 5 min homework practice of CDI skills, when stressed. The therapist used motivational interviewing techniques to help her recognize the priority she placed on her son's behavioral adjustment, and together she and the therapist carefully reviewed her schedule to identify a time in each day that she could successfully commit 5 min to her son's treatment. She selected the morning, before Sascha woke up, as a predictable time to fit in 5 min with Mickey, and she was pleased to discover that this early playtime seemed to improve his mood on the school bus, with fewer complaints about aggressive behaviors.

Mickey's aggressive behavior in the CDI sessions was another problem early in treatment. It was necessary to stop CDI on several occasions during coaching and restart it after a few minutes, because he initially pushed or hit his mother when she ignored his aggressive toy play or whiney behavior. At home, his mother stopped the CDI special time for the day whenever Mickey became aggressive during their CDI practice. However, she was instructed not to withhold special time as a disciplinary tactic, because it was treatment for Mickey, not a reward.

After Ms. A began more regular homework practice, she was able to decrease her questions fairly quickly, and her positive attention became more genuine and enthusiastic. In addition, her ability to switch between positive attention and ignoring steadily improved and appeared seamless and automatic by the time she met the CDI mastery criteria at the seventh CDI Coach session. The changes she had made in the CDI were reflected in Mickey's behavior in session. Gradually he stayed by her side at the play table for longer periods of play with a single toy, and his play became less boisterous and more conversationally interactive. Mickey now clearly enjoyed the special time with his mother, and she expressed surprise at how much she now looked forward to spending this time each morning with Mickey. As a result, she had started practicing CDI with her daughter, too, after Mickey left for school.

Even though improved during the CDI phase of treatment, Mickey's ECBI Intensity score of 150 at the seventh CDI Coach session was still above the clinical cutoff, and several presenting problems remained. Mickey's angry defiance toward his mother had lessened, and he no longer hit or yelled at her, but he continued to resist her redirection, especially about bedtime. He also continued to provoke his sister.

The PDI Teach session began with an introduction to the eight "Rules for Effective Commands" (Table 6.2), and Ms. A seemed to understand easily the principles of giving good direct commands. The therapist then modeled the parent responses to compliance and noncompliance, illustrating use of the timeout chair and the backup timeout room. After demonstrating the skills, the therapist engaged Ms. A in role-playing the parent responses to a range of potential child behaviors following direct commands. Ms. A quickly learned the basic steps of the procedure and was able to apply them correctly in role-play. She expressed concern about how Mickey would handle instructions to stay on the chair, and the therapist integrated the anticipated child behaviors into the role-play to teach ways of handling them effectively. Ms. A was relieved to learn that she was not expected to practice PDI by herself until she had an in-session coaching experience. The therapist stressed the importance of continuing daily CDI practice in the coming week, so that Mickey's first exposure to the timeout procedure would represent removal from a strong positive reinforcement – the enjoyable play with his mother.

As Ms. A anticipated, the first PDI coaching session (PDI Coach 1) was taxing and required repeated timeout chair/timeout room sequences because Mickey resisted following his mother's directions in the play. When placed in timeout, Mickey shouted at his mother and accused her of being mean and unloving. The therapist provided continuous supportive coaching to Ms. A to reduce her anxiety and fear that Mickey would become totally unmanageable if not given his way. Mickey required four episodes of returning to the timeout room for chair escapes before he completed his first chair timeout and complied with the initial command. His mother was surprised to see how quickly he re-entered into warm CDI interactions with her after the timeout experience, and she commented later that it appeared to have been harder on herself than on Mickey. Despite her successful experience during PDI Coach 1, Ms. A wanted to wait until after the next session before practicing PDI at home. After processing her feelings of anxiety about independent PDI practice, the therapist supported her preferences, and the homework assignment consisted of continuing the 5 min CDI practice each day.

At PDI Coach 2, Mickey needed only one timeout room experience before learning to stay on the chair until given permission to get off. He had a second incident of noncompliance that resulted in timeout on the chair, and although he slouched upside down with his feet over the armrests and yelled a barrage of accusations at his mother, he remaining on the chair until she gave him permission to get off. During this second chair timeout, Ms. A was much calmer when giving the instructions than previously and, with support from the coach, was able to ignore his behaviors on the chair. Buoyed by her success in managing his behavior in this second coach session, she felt ready to practice the PDI at home. She selected a time to practice that would be sufficient if she had to follow-through with a lengthy timeout sequence, and for a back-up timeout room she chose a small guest bathroom in her apartment that could be temporarily child-proofed.

Ms. A was cheerful when she and Mickey arrived at PDI Coach 3. She had attended the first parent–teacher conference at Mickey's new school and was happy to learn that Mickey seemed to be calming down over the past few weeks, although the teacher reported he was still provoking other children with intrusive behaviors such as poking or pushing them. Ms. A was also happy about her practice of PDI at home. Her homework sheet indicated that Mickey had required use of the timeout room only twice, once on the first day she practiced and once on the second. He had required two or three chair timeouts each day, which by the week's end he completed quietly without fuss. In the session, both CDI and PDI interactions were coded before coaching began. Ms. A remained at mastery level on CDI skills, and was close to mastery of the PDI skills, using clear direct commands and correct follow-through with labeled praise after Mickey obeyed. Mickey did not require the timeout chair in this session but required three chair warnings during coaching when he did not obey right away. During coaching, the therapist focused on decreasing Ms. A's use of extra words or comments to Mickey when he tested limits by "almost but not quite" doing what he was told to do. After coaching, Ms. A noted she could see Mickey's compliance improve in the session after she matter-of-factly stated only the warning when he started testing limits, and she determined that would be her focus during homework practice the next week. The therapist also described a school–home-notes procedure (not a standard PCIT procedure) for decreasing Mickey's negative touching of other children at school, which Ms. A planned to discuss with his teachers in the next week.

During the next two sessions, the family's progress was steady. After a slight rise following the first PDI Coach session, Mickey's ECBI scores declined to 140 at PDI Coach 4 and 120 at Coach 5. Ms. A's PDI skills reached mastery during PDI Coach 5 and were becoming as automatic as her CDI skills.

When the therapist graphed the ECBI before PDI Coach 6, she noted an unexpected increase in the frequency of reported behavior problems. Notably, there were increases on temper tantrums, fighting, sassing, and whining. The therapist learned that Mickey's father had visited unexpectedly, intoxicated, and demanded to take the children for an unsupervised visit. The parents argued heatedly about such a visit and about the father's drinking and delinquent child support payments. Ms. A stayed firm in her refusal to let the father take the children and threatened to call the police. After the father stormed off, Mickey had yelled that he wanted to visit his father, that Ms. A was a mean mother, and that he did not want to have any more special times with her. Ms. A described being overwhelmed by the experience and stopping her homework practice until this session. The therapist praised her for handling the threatening situation with her ex-husband in an effective manner and reminded her that she could call between sessions with any urgent questions or concerns. While processing ways that Ms. A could help Mickey recover from the event, Ms. A determined she needed to increase her dose of "loving therapy," referring to CDI, while keeping up expectations that Mickey would listen to her when told to do something. The therapist praised Ms. A for her increasing understanding of the PCIT principles, and agreed with her plan to lengthen the CDI sessions to 10 min in the morning temporarily, to help get Mickey off to a good start for the day. The discussion of the event with the father took more than the usual few minutes of checking on potential stressors allocated in sessions, but the therapist made certain to preserve enough session time to provide coaching and to end the session with positive feedback for Ms. A's strong CDI and PDI skills.

Ms. A returned to PDI Coach 7 reporting that she had practiced consistently, using extra CDI time, and that Mickey seemed back on track with minding. However, he was still easily irritated with Sascha and would push or hit her if she got close to his things. The therapist determined that this was an appropriate point in treatment to introduce the House Rule procedure, and suggested that "no hitting or pushing" would be a good house rule for Mickey. After working out a detailed plan for Mickey, Ms. A wondered whether it was really fair not also to discipline Sascha when she provoked Mickey's hitting. She asked whether a 3-year-old was too young to have her own house rules. The therapist lauded Ms. A for her insightfulness and informed her that PCIT had been used successfully with children even younger than her daughter, but that before implementing house rules with Sascha, it would be important to have her learn the basic PDI procedure. Because Ms. A had already begun using CDI with her daughter, they decided to schedule a sibling session for PDI Coach 8.

The sibling session gave Ms. A the opportunity to practice PDI with Sascha when she grabbed toys from Mickey and refused to give them back when instructed. Mickey appeared pleased that Sascha was held to the same behavioral expectations he was, and he did not challenge his mother while his sister was in timeout. Ms. A was coached in alternating her

CDI "do" skills between the children, using direct commands to reign in potential aggressive behavior, and using labeled praises for cooperative behaviors. Ms. A was eager to add a brief practice time with both children to her homework sheet, and said she felt confident that she could manage sibling fighting that occurred in the future by making it a house rule for both children. The therapist reinforced her confidence by pointing out the many potential sibling conflicts she had averted on her own during coaching, and noted how her PCIT skills seemed to have become second nature. The therapist commented that treatment seemed very close to a successful conclusion.

At PDI Coach 9, the therapist looked at the completed ECBI in the waiting room and could tell it was likely in the range required for treatment completion, which she confirmed by quickly scoring it on the way to the playroom. The therapist began the session by coding the two parent–child interactions to be certain that Ms. A's skills were still at mastery, and then reviewed with Ms. A the charts graphing her weekly progress on the CDI and PDI skills and the weekly ECBI scores over the course of treatment. Ms. A reported that Mickey had received very good school–home notes all week, and Mickey proudly added that he hadn't hit Sascha – and that she wasn't grabbing his stuff. Ms A praised Mickey, and expressed delight with his rapid response to the house rule. She acknowledged that the children were both learning to play better together. The therapist asked Ms. A if she felt ready to manage things on her own. It was clear by Ms. A's confident demeanor that she was ready. The therapist and Ms. A spent some time talking about how Ms. A would handle new problems that might arise in the future. At the end of the session, Ms. A expressed pride in knowing how to handle unforeseen problem situations, and felt safe because she knew she could ask for additional help if she really needed it. The therapist congratulated her and Mickey for their great work together, and Mickey was pleased to get his own graduation ribbon. He and his mother were smiling as they waved goodbye on the way out.

CONCLUSIONS

This chapter has described parent–child interaction therapy for young children with conduct disorders and their families. Key elements of the treatment have been illustrated, such as involving the parents and child together in treatment, using assessment to guide the families' progress, actively coaching the parents in relationship and behavior change skills, and continuing treatment until the parents mastered the skills and their child's behavior was within the normal range. These treatment elements draw on both attachment and social learning principles to produce lasting improvements in the parent–child bond as well as reductions in the child's disruptive behavior.

Studies have been presented that document treatment efficacy and generalization of its effects across cultures, settings, and time, for the majority of families who complete treatment. Further research is needed to address the role of parent psychopathology on treatment adherence and to examine efficacy and cost effectiveness of PCIT in individual versus group modalities, to guide further dissemination of PCIT into community clinics. In view of the high risk of poor lifetime outcomes for young children with conduct disorders, the need for more effectiveness studies in real world settings is critical. Early intervention has the power to alter the dismal prognosis for these children; however, in disseminating PCIT to a wider range of mental health providers, we cannot overlook the need to ensure proper training and close adherence to essential treatment elements. This challenge – balancing the drive to assist families with the preservation of treatment integrity – demands further study of necessary treatment elements and the training resources necessary to become an effective PCIT therapist.

REFERENCES

Azar, S. T., & Wolfe, D. A. (1989). Child abuse and neglect. In E. J. Mash & R. A. Barkley (Eds.), *Treatment of childhood disorders* (pp. 451–489). New York: Guilford.

Bagner, D. M., & Eyberg, S. M. (2007). Parent–child interaction therapy for disruptive behavior in children with mental retardation: A randomized controlled trial. *Journal of Clinical Child and Adolescent Psychology, 36*, 418–429.

Baumrind, D. (1966). Effects of authoritative control on child behavior. *Child Development, 37*, 887–907.

Baumrind, D. (1991). The influence of parenting style on adolescent competence and substance use. *Journal of Early Adolescence, 11*, 56–96.

Boggs, S. R., Eyberg, S. M., Edwards, D., Rayfield, A., Jacobs, J., Bagner, D., et al. (2004). Outcomes of parent–child interaction therapy: A comparison of dropouts and treatment completers one to three years after treatment. *Child & Family Behavior Therapy, 26*(4), 1–22.

Brinkmeyer, M. Y. (2006). *Conduct disorder in young children: A comparison of clinical presentation and treatment outcome in preschoolers with conduct disorder versus oppositional defiant disorder. Unpublished Doctoral Dissertation.*. Gainesville, FL: University of Florida.

Campbell, S. B. (1997). Behavior problems in preschool children: Developmental and family issues. *Advances in Clinical Child Psychology, 19*, 1–26.

Chaffin, M., Silovsky, J.F., Funderburk, B., Valle, L.A., Brestan, E.V., et al. (2004). Parent–child interaction therapy with physically abusive parents: Efficacy for reducing future abuse reports. *Journal of Consulting and Clinical Psychology, 72*, 500–510.

Chase, R. M., & Eyberg, S. M. (2008). Clinical presentation and treatment outcome for children with comorbid externalizing and internalizing symptoms. *Journal of Anxiety Disorders, 22*, 273–282.

Choate, M., Pincus, D., Eyberg, S. M., & Barlow, D. (2005). Adapting parent–child interaction therapy for young children with separation anxiety disorder. *Cognitive and Behavioral Practice, 12*, 126–135.

Coie, J. D., Watt, N. F., West, S. G., Hawkins, J. D., Asarnow, J. R., Markman, H. J., et al. (1993). The science of prevention. A conceptual framework and some directions for a national research program. *American Psychologist, 48*, 1013–1022.

Dishion, T. J., & Patterson, G. R. (1992). Age effects in parent training outcome. *Behavior Therapy, 23*, 719–729.

Earls, F. (1980). Prevalence of behavior problems in 3-year-old children. A cross-national replication. *Archives of General Psychiatry, 37*, 1153–1157.

Eisenstadt, T. H., Eyberg, S. M., McNeil, C. B., Newcomb, K., & Funderburk, B. W. (1993). Parent–child interaction therapy with behavior problem children: Relative effectiveness of two stages and overall treatment outcome. *Journal of Clinical Child & Adolescent Psychology, 22*, 42–51.

Eyberg, S. M., Edwards, D., Boggs, S., & Foote, R. (1998). Maintaining the treatment effects of parent training: The role of booster sessions and other maintenance strategies. *Clinical Psychology: Science and Practice, 5*, 544–554.

Eyberg, S. M., Nelson, M. M., Duke, M., & Boggs, S. R. (2004). *Manual for the Dyadic Parent–Child Interaction Coding System* (3rd ed.). Retrieved January 4, 2009 from http://pcit.phhp.ufl.edu/Measures/DPICS%20Manual%20Draft%203.06.pdf

Eyberg, S. M., & Pincus, D. (1999). *Eyberg Child Behavior Inventory and Sutter–Eyberg Student Behavior Inventory – revised: Professional manual.* Odessa, FL: Psychological Assessment Resources.

Eyberg, S. M., Funderburk, B. W., Hembree-Kigin, T. L., McNeil, C. B., Querido, J. G., & Hood, K. (2001). Parent–child interaction therapy with behavior problem children: One and two year maintenance of treatment effects in the family. *Child & Family Behavior Therapy, 23*, 1–20.

Eyberg, S. M., Nelson, M. M., & Boggs, S. R. (2008). Evidence-based treatments for child and adolescent disruptive behavior disorders. *Journal of Clinical Child and Adolescent Psychology, 37*, 213–235.

Fernandez, M., & Eyberg, S. M. (2009). Predicting treatment and follow-up attrition in parent–child interaction therapy. *Journal of Abnormal Child Psychology, 37*, 431–441.

Fernandez, M., Butler, A. M., & Eyberg, S. M. (in press). Treatment Outcome for Low Socioeconomic Status African American Families in Parent–Child Interaction Therapy: A Pilot Study. *Child and Family Behavior Therapy.*

Floyd, E. (2005). *Treatment of oppositional defiant disorder in preschoolers with or without comorbid attention deficit hyperactivity disorder. Unpublished Doctoral Dissertation.*. Florida: University of Florida.

Guerney, B. G., Jr. (1964). Filial therapy: Description and rationale. *Journal of Consulting and Clinical Psychology, 28*, 304–310.

Hood, K., & Eyberg, S. M. (2003). Outcomes of parent–child interaction therapy: Mothers' reports on maintenance three to six years after treatment. *Journal of Clinical Child and Adolescent Psychology, 32*, 419–429.

Jacobs, J. R., Boggs, S. R., Eyberg, S. M., Edwards, D., Durning, P., Querido, J. G., et al. (2000). Psychometric properties and reference point data for the Revised Edition of the School Observation Coding System. *Behavior Therapy, 31*, 695–712.

Leung, C., Tsang, S., Heung, K., & Yiu, I. (2009). Effectiveness of parent–child interaction therapy (PCIT) among Chinese families. *Research on Social Work Practice, 19*, 304–313. doi: 10.1177/1049731508321713

Loeber, R., Burke, J. D., Lahey, B. B., Winters, A., & Zera, M. (2000). Oppositional defiant and conduct disorder: A review of the past 10 years, part I. *Journal of the American Academy of Child & Adolescent Psychiatry, 39*, 1468–1484.

Loeber, R., & Dishion, T. (1983). Early predictors of male delinquency: A review. *Psychological Bulletin, 94*, 68–99.

Matos, M., Bauermeister, J. J., & Bernal, G. (2009). Parent–child interaction therapy for Puerto Rican preschool children with ADHD and behavior problems: A pilot efficacy study. *Family Process, 48*, 232-252. doi: 10.1111/j.1545-5300.2009.01279.x.

McCabe, K. M., & Yeh, M. (2009). Parent-child interaction therapy for Mexican Americans: A randomized clinical trial. *Journal of Clinical Child & Adolescent Psychology, 38*, 753–759.

Niec, L. N., Hemme, J. M., Yopp, J. M., & Brestan, E. V. (2005). Parent–child interaction therapy: The rewards and challenges of a group format. *Cognitive and Behavioral Practice, 12*, 113–125.

Nixon, R. D. V., Sweeney, L., Erickson, D. B., & Touyz, S. W. (2003). Parent–Child Interaction Therapy: A comparison of standard and abbreviated treatments for oppositional defiant preschoolers. *Journal of Consulting and Clinical Psychology, 71*, 251–260.

Olweus, D. (1979). Stability of aggressive reaction patterns in males: A review. *Psychological Bulletin, 86*, 852–875.

Patterson, G. R. (1974). Interventions for boys with conduct problems: Multiple settings, treatments, and criteria. *Journal of Consulting and Clinical Psychology, 42*, 471–481.

Patterson, G. R. (1982). *A social learning approach to family intervention. III. Coercive family process.* Eugene, OR: Castalia.

Phillips, J., Morgan, S., Cawthorne, K., & Barnett, B. (2008). Pilot evaluation of Parent–Child Interaction Therapy delivered in an Australian community early childhood clinic setting. *Australian and New Zealand Journal of Psychiatry, 42*, 712–719.

Pincus, D. B., Santucci, L. C., Ehrenreich, J. T., & Eyberg, S. M. (2008). The implementation of modified parent–child interaction therapy for youth with separation anxiety disorder. *Cognitive and Behavioral Practice, 15*, 118–125.

Querido, J. G., Warner, T. D., & Eyberg, S. M. (2002). The cultural context of parenting: An assessment of parenting styles in African American families. *Journal of Clinical Child and Adolescent Psychology, 31*, 272–277.

Reid, M. J., Webster-Stratton, C., & Hammond, M. (2003). Follow-up of children who received the Incredible Years intervention for oppositional defiant disorder. *Behavior Therapy, 42*, 471–491.

Schuhmann, E. M., Foote, R., Eyberg, S. M., Boggs, S., & Algina, J. (1998). Parent–child interaction therapy: Interim report of a randomized trial with short-term maintenance. *Journal of Clinical Child Psychology, 27*, 34–45.

Webster-Stratton, C., & Herbert, M. (1994). *Troubled families – problem children*. Chichester: Wiley.

Werba, B. E., Eyberg, S. M., Boggs, S. R., & Algina, J. (2006). Predicting outcome in parent–child interaction therapy: Success and attrition. *Behavior Modification, 30*, 618–646.

White, J., Moffitt, T. E., Earls, F., Robins, L. N., & Silva, P. A. (1990). How early can we tell? Preschool predictors of boys' conduct disorder and delinquency. *Criminology, 28*, 507–528.

Wierzbicki, M., & Pekarik, G. (1993). A meta-analysis of psychotherapy dropout. *Professional Psychology: Research & Practice, 24*, 190–195.

7

Parent Training for the Treatment of Oppositional Behavior in Young Children: Helping the Noncompliant Child

ROBERT J. McMAHON, NICHOLAS LONG, and REX L. FOREHAND

CONCEPTUAL MODEL/OVERVIEW OF PROGRAM

Noncompliance (i.e., excessive disobedience to adults) is consistently reported to be the most prevalent behavior problem for clinic-referred and non-referred "normal" children alike, and is currently viewed as a keystone behavior in the development and maintenance of conduct disorders. "Helping the Noncompliant Child" (HNC) (Forehand & McMahon, 1981; McMahon & Forehand, 2003) is based on a parent training program originally developed by Hanf at the University of Oregon Medical School in the late 1960s (e.g., Hanf & Kling, 1973) to treat noncompliance in young (3–8 years of age) children with a range of developmental disabilities (see Reitman & McMahon, 2010). While several independent groups of clinical

ROBERT J. McMAHON • University of Washington
NICHOLAS LONG • University of Arkansas for Medical Sciences
REX L. FOREHAND • University of Vermont

R.C. Murrihy et al. (eds.), *Clinical Handbook of Assessing and Treating Conduct Problems in Youth*, DOI 10.1007/978-1-4419-6297-3_7,

researchers have adapted Hanf's original program, the adaptation by the current authors (Forehand & McMahon, 1981; McMahon & Forehand, 2003) is one of the most formally operationalized and evaluated versions of this approach to working with young children with conduct problems. The purpose of this chapter is to provide a description of the theoretical assumptions that underlie HNC, an overview of the program, and a summary of its empirical support. We also provide a description of a typical HNC case, and conclude with remarks concerning future directions.

Longitudinal studies have shown that there are multiple pathways that lead to the development of conduct problems (e.g., Moffitt, 1993, see Chap. 3). The "early-starter" (Patterson, Capaldi, & Bank, 1991) pathway is characterized by the onset of conduct problems in the preschool and early school-age years, and by a high degree of continuity throughout childhood and into adolescence and adulthood. It is thought that these children progress from relatively less serious (e.g., noncompliance, temper tantrums) to more serious (e.g., aggression, stealing, substance abuse) conduct problem behaviors over time; that overt behaviors (e.g., defiance, fighting) appear earlier than covert behaviors (e.g., lying, stealing); and that later conduct problem behaviors expand the children's behavioral repertoire rather than replace earlier behaviors (e.g., McMahon, Wells, & Kotler, 2006; Patterson, Reid, & Dishion, 1992). Furthermore, there is an expansion of the settings in which the conduct problem behaviors occur over time, from the home to other settings such as the school and the broader community.

The primary role of family socialization processes in the development of the early-starter pathway has been described and empirically demonstrated by Patterson and his colleagues (e.g., Chamberlain & Patterson, 1995; Patterson, 1982; Patterson et al., 1992). Patterson emphasizes the coercive, or controlling, nature of conduct problem behaviors and has developed the coercion model to account for their development and maintenance (see Fig. 7.1 for an example). The model describes a process of "basic training" in conduct problem behaviors that occurs in the context of an escalating cycle of coercive parent–child interactions in the home that begins prior to school entry. The proximal cause for entry into the coercive cycle is thought to be ineffective parental management strategies, particularly in regard to child compliance with parental commands or instructions during the preschool period. As this process continues over long periods, significant increases in the rate and intensity of these coercive behaviors occur as family members are reinforced by engaging in aggressive behaviors, which temporarily decrease or even appear to halt the child's inappropriate behaviors. Furthermore, the child also observes his or her parents engaging in coercive responses, and this provides the opportunity for modeling of aggression to occur over time (Patterson, 1982).

Upon school entry, the child's coercive style of interaction is likely to extend to interactions with teachers and peers, resulting in frequent disciplinary confrontations with school personnel, rejection by peers, and continued coercive interchanges with parents (e.g., Patterson et al., 1992). By age 10 or 11, this recurrent constellation of negative events places the child at increased risk for association with deviant peer groups

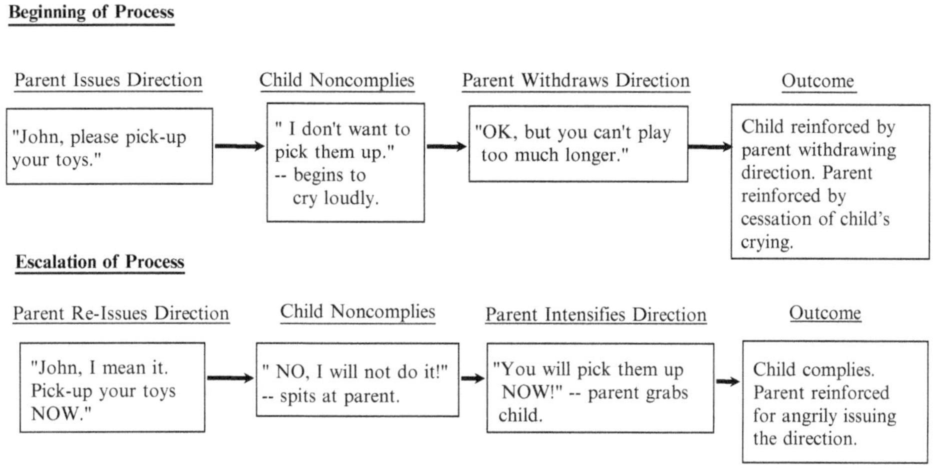

Fig. 7.1. The coercive process between a parent and child. From Forehand, R., & Long, N. (2002). *Parenting the strong-willed child: The clinically-proven five-week program for parents of two-to six-year-olds* (2nd ed.), New York: McGraw-Hill.

in middle school and high school (with a likely escalation in conduct problem behaviors). Adolescents who have progressed along the early-starter pathway are not only at significant risk for continuing to engage in more serious conduct problem behaviors throughout adolescence (e.g., delinquency, substance abuse) and into early adulthood, but as adults they are also at increased risk for other psychiatric diagnoses and a variety of negative life outcomes (e.g., lower occupational adjustment and educational attainment, poorer physical health) (e.g., Farrington, 2003; Kratzer & Hodgins, 1997).

Noncompliance appears to be a keystone behavior in the development of conduct problems. It appears early in the progression of conduct problems and continues to be manifested in subsequent developmental periods (e.g., Chamberlain & Patterson, 1995), playing a role in later academic and peer relationship problems. Low levels of compliance are also associated with referral for mental health services in children with conduct problems (Dumas, 1996). Furthermore, intervention research has shown that when child noncompliance is targeted, there is often concomitant improvement in other conduct problem behaviors as well (Russo, Cataldo, & Cushing, 1981; Wells, Forehand, & Griest, 1980). All of these findings support the key role that noncompliance plays in conduct problems.

Because of the significant role of early parent–child interaction in the development of conduct problems, family-based interventions have been widely employed. Such approaches have typically been based on a social learning-based "parent training" model of intervention (e.g., Miller & Prinz, 1990). The underlying assumption of this model is that a parenting skills deficit has been at least partly responsible for the development and/or maintenance of the conduct problem behaviors. This type of intervention has been shown to be very effective in working with this population (e.g., Maughan, Christiansen, Jenson, Olympia, & Clark, 2005; McMahon, 2006). Furthermore, parent training may have significant preventive effects, especially if it is applied during the preschool period (e.g., Reid, 1993), or is a component of broader preventive interventions for school-age children at risk of conduct problems (e.g., Conduct Problems Prevention Research Group, 1992).

DESCRIPTION OF HNC

Objectives

The long-term goals of HNC are the secondary prevention of serious conduct problems in preschool and early elementary school-aged children and the primary prevention of subsequent juvenile delinquency and related problems (e.g., substance use, school dropout). Consistent with the developmental and social-learning based assumptions on which HNC is predicated, the short-term and intermediate objectives include: (a) disruption of the coercive style of parent–child interaction which characterizes these families and the establishment of more positive, prosocial interaction patterns; (b) improved parenting skills in terms of more accurate tracking and attending to the child's appropriate behavior, increased use of praise and other positive verbal statements to the child, ignoring of minor inappropriate child behaviors, provision of clear and appropriate instructions to the child, and provision of appropriate consequences for child compliance, noncompliance, and other behaviors; and (c) increased child prosocial behaviors and decreased conduct problem behaviors, especially noncompliance. It has been shown that increased compliance to parental instructions results in a decrease in other conduct problem behaviors such as physical and verbal aggression, temper tantrums, and inappropriate talk (e.g., sassiness); furthermore, children's competencies increase as they learn more prosocial ways of interacting with their parents, siblings, teachers, and peers (McMahon & Forehand, 2003).

Targeted Population

HNC is designed for parents and their 3–8-year-old children who are demonstrating noncompliance and other conduct problems. There are no specific inclusion or exclusion criteria for parent participation. Involvement of both mothers and fathers is actively encouraged, but participation by both parents is not mandatory. While families from lower socioeconomic backgrounds are more likely to drop out than other families (McMahon, Forehand, Griest, & Wells, 1981), HNC is as effective with lower socioeconomic families who complete the program as it is for families in other socioeconomic brackets (Rogers, Forehand, Griest, Wells, & McMahon, 1981).

Although HNC has been most extensively evaluated with populations of children with conduct problems, it has also been successfully adapted and employed with several other high-risk populations of children and parents, including children with developmental disabilities (Breiner, 1989; Breiner & Forehand, 1982; Forehand, Cheney, & Yoder, 1974; Hanf & Kling, 1973), children with attention-deficit/hyperactivity disorder (ADHD; e.g., Long, Rickert, & Ashcraft, 1993; Pisterman et al., 1989), as a component of interventions for mothers at risk for child abuse and neglect (e.g., Lutzker, 1984; Wolfe, Edwards, Manion, & Koverola, 1988), and as a preventive intervention for children of substance abusing parents of various ethnicities (Kumpfer & DeMarsh, 1987; Kumpfer, Molgaard, & Spoth, 1996). In addition, HNC may be beneficial as part of a broader treatment plan when working with children who (a) are enuretic or encopretic, (b) fail to adhere to medical regimens, and (c) are hospitalized in inpatient psychiatric units (see Wells, 2003). Portions of HNC have been successfully adapted for the parent group component of the Fast Track program (Conduct Problems Prevention Research Group, 1992; McMahon, Slough, & the Conduct Problems Prevention Research Group, 1996) and the Multimodal Treatment Study for ADHD (MTA; Wells et al., 2000). Fast Track and the MTA are large, multisite studies that investigated the effectiveness of multicomponent interventions (both of which included parent training) for preventing the development of serious conduct problems in young at-risk school-aged children and children with ADHD, respectively.

HNC is best suited for indicated (i.e., manifest conduct problems) and selected (i.e., at-risk) populations. Reducing child noncompliance and other conduct problems and improving parent–child interactions are important because of their immediate effects on the family (indicated) and for reducing the risk for the development of more serious forms of conduct problems in later childhood and adolescence (selected).

Assessment

An important aspect of HNC is a thorough assessment of the parent–child relationship (McMahon & Forehand, 2003). The multimethod assessment process used to accomplish this consists of an interview, observations of parent and child interactions, questionnaires completed by the parent, and parent-recorded data. Daily situations, which frequently are problematic for noncompliant children, are assessed during the interview (e.g., going to bed at night, taking a bath, disrupting the parent during a telephone conversation). If a parent experiences a problem in any area, a detailed description is requested regarding how he or she handles the situation, how the child responds, and how often the problem occurs.

After the interview, which typically lasts 45 min, the parent and child are observed in two structured toy play situations, labeled "Child's Game" and "Parent's Game." These observations last from 5 to 10 min each. The Child's Game consists of a parent following rules and activities determined by the child; The Parent's Game requires the parent to engage the child in activities according to rules of the parent's choosing. These brief interactions give the clinician an idea of how the parent and child interact. (When feasible, observational data can also be collected in the home setting, preferably at a time when child problem behaviors typically occur.)

The questionnaires focus on the parents' report of the child's functioning (e.g., Achenbach and Rescorla's [2000, 2001] Child Behavior Checklist) and on the parents' personal and marital functioning (e.g., Beck, Steer, & Brown's [1996] Beck Depression Inventory-II; Porter & O'Leary, 1980 O'Leary-Porter Scale). Questionnaires can identify problems that the therapist may have inadvertently missed during the interview, as well as supplemental information gained from the interview, observations, and parent-recorded data. Furthermore, the questionnaires that address parental functioning can identify problems causing severe distress that may impede parents' implementation of the parenting program.

Finally, parents identify the three child behaviors that are of greatest concern and record their occurrence for 4 consecutive days. This provides specific information concerning the frequency of various problematic child behaviors in the home setting. If the initial assessment indicates that child behavior problems are also occurring in the preschool or school setting, then similar methods are used to gather information from that setting to determine whether school-based intervention is also warranted.

With the information gathered from interviews, observations, questionnaires, and parent-recorded data, the therapist can re-examine the following issues: Is child noncompliance in multiple situations the primary issue? Can parenting practices be modified to influence the child's behavior? Is family stress, other than that caused by the child's behavior, relatively low, or addressable through other interventions? If the answer to each of these questions is yes, then HNC is a reasonable choice for intervention.

In our experience, there are some situations in which HNC is contraindicated. For example, HNC may not be appropriate for some children with disorders on the autism spectrum since this parenting intervention relies upon parental attention to help change behavior. If such attention is aversive to the child, then HNC (in its complete package) is probably not an appropriate intervention. Parental psychosis, other serious mental illnesses, and/or significant substance use problems that are not being effectively treated may preclude successful involvement in HNC if they interfere with the parent's ability to follow through with this intervention.

Format

The primary format for HNC is sessions conducted by a therapist with the parent(s) and child. We employ a controlled learning environment in which to teach the parent to change maladaptive patterns of interaction with the child. Sessions are typically conducted with individual families rather than in groups, although the program has been adapted for use in a group format (e.g., Baum, Reyna-McGlone, & Ollendick, 1986; Conners, Edwards, & Grant, 2007; Long & Forehand, 2000a, 2000b; McMahon et al., 1996; Pisterman et al., 1989) as well as a self-directed format (e.g., Forehand & Long, 2010; Long et al., 1993). Ideally, intervention occurs in playrooms equipped with one-way mirrors for observation, sound systems, and unobtrusive one-way radio devices (e.g., "bug-in-the-ear") by which the therapist can communicate unobtrusively with the parent; however, these accouterments are *not* necessary for the successful implementation of HNC.

The number of sessions necessary for the completion of each phase of HNC depends upon the speed with which the parent demonstrates competence in the skills being taught and the child's response to this intervention. The mean number of sessions necessary to complete HNC has been approximately 8–10 sessions, with a range of 5–14 sessions. Sessions are typically held once or twice per week, and each session is 75–90 min in length.

Session Content

After completion of the assessment, the therapist presents a conceptualization of the child's noncompliance and other conduct problems in the context of Patterson's (1982) coercion theory and presents the rationale for HNC (e.g., the role of parent–child interaction in the development and maintenance of the conduct problems; the focus on changing child noncompliance). An overview of the content (i.e., the various parenting skills) and the process (e.g., the use of didactic instruction, modeling, rehearsal, practice with the child in session and in the home, behavioral criteria) of the program is then presented.

HNC consists of two phases. In each phase, a series of parenting skills are taught in a sequential manner. During the Differential Attention phase (Phase I), the parent learns to increase the frequency and range of social attention to the child and reduce the frequency of competing verbal behavior. A major goal is to break out of the coercive cycle by establishing a positive, mutually reinforcing relationship between the parent and child.

The parent is first taught to attend to and describe the child's appropriate behavior (Attends) while eliminating commands, questions, and criticisms. The second segment of Phase I consists of teaching the parent to use verbal (e.g., praise) and physical (e.g., hugs) attention contingent upon appropriate behaviors (Rewards) and to actively ignore minor inappropriate behaviors (Ignoring). The parent then learns to develop programs to simultaneously increase desirable child behaviors and decrease less appropriate competing behaviors through the systematic use of contingent attention and ignoring (i.e., differential attention). (See Table 7.1 for a description of Phase I parenting skills.)

In Phase II of HNC (Compliance Training), the primary parenting skills are taught in the context of the Clear Instructions Sequence (see Fig. 7.2). The Clear Instructions Sequence consists of three paths. The therapist first teaches the parent to use appropriate commands (Clear Instructions) to increase the likelihood of child compliance. The parent is taught to give direct, concise instructions one at a time, and to allow the child sufficient time to comply (see Table 7.2). If compliance is initiated within 5 s of the clear instruction, the parent is taught to praise or attend to the child within 5 s of the compliance initiation (Path A). If compliance is not initiated, then the parent gives the child a warning ("If you don't ..., then you will have to go to time out."). If the child initiates compliance within 5 s, the parent praises and attends to the child (Path B). However, if the child does not comply with the warning, then the parent is taught to implement a brief time-out procedure that involves placing the child in a chair for

Table 7.1. Phase 1 skills (Adapted from McMahon & Forehand, 2003)

The skill of attending

- Follows, rather than leads, the child's activity (by a running verbal commentary)
- Used to acknowledge and reinforce appropriate behaviors
  - Two basic types
  - Describe overt behavior ("You just put the red block on top of the green block")
  - Emphasize desired prosocial behavior ("You're talking in a regular voice")
- "Volume control" feature allows parent to raise or lower the intensity and frequency of the positive attention
- Do *not*:
  - Ask questions
  - Give commands
  - Try to teach

The skill of rewarding

- Three types
  - Physical rewards (e.g., hug, kiss, pat on the back)
  - Unlabeled verbal rewards (e.g., "Great!" "Nice job!")
  - Labeled verbal rewards (e.g., "Thank you for picking up the toys like I asked")
- Guidelines for using rewards
  - Be specific
  - Give immediately
  - Focus on improvement
  - Use consistently

The skill of ignoring

- Attention-seeking behaviors (e.g., whining, nagging, temper tantrums, interrupting) can be ignored. Behaviors that are potentially harmful to people or property (e.g., fighting) should *not* be ignored
- Ignoring is an active process
  - Decide ahead of time which inappropriate behaviors to ignore
  - When ignoring, actively avoid giving attention to the child
- Three components:
  - No eye contact or nonverbal cues ("Don't look!")
  - No verbal contact ("Don't talk!")
  - No physical contact ("Don't touch!")
- Ignoring *starts* as soon as inappropriate behavior begins. Ignoring *stops* soon after (10–15 s) the inappropriate behavior ceases
- The inappropriate behavior must be ignored *every* time that it occurs; otherwise the behavior will get worse instead of better
  - Ignoring is never used alone. It always should be combined with positive attention (attends and rewards) for the alternative appropriate behavior

From McMahon, R.J., & Forehand, R.L. (2003). *Helping the noncompliant child: Family-based treatment for oppositional behavior* (2nd ed.). New York: Guilford Press. Reprinted with permission.

3 min (Path C) (see Table 7.3). If the child does not remain in the chair, then one or more back-up procedures are used, including additional time, response cost, and/or removal to a different room. Following time out, the command that originally elicited noncompliance is repeated. Compliance (Path A) is followed by contingent attention from the parent. Noncompliance is followed by implementation of Path B, and if necessary, Path C.

When using the Clear Instructions Sequence successfully at home, the parent is taught to use Standing Rules as a supplement to this sequence. Standing Rules are "if... then" statements ("If you hit your brother, then you must go to time out.") that, once stated and explained to the child, are permanently in effect. Because Standing Rules provide an immediate

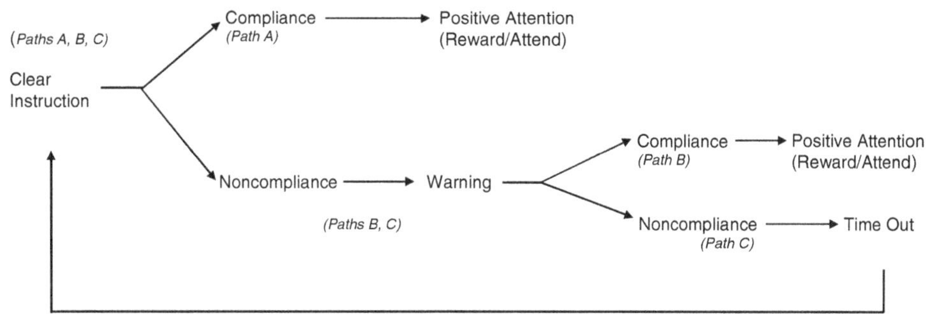

Fig. 7.2. Flowchart of the Clear Instructions Sequence. From McMahon, R.J., & Forehand, R.L. (2003). *Helping the noncompliant child: Family-based treatment for oppositional behavior* (2nd ed.). New York: Guilford Press. Reprinted with permission.

Table 7.2. Clear instructions (From McMahon & Forehand, 2003)

How to give clear instructions

- Get child's attention
  - Move close
  - Say the child's name (maximum of two times)
  - Establish eye contact
- State the instruction clearly
  - Give one instruction at a time
  - Use firm voice
  - Phrase as "do" command
  - Use simple language
  - Use gestures as appropriate
  - Rationale (if given) *precedes* the clear instruction
- Wait 5 s
  - Count silently
  - No verbalization to child

From McMahon, R.J., & Forehand, R.L. (2003). *Helping the noncompliant child: Family-based treatment for oppositional behavior* (2nd ed.). New York: Guilford Press. Reprinted with permission.

consequence for the child's inappropriate behavior, they can be particularly useful for situations in which there is a danger to the child, someone else, or property. Finally, the therapist teaches the parent to implement the Phase I and Phase II parenting skills in situations outside the home (e.g., riding in the car, shopping, visiting others). Although booster sessions are not a formal part of HNC, many clinicians have found it helpful to schedule at least one follow-up booster session 1–2 months after the last regular treatment session.

Adjuncts to the basic HNC program have been developed for teaching maternal self-control procedures (Wells, Griest, & Forehand, 1980); the social learning procedures underlying the parent training program (McMahon, Forehand, & Griest, 1981); and procedures to enhance general family functioning, especially with regard to developmentally appropriate parental perceptions of the child's behavior, marital adjustment, parental personal adjustment, and the parents' extrafamilial relationships

Table 7.3. The Clear Instructions Sequence (From McMahon & Forehand, 2003)

The Clear Instructions Sequence for noncompliance

- Issue a single clear instruction (e.g., "Please pick-up your toys now")
- If the child initiates compliance to the clear instruction within 5 s, provide positive attention (i.e., rewards, attends) (e.g., "Thank you so much for playing quietly. I really appreciate it when you do what I ask.") (Path A)
- If the child does *not* initiate compliance to the clear instruction within 5 s, issue a warning: "If you do not [blank], you will have to go to time out"
- If the child initiates compliance to the warning within 5 s, provide positive attention (i.e., rewards, attends) (Path B)
- If the child does *not* initiate compliance to the warning within 5 s, lead the child to the time-out chair without lecturing, scolding, or arguing (Path C)
- Tell the child: "Because you did not [blank], you have to sit in the chair until I say you can get up"
- Ignore the child's shouting, protesting, and promises to comply
- Leave child in time out for 3 min (including being quiet for the last 15 s)
- When the time out is completed, remove the child from the chair and return to the situation that elicited noncompliance
- Restate the original clear instruction
- Follow the clear instructions sequence (positive attention for complying with your instruction; warning and time out as necessary)

From McMahon, R.J., & Forehand, R.L. (2003). *Helping the noncompliant child: Family-based treatment for oppositional behavior* (2nd ed.). New York: Guilford Press. Reprinted with permission.

(Griest et al., 1982). Instruction in these adjunctive procedures can be integrated into the basic parent training program or, in the case of the maternal self-control procedures, immediately following completion of the parent training program.

Teaching Methods

HNC is an active intervention that places substantial emphasis on helping the parent to become competent and comfortable with the various parenting skills taught in the program. For each skill, the following procedures are used:

1. The procedure and rationale for each skill are explained, and the underlying social learning principles on which the skill is based are briefly presented.
2. The therapist demonstrates the skill via modeling and role playing.
3. The parent practices the skills with the therapist, who role plays the child.
4. The child is taught the procedure. First, a developmentally appropriate explanation of the procedure is given to the child by the parent and therapist. The child repeats the procedure verbally and participates in role plays of situations involving the procedure.
5. The parent practices with the child in the intervention setting. The therapist observes and coaches.
6. The parent practices with the child in the intervention setting but without ongoing feedback from the therapist.
7. Specific homework is assigned to practice the skills on a daily basis at home, both in structured practice sessions with the child and,

as the parent progresses through the program, at various times throughout the day (e.g., in Phase I, the parent develops programs to increase at least three child behaviors using the new skills).

8. Parents are given handouts specific to each parenting skill for reference in the home setting, and data sheets to record practice sessions and use of the new parenting skills in the home.

An optional activity (that has not been part of the formal evaluation studies) is referring parents to relevant sections of the self-guided program for parents presented in Forehand and Long (2010) (see below).

Progression to each new skill in HNC is determined by the use of behavioral and temporal (number of sessions) criteria. The therapist uses observational data collected during each session to determine whether the parent–child pair has attained the behavioral criteria necessary for movement to the next step of the program. The behavioral criteria ensure that the parent has attained an acceptable degree of competence in a particular skill before being taught additional parenting techniques. This is critical since the parenting skills build on one another. In addition, these criteria allow for the individualization of HNC by allocating training time more efficiently since they allow the therapist to concentrate his or her attention on the more serious parenting skill deficiencies. Because HNC is typically conducted with individual families and because of the competency-based approach to intervention, there is ample opportunity for family members to discuss other issues of personal concern.

Staffing

A single therapist per family is sufficient to conduct HNC successfully. However, if resources permit, use of a co-therapist can increase the therapist's flexibility in demonstrating various skills to the parent (e.g., the therapist role-plays the parent while the co-therapist role-plays the child), and can serve as a useful in vivo training experience for new therapists.

Evaluations of the HNC program have been based on implementation by individuals with at least a bachelor's degree in psychology, most typically clinical psychology graduate students. Implementation by others may be appropriate with adequate training and supervision. Ideally, the therapist should have a background in psychology or education, and should be familiar with social learning principles and their application to child behavior.

Program Materials

A comprehensive presentation of the theoretical assumptions; assessment procedures; format, content, and teaching methods; and empirical support for HNC is contained in the therapist's manual (*Helping the Noncompliant Child: Family-Based Treatment for Oppositional Behavior*; McMahon & Forehand, 2003). This manual, available from Guilford Press (www.guilford.com), also contains copies of program-specific assessment materials, parent handouts, and charts. A 70 min videotape (Forehand, Armistead, Neighbors, & Klein, 1994) that portrays the intervention procedures employed in the program is available for training therapists from ChildFocus (500 Crosswind Drive, Charlotte, VT 05445). A supplemental self-help book for parents that employs similar skills and teaching techniques (*Parenting the Strong-Willed Child*; Forehand & Long, 2010) is available from McGraw-Hill (http://books.mcgraw-hill.com). A leader's guide for a 6-week parenting class curriculum program (*Parenting the Strong-Willed Child* (*PSWC*); Long & Forehand, 2000a), based on the Forehand and Long (2010) book, is available from Dr. Nicholas Long, UAMS Department of Pediatrics, Slot 512-21, 1 Children's Way, Little Rock, AR 72202.

EMPIRICAL SUPPORT

HNC has been extensively evaluated. See Table 7.4 for a listing of evaluation studies concerning outcome and generalization. The following section summarizes this body of research (also see McMahon & Forehand, 2003, Chap. 10, for a more detailed summary).

Research Design/Sampling Strategy Used to Evaluate HNC

The samples of children who participated in evaluations of the different aspects of HNC were referred to outpatient mental health clinics for excessive levels of noncompliance and other conduct problem behaviors. Various designs have been employed to examine different questions related to the outcome, generalization, and social validity of HNC. Comparison conditions that have been employed in these studies include waiting-list control (Peed, Roberts, & Forehand, 1977), non-referred "normal" samples (e.g., Wells, Forehand, & Griest, 1980), variations of the basic parent training program including component analyses (e.g., McMahon, Forehand, & Griest, 1981), and alternative interventions (Baum et al., 1986; Long et al., 1993; Wells & Egan, 1988). Excluding studies employing single-subject designs, sample sizes with clinic-referred or risk samples have ranged from 8 to 71 families. Attrition has been minimal in the treatment outcome studies at post-intervention assessments (i.e., <20% dropout; Furey & Basili, 1988; McMahon, Forehand, Griest, & Wells, 1981). However, it was significantly higher (38–50%) in three longer-term (8 months; 4.5–10.5 years; 14 years) follow-up studies (Forehand & Long, 1988; Griest, Forehand, & Wells, 1981; Long, Forehand, Wierson, & Morgan, 1994). Studies of component analyses of HNC usually involved non-referred samples of children and/or parents. (See McMahon & Forehand, 2003, Chap. 10, for a description of these studies.)

Outcome Measures

Two primary types of measures have been employed in the outcome evaluation studies: direct observation and parent-report measures. These measures have been collected immediately prior to and after the intervention, as well as at various follow-up assessments. With respect to direct observation, trained observers collected these data in the home

Table 7.4. Outcome-related investigations of HNC (Adapted and expanded from McMahon & Forehand, 2003)

Study	Sample size	Comparison/ control group	Outcome data	Follow-up	Focus	Miscellaneous
Immediate outcome						
Forehand & King (1974)	8	–	CO	–	Clinic outcome	
Forehand & King (1977)	22	NON	CO, Q	3 months	Clinic outcome	
Breiner & Forehand (1982)	10	ATT	HO, PR, Q	–	Developmentally disabled sample	
Conners, Edwards, & Grant (2007)	71	–	Q	6 months	Head Start sample	
Forehand et al. (1974)	1	–	CO, Q	3 months	Case study of developmentally disabled child	
Generalization/social validity						
Peed et al. (1977)	12	WLC	CO, HO, Q	–	Home generalization	
Forehand, Griest, & Wells (1979)	20	–	HO, PR, Q	–	Home generalization	Relationship of multiple outcome measures
Rogers, Forehand, Griest, Wells, & McMahon (1981)	31	–	HO, Q	–	Home generalization	SES
McMahon, Forehand, & Tiedemann (1985)	55	Different age groups	HO, Q	2 months	Home generalization	Child age
Breiner & Forehand (1981)	32	NON	HO, SO	–	School generalization	
Forehand, Sturgis, et al. (1979) – Study 2	16	NON	HO, SO, Q	–	School generalization	
Forehand, Breiner, McMahon, & Davies (1981)	16	–	HO, SO	–	Prediction of cross-setting change in school behavior	
Forehand, Sturgis, et al. (1979) – Study 1	11	–	HO, Q	6 and 12 months	Temporal generalization	
Baum & Forehand (1981)	34	–	HO, Q	1–4.5 years	Temporal generalization, social validity	
Forehand, Rogers, McMahon, Wells, & Griest (1981)	18	–	HO, Q	8 months	Temporal generalization	

(continued)

Table 7.4 (continued)

Study	Sample size	Comparison/ control group	Outcome data	Follow-up	Focus	Miscellaneous
Forehand, Steffe, Furey, & Walley (1983)	34	–	Q	11–86 months (3.6 years)	Temporal generalization	
Forehand & Long (1988)	42	NON	CO, Q (P,T,C)	4.5–10.5 years (7.5 years)	Temporal generalization, social validity	
Long, Forehand, Wierson, & Morgan (1994)	52	NON	Q (P,C)	≥14 years	Temporal generalization	
Humphreys, Forehand, McMahon, & Roberts (1978)	8	–	HO	–	Sibling generalization	
Wells, Forehand, & Griest (1980)	24	NON	HO	–	Behavioral generalization	
Forehand, Wells, & Griest (1980)	30	NON	HO, Q	2 and 15 months[a]	Social validity, positive side effects	
Cross Calvert & McMahon (1987)	90 mothers	PTA, PR, PRM	Q	–	Social validity	Nonreferred sample
McMahon, Johnson, & Robbins (2010)	96 students, 57 mothers	TAD, WI, TAD + WI	Q	–	Social validity	Nonreferred samples
McMahon, Tiedemann, Forehand, & Griest (1984)	20	TA, SL	Q	2 months	Social validity	
Positive side effects						
Brody & Forehand (1985)	24	MD, non-MD	HO, Q	–	Marital satisfaction	
Forehand, Griest, Wells, & McMahon (1982)	27	High, medium, low marital satisfaction	HO, Q	2 months	Marital satisfaction	
Roberts, Joe, & Rowe-Hallbert (1992) – Study 3	39	–	Q	–	Parenting locus of control	
Enhancement of generalization						
Wells, Griest, & Forehand (1980)	16	PTA, PT + SC	HO, PR	2 months	Maternal self-control adjunct	
McMahon, Forehand, & Griest (1981)	20	TA, SL	HO, Q	2 months	Social learning principles adjunct	
Griest et al. (1982)	32	PTA, PET, NON	HO, Q	2 months	PET adjunct	

Self-administered interventions						
McMahon & Forehand (1978)	3	Multiple baseline across subjects	HO	6 weeks	Self-administered	Mealtime behavior
McMahon & Lehman (2010)	40	TAD, WI, TAD+WI, NTC	CO, Q	–	Self-administered/clear instructions	Nonreferred sample
Long, Rickert, & Ashcraft (1993)	32	WI+meds, meds	Q (P,T)	–	Self-administered	Children with ADHD
Comparisons with other interventions						
Wells & Egan (1988)	19	PTA, SFT	CO, Q	–	Comparative	
Baum, Reyna McGlone, & Ollendick (1986)	34	PT+CSC, PT+C-ATT, STEP+C-ATT	CO, Q (P,C)	6–8 months	Comparative	
Prediction of dropout/follow-up participation						
McMahon, Forehand, Griest, & Wells (1981)	48	–	HO, Q	–	Dropout	
Furey & Basili (1988)	53	–	HO, Q	–	Dropout	
Griest, Forehand, & Wells (1981)	16	–	HO, Q	8 months	Participation in follow-up	

Note. Sample size is total. *Control/comparison group:* NON, nonreferred; ATT, attention control; WLC, waiting-list control; PTA, parent training alone; PR, parent training plus verbal rationale; PRM, parent training plus verbal rationale and modeling; TAD, therapist administered; WI, written instructions; TAD+WI, therapist administration plus written instructions; TA, technique alone; SL, social learning principles adjunct; MD, maritally distressed; non-MD, non-maritally distressed; PT+SC, parent training plus maternal self-control adjunct; PET, parent training plus Parent Enhancement Therapy; NTC, no-training control; SFT, systems family therapy; PT+CSC, parent training plus child self-control; PT+C-ATT, parent training plus child attention control; STEP+C-ATT, Systematic Training for Effective Parenting plus child attention control. *Outcome data:* CO, clinic observation; HO, home observation; PR, parent-recorded data; Q, questionnaire; P, parent report; T, teacher report; C, child report.[a]Consumer satisfaction/social acceptability data only at 15-month follow-up

From McMahon, R.J., & Forehand, R.L. (2003). *Helping the noncompliant child: Family-based treatment for oppositional behavior* (2nd ed.). New York: Guilford Press. Reprinted with permission.

(and, in some studies, in the school) setting, usually in blocks of four 40 min observations conducted on different days. The Behavioral Coding System (Forehand & McMahon, 1981) includes both parent (e.g., commands, rewards, attends) and child (e.g., compliance, noncompliance, inappropriate behavior) behaviors. The Behavioral Coding System has been shown to have adequate psychometric properties and to be sensitive to treatment effects. Parent-report measures included questionnaires designed to assess parental perceptions of the child's behavior/adjustment (e.g., Parent Attitudes Test [Cowen, Huser, Beach & Rappaport, 1970]; Becker Bipolar Adjective Checklist [Becker, 1960]) and the parent's personal/marital adjustment (e.g., Beck Depression Inventory [Beck, Rush, Shaw, & Emery, 1979]; Marital Adjustment Test [Kimmel & VanderVeen, 1974]).[1] The Parent's Consumer Satisfaction Questionnaire (Forehand & McMahon, 1981; McMahon & Forehand, 2003) assesses parental satisfaction with the overall program, the teaching format and parenting techniques, and the therapist. It has been administered immediately following intervention and at subsequent follow-ups. Various other measures have been employed in different studies.

Evaluation Results/Program Efficacy

HNC has been extensively evaluated in terms of its efficacy, generalization, and social validity. Short-term efficacy and setting generalization from the clinic to the home have been demonstrated for both parent and child behaviors, as well as parents' perceptions of their children (e.g., Peed et al., 1977). Furthermore, these improvements occur regardless of families' socioeconomic status (Rogers et al., 1981) or age of the children (within the 3–8 year-old range; McMahon, Forehand, & Tiedemann, 1985), suggesting these two variables do not moderate treatment outcome. Two studies have failed to find evidence for setting generality to the classroom, but there was also no evidence of a behavioral contrast effect, since there were no systematic increases or decreases in child inappropriate behavior in the classroom (Breiner & Forehand, 1981; Forehand et al., 1979).

Maintenance of the effects of HNC has been documented in several studies (e.g., Baum & Forehand, 1981; Forehand & Long, 1988; Forehand et al., 1979; Long et al., 1994), with follow-up assessments ranging from 2 months to 14 years after treatment termination. Forehand and Long (1988) demonstrated that relative to a non-referred "normal" sample, a sample of children who had participated in HNC 4.5–10.5 years earlier (and who were now between the ages of 11 and 14) were functioning well. Long et al. (1994) reported similar findings at a 14-year follow-up. The young adults (17–22 years old; M = 20 years) who had participated in HNC as children reported comparable levels of delinquency, drug use, psychopathology, self-esteem,

[1] As noted above, we currently employ the CBCL (Achenbach & Rescorla, 2000, 2001) to assess parental perceptions of the child's adjustment, and the O'Leary-Porter Scale (Porter & O'Leary, 1980) to assess marital conflict.

academic progress, and quality of relationship with parents to those reported by young adults in the "normal" community comparison group. Sibling generalization has been demonstrated by Humphreys, Forehand, McMahon, and Roberts (1978), who showed that mothers employed the skills they had learned in HNC with untreated siblings who responded by being more compliant to maternal directives. Finally, improvement in child compliance has been shown to be accompanied by decreases in other overt conduct problem behaviors, such as aggression, tantrums, whining, and inappropriate verbal behavior, thereby supporting behavioral generalization of HNC (Wells, Forehand, & Griest, 1980).

With respect to the social validity of HNC, child compliance and inappropriate behavior have improved to within the normal range by the end of treatment, although mothers' perceptions of the children's adjustment appear to lag slightly behind the children's behavioral improvements. However, by 2 months after the conclusion of treatment, mothers' perceptions are consistent with the children's improved behavior and are comparable to those of mothers of "normal" children (Forehand, Wells, & Griest, 1980). High parental ratings of the acceptability of, and satisfaction with, HNC in general and its components have also been documented (e.g., Baum & Forehand, 1981; Cross Calvert & McMahon, 1987; Forehand et al., 1980; McMahon, Tiedemann, Forehand, & Griest, 1984). There is also evidence that parental participation in HNC can have positive effects on parents' levels of depressive symptoms (extending at least 2 months beyond the end of the intervention) (Forehand et al., 1980; Forehand, Furey, & McMahon, 1984) and a shorter-term effect on marital satisfaction (Brody & Forehand, 1985; Forehand, Griest, Wells, & McMahon, 1982).

Several procedures have been evaluated as adjuncts to the basic parent training program. These include maternal self-control procedures (Wells, Griest, & Forehand, 1980); training the parents in the social learning principles underlying the parent training program (McMahon, Forehand, & Griest, 1981); and a multimodal package ("parent enhancement therapy") designed to enhance general family functioning, which includes components related to parental perceptions of the child's behavior, marital adjustment, parental personal adjustment, and the parents' extrafamilial relationships (Griest et al., 1982). In general, these studies have supported the efficacy of these adjunctive procedures in enhancing the generalization and/or maintenance of effects, over and above those gains obtained in the basic HNC program.

Two studies have compared the effects of HNC with other interventions for children with conduct problems. Wells and Egan (1988) found that HNC was more effective than systems family therapy on observational measures of parent and child behaviors. The two treatment groups did not differ on parental self-report measures of personal (depression, anxiety) or marital adjustment. Baum et al. (1986) reported that a group version of HNC was more effective at post treatment and at a 6–8-month follow-up than a parent discussion group based on the Systematic Training for Effective Parenting (STEP) program (Dinkmeyer & McKay, 1976).

In addition, Long et al. (1993) reported that parents of children with ADHD who received a self-guided written booklet explaining the HNC parenting skills reported less intensive oppositional behavior than did the parents of children with ADHD who did not receive the booklet. (All of the children were receiving medication to address the ADHD symptoms.) Finally, Conners et al. (2007) evaluated the effects of the *Parenting the Strong-Willed Child* (*PSWC*) parenting class curriculum program with 71 Head Start parents. Parents reported significant decrements in both the frequency and intensity of child behavior problems, reductions in parenting stress, and improvements in their parenting behaviors. All changes were sustained 6 months later.

External Reviews

Several external reviews of child mental health or parenting programs have resulted in the HNC program being identified as an evidence-based intervention. In a review of "best practices" lists (Metzler, Eddy, & Taylor, 2002), HNC was included as 1 of the top 21 evidence-based family-focused programs. It has been included on lists of the most effective programs focusing on the treatment of conduct problems (Brestan & Eyberg, 1998; Eyberg, Nelson, & Boggs, 2008), intrafamilial child abuse (e.g., Saunders, Berliner, & Hanson, 2001), the prevention of substance abuse and delinquency (Alvarado, Kendall, Beesley, & Lee-Cavaness, 2000; Webster-Stratton & Taylor, 2001), and "mental disorders" (Greenberg, Domitrovich, & Bumbarger, 1999). For example, the Strengthening America's Families Project (sponsored by the Office of Juvenile Justice and Delinquency Prevention and the Center for Substance Abuse Prevention) identified HNC as one of seven Exemplary I Programs (out of more than 500 programs examined) (Alvarado et al., 2000). Most recently, HNC has been listed as one of only 16 evidence-based psychosocial treatments for youth with conduct problems (Eyberg et al., 2008), and received top ratings from the National Academy for Parenting Practitioners' listing of evidence-based parenting programs in the U.K. Training sessions have been conducted in multiple states and provinces (e.g., Arkansas, Colorado, Florida, Georgia, Idaho, Massachusetts, Michigan, New Hampshire, New York, Ohio, Oklahoma, Vermont, Washington, Alberta, and British Columbia,) in North America, and HNC is being implemented widely in Illinois through the Illinois Department of Mental Health and in New Hampshire by state-funded community mental health agencies.

CASE STUDY

When Michael was 2-years old, his parents started worrying that his behavior was more difficult to manage than most children his age. Michael's parents indicated that he was "very stubborn" and that "he had a mind of his own." At the time, however, his parents did not become overly concerned because they were told frequently by friends and family members that "he's just all boy," and that "it's just the terrible twos – he'll grow out of it." Unfortunately, Michael's behavior did not improve as he became older. By the time he was 4-years old, he was described as "defiant." His parents stated that he would rarely follow their instructions and that typically he "only wants to do what he wants, when he wants, and how he wants." In their attempts to increase Michael's compliance, they often resorted to yelling and threatening him, even though they realized that this was not very effective. They also were concerned that their general relationship with Michael was steadily deteriorating. At the urging of his preschool teacher, the parents spoke to their pediatrician about Michael's behavior and the pediatrician referred them to a psychologist. At this time, Michael was almost 5 years old.

The psychologist conducted an evaluation that included a parent interview, behavioral questionnaires, and a clinic observation of Child's Game and Parent's Game. On the basis of this evaluation, the psychologist concluded that the primary problems were Michael's noncompliance and related negative parent–child interactions. Michael was reported, and observed, to ignore most of the instructions his parents gave him, resulting in his parents becoming very frustrated. Also, the parents were observed to give numerous vague, unclear instructions to Michael. On the basis of her assessment, the psychologist made the DSM-IV diagnosis of oppositional defiant disorder (ODD) and recommended the HNC treatment program. The therapist discussed the rationale for HNC and presented an overview of the treatment. The therapist explained the primary goals of HNC, which were to: (a) change the coercive cycle of their interactions with Michael, (b) enhance the positive quality of their interactions with him through increased use of positive attention, ignoring minor inappropriate behaviors, and providing clear and appropriate instructions and consequences for his behavior; and (c) increased prosocial behaviors and fewer conduct problem behaviors, especially noncompliance, from Michael. An overview of the different skills involved in the two phases of HNC was provided (Phase 1 – Differential Attention, and Phase 2 – Compliance Training). Also, the structure of how the parents would learn these skills was explained (i.e., didactic presentation by the therapist, discussion, demonstration, role playing, practicing with Michael – with feedback provided by the therapist, handouts reviewing the content of the program, and homework/practice assignments). The parents then were asked to discuss whether they wished to participate in HNC, and to let the therapist know of their decision within the week. The parents decided to participate in HNC, and the first treatment session was scheduled.

Session 1

The first treatment session started with Michael being given a setting instruction. He was told to play quietly by himself and that if he interrupted the therapist and his parents while they were talking, they would ignore him. The therapist then demonstrated the ignoring procedure to Michael. During the session, the parents were also prompted to praise him for complying with the setting instruction. By the end of the session, the parents were beginning to praise Michael at appropriate intervals without a prompt from the therapist.

The bulk of the session was devoted to introducing the skill of attending (which is the first skill in Phase 1). The therapist explained that attending is a skill that is used to let Michael know that his appropriate behavior is noticed, and behavior that receives attention from his parents typically increases. The parents were told that attending involves describing Michael's appropriate behavior, and it is practiced within what is called the Child's Game. The Child's Game involves the parent letting the child take the lead in playing and the parent takes a non-directive role during these practice sessions (e.g., the parent does not give directions or ask questions during the Child's Game). After explaining attending, the therapist modeled the skill of attending with the parents playing the role of the child. The parents then practiced attending with the therapist playing the role of the child. Throughout this practice, Michael watched attentively. The therapist took opportunities to include Michael in the activity, first by making explanatory statements about what his parents were doing, and then by gradually including Michael in the Child's Game activity. The therapist then had the parents practice attending only with Michael, while the therapist observed and provided feedback. The parents had a difficult time, as do many parents, with being non-directive. They had a tendency to ask Michael questions (e.g., "What are you making?") and to give indirect directions (e.g., "Why don't you build a tower?"). The therapist pointed out their questions and directions and made suggestions of appropriate attending statements that could be used in their place (e.g., "You're putting the round block on top of the square block .... You're making it higher and higher."). At the end of the session, the parents were given handouts reviewing what had been covered in the session and the homework assignment was discussed (i.e., daily 10–15 min practice of attending within the Child's Game).

Session 2

At the beginning of the session, the therapist had Michael's parents each spend 5 min practicing attending with Michael within the Child's Game. The therapist observed and coded these interactions and noted that both parents were still giving too many instructions and asking too many questions during the Child's Game. Also, although they were giving some appropriate attending statements, the rate of attending was still relatively low. Michael's parents reported that they had practiced attending on all but one day and that Michael seemed to enjoy their attention during the Child's Game. The therapist gave the parents feedback based on the observed/coded interactions. The remainder of the session was devoted to the parents practicing attending with Michael (with the therapist coaching the parents; i.e., providing prompts/feedback). The parents were instructed to continue daily practice of attending with Michael within the Child's Game.

Session 3

This session, as did all subsequent sessions, started with an observation of the Child's Game that was coded by the therapist. The parents were observed to be improving in their use of attending, but they had not yet met the behavioral criteria to move on to learning the next skill in Phase I. The therapist and parents discussed the daily practice sessions and the therapist answered the parents' questions about attending. The remainder of this session was spent with the therapist coaching the parents (in the skill of attending) while they practiced with Michael within the Child's Game. The parents were instructed to continue daily practice of attending within the Child's Game.

Session 4

During the observation at the beginning of the session, the parents met the behavioral criteria for attending. Therefore, the therapist introduced the next Phase I skill of rewarding. The therapist discussed the different types of rewards as well as the characteristics of effective rewards. The therapist then modeled the skill of rewarding with one of the parents playing the role of the child. The parents then practiced rewarding as the therapist played the role of Michael. As with attending, the therapist gradually included Michael in the practice activity, after providing him with verbal explanations and demonstrations about rewards. Michael's parents spent the remainder of the session practicing rewarding and attending with Michael and the therapist provided feedback and coaching. The parents learned effective rewarding much more easily than they had learned attending. At the end of the session, the parents were instructed to practice both attending and rewarding daily with Michael within the Child's Game.

Session 5

The parents met the behavioral criteria for rewarding during the observation period at the beginning of this session. The parents also reported that Michael was enjoying the Child's Game and was responding well to both the attending and rewarding. In this session, the skill of ignoring was introduced as an active procedure. The therapist discussed the characteristics of effective ignoring as well as appropriate and inappropriate behaviors to ignore. The therapist then modeled ignoring and had the parents role play ignoring with her. After explaining and demonstrating ignoring to Michael, the parents practiced attending, rewarding, and ignoring while the therapist provided prompts and feedback. At the end of this session, the therapist helped the parents develop a differential attention plan using attending and rewarding to increase Michael's use of age-appropriate language and ignoring to decrease his use of baby-talk.

Session 6

The parents reported that the differential attention plan was working in that Michael had been using less baby-talk in the last few days. The therapist then helped the parents develop a second differential attention plan. This time the therapist let the parents take more of the lead in developing the plan. That plan focused on increasing Michael's use of appropriate table manners. During the remainder of this session, Phase II of the program (Compliance Training) was introduced. The therapist discussed the importance of giving Michael clear instructions and their relationship to compliance. The therapist then reviewed and discussed the characteristics of clear instructions and gave examples of both unclear and clear instructions. Next, the parents were presented with a series of clear and unclear instructions to see if they could accurately differentiate them. Once the parents understood the importance and characteristics of clear instructions, the therapist introduced Path A of the Clear Instructions Sequence. Path A involves attending/rewarding compliance to clear instructions. The concept of the Parent's Game (the parent directs the play) was then introduced for the practice of Phase II skills. The parents role played Path A with the therapist, and the therapist explained and demonstrated Path A with Michael. Finally, the parents practiced Path A with Michael while the therapist provided prompts and feedback. The parents were then given their homework assignment, which involved practicing Path A with Michael.

Session 7

The remaining pathways (Paths B and C) of the Clear Instructions Sequence were introduced and discussed. Path B (warning following noncompliance to a clear instruction) was role played with the therapist playing the role of the child; subsequently, the process was explained to and demonstrated for Michael. Time out was discussed and the specific procedure was presented to the parents. The parents had used a different time-out procedure unsuccessfully in the past with Michael. Therefore, the therapist stressed the importance of following the HNC time-out procedure guidelines. The therapist discussed the rationale for certain characteristics of the time-out procedure that were different from how the parents had used it in the past (e.g., they had talked to Michael during time out; they had not used a quiet contingency). The therapist then helped the parents problem-solve issues related to time out such as the best location for time out in their home. Next, Path C (use of time out for noncompliance) was role played. The therapist and parents then discussed and role played some specific challenges to time out, including tardy compliance, refusal to stay in time out, and compliance only to the warning. After explaining and demonstrating Path C to Michael, the remainder of the session involved the parents practicing the Clear Instructions Sequence (Paths A, B, C) within the Parent's Game with Michael (while the therapist provided prompts and feedback). Michael was issued a warning (Path B) during the practice, but he complied with the warnings so he did not have to go to time out (Path C).

Session 8

The parents and therapist discussed how the Clear Instructions Sequence and time out had been going at home. The parents reported that Michael had been to time out on three separate occasions since the last session; on one of those occasions, the parents had to cycle through the Clear Instructions Sequence (including time out) twice before Michael complied with the original instruction. Utilizing the Parent's Game, the parents spent the majority of this session practicing the Clear Instructions Sequence (all three pathways) while receiving prompts and feedback from the therapist.

Session 9

The therapist and parents discussed issues related to the Clear Instructions Sequence and time out that had come up at home since the last session. The parents reported that Michael's noncompliance was decreasing, as he had only had to go to time out once during the last few days. The parents practiced the Clear Instructions Sequence within the Parent's Game with the therapist providing feedback. The remaining focus of this session was on introducing Standing Rules ("if ... then" statements) to the parents and Michael, and how they are used to supplement the Clear Instructions Sequence. The therapist helped the parents generate one Standing Rule: If Michael hit anyone (e.g., his sister, the parents, peers), then he went immediately to time out.

Session 10

The parents reported that Michael was much more compliant and had been following the Standing Rule. During the past week, they reported that he only had to go to time out twice (once for noncompliance and once for breaking the Standing Rule). The primary focus of this session was on generalization. The therapist helped the parents learn how they could use both Phase I and Phase II skills to help deal with situations outside of the home. They discussed the situations outside the home that the parents indicated were most likely to be problematic (e.g., stores, restaurants, and the car). For example, when taking Michael to the grocery store, the therapist emphasized the importance of involving Michael in shopping (e.g., having him place items in the cart) and using attending and rewarding to reinforce his cooperative involvement. The parents were advised to issue clear "do" instructions (such as "keep your hands in the cart"), as needed, to which they could then attend and reward compliance. Finally, the parents were also advised to think in advance about an appropriate setting for time out (e.g., in the store or removing the child to the car) should it become necessary while they were shopping.

Session 11

This session involved discussing situations that had occurred outside the home over the past week and how the parent used Phase I and Phase II skills. The parents reported that the week had gone well, including trips to stores and a meal at a restaurant. The therapist discussed the progress they had made with Michael and pointed out that they now had a set of skills that they could use not only to maintain Michael's improved behavior but also to address future behavior problems. The remainder of the session was spent reviewing the various skills, stressing the importance of consistency, encouraging the continued use of Phase I skills, and answering questions from the parents. The therapist said that she would check in with the parents by phone in 1 month to see how things were going with Michael.

CONCLUSIONS/FUTURE DIRECTIONS

In this chapter, we have provided an overview of the theoretical and conceptual basis for family-based interventions with children who present with excessive noncompliance; a description of the HNC intervention; a summary of its empirical support; and a case study describing a typical progression through the program. As we move forward in the years ahead, we plan to focus our activities in two separate yet interrelated areas: (a) further dissemination of HNC to "real-life" settings and other populations of children, and (b) expanded research efforts. With respect to the former, we are working with colleagues who are implementing HNC through the community mental health system in New Hampshire (Dr. Sarah Stearns); adapting HNC to children with ADHD (Drs. Howard Abikoff and Laurie Miller-Brotman at New York University); and implementing (and possibly adapting) HNC with Mexican immigrant families in Illinois (Dr. Ane Marinez-Lora at the University of Illinois-Chicago). The latter two ventures are being conducted in the context of research trials; in addition, we hope to expand the research base on HNC by conducting both large-scale efficacy trials as well as effectiveness trials focused on the dissemination and implementation of HNC in community settings. We are currently in the process of conducting a randomized-controlled study of the self-directed version of this program (Forehand & Long, 2010). We also plan to further evaluate the parenting class version (Conners et al., 2007), which involves six 2-h class sessions focused on the key elements of the HNC program. These HNC-based interventions are intended for use with selected populations (i.e., those families who have children who have less severe disruptive behavior and are at risk for the development of conduct problems). Through the development and evaluation of these other service delivery approaches, we hope to positively impact a broader population of families who could benefit from learning the skills taught in HNC. Finally, we plan to continue to conduct component analyses of HNC to identify mechanisms of action and to "fine-tune" the effects of the intervention.

REFERENCES[2]

Achenbach, T. M., & Rescorla, L. A. (2000). *Manual for the ASEBA preschool forms and profiles*. Burlington, VT: University of Vermont Department of Psychiatry.

Achenbach, T. M., & Rescorla, L. A. (2001). *Manual for the ASEBA school-age forms and profiles*. Burlington, VT: University of Vermont, Research Center for Children, Youth, & Families.

---

[2]References marked with an asterisk (*) indicate studies included only in Table 7.4 and which are not cited in the text.

Alvarado, R., Kendall, K., Beesley, S., & Lee-Cavaness, C. (2000). *Strengthening America's families: Model family programs for substance abuse and delinquency prevention.* Salt Lake City, UT: University of Utah.

Baum, C. G., & Forehand, R. (1981). Long-term follow-up assessment of parent training by use of multiple-outcome measures. *Behavior Therapy, 12*, 643–652.

Baum, C. G., Reyna-McGlone, C. L., & Ollendick, T. H. (1986, November). *The efficacy of behavioral parent training: Behavioral parent training plus clinical self-control training, and a modified STEP program with children referred for noncompliance.*. Chicago, IL: Paper presented at the meeting of the Association for Advancement of Behavior Therapy.

Beck, A. T., Rush, A. J., Shaw, B. F., & Emery, G. (1979). *Cognitive therapy of depression.* New York: Guilford Press.

Beck, A. T., Steer, R. A., & Brown, G. K. (1996). *Beck Depression Inventory manual* (2nd ed.). San Antonio, TX: The Psychological Corporation.

Becker, W. C. (1960). The relationship of factors in parental ratings of self and each other to the behavior of kindergarten children as rated by mothers, fathers, and teachers. *Journal of Consulting and Clinical Psychology, 24*, 507–527.

Breiner, J. L. (1989). Training parents as change agents for their developmentally disabled children. In C. E. Schaefer & J. M. Briesmeister (Eds.), *Handbook of parent training: Parents as co-therapists for children's behavior problems* (pp. 269–304). New York: Wiley.

Breiner, J. L., & Forehand, R. (1981). An assessment of the effects of parent training on clinic-referred children's school behavior. *Behavioral Assessment, 3*, 31–42.

Breiner, J., Forehand, R. (1982, November). *Training groups of parents in the management of their developmentally and language delayed children.* Paper presented at the meeting of the Association for Advancement of Behavior Therapy, Los Angeles

Brestan, E. V., & Eyberg, S. M. (1998). Effective psychosocial treatments of conduct-disordered children and adolescents: 29 years, 82 studies, and 5, 272 kids. *Journal of Clinical Child Psychology, 27*, 180–189.

Brody, G., & Forehand, R. (1985). The efficacy of parent training with maritally distressed and non-distressed mothers: A multimethod assessment. *Behaviour Research and Therapy, 23*, 291–296.

Chamberlain, P., & Patterson, G. R. (1995). Discipline and child compliance in parenting. In M. H. Bornstein (Ed.), *Handbook of parenting (Applied and practical parenting)* (pp, Vol. 4, pp. 205–225). Hillsdale, NJ: Erlbaum.

Conduct Problems Prevention Research Group. (1992). A developmental and clinical model for the prevention of conduct disorders: The FAST Track program. *Development and Psychopathology, 4*, 509–527.

Conners, N. A., Edwards, M. C., & Grant, A. S. (2007). An evaluation of a parenting class curriculum for parents of young children: Parenting the Strong-Willed Child. *Journal of Child and Family Studies, 16*, 321–330.

Cowen, E. L., Huser, J., Beach, D. R., & Rappaport, J. (1970). Parental perceptions of young children and their relation to indexes of adjustment. *Journal of Consulting and Clinical Psychology, 34*, 97–103.

Cross Calvert, S., & McMahon, R. J. (1987). The treatment acceptability of a behavioral parent training program and its components. *Behavior Therapy, 18*, 165–179.

Dinkmeyer, D., & McKay, G. D. (1976). *Systematic training for effective parenting.* Circle Pines, MN: American Guidance Service.

Dumas, J. E. (1996). Why was this child referred? Interactional correlates of referral status in families of children with disruptive behavior problems. *Journal of Clinical Child Psychology, 25*, 106–115.

Eyberg, S. M., Nelson, M. M., & Boggs, S. R. (2008). Evidence-based psychosocial treatments for children with disruptive behavior. *Journal of Clinical Child and Adolescent Psychology, 37*, 215–237.

Farrington, D. P. (2003). Key results from the first forty years of the Cambridge Study in Delinquent Development. In T. P. Thornberry & M. D. Krohn (Eds.), *Taking stock of delinquency: An overview of findings from contemporary longitudinal studies* (pp. 137–183). New York: Kluwer Academic/Plenum Publishers.

Forehand, R., Armistead, L., Neighbors, B., & Klein, K. (1994). *Parent training for the noncompliant child: A guide for training therapists.* Charlotte, VT: ChildFocus.

*Forehand, R., Breiner, J., McMahon, R. J., & Davies, G. (1981). Predictors of cross setting behavior change in the treatment of child problems. *Journal of Behavior Therapy and Experimental Psychiatry, 12,* 311–313.

Forehand, R., Cheney, T., & Yoder, P. (1974). Parent behavior training: Effects on the non-compliance of a deaf child. *Journal of Behavior Therapy and Experimental Psychiatry, 5,* 281–283.

Forehand, R., Furey, W., & McMahon, R. J. (1984). The role of maternal distress in a parent training program to modify child noncompliance. *Behavioural Psychotherapy, 12,* 93–108.

*Forehand, R., Griest, D. L., & Wells, K. C. (1979). Parent behavioral training: An analysis of the relationship among multiple outcome measures. *Journal of Abnormal Child Psychology, 7,* 229–242.

Forehand, R., Griest, D. L., Wells, K., & McMahon, R. J. (1982). Side effects of parent counseling on marital satisfaction. *Journal of Counseling Psychology, 29,* 104–107.

*Forehand, R., & King, H. E. (1974). Pre-school children's non-compliance: Effects of short-term behavior therapy. *Journal of Community Psychology, 2,* 42–44.

*Forehand, R., & King, H. E. (1977). Noncompliant children: Effects of parent training on behavior and attitude change. *Behavior Modification, 1,* 93–108.

Forehand, R., & Long, N. (1988). Outpatient treatment of the acting out child: Procedures, long term follow-up data and clinical problems. *Advances in Behaviour Research and Therapy, 10,* 129–177.

Forehand, R., & Long, N. (2010). *Parenting the strong-willed child: The clinically-proven five-week program for parents of two- to six-year-olds* (3rd ed.). New York: McGraw-Hill.

Forehand, R. L., & McMahon, R. J. (1981). *Helping the noncompliant child: A clinician's guide to parent training.* New York: Guilford Press.

*Forehand, R., Rogers, T., McMahon, R. J., Wells, K. C., & Griest, D. L. (1981). Teaching parents to modify child behavior problems: An examination of some follow-up data. *Journal of Pediatric Psychology, 6,* 313–322.

*Forehand, R., Steffe, M., Furey, W. M., & Walley, P. M. (1983). Mothers' evaluation of a parent training program completed three and one-half years earlier. *Journal of Behavior Therapy and Experimental Psychiatry, 14,* 339–342.

Forehand, R., Sturgis, E. T., McMahon, R. J., Aguar, D., Green, K., Wells, K., et al. (1979). Parent behavioral training to modify child noncompliance: Treatment generalization across time and from home to school. *Behavior Modification, 3,* 3–25.

Forehand, R., Wells, K. C., & Griest, D. L. (1980). An examination of the social validity of a parent training program. *Behavior Therapy, 11,* 488–502.

Furey, W. M., & Basili, L. A. (1988). Predicting consumer satisfaction in parent training for noncompliant children. *Behavior Therapy, 19,* 555–564.

Greenberg, M. T., Domitrovich, C., & Bumbarger, B. (1999). *Preventing mental disorders in school-age children: A review of the effectiveness of prevention programs.* Report to the Center for Mental Health Services; Substance Abuse Mental Health Services Administration, U.S. Department of Health and Human Services. [Available at http://www.prevention.psu.edu/CMHS.html]

Griest, D. L., Forehand, R., Rogers, T., Breiner, J. L., Furey, W., & Williams, C. A. (1982). Effects of parent enhancement therapy on the treatment outcome and generalization of a parent training program. *Behaviour Research and Therapy, 20,* 429–436.

Griest, D. L., Forehand, R., & Wells, K. C. (1981). Follow-up assessment of parent behavioral training: An analysis of who will participate. *Child Study Journal, 11,* 221–229.

Hanf, C., & Kling, J. (1973). *Facilitating parent-child interactions: A two-stage training model.* Unpublished manuscript. University of Oregon Medical School.

Humphreys, L., Forehand, R., McMahon, R. J., & Roberts, M. (1978). Parent behavioral training to modify child noncompliance: Effects on untreated siblings. *Journal of Behavior Therapy and Experimental Psychiatry, 9,* 235–238.

Kimmel, D. C., & VanderVeen, F. (1974). Factors of marital adjustment in Locke's Marital Adjustment Test. *Journal of Marriage and the Family, 36,* 57–63.

Kratzer, L., & Hodgins, S. (1997). Adult outcomes of child conduct problems: A cohort study. *Journal of Abnormal Child Psychology, 25*, 65–81.

Kumpfer, K. L., & DeMarsh, J. (1987). *Prevention services for children of substance-abusing parents*. National Institute on Drug Abuse Final Technical Report. (R18 DA 02758-01/02 and DA 03888-01).

Kumpfer, K. L., Molgaard, V., & Spoth, R. (1996). The Strengthening Families Program for the prevention of delinquency and drug use. In R.DeV. Peters & R. J. McMahon (Eds.), *Preventing childhood disorders, substance abuse, and delinquency* (pp. 241–267). Thousand Oaks, CA: Sage.

Long, N., & Forehand, R. (2000a). *Parenting the Strong-willed child: Leader's guide for the six-week parenting class*. (Request from Dr. Nicholas Long, UAMS Department of Pediatrics, Slot 512-21, 1 Children's Way, Little Rock, AR 72202).

Long, N., & Forehand, R. (2000b). Modifications of a parental training program for implementation beyond the clinical setting. In N. N. Singh, J. P. Leung, & A. N. Singh (Eds.), *International perspectives on child and adolescent mental health* (pp. 293–310). New York: Elsevier.

Long, P., Forehand, R., Wierson, M., & Morgan, A. (1994). Moving into adulthood: Does parent training with young noncompliant children have long-term effects? *Behaviour Research and Therapy, 32*, 101–107.

Long, N., Rickert, V., & Ashcraft, E. (1993). Bibliotherapy as an adjunct to stimulant medication in the treatment of attention-deficit hyperactivity disorder. *Journal of Pediatric Health Care, 7*, 82–88.

Lutzker, J. R. (1984). Project 12-Ways: Treating child abuse and neglect from an ecobehavioral perspective. In R. F. Dangel & R. A. Polster (Eds.), *Parent training: Foundations of research and practice* (pp. 260–297). New York: Guilford Press.

Maughan, D. R., Christiansen, E., Jenson, W. R., Olympia, D., & Clark, E. (2005). Behavioral parent training as a treatment for externalizing behaviors and disruptive behavior disorders: A meta-analysis. *School Psychology Review, 34*, 267–286.

McMahon R. J. (2006). Parent training interventions for preschool-age children. In R.E. Tremblay, R.G. Barr, & R.DeV. Peters (Eds.), *Encyclopedia on early childhood development* [online]. Montreal, Quebec: Centre of Excellence for Early Childhood Development; 1–8. Available at http://www.excellence-earlychildhood.ca/documents/McMahonRJANGxp.pdf

*McMahon, R. J., & Forehand, R. (1978). Nonprescription behavior therapy: Effectiveness of a brochure in teaching mothers to correct their children's inappropriate mealtime behavior. *Behavior Therapy, 9*, 814–820.

McMahon, R. J., & Forehand, R. L. (2003). *Helping the noncompliant child: Family-based treatment for oppositional behavior* (2nd ed.). New York: Guilford Press.

McMahon, R. J., Forehand, R., & Griest, D. L. (1981). Effects of knowledge of social learning principles on enhancing treatment outcome and generalization in a parent training program. *Journal of Consulting and Clinical Psychology, 49*, 526–532.

McMahon, R. J., Forehand, R., Griest, D. L., & Wells, K. C. (1981). Who drops out of treatment during parent behavioral training? *Behavioral Counseling Quarterly, 1*, 79–85.

McMahon, R.J., Forehand, R., & Tiedemann, G.L. (1985, November). *Relative effectiveness of a parent training program with children of different ages*. Poster presented at the Association for Advancement of Behavior Therapy, Houston.

*McMahon, R.J., Johnson, K.K., & Robbins, K.H. (2010). *Acceptability of written instructions versus therapist administration of a parent training program*. Manuscript submitted for publication.

*McMahon, R.J., & Lehman, K. (2010). *Effectiveness of written instructions in teaching mothers to give clear instructions to their children*. Manuscript submitted for publication.

McMahon, R. J., Slough, N. M., & the Conduct Problems Prevention Research Group. (1996). Family-based intervention in the Fast Track program. In R.Dev. Peters & R. J. McMahon (Eds.), *Preventing childhood disorders, substance abuse, and delinquency* (pp. 90–110). Thousand Oaks, CA: Sage.

McMahon, R. J., Tiedemann, G. L., Forehand, R., & Griest, D. L. (1984). Parental satisfaction with parent training to modify child noncompliance. *Behavior Therapy, 15*, 295–303.

McMahon, R. J., Wells, K. C., & Kotler, J. S. (2006). Conduct problems. In E. J. Mash & R. A. Barkley (Eds.), *Treatment of childhood disorders* (3rd ed., pp. 137–268). New York: Guilford Press.

Metzler, C., Eddy, M., & Taylor, T. K. (2002, May). The evidence standards of ten "best practices" lists and the evidence base of the top family-focused programs. In C. Metzler (Chair), *Finding common ground among "best practices" lists: The evidence base and program elements of top family focused and school-based programs.* Symposium conducted at the meeting of the Society for Prevention Research, Seattle, WA.

Miller, G. E., & Prinz, R. J. (1990). Enhancement of social learning family interventions for childhood conduct disorder. *Psychological Bulletin, 108*, 291–307.

Moffitt, T. E. (1993). "Adolescence-limited" and "life-course-persistent" antisocial behavior: A developmental taxonomy. *Psychological Review, 100*, 674–701.

Patterson, G. R. (1982). *Coercive family process*. Eugene, OR: Castalia.

Patterson, G. R., Capaldi, D., & Bank, L. (1991). An early starter model for predicting delinquency. In D. J. Pepler & K. H. Rubin (Eds.), *The development and treatment of childhood aggression* (pp. 139–168). Hillsdale, NJ: Erlbaum.

Patterson, G. R., Reid, J. B., & Dishion, T. S. (1992). *Antisocial boys*. Eugene, OR: Castalia.

Peed, S., Roberts, M., & Forehand, R. (1977). Evaluation of the effectiveness of a standardized parent training program in altering the interactions of mothers and their noncompliant children. *Behavior Modification, 1*, 323–350.

Pisterman, S., McGrath, P., Firestone, P., Goodman, J. T., Webster, I., & Mallory, R. (1989). Outcome of parent-mediated treatment of preschoolers with attention deficit disorder with hyperactivity. *Journal of Consulting and Clinical Psychology, 57*, 628–635.

Porter, B., & O'Leary, K. D. (1980). Marital discord and childhood behavior problems. *Journal of Abnormal Child Psychology, 8*, 287–295.

Reid, J. B. (1993). Prevention of conduct disorder before and after school entry: Relating interventions to developmental findings. *Development and Psychopathology, 5*, 243–262.

Reitman, D., & McMahon, R. J. (2010). *Constance "Connie" Hanf: The mentor and the model.* Manuscript submitted for publication.

*Roberts, M. W., Joe, V. C., & Rowe-Hallbert, A. L. (1992). Oppositional child behavior and parental locus of control. *Journal of Clinical Child Psychology, 21*, 170–177.

Rogers, T. R., Forehand, R., Griest, D. L., Wells, K. C., & McMahon, R. J. (1981). Socioeconomic status: Effects on parent and child behaviors and treatment outcome of parent training. *Journal of Clinical Child Psychology, 10*, 98–101.

Russo, D. C., Cataldo, M. F., & Cushing, P. J. (1981). Compliance training and behavioral covariation in the treatment of multiple behavior problems. *Journal of Applied Behavior Analysis, l4*, 209–222.

Saunders, B. E., Berliner, L., & Hanson, R. F. (2001). *Guidelines for the psychosocial treatment of intrafamilial child physical and sexual abuse (Final draft report: July 30, 2001).* Charleston, SC: Authors. [Available at http://www.musc.edu/cvc/]

Webster-Stratton, C., & Taylor, T. (2001). Nipping early risk factors in the bud: Preventing substance abuse, delinquency, and violence in adolescence through interventions targeted at young children (0–8 years). *Prevention Science, 2*, 165–192.

Wells, K. C. (2003). Adaptations for special populations. In R. J. McMahon & R. L. Forehand, *Helping the noncompliant child: Family-based treatment for oppositional behavior* (2nd ed., pp. 182–200). New York: Guilford Press.

Wells, K. C., & Egan, J. (1988). Social learning and systems family therapy for childhood oppositional disorder: Comparative treatment outcome. *Comprehensive Psychiatry, 29*, l38–l46.

Wells, K. C., Forehand, R., & Griest, D. L. (1980). Generality of treatment effects from treated to untreated behaviors resulting from a parent training program. *Journal of Clinical Child Psychology, 9*, 217–219.

Wells, K. C., Griest, D. L., & Forehand, R. (1980). The use of a self-control package to enhance temporal generality of a parent training program. *Behaviour Research and Therapy, 18*, 347–353.

Wells, K. C., Pelham, W. E., Kotkin, R. A., Hoza, B., Abikoff, H. B., Abramowitz, A., et al. (2000). Psychosocial treatment strategies in the MTA study: Rationale, methods, and critical issues in design and implementation. *Journal of Abnormal Child Psychology, 28*, 483–505.

Wolfe, D. A., Edwards, B., Manion, I., & Koverola, C. (1988). Early intervention for parents at risk of child abuse and neglect: A preliminary investigation. *Journal of Consulting and Clinical Psychology, 56*, 40–47.

8

Collaborative Problem Solving

ROSS W. GREENE

INTRODUCTION

Collaborative Problem Solving (CPS) is an evidence-based, cognitive-behavioral psychosocial treatment approach first described in the book *The Explosive Child* (Greene, 1998). The model blends many different lines of theory and research, including developmental theory, systems theory, social learning theory, and research in the neurosciences. CPS has been applied predominantly to youth with externalizing behavior problems, and has been implemented in a wide range of settings, including families, general and special education schools, inpatient psychiatry units, and residential and juvenile correction facilities. This chapter describes the most current rendition of the model, along with research findings to date.

KEY THEMES

The CPS model relies heavily on transactional or reciprocal models of development (e.g., Bell, 1968; Belsky, 1984; Chess & Thomas, 1984; Cicchetti & Lynch, 1993, 1995; Gottlieb, 1992; Sameroff, 1975, 1995) which posit that outcome is a function of the degree of "fit" or "compatibility" between characteristics of the child and characteristics of his or her environment, including parents, teachers, siblings, peers, neighborhoods, and so forth. When there is compatibility between characteristics of a child and his or her environment – what may be referred to as *child–environment compatibility* – outcomes are expected to be advantageous. When there

ROSS W. GREENE • Harvard Medical School

R.C. Murrihy et al. (eds.), *Clinical Handbook of Assessing and Treating Conduct Problems in Youth*, DOI 10.1007/978-1-4419-6297-3_8,

is child–environment *incompatibility*, disadvantageous outcomes would be predicted. Compatibility is not an all-or-none construct; there may be greater compatibility in one environment (e.g., school) as compared to another (e.g., home), and there may be varying degrees of compatibility within the same environment depending on the specific demands being imposed at a given time.

There are a variety of child characteristics that may confer a vulnerability to child–environment incompatibility, and along these lines, the CPS model draws upon research demonstrating that children compromised in the general skills of flexibility/adaptability, frustration tolerance, and problem solving – and in more specific domains such as executive skills, language/communication skills, emotion regulation skills, cognitive flexibility skills, and social skills – are at significant risk for social, emotional, and behavioral challenges (Greene, 1998; Greene & Doyle, 1999). These lagging skills have typically been documented and studied in the context of various psychiatric disorders, such as attention-deficit/hyperactivity disorder (ADHD), mood and anxiety disorders, oppositional defiant disorder (ODD), conduct disorder (CD), and autism spectrum disorders. However, lagging skills do not guarantee that challenging behavior will occur. Consistent with a transactional perspective, the risk for challenging behavior is also heavily influenced by the demands of the environment, the manner in which caregivers understand and respond to a child's lagging skills, and the extent to which key interaction partners are also lacking such skills.

While the CPS model relies, by necessity, on research documenting the cognitive characteristics of youth who meet criteria for various psychiatric disorders, the utilization of and enthusiasm for diagnoses pretty much ends there. Diagnoses pathologize individuals, and cannot possibly convey the complex interplay of characteristics of a child and his or her environment(s) and the degree of compatibility between them. Further, diagnoses are oriented toward clusters of *behavior* and do not typically specify the lagging *cognitive* skills that may be contributing to child–environment incompatibility in individual children; nor do they convey the manner in which a child's environment is responding to these lagging skills (Greene, 2008, 2010).

Along these lines, the CPS model places a major emphasis on *cognition* (i.e., lagging skills that confer a vulnerability to the manifestation of challenging behaviors) rather than on the behaviors themselves. Because almost all challenging behaviors occur under the same conditions – *when the demands of the environment exceed a child's capacity to respond adaptively* – such behaviors are distinguished primarily by their degree of severity. At the mild end of the "severity spectrum" are behaviors such as whining, crying, pouting, sulking, and withdrawing; in the moderate range are behaviors such as screaming, swearing, hitting, spitting, biting, kicking, destroying property, and the like; and at the severe end of spectrum are behaviors that are severely injurious (and sometimes fatal) to oneself or others. Where a child's challenging behavior falls on this spectrum is a consideration, but not the most important one. Far more important – for purposes of understanding *why* the behavior is occurring – is the identification of the specific lagging cognitive skills that confer the vulnerability to the manifestation of these behaviors and the manner in which the environment is responding to these lagging skills. Equally crucial – for purposes of identifying potential targets of intervention – is the identification of the predictable conditions precipitating challenging behavior in individual children (and in which, by definition, a child's lagging skils are being demanded). There are various synonyms for "conditions" – triggers, antecedents, situations, circumstances – but in the parlance of the CPS model they are referred to as *unsolved problems* (Greene, 2008, 2009, 2010).

Conceptually, unsolved problems reside at the intersection between a child's lagging skills and environmental demands for those very skills. For example, if a child lacks the skills to complete a particular homework assignment, and a caregiver is demanding that the homework assignment be completed, and one or both interaction partners are responding to this scenario in a manner that contributes to disadvantageous behavior in one or both interaction partners, then that homework assignment is an unsolved problem that is reliably and predictably precipitating incompatibility episodes. The disadvantageous behavior will persist until the problem is solved.

The goal of treatment is to *understand, address, and resolve factors contributing to* child – environment *incompatibility*. This is accomplished by helping adult caregivers (1) understand the specific child and environmental characteristics contributing to the development of disadvantageous behavior in the child and/or his interaction partners; (2) become cognizant of three basic strategies for handling unmet expectations – unilateral problem-solving, collaborative problem-solving, and removing the expectation – and recognize the impact of each of these three approaches on child–environment compatibility; and (3) become proficient, along with the child, at collaboratively resolving problems as a means of handling situations that are reliably and predictably precipitating challenging episodes so as to improve child–environment compatibility and reduce disadvantageous behavior.

Finally, the *collaborative* aspect of Collaborative Problem Solving is crucial. Adults often resolve problems with children in a unilateral fashion, typically through imposition of adult will, sometimes with incentives added to the mix to enhance the child's motivation to comply with the adult's solution. Solutions arrived at in this fashion are viewed, at best, as unreliable and short-lived and, at worst, as precipitants to challenging behavior. By contrast, problems solved collaboratively tend to be more durable, and because such an approach involves the child in the crucial processes of defining a problem, identifying concerns, taking another's concerns into account, generating alternative solutions, and anticipating and monitoring outcomes, the child is indirectly trained in skills that he or she is lacking. Solving a problem durably requires three ingredients: gathering information so as to achieve the clearest possible understanding of a child's concern or perspective on a given unsolved problem; having adults clarify and articulate their own concern or perspective; and having the two parties brainstorm and implement solutions so as to address the concerns of both parties and then monitor the reliability and durability of an agreed-upon solution so as to assess its success in durably solving the problem. These are the three ingredients of what is known, in the CPS model, as "Plan B."

LAGGING SKILLS

Let us consider in somewhat greater (but by no means exhaustive) depth the notion that lagging skills confer a vulnerability to child–environment incompatibility. Support for this notion can be drawn from research on the psychiatric disorder (ODD) to which the CPS model has primarily been applied to date. According to the current rendition of the DSM (APA, 1994), ODD refers to a recurrent childhood pattern of developmentally inappropriate levels of negativistic, defiant, disobedient, and hostile behavior toward authority figures, and may include temper outbursts, persistent stubbornness, resistance to directions, unwillingness to compromise, give in, or negotiate with adults or peers, deliberate or persistent testing of limits, and verbal (and minor physical) aggression. According to the CPS model, ODD is perhaps the quintessential example of child–environment incompatibility (it clearly takes two to tango), and its core feature – *noncompliance* – merely one of many possible manifestations of such incompatibility.

Compliance refers to a child's capacity to defer or delay his or her own goals in response to the imposed goals or standards of an authority figure, and develops in a sequence that includes, in infancy, managing the discomfort that can accompany hunger, cold, fatigue, and pain; modulating arousal, and communicating with caregivers to signal that assistance is needed (e.g., Gottman, 1986; Kopp, 1989). In the toddler years, emerging language-processing and communication skills set the stage for the development of increasingly sophisticated mechanisms for self-regulation and affective modulation (e.g., Kopp, 1989; Mischel, 1983). Like other maladaptive behaviors, noncompliance occurs when there is a mismatch between demands from the environment and a child's capacity to respond adaptively to those demands. This perspective points intervention, first and foremost, down the path of identifying and understanding characteristics of the child and the environment that are setting the stage for incompatibility. Characterizing a child as "having ODD" is distinctly unidirectional, connotes that the problem resides within the child (unless a different unidirectional explanation – that the parents of the child are passive, permissive, inconsistent, noncontingent disciplinarians – is invoked instead), and can be expected to point intervention down a distinctly unidirectional path.

What evidence is there to suggest that lagging skills – in the child, adult, or both – contribute to the development of noncompliance? The evidence for lagging skills is, at least at this point, more compelling in the case of the child, so we'll begin there. Much of this evidence comes from research documenting the various disorders that are commonly comorbid with ODD. For example, there is a significant overlap between ODD and ADHD (Abikoff & Klein, 1992; Greene et al., 2002; Hinshaw et al., 1993; Lahey & Loeber, 1994), the latter referring to a profile of compromised skills (often referred to as executive skills) in a wide range of domains, including self-regulation, working memory, higher-order problem-solving, shifting cognitive set, and flexibility (Barkley, 1997a; Denckla, 1996; Milner, 1995; Pennington & Ozonoff, 1996). These lagging skills may heighten the likelihood of various adverse outcomes, and certainly noncompliance is high on the list. For instance, a disorganized, impulsive child might have difficulty pinpointing the specific problem he is trying to solve (e.g., wanting to continue watching television after having been directed to come to dinner), generating alternative solutions to the problem (at least in part by reflecting on past solutions), projecting potential solutions into the future so as to anticipate likely outcomes, and delaying responding until potential courses of action and their likely outcomes have been considered. While it is true that learning history may influence response selection, it is clearly not the only variable coming into play.

The overlap between ODD and disorders of mood (Angold & Costello, 1993; Geller & Luby, 1997) and anxiety (Garland & Weiss, 1996; Greene et al., 2002) is also reasonably well-established. Indeed, it has been shown that ODD youth with comorbid mood disorders are at particular risk for the development of CD (Greene et al., 2002). Skills related to regulation of emotions develop in early infancy and increase in complexity and sophistication as a child matures. Children who fail to develop such skills at an expected or advantageous pace may be over- or under-reactive to a wide range of affectively charged situations, including demands for compliance (Stifter et al., 1999; Greene & Doyle, 1999). Children whose tendency is to over-react to affectively charged situations may find the physiological and emotional arousal associated with such situations difficult to regulate, and may become cognitively debilitated in the midst of such arousal (a phenomenon referred to as "cognitive incapacitation" by Zillman [1988]). Thus, a child compromised in the capacity to regulate emotion and arousal might respond to the frustration that occurs in the context of imposed demands for compliance with a high level of emotional reactivity (e.g., screaming, crying, swearing, physical aggression) rather than reflection, reason, and rational problem solving. Children who tend to under-react to affectively charged situations may have difficulty mustering the requisite emotional and cognitive resources to respond to such situations adaptively and may respond to these situations in ways (e.g., crying, withdrawing) that reflect a similar level of debilitation.

There is also a clear overlap between ODD and impairments in language processing and communication skills (Baker & Cantwell, 1987; Beitchman et al., 1989, 1990; Moffitt & Lynam, 1994). This overlap is not surprising, as skills such as problem-solving, frustration tolerance, and flexibility are mediated by language-based skills, including labeling, categorizing, and communicating feelings and needs and identifying and selecting corresponding behavioral strategies (e.g., Bretherton, Fritz, Zahn-Waxler, & Ridgeway, 1986). Language permits children to obtain verbal feedback about the appropriateness of the behavioral strategies they select, thereby facilitating thinking about and reflecting on previous and future actions (e.g., Kopp, 1989). Those children compromised in the capacity to label emotions (such as frustration or anger) may have difficulty identifying and internalizing an adaptive repertoire of behavior strategies for responding to such emotions. Children limited in their communication skills may be inefficient in reflecting on previous and future actions, may fail to expand response repertoires, and may consequently respond to conflict or disagreements in a manner reflective of a very narrow range of response options.

Having veered into unidirectional waters for the preceding three paragraphs, it is worth reiterating that, while these and numerous other lagging skills heighten the likelihood of child–environment incompatibility, the compatibility equation is incomplete without consideration of key aspects of the environment. Regrettably, environmental factors haven't often been studied from a transactional perspective, so there is a similarly unidirectional feel to this discussion as well. Various environmental factors have been associated with conduct problems in children, including pregnancy complications (such as viral infections or poor maternal nutrition), delivery complications (such as hypoxia or lack of oxygen to the fetus during labor; see Brennan, Grekin, & Mednick, 2003, for a review), and low SES (see Harnish, Dodge, & Valente, 1995).

However, it is parental disciplinary practices that have perhaps received the greatest attention, influenced strongly by the social interactional model (e.g., Patterson & Gullion, 1968; Patterson, Reid, & Dishion, 1992; see Taylor & Biglan, 1998). This model focuses on patterns of parental discipline that contribute to the development of "coercive" parent–child exchanges. As described by Chamberlain and Patterson (1995), four subtypes of "parent inadequate discipline" have been identified as contributing to the development of coercive parent–child interchanges. These subtypes include *inconsistent discipline* (parents who respond indiscriminately to a child's positive and negative behaviors, evidence poor or inconsistent follow through with commands, give in when a child argues, and unpredictably change expectations and consequences for rule violations); *irritable explosive discipline* (parents who issue high rates of direct commands; frequently use high intensity, high-amplitude strategies such as hitting, yelling, and threatening; and frequently make humiliating or negative statements about the child); *low supervision and involvement* (parents who are unaware of their child's activities outside of their direct supervision, do not know with whom the child is associating, are unaware of their child's adjustment at school, rarely engage in joint activities with their child, and are unwilling or unable to provide supervision even when aware of the child's association with antisocial peers), and *inflexible rigid discipline* (parents who rely on a single or limited range of discipline strategies for all types of transgressions, fail to take contextual or extenuating factors into account, consistently fail to provide rationales or to use other induction techniques in the context of discipline confrontations, and fail to adjust the intensity of the discipline reaction to the severity of the child's infraction). As a side note, these disciplinary patterns may well apply to other important caregivers, such as teachers, but this possibility has been poorly studied (see Greene 1995, 1996; Greene et al., 1997).

Also poorly studied is the possibility that many of the same skills found lacking in challenging children – disorganization, poor impulse control, irritability, anxiety, poor affective modulation, communication skill deficits, and so forth – may have equal relevance to their adult caregivers and contribute to the above patterns of discipline. Indeed, my experience is that the child is not the only interaction partner in "incompatibility episodes" who is lacking crucial cognitive skills; adult caretakers are often lacking skills as well. For example, some adults have difficulty prioritizing (perhaps because of an obsessive cognitive style or high level of anxiety) and deciding the relative importance of their goals for a child. Thus, they may consider all of their goals to be of equal and critical importance, pursue these goals with unrelenting energy, and may over-react to child behaviors that might not fall outside of what would be considered developmentally appropriate. Other adults may bring very rigid definitions regarding adult "authority" to parent–child interactions, leaving little room for discussion, processing, working toward mutually satisfactory solutions, or involving a child in the resolution of adult–child disagreements. Still others have a limited repertoire of strategies for pursuing the goals they have set for a child. Yet others parents manage a household in a manner that is disorganized and unstructured, contributing to impulsive, poorly planned discipline decisions. Others may be depressed or highly irritable, leaving little energy and patience for routine disciplinary issues. In other words, disadvantageous behavior in adult caregivers occurs under the exact same conditions as disadvantageous behavior in challenging children: when the demands of the environment exceed the individual's capacity to respond adaptively.

This being the case, the goal of assessment is to achieve an understanding of the incompatibilities giving rise to disadvantageous behaviors in children and their adult caregivers and other aspects of their environments and, based on this understanding, to pinpoint potential factors to be addressed by intervention.

ASSESSMENT

The quality, specificity, and comprehensiveness of assessment should contribute directly to the effectiveness of treatment (Greene & Ollendick, 2000; Hayes, Nelson, & Jarrett, 1987). If assessment is narrow and unidirectional, intervention is likely to be narrow and unidirectional.

In the CPS model, the primary assessment instrument used to assess lagging skills and unsolved problems is the Assessment of Lagging Skills and Unsolved Problems (ALSUP; see Fig. 8.1). Though the ALSUP has the appearance of a checklist – indeed, it has also been configured in a Likert-scale format (see Fig. 8.2) – it is best thought of as a discussion guide. A comprehensive understanding of a child's challenging behavior cannot be achieved through checking or tabulating items, but rather through discussion, information gathering, and achieving a consensus on the lagging skills and unsolved problems contributing to incompatibility episodes. Along these lines, the ALSUP has not been developmentally normed. Whether a lagging skill is within or outside the norm for a child of a given age is of little relevance; if a lagging skill is contributing to challenging behavior in a given child, it is relevant. In other words, the goal is not to determine whether a child "has a problem" based on a specific score or comparison to individuals of the same age, grade, or gender. If a child is, for example, having difficulty communicating his needs or concerns to those around him, and if this difficulty is contributing to incompatibility episodes, then there is most assuredly "a problem," whether the child is a 2-year-old female or a 17-year-old male.

ASSESSMENT OF LAGGING SKILLS AND UNSOLVED PROBLEMS (Rev. 12/5/08)

Child's Name ________________________________ Date______________

LAGGING SKILLS

_____Difficulty handling transitions, shifting from one mindset or task to another
_____Difficulty doing things in a logical sequence or prescribed order
_____Difficulty persisting on challenging or tedious tasks
_____Poor sense of time
_____Difficulty reflecting on multiple thoughts or ideas simultaneously
_____Difficulty maintaining focus
_____Difficulty considering the likely outcomes or consequences of actions (impulsive)
_____Difficulty considering a range of solutions to a problem
_____Difficulty expressing concerns, needs, or thoughts in words
_____Difficulty understanding what is being said
_____Difficulty managing emotional response to frustration so as to think rationally
_____Chronic irritability and/or anxiety significantly impede capacity for problem- solving or heighten frustration
_____Difficulty seeing the "grays"/concrete, literal, black-and-white, thinking
_____Difficulty deviating from rules, routine
_____Difficulty handling unpredictability, ambiguity, uncertainty, novelty
_____Difficulty shifting from original idea, plan, or solution
_____Difficulty taking into account situational factors that would suggest the need to adjust a plan of action
_____Inflexible, inaccurate interpretations/cognitive distortions or biases (e.g., "Everyone's out to get me," "Nobody likes me," "You always blame me, "It's not fair," "I'm stupid")
_____Difficulty attending to or accurately interpreting social cues/poor perception of social nuances
_____Difficulty starting conversations, entering groups, connecting with people/lacks other basic social skills
_____Difficulty seeking attention in appropriate ways
_____Difficulty appreciating how his/her behavior is affecting other people
_____Difficulty empathizing with others, appreciating another person's perspective or point-of-view
_____Difficulty appreciating how s/he is coming across or being perceived by others

UNSOLVED PROBLEMS

HOME

_____ Waking up/getting out of bed in the morning
_____ Completing morning routine/getting ready for school
_____ Sensory hypersensitivities
_____ Starting or completing homework or a particular academic task
_____ Food quantities/choices/preferences/timing
_____ Time spent in front of a screen (TV, video games, computer)
_____ Going to/getting ready for bed at night
_____ Boredom
_____ Sibling interactions
_____ Cleaning room/completing household chores
_____ Taking medicine
_____ Riding in car/wearing seatbelt

SCHOOL

_____ Shifting from one specific task to another (specify)
_____ Getting started on/completing class assignment (specify)
_____ Interactions with a particular classmate/teacher (specify)
_____ Behavior in hallway/at recess/in cafeteria/on school bus/waiting in line (specify)
_____ Talking at appropriate times
_____ Specific academic tasks/demands, e.g., writing assignments (specify)
_____ Handling disappointment/losing at a game/not coming in first/not being first in line (specify)

OTHERS (list)

Fig. 8.1. Assessment of lagging skills and unsolved problems.

Upon examining the ALSUP, and in reflecting upon the preceding discussion, the astute reader might well ask why the ALSUP doesn't include a section for identifying the lagging skills of adult caretakers as well. The answer: it should, but doing so might not be the ideal strategy. As I have noted elsewhere (Greene, 2009), adults who live or work with children who exhibit challenging behaviour are typically quite convinced that it is the child who is the "identified patient" who has "the problem." Trying to dissuade adults from this perspective too quickly can cause them to precipitously abandon the therapeutic ship. While adult caretakers will doubtless need to be convinced of their role in incompatibility episodes, timing is everything. Let there be no doubt: the lagging skills of key interaction partners are an indispensable, though often informal, focus of assessment.

ASSESSMENT OF LAGGING SKILLS & UNSOLVED PROBLEMS (Rev. 12/5/08)

Child's Name ______________________ Date__________ Person Completing Form____________

LAGGING SKILLS

	Never	Sometimes	Often	Very often
1. Difficulty handling transitions, shifting from one mindset or task to another	0	1	2	3
2. Difficulty doing things in a logical sequence or prescribed order	0	1	2	3
3. Difficulty persisting on challenging or tedious tasks	0	1	2	3
4. Poor sense of time	0	1	2	3
5. Difficulty reflecting on multiple thoughts or ideas simultaneously	0	1	2	3
6. Difficulty maintaining focus	0	1	2	3
7. Difficulty considering the likely outcomes or consequences of actions (impulsive)	0	1	2	3
8. Difficulty considering a range of solutions to a problem	0	1	2	3
9. Difficulty expressing concerns, needs, or thoughts in words	0	1	2	3
10. Difficulty understanding what is being said	0	1	2	3
11. Difficulty managing emotional response to frustration so as to think rationally	0	1	2	3
12. Chronic irritability and/or anxiety significantly impede capacity for problem-solving or heighten frustration	0	1	2	3
13. Difficulty seeing the "grays"/concrete, literal, black-and-white, thinking	0	1	2	3
14. Difficulty deviating from rules, routine	0	1	2	3
15. Difficulty handling unpredictability, ambiguity, uncertainty, novelty	0	1	2	3
16. Difficulty shifting from original idea, plan, or solution	0	1	2	3

Fig. 8.2. (continued)

17. Difficulty taking into account situational factors that would suggest the need to adjust a plan of action	0	1	2	3
18. Inflexible, inaccurate interpretations/cognitive distortions or biases (e.g., "Everyone's out to get me," "Nobody likes me," "You always blame me, "It's not fair," "I'm stupid")	0	1	2	3
19. Difficulty attending to or accurately interpreting social cues/poor perception of social nuances	0	1	2	3
20. Difficulty starting conversations, entering groups, connecting with people/lacking other basic social skills	0	1	2	3
21. Difficulty seeking attention in appropriate ways	0	1	2	3
22. Difficulty appreciating how his/her behavior is affecting other people	0	1	2	3
23. Difficulty empathizing with others, appreciating another person's perspective or point of view	0	1	2	3
24. Difficulty appreciating how s/he is coming across or being perceived by others	0	1	2	3

UNSOLVED PROBLEMS

HOME	Never	Sometimes	Often	Very often
1. Waking up/getting out of bed in the morning	0	1	2	3
2. Completing morning routine/getting ready for school	0	1	2	3
3. Sensory hypersensitivities	0	1	2	3
4. Starting or completing homework or a particular academic task	0	1	2	3
5. Food quantities/choices/preferences/timing	0	1	2	3
6. Time spent in front of a screen (TV, video games, computer)	0	1	2	3
7. Going to/getting ready for bed at night	0	1	2	3
8. Boredom	0	1	2	3
9. Sibling interactions	0	1	2	3
10. Cleaning room/completing household chores	0	1	2	3
11. Taking medicine	0	1	2	3
12. Riding in car/wearing seatbelt	0	1	2	3

SCHOOL	Never	Sometimes	Often	Very often
1. Shifting from one specific task to another (specify)	0	1	2	3
2. Getting started on/completing class assignments (specify)	0	1	2	3
3. Interactions with a particular classmate/teacher (specify)	0	1	2	3
4. Behavior in hallway/at recess/in cafeteria/on school bus/waiting in line (specify)	0	1	2	3
5. Talking at appropriate times	0	1	2	3
6. Academic tasks/demands, e.g., writing assignments (specify)	0	1	2	3
7. Handling disappointment/losing at a game/not coming in first/not being first in line (specify)	0	1	2	3

OTHERS (list)	Never	Sometimes	Often	Very often
1.	0	1	2	3
2.	0	1	2	3
3.	0	1	2	3
4.	0	1	2	3

Fig. 8.2. Assessment of lagging skills and unsolved problems (Likert-scale format).

The ALSUP also contains a section to assist in the identification of unsolved problems which, as described above, refers to the conditions under which the demands of the environment exceed a child's capacity to respond adaptively, thereby heightening the likelihood of challenging behavior. This section of the ALSUP is more in keeping with the transactional theme of the CPS model. Returning to an earlier example, if a child lacks the skills to complete a particular homework assignment, and the adult caregiver overseeing completion of the assignment is intervening in ways that exacerbate the problem, then the unsolved problem does not reside within either the child or the adult; they're both contributing to the incompatibility episodes arising from this unsolved problem.

A tried and true assessment practice – the *situational analysis* – can be helpful in the completion of this section of the ALSUP. The goal is to identify with *whom* (mother, father, peers, sibling, teacher, soccer coach), over *what* (difficult academic tasks, time spent in front of a screen, taking medicine, diet, homework), *where* (at a peer's apartment, in his own home, between classes at school, in math class, on the school bus), and *when* (when hanging out with peers outside of adult supervision, when being awakened for school in the morning, when told to go to bed at night, when sitting next to a sibling in the car) incompatibility episodes are reliably and predictably occurring. Embedded within every incompatibility episode is information about the lagging skills, temperament, expectations, cognitive biases and distortions, belief systems of the interaction partners, and responses of the adult caregivers.

Fair warning: often those upon whom the assessor is relying upon for such information may not be highly skilled at thinking about behavior in situational terms (they may be more naturally inclined to view behaviors as reflective of unwavering "traits"). A useful strategy here is to ask reporters to recount (in story form) instances in which challenging conduct problems occurred can be a useful device. More fair warning: the stories are likely to begin at the end with a description of a child's challenging behaviors (understandable, since the behaviors are usually the primary concern of the reporters) rather than a description of the conditions (unsolved problems) that preceded the behaviors (this information should be much more important to assessors). Thus, it is often necessary to ask reporters to "rewind the tape" so as to uncover the actual circumstances leading up to the problematic behavior, which are usually more complicated than originally presented.

Because incompatibility episodes do not occur in a developmental vacuum, a *developmental history* is usually a worthwhile assessment component, for it provides a mechanism through which information about lagging skills, temperament, expectations, cognitive biases and distortions, belief systems of the interaction partners, and disciplinary practices of the adult caregivers can be placed in an historical context and a general sense can be obtained of the duration of child–environment incompatibility. What was the child like as an infant? What were the subjective and overt responses of the adult caregivers? When did the caregivers first notice "behavior problems" in their child? What was their reaction to, understanding of, and response to these behavior problems? Were there any extenuating circumstances affecting the caregivers or family at the time behavior problems emerged or at any other point in the child's development (see Greene, 2009)?

Since school is an environment in which children and adolescents tend to spend a fair amount of time, a *school history* will also be crucial.

Anecdotally, but not unexpectedly, when incompatibility occurs cross-situationally (i.e., at home *and* at school), treatment is more difficult than in cases where incompatibility is confined to one environment, for such a scenario often suggests a more severe profile of lagging skills in the child and/or that the caregivers in the different environments are responding in ways that heighten the likelihood of challenging episodes. Are such episodes occurring at school? Under what conditions and with what interaction partners are these episodes occurring? What are the unsolved problems reliability and predictably precipitating such episodes? Is the child accessing the school discipline program, and to what degree has the program been effective? If, as is often the case, the child is accessing the school discipline program frequently, then the ineffectiveness of the program is probably self-evident.

It will also be important to gather information about the *treatment history* of the child and key adult caregivers. Ineffective prior treatment can fuel alienation, hopelessness, and cynicism and can color an individual's perspective on the prospects for current treatment and must be taken into account in formulating treatment plans (some of the most difficult-to-treat children have bounced from one professional and treatment program to another, and have lost faith that the "system" will ever be helpful). What was the nature of the prior treatment? Individual therapy? Family therapy? Parent management training? Medication? Was the treatment effective or did it exacerbate or increase the frequency of incompatibility episodes? Why was it terminated? What does this tell us about the expectations of those involved and the degree to which they were able to participate in treatment and execute treatment recommendations? Have any diagnoses been rendered? How do the different interaction partners understand the meaning of the diagnoses?

The assessor should also inquire about prior *formal assessment* that may have been conducted, both for the purposes of recommending such assessment (if it is needed) and for obtaining additional information about general cognitive skills, executive skills, language processing skills, social skills, and other cognitive factors that may have bearing on interactions between a child and key people in his or her environment.

The behavior checklist is a very common tool for assessing children, and while such "objective" instruments do provide an efficient overview of the problematic behaviors a child is exhibiting, there are important limitations to their use. They tend to focus on only one element of child–environment incompatibility (the child) and therefore tend to steer assessment in a direction that pathologizes children (rather than in the direction of examining incompatibilities between characteristics of a child and his environments). Thus, they tend to provide very little formal information about the expectations, biases, disciplinary practices, and other characteristics of the important adult caregivers doing the "checking" and how these characteristics influence, and are influenced by, characteristics of the child.

Another common assessment practice, perhaps especially in schools, is the "functional assessment," which is based on the belief that a given behavior is "working" at (or serves the function of) getting a child something he wants (for example, attention) or enabling the child to escape or avoid something unpleasant, difficult, tedious, or uncomfortable (for example, homework). However, this definition of function tends to lead to interventions aimed at convincing a child that his behavior will not work (this is usually accomplished through use of punishment) or trying to encourage the performance of replacement behaviors that adults believe will work better (this is usually accomplished through use of incentives). Interestingly, such interventions are sometimes characterized as being reflective of transactional thinking, perhaps because they involve both interaction partners (the child, who is now on the receiving end of formal, imposed consequences, and the adults, who are now on the administering end). Yet, the logic of this form of assessment and intervention could well be called into question if the goal was to understand and address the transactional processes and host of other factors known to contribute to incompatibility episodes.

Elsewhere (Greene, 2008, 2009), I have recommended a revised conceptualization of function, flowing from the following questions: If a child had the skills to go about getting, escaping, and avoiding in an adaptive fashion, then why is s/he going about getting, escaping, and avoiding in a maladaptive fashion? Isn't the fact that the child is going about getting, escaping, and avoiding in a maladaptive fashion evidence of the fact that s/he does not have the skills to go about getting, escaping, and avoiding in an adaptive fashion? As described below, this definition of function leads to interventions aimed at solving the problems that are giving rise to child–environment incompatibility in ways that are realistic and mutually satisfactory and also teach lagging skills.

TREATMENT

Consistent with a transactional perspective and with the above discussion, intervention options can be expected to be most effective when they are compatible with the needs and capacities of those persons to whom intervention is being applied (Greene & Ollendick, 2000), an equation we could refer to as *person–treatment compatibility* (Greene, 1995, 1996). Diverse psychosocial treatment approaches have been applied to children's social, emotional, and behavioral challenges, many with a distinctly unidirectional orientation. Must interventions aimed at improving child–environment compatibility address all facets of the compatibility equation to be effective? Not necessarily. But aspects of the equation that are left unaddressed certainly have the potential to impede or undercut treatment gains.

For example, pharmacotherapy is a very popular approach to externalizing problems in children and – even though it is a distinctly unidirectional intervention – can have a significant impact on child–environment incompatibility (both positive and negative). On the positive side, if factors thought to be residing within the *child* – for example, hyperactivity and poor impulse control – are contributing to child–environment incompatibility and are addressed through the use of medication, compatibility would be expected to improve and incompatibility episodes would be reduced.

However, if it is also the case that adult caregivers have, for instance, unreasonable academic and behavioral expectations or unrealistic notions about changes that will be achieved through administration of stimulant medication, then this aspect of the compatibility equation would not be addressed through administration of medication to the child and could offset the positive effects of the medication. Treatment would then need to be expanded to other aspects of the equation.

Diverse forms of psychosocial treatment have been applied to children's externalizing behavior problems as well, and many of these interventions have also had a unidirectional orientation. Some psychosocial treatment models have focused on training cognitive skills to challenging children (see Coie & Dodge, 1998; Kendall, 1985, 1991; Kendall & MacDonald, 1993), and several such models have been identified as "probably efficacious," including those focusing on training problem-solving skills (e.g., Kazdin, Esveldt-Dawson, French, & Unis, 1987; Kazdin, Siegel, & Bass, 1992) and anger management skills (e.g., Feindler, 1990, 1991, 1995; Lochman, 1992; Lochman, Burch, Curry, & Lampron, 1984; Lochman, Lampron, Gemmer, & Harris, 1987). However, similar to medication, such interventions aim to change factors residing within the *child* to improve child–environment transactions and would therefore not be expected to address the transactional processes giving rise to challenging behavior. Nor would such interventions be well-suited to addressing the unsolved problems precipitating incompatibility episodes.

Other psychosocial interventions have focused primarily on addressing factors thought to be residing in *parents*. Various parent-training (PT) models have been disseminated and utilized, and focus primarily on training parents of challenging children to be less passive, less permissive, more contingent, and more consistent, usually through application of strategies such as positive attending; use of appropriate commands; contingent attention and reinforcement; and use of a time-out procedure (see McMahon & Wells, 1998). In general, research has also documented the efficacy of these procedures (see Brestan & Eyberg, 1998, for a comprehensive review), and several intervention programs emanating from these models have been identified as either "well-established" or as "probably efficacious."

However, as with any treatment paradigm, there are a variety of limitations associated with parent-training models, perhaps suggesting some issues related to person–treatment compatibility and to the limited scope of this intervention. First, a substantial number of parents who receive PT do not fully comply with implementation or drop out of treatment altogether (e.g., Prinz & Miller, 1994). Most studies examining the efficacy of PT have presented data only for those who remained in treatment rather than those who began treatment. Among those who remain in treatment, PT has been shown to produce statistically significant changes in oppositional behavior, but very few studies have reported clinically significant changes (Kazdin, 1997). Indeed, 30–40% of those children remaining in treatment continue to evidence behavior problems in the clinical range at follow-up (e.g., Kazdin, 1993; Webster-Stratton, 1990). Data have shown that a significant percentage of children – perhaps higher than 50% – are not functioning within the normal range when such treatment is completed

(Dishion & Patterson, 1992). Finally, the vast majority of studies examining the efficacy of PT has not included clinically referred youth (Kazdin, 1997; Patterson & Chamberlain, 1994), and has typically failed to examine long-term treatment effects (Kazdin, 1993; 1997). In view of these limitations, it may be reasonable to conclude that, in focusing primarily on altering parental discipline patterns, PT does not address the range of transactional processes giving rise to challenging behavior; nor would PT be expected to address the unsolved problems and lagging skills giving rise to incompatibility episodes.

As a side note, most school discipline programs also place a strong emphasis on the use of operant procedures. While it is not unusual to hear school personnel invoke parental inadequacies as the root cause of children's challenging behavior, when used in schools, such procedures are typically employed to address problems said to reside in the child, such as poor motivation, attention-seeking, and limit-testing (Greene, 2008).

Collaborative Problem Solving is a relative newcomer to the psychosocial treatment realm. As noted earlier, CPS is something of a "hybrid" model, incorporating facets of transactional, systems, and social learning theories. The goal of treatment in CPS is to *understand, address, and resolve factors contributing to child-environment incompatibility*, and this goal is achieved by helping adult caregivers (1) understand the specific child and environmental characteristics contributing to the development of disadvantageous behavior in the child and other individuals; (2) become cognizant of three basic strategies for handling unmet expectations and unsolved problems – imposition of adult will, solving problems collaboratively, and removing the expectation and unsolved problems – and recognize the impact of each of these three approaches on child–environment compatibility; and (3) become proficient, along with the child at collaboratively resolving problems as a means of resolving disagreements and defusing potentially conflictual situations so as to improve child–environment compatibility and reduce disadvantageous behavior. Let us consider each of these goals in greater detail.

Achieve an Understanding of Challenging Behavior. In pursuing this goal, adults are helped to understand that lagging skills are what leaves a child vulnerable to challenging behavior, and are then helped to identify the specific lagging skills coming into play for an individual child. For many adults, this process sets in motion a paradigm shift, and this shift can, in and of itself, help adults respond to challenging behavior in a less personalized, less punitive less reactive, and more empathic manner, and is crucial to helping adults understand the necessity for an alternative approach that takes a child's lagging skills into account.

As I have noted elsewhere (Greene, 2009), adults often bring children who are exhibiting challenging behavior into treatment asking the question, "What should I do?" The first goal is help adults shift, at least initially, to a different set of questions ("Why is this child acting this way and why is it that what seems to work with other children is not working with this one?"). In schools and treatment facilities, unidirectional explanations that imply intent (e.g., attention-seeking, manipulative, coercive, limit-testing, unmotivated), labels that imply fixed character (e.g., sociopath, psychopath, conduct disordered), and explanations that elevate some of the facts that are known about a child to "causal status" ("he was exposed to substances in utero," "his mother's crazy," "his father's in jail," "you know what neighborhood he lives in," "his brother's the same way") often color the perspectives of those responsible for intervention. Moreover, children who have evidenced challenging behavior for many years often come with large "portfolios" filled with massive and overwhelming amounts of information, prior testing, and past treatment plans.

As you've read, in CPS, there are two important "filters" for sorting through this information: *lagging skills* and *unsolved problems*. While much of a child's history is interesting as background information – typically providing countless sobering examples of child–environment incompatibility and child–treatment incompatibility – the goal is to identify "actionable" information. The advantage of focusing on lagging skills and unsolved problems is that the skills can be taught and the problems solved; thus, these filters may be more likely to set the stage for productive, systematic intervention than focusing on past events about which the child, and those trying to help him, can do little to change.

Each child has a unique profile of lagging skills and unsolved problems; it is crucial for the key adults who interact with a child to come to a consensus about his or her specific lagging skills and unsolved problems and, as part of this process, to establish priorities for what to begin working on first (because it will not be possible to fix everything in one fell swoop). The ALSUP will be an important tool for these purposes. This process, and the consensus that emerges from it, propel CPS treatment into its next phase.

Yet, this consensus can be particularly difficult to achieve in schools and treatment facilities, where communication can be challenging across classes and shifts and where it can be extremely difficult to intervene in a cohesive, consistent manner in which the "left hand knows what the right hand is doing." Of course, CPS is not the only model of intervention requiring good communication; any *effective* model of care has the same requirement. Thus, while the creation of mechanisms for effective communication is not an ingredient specific to the CPS model, it is typically an extremely important focal point when the model is being implemented.

This treatment ingredient helps adults recognize that incompatibility episodes occur in the context of specific unsolved problems, and promotes the understanding that, if a problem can be solved, it won't precipitate challenging behavior any longer. Solved problems do not precipitate challenging behavior, only unsolved problems do.

The role of *adult* characteristics in contributing to incompatibility episodes is typically not a major emphasis early in treatment, but increases in importance as treatment progresses. The manner in which adults respond to problems and unmet expectations is typically the first adult characteristic to be examined. This leads us to our next goal.

Delineate Three Response Options. This goal speaks to the need to help adults understand that the manner by which they try to solve problems and pursue unmet expectations with the child is a major factor influencing the frequency and intensity of incompatibility episodes. Imposition of adult will (in the parlance of CPS, this approach is referred to as

"Plan A") is one way to pursue unmet expectations and solve problems, but is also the most common precipitant of acute (but highly predictable) incompatibility episodes. Removing an expectation (known as "Plan C") is effective at reducing tension between child and adult, but not effective at helping adults pursue unmet expectations. Collaborative Problem Solving ("Plan B") is an effective way to pursue expectations without increasing the likelihood of incompatibility episodes while simultaneously training and practicing emotion regulation, frustration tolerance, problem-solving, flexibility, and a host of other lagging skills (in both interaction partners).

The three Plans can serve as useful "shorthand" for helping adults communicate and think about how they are approaching problems. The ultimate goal is to help adults reduce their use of Plan A (thereby reducing incompatibility episodes), determine which unsolved problems are to be the current focus of intervention and which are not (this is where Plan C comes in), and dramatically increase their use of Plan B so that problems are resolved in a realistic, mutually satisfactory, durable manner and incompatibility episodes are dramatically reduced. Over time, this combination of ingredients sets the stage for new interaction patterns in which adult caregivers are imposing their will less frequently, collaboratively solving problems more frequently (and preferably proactively), communicating more effectively, and improving various facets of child–environment compatibility.

It is quite common for adult caregivers – who have historically been relying heavily on some combination of imposed consequences and problem avoidance, have had only two options in their repertoires (Plan A and Plan C), and have therefore been engaged in the practice of "battle picking" – to conclude that Plan B is the equivalent of "giving in," to feel that they are relinquishing authority by using Plan B, and to believe that the CPS model involves dropping all adult expectations. The clinician takes the time to inquire about these concerns and helps caregivers talk about and move beyond them. Adults are pursuing expectations and "setting limits" with both Plan A and Plan B and are not dropping all their expectations, and Plan B has a significantly greater upside (and significantly less downside) than Plan A.

Help Adults Become Proficient at Plan B. This goal involves helping adult caregivers begin effectively using Plan B to solve, in a realistic and mutually satisfactory manner, predictable, longstanding issues of conflict or disagreement so as to reduce the likelihood of incompatibility episodes, create new interaction patterns, and increase child–environment compatibility. Plan B often involves a child and adult caregiver, but also has application to interactions between two individual children, to groups of children, and to problems that occur between adults (Greene, 2008). For purposes of this chapter, Plan B will be described primarily in the context of adult–child interactions.

Key to the creation of these new patterns is to help adults and children solve problems *proactively* rather than *emergently*. Adult caregivers (and many children) are surprised to learn that most of the problems precipitating incompatibility episodes are actually highly predictable and can therefore be discussed in a planful manner. The reality is that "Emergency Plan

B" tends to be far less productive than "Proactive Plan B," the former being more of a crisis management tool and the latter reflective of a crisis prevention mindset. The primary disadvantage of emergent Plan B is heat (as in "the heat of the moment"), which makes solving problems far more challenging. Incompatibility episodes are merely a signal that there is a problem that has not yet been solved. Upon reflection, it is almost always the case that the problems causing incompatibility episodes were already highly predictable.

Plan B consists of three ingredients. The first, historically referred to as the "Empathy step," involves having adult caregivers *gather information* from a child so as to achieve the clearest possible *understanding* of the child's concern or perspective on a given problem. This is not easy for many adults, who often have preconceived notions about the child's concerns, have difficulty accepting children's concerns as legitimate, and may not be skilled at gathering highly specific information. This ingredient may also present significant challenges for children, who may never have given their concerns much thought (often because they have never been asked) and may also, in some instances, lack the communication skills to express their concerns. The second ingredient, known as the "Define the Problem" step, involves having the adult be highly specific about his or her concern or perspective on the same problem. This presents challenges as well, for many adults are much more certain about their solutions than they are about their concerns. Having now entered two concerns (but no solutions, yet) into consideration, the third ingredient, called the "Invitation" step, is where adult and child *brainstorm solutions* that will address the concerns of both parties. This ingredient, too presents significant challenges to adults and children, who may not have had much practice at considering solutions that are mutually satisfactory.

Becoming proficient at these three ingredients is hard work for both children and their adult caregivers. In an outpatient context, an overview of the three ingredients is provided once the clinician has introduced the philosophical and theoretical underpinnings of the CPS model, a profile of lagging skills and unsolved problems has been formulated (taking into account lagging skills and characteristics of the environment), and priorities established (drawing from the list of unsolved problems). Treatment then continues with the clinician instructing adult caregivers in the use of Plan B and being directly involved in the first few in-session Plan B discussions between adult caregivers and the child, moves on with the caregivers attempting Plan B in session (with guidance and feedback from the clinician), and continues with the caregivers engaging the child in Plan B discussions outside of the clinical setting, with increasing independence and, over time, decreased reliance on the clinician for feedback.

Clinicians implementing CPS do not take sides; instead they adopt the stance that the concerns of both parties are legitimate and need to be addressed for a problem to be durably solved. Adults often find the clinician's neutrality to be a bit disarming, as they may be accustomed to therapies (or general child-rearing trends in society) in which adult concerns take priority over the concerns of children. The adults are reassured that their concerns are legitimate and will be addressed through the process of collaboratively resolving problems. Children tend to be receptive to finally having their concerns heard and legitimized, but have often had little practice at generating alternative solutions and contemplating the degree to which the solutions are mutually satisfactory. The clinician helps the child appreciate the legitimacy of the adult concerns (or at least take the adult concerns into account). The ultimate goal is to help children and adults work toward solutions that address the concerns of both parties, and it is the children and adults, rather than the therapist, who determine whether a proposed solution is indeed mutually satisfactory.

The process is similar in schools and therapeutic facilities, where it is equally important to begin with philosophical and theoretical underpinnings. Unevenness in acceptance of the CPS philosophy across staff is to be expected. Thus, mechanisms must be in place to provide opportunities for staff to express concerns about the model, have misperceptions clarified, and then practice and receive feedback on their use of Plan B.

As described elsewhere (Greene, 2009), implementing CPS in an outpatient setting requires an array of clinical skills, including (a) knowledge of the lagging skills setting the stage for challenging behavior; (b) the ability to transmit this knowledge to adult caregivers in a way that is persuasive but not dogmatic; (c) the ability to develop therapeutic alliances with adult caretakers and challenging children so as to keep them engaged in the process (even when the going gets rough) and maintain a sense of realistic optimism; (d) the ability to empathize with each party about what they have gone through and are going through (even when the child is not a willing participant in treatment) and deal effectively with each party's misgivings and conceptions about this form of intervention; (e) the ability to take complex scenarios and reduce them to their basic ingredients: lagging skills and unsolved problems; (f) a capacity for neutrality, for it is not the role of the clinician to take sides or serve as judge and jury; (g) the ability to keep bringing participants back to the key themes of the intervention when they go astray, recognize when participants are having difficulty with key aspects of Plan B, and provide feedback and guidance on these aspects; (h) a sense of whether and when family members are able to converse directly with each other and the ability to prevent discussions from spinning out of control; (i) patience and persistence, because longstanding problems and patterns of interaction tend not to resolve quickly; (j) flexibility and creativity, because adult caretakers have typically been bumping up against inflexible systems for a very long time and have problems that often are not readily resolved through conventional solutions; and (k) energy, an "activist" mentality, and an understanding of how systems work, because the participants may well need someone to advocate on their behalf in a society where Plan A is still quite popular.

Implementation of CPS in schools and therapeutic facilities requires some additional skills, including (a) knowledge of the politics of larger systems, an awareness of the need to understand the politics and hierarchy within each individual system prior to beginning training in CPS, and strategies for helping large systems bring people on board and deal effectively with the "politics of change"; (b) knowledge of the difficulties in communication inherent in large systems and of ways to help such systems establish optimal mechanisms for communication; and (c) recognition that things are likely to get worse before they get better.

Moreover, in such facilities, the individuals with whom (or situations in which) a child typically has difficulty in the outside world may not be readily accessible. This does not mean that Plan B cannot occur, but simply that staff may have to serve as the mouthpiece for those individuals. Fortunately, interactions and problems in restrictive facilities often imitate real life; the skills the children are lacking and problems they are having in the facility are the same as those that they were having in the "real world" (and that prompted their placement), so solving problems and teaching skills in the facility is not pretense, it is the real deal.

CPS is not a passive model of intervention. Pre-existing belief systems and practices do not change quickly. Adults have legitimate concerns about whether they will still be in control, whether they (and perhaps their other children, students, or residents) will be safe, and whether chaos will ensue when one is implementing the CPS model. Fortunately, data (see below) suggest that parents feel significantly more competent, set limits more effectively, and feel significantly better about their relationship with their child after CPS treatment. Noncompliance and other conduct problems are significantly reduced in response to CPS; and, in restrictive facilities, use of chemical, physical, mechanical restraint, and locked-door seclusion are significantly reduced (along with staff and patient injuries) when CPS is implemented.

Is CPS a transactional model of intervention? The approach involves key interaction partners (rather than targeting only one), incorporates (in both assessment and treatment) characteristics of child and environment giving rise to child–environment incompatibility, and – in working toward realistic and mutually satisfactory solutions to the unsolved problems precipitating incompatibility episodes –teaches lagging cognitive skills to all interaction partners.

As described below, the model has been shown to be an effective means of reducing oppositional behavior in children, improving adult–child interactions, and improving parental feelings of competence. The skills-training aspect of the model has yet to be documented, but is presently being evaluated in a 5-year NIMH-funded study at the Virginia Tech Child Study Center.

RESEARCH

Empirical evaluation of CPS has provided evidence of its effectiveness (Greene et al., 2004). An initial outpatient study of CPS (funded by the Stanley Foundation) involved 50 clinically referred youth (boys and girls) with ODD between the ages of 4 and 13 years. In addition to ODD, all children receiving treatment also had at least subthreshold symptoms of either bipolar disorder or severe major depression. The 50 children were randomly assigned (using a 3:2 randomization scheme) to either CPS or PT; 47 children completed treatment (CPS $n = 28$, PT $n = 19$).

Parents receiving PT were treated using Barkley's (1997b) program for defiant youth. All participants in this condition received 10 weeks of treatment (9 consecutive weeks and a 1-month follow-up). The length of treatment for participants in the CPS condition was variable, and ranged from 6 to 16 weeks, depending on clinicians' assessment of the needs of each child and family. However, the average length of treatment in the CPS condition was also 10 weeks.

A variety of instruments were used to assess treatment response at the beginning and end of treatment and at 4-month follow-up, including clinical global impression (CGI) ratings by therapists and parents; parent ratings of the frequency and severity of their children's oppositional behavior; parenting stress; and parent–child relationship. Comprehensive results from this study are presented elsewhere (Greene et al., 2002) but summarized here. Briefly, the two groups did not differ significantly at baseline on any measures of treatment outcome. As noted above, while average length of treatment for both groups was 10 weeks, duration of treatment was constant in the PT condition but variable in the CPS condition. To protect against the potential confounds this presented, we assessed the degree to which treatment duration was a significant predictor of outcome for all outcome variables; it was not.

The CPS condition produced significant improvement in parents' ratings of their children's oppositional behavior from baseline to post-treatment and from baseline to 4-month follow-up. No significant differences were found between the two treatment groups at either point in time, nor were time by group interactions significant from pre-treatment to post-treatment or from pre-treatment to 4-month follow-up. Large effect sizes were found for both CPS (1.19) and PT (0.80) from baseline to post-treatment; from baseline to 4-month follow-up, a large effect size was found for CPS (1.19) and a moderate effect size for PT (0.48).

The CPS condition produced borderline significant improvement from baseline to post-treatment in global parenting stress. No significant differences were found between the two treatment groups, nor was the time by group interaction significant. The CPS condition produced borderline significant improvement in a variety of domains of parenting stress, including child adaptability and parent competence. The time by group interaction was not significant on any subscale. With regards to the parent–child relationship, the CPS condition produced significant improvement in limit-setting and borderline significant improvement in parent–child communication. There was a borderline significant time by group interaction on the child autonomy subscale, with children in the PT condition evidencing deterioration, and the children in the CPS condition evidencing improvement, in this domain from pre-treatment to post-treatment.

We next examined ratings of the two treatment conditions on the therapist-completed (at post-treatment) and parent-completed (at 4-month follow-up) clinical global impression (CGI) instrument, entering treatment group as a predictor in regression models. At post-treatment, treatment group emerged as a significant predictor, with the behavior of children in the CPS condition rated as having improved to a significantly greater degree as compared to children in the PT condition. Treatment group also emerged as a significant predictor on parent ratings on the CGI at 4-month follow-up, with children in the CPS condition rated as having improved to a significantly greater degree as compared with children in the PT condition.

We identified children who evidenced an "excellent response to treatment" as those whose behavior was, at post-treatment (rated by therapists) and at 4-month follow-up (rated by mothers) as "very much improved" or "much improved" on the CGI. Treatment group was not a significant predictor of an excellent response to treatment at post-treatment, although 71% of children in the CPS condition evidenced an excellent response to treatment at post-treatment, as compared with 47% of those in the PT condition. At 4-month follow-up, treatment group was a borderline significant predictor of excellent response to treatment; 80% of children in the CPS condition evidenced an excellent response to treatment at this data point, as compared with 44% of those in the PT condition.

Clinical significance was defined as an improvement of 30% or greater in ODD-related behaviors (as measured by the Oppositional Defiant Disorder Rating Scale) between baseline and post-treatment and between baseline and 4-month follow-up. No significant differences were found between the two groups in rates of children evidencing clinically significant change. At post-treatment, 52% of children in the CPS condition were rated as having evidenced clinically significant improvement, as compared with 32% of those in the PT condition. At 4-month follow-up, 46% of children in the CPS condition were rated as having evidenced clinically significant improvement, as compared with 32% of those in the PT condition.

As noted above, a large-scale 5-year replication of the above study is currently underway at Virginia Tech. In addition, two published studies have documented the effectiveness of the model in inpatient settings (Greene et al., 2006; Martin et al., 2008). Reports documenting the effectiveness of the model in juvenile detention and public school settings are currently in preparation.

CASE STUDY

Given the wide range of settings in which the CPS model has been implemented, it is hard to choose one in which to provide an illustration of Plan B in both principle and action. Fortunately, Plan B looks fairly similar regardless of setting, so the following example will have relevance to all of them.

Maggie is a 13-year old seventh-grader. The use of Plan B described here occurred at school, where there are numerous examples of child–environment incompatibility. For example, Maggie frequently fails to begin her assignments (especially in math) when instructed to (at which times, she sometimes distracts her classmates with conversation or attempts at humor), engages in "horseplay" in the hallways between classes, has a reputation for hanging out with other kids who get into trouble, sometimes violates the school's dress code, and often responds to corrective feedback from adults with a "bad attitude" and "disrespect." Her teachers and the school administration are aware of her troubled family history (her father left home when Maggie was in preschool), and Maggie and her mother have a well-known volatile relationship. Indeed, when school personnel try talking with Maggie about her problems at school, she often invokes her interactions with her mother as the cause. This has historically caused school personnel to feel that they cannot help Maggie much – beyond recommending to her mother that counseling be sought – since her problems seem related to factors outside the school setting and beyond their control.

Maggie is a frequent visitor to the assistant principal's office and a frequent recipient of detentions and suspensions. This causes her mother great frustration; each time Maggie is sent home from school, Maggie's mother misses work, exacerbating their already-tenuous financial situation and increasing the likelihood of episodes of child–parent incompatibility. Moreover, after many years of such interventions, Maggie's mother has become skeptical about their effectiveness and has come to feel that school staff blames her for Maggie's difficulties at school. School personnel patiently explain to the mother that the system they use for discipline was set in stone by the school board and that they have little flexibility in its application.

Yet, recently when the teachers and administrators met to discuss Maggie, the assistant principal suggested using the ALSUP as their discussion guide. They were able to identify a variety of lagging skills and predictable unsolved problems contributing to her difficulties. Foremost among Maggie's lagging skills were difficulty handling transitions, shifting from one mindset or task to another, persisting on challenging or tedious tasks, difficulty maintaining focus, managing emotional response to frustration so as to think rationally, and taking into account situational factors that would suggest the need to adjust a plan of action. The list of unsolved problems included being in hallways between classes, difficulty in starting and completing assignments, and issues in handling teacher's feedback. Then the assembled educators discussed their priorities, and identified the unsolved problems that were to be the focus of their first Plan B discussions with Maggie, as well as on who would be initiating these discussions with her.

Members of the discussion group were mixed in their views of how Maggie would respond to Plan B. Several teachers commented that they had "talked" and "processed" things with Maggie on dozens of occasions (while acknowledging that the talking and processing had not included the ingredients of Plan B). Others predicted that Maggie wouldn't participate at all. Still others suggested that they really had nothing to lose, since their standard approach had not achieved appreciable success. Maggie's science teacher, with whom she had a good relationship, volunteered to try Plan B with Maggie on the issue of handling teacher feedback, and Maggie not only participated willingly but was also rather forthcoming about how some of her teachers (especially her math teacher) were treating her, how she often entered school in the morning "in a mood" because of adversarial interactions with her mother before school (math was her first class), and about her frustrations with various academic assignments (especially math) on which she believed she was not receiving enough help. The teacher's initial Plan B conversation with Maggie – which took place during the teacher's prep time – didn't make it past the Empathy step and lasted about 30 minutes, but Maggie was agreeable to continuing the conversation, this time with her math teacher joining in. The math teacher received advanced preparation on the necessity of listening, nondefensively, to Maggie's concerns; Maggie was prepped on the need to express her concerns in a way that would not cause the math teacher to stop listening. The math teacher was able to both tolerate and understand Maggie's concerns; Maggie was able to tolerate and comprehend the teacher's concerns. Then the consideration of mutually satisfactory solutions commenced and an initial action plan was put in place. The action plan included several components: (a) a mechanism for Maggie to signal to the math teacher if it had been a difficult morning at home; (b) how the teacher would respond if Maggie was too agitated to begin work immediately; (c) how to ensure that Maggie received the academic help she felt she needed; (d) how the teacher could deliver feedback in ways that were not embarrassing to Maggie; and (e) an agreement to meet again to consider how the plan was working and to continue the problem-solving process if any facets of the plan were not achieving durable success.

This process was replicated, with different teachers initiating Plan B, on the various additional unsolved problems affecting Maggie at school. Some went better than others, but as the school year continued, teachers began commenting on their new understanding of Maggie, their appreciation of her willingness to work with them to solve problems, and the uneven but appreciable progress she was making on the unsolved problems they had addressed. They also noted that the time they spent doing Plan B with Maggie was significantly less than the time they'd spent dealing with her when they were using Plan A. Over time, use of punitive interventions with Maggie declined precipitously; as progress was made on solving problems and incompatibility episodes were reduced, the teachers and assistant principal came to feel that such interventions would do her more harm than good. They began informally applying CPS to other "frequent flyers" in the school discipline program and began developing formal mechanisms for ensuring that CPS was used in the school's assessment and intervention practices.

CONCLUSION

Collaborative Problem Solving is a relatively new cognitive–behavioral psychosocial treatment approach that has been applied, predominantly to youth with externalizing behavior problems, in a variety of contexts, including families, general and special education schools, inpatient psychiatry units, residential and juvenile detention facilities, and in law enforcement agencies. Relying heavily on transactional theories of development, systems theory, social learning theory, and research in the neurosciences, the model posits that lagging cognitive skills and unsolved problems set the stage for child–environment incompatibility and applies a collaborative approach to problem-solving as the primary tool for improving compatibility. Initial studies have documented the effectiveness of the model in outpatient and inpatient settings, and forthcoming papers document its effectiveness in schools and juvenile detention settings.

REFERENCES

H. Abikoff, R.G. Klein, Attention-deficit hyperactivity disorder and conduct disorder: Comorbidity and implications for treatment. Journal of Consulting and Clinical Psychology **60**, 881–892 (1992)

American Psychiatric Association, *Diagnostic and statistical manual of mental disorders*, 4th edn. (Author, Washington, DC, 1994)

A. Angold, E.J. Costello, Depressive comorbidity in children and adolescents: Empirical, theoretical, and methodological issues. American Journal of Psychiatry **150**, 1779–1791 (1993)

L. Baker, D.P. Cantwell, A prospective psychiatric follow-up of with speech/language disorders. Journal of the American Academy of Child and Adolescent Psychiatry **26**, 546–553 (1987)

R.A. Barkley, Behavioral inhibition, sustained attention, and executive functions: Constructing a unifying theory of ADHD. Psychological Bulletin **121**(1), 65–94 (1997a)

R.A. Barkley, *Defiant children: A clinician's manual for assessment and parent training*, 2nd edn. (Guilford Press, New York, 1997b)

J.H. Beitchman, J. Hood, A. Inglis, Psychiatric risk in children with speech and language disorders. Journal of Abnormal Child Psychology **18**, 283–296 (1990)

J.H. Beitchman, J. Hood, J. Rochon, M. Peterson, Empirical classification of speech/ language impairment in. II. Behavioral characteristics. Journal of the American Academy of Child and Adolescent Psychiatry **28**, 118–123 (1989)

R. Bell, A reinterpretation of the direction of effects in socialization. Psychological Review **75**, 81–95 (1968)

J. Belsky, The determinants of parenting: A process model. Child Development **55**, 83–96 (1984)

P.A. Brennan, E.R. Grekin, S.A. Mednick, Prenatal and perinatal influences on conduct disorder and serious delinquency, in *Causes of conduct disorder and juvenile delinquency*, ed. by B.B. Lahey, T.E. Moffitt, A. Caspi (Guilford, New York, 2003), pp. 319–344

E.V. Brestan, S.M. Eyberg, Effective psychosocial treatment of conduct-disordered children and adolescents: 29 years, 82 studies, and 5, 272 kids. Journal of Clinical Child Psychology **27**(2), 180–189 (1998)

I. Bretherton, J. Fritz, C. Zahn-Waxler, D. Ridgeway, Learning to talk about emotions: A functionalist perspective. Child Development **57**, 529–548 (1986)

C.L. Budman, R.D. Bruun, K.S. Park, M.E. Olson, Rage attacks in children and adolescents with Tourette's disorder: A pilot study. Journal of Clinical Psychiatry **59**(11), 576–580 (1998)

P. Chamberlain, G.R. Patterson, Discipline and child compliance in parenting, in *Handbook of parenting (Vol.4): Applied and practical parenting*, ed. by M.H. Bornstein (Lawrence Erlbaum, Mahwah, NJ, 1995)

S. Chess, A. Thomas, *Origins and evolution of behavior disorders: From infancy to early adult life* (Brunner/Mazel, New York, 1984)

D. Cicchetti, M. Lynch, Toward and ecological/transactional model of community violence and child maltreatment. Psychiatry **56**, 96–118 (1993)

D. Cicchetti, M. Lynch, Failures in the expectable environment and their impact on individual development: The case of child maltreatment, in *Developmental psychopathology*, ed. by D. Cicchetti, D.J. Cohen. Risk, disorder, and adaptation, vol. 2 (Wiley, New York, 1995), pp. 32–71

Coie, J. D., & Dodge, K. A. (1998). Aggression and anti-social behavior. In W. Damon (Ed.), *Handbook of child psychology* (5th ed.): Vol. 3. Social, emotional, and personality development (pp. 779–862). New York: Wiley

M.B. Denckla, A theory and model of executive function: A neuropsychological perspective, in *Attention, memory, and executive function*, ed. by G.R. Lyon, N.A. Krasnegor (Paul H. Brookes, Baltimore, MD, 1996), pp. 263–278

T.J. Dishion, G.R. Patterson, Age affects in parent training outcomes. Behavior Therapy **23**, 719–729 (1992)

Feindler, E. L. (1990). Adolescent anger control: Review and critique. In M. Hersen, R. M. Eisler, & P. M. Miller (Eds.), *Progress in behavior modification* (Vol. 26, 00. 11–59). Newbury Park, CA: Sage.

E.L. Feindler, Cognitive strategies in anger control interventions for children and adolescents, in *Child and adolescent therapy: Cognitive-behavioral procedures*, ed. by P.C. Kendall (Guilford Press, New York, 1991), pp. 66–97

E.L. Feindler, An ideal treatment package for children and adolescents with anger disorders, in *Anger disorders: Definition, diagnosis, and treatment*, ed. by H. Kassinove (Taylor & Francis, Washington, DC, 1995), pp. 173–195

E.J. Garland, M. Weiss, Case study: Obsessive difficult temperament and its response to serotonergic medication. Journal of the American Academy of Child and Adolescent Psychiatry **35**(7), 916–920 (1996)

B. Geller, J. Luby, Child and adolescent bipolar disorder: Review of the past 10 years. Journal of the American Academy of Child and Adolescent Psychiatry **36**(9), 1–9 (1997)

G. Gottlieb, *Individual development and evolution: The genesis of novel behavior* (Oxford University Press, New York, 1992)

J. Gottman, The world of coordinated play: Same and cross-sex friendship in children, in *Conversations of friends: Speculations on affective development*, ed. by J.M. Gottman, J.G. Parker (Cambridge University Press, Cambridge, England, 1986), pp. 139–191

R.W. Greene, Students with ADHD in school classrooms: Teacher factors related to compatibility, assessment, and intervention. School Psychology Review **24**(1), 81–93 (1995)

R.W. Greene, Students with ADHD and their teachers: Implications of a goodness-of-fit perspective, in *Advances in clinical child psychology*, ed. by T.H. Ollendick, R.J. Prinz (Plenum, New York, 1996), pp. 205–230

R.W. Greene, *The explosive child: Understanding and parenting easily frustrated, "Chronically Inflexible" children* (HarperCollins, New York, 1998)

R.W. Greene, *Lost at school: Why our kids with behavioral challenges are falling through the cracks and how we can help them* (Scribner, New York, 2008)

Greene, R.W. (2010). Conduct disorder and oppositional defiant disorder. In J. Thomas & M. Hersen (Eds.), *Handbook of Clinical Psychology Competencies*. New York: Springer Publishing, 1329–1350

Greene, R.W. (2010). *Collaborative problem solving: The model and its application across settings*. New York: Guilford (in press)

R.W. Greene, R.R. Abidin, C. Kmetz, The index of teaching stress: A measure of student-teacher compatibility. Journal of School Psychology **35**(3), 239–259 (1997)

R.W. Greene, S.A. Ablon, A. Martin, Innovations: Child psychiatry: Use of collaborative problem solving to reduce seclusion and restraint in child and adolescent inpatient units. Psychiatric Services **57**(5), 610–616 (2006)

R.W. Greene, J.S. Ablon, M. Monuteaux, J. Goring, A. Henin, L. Raezer, G. Edwards, J. Markey, S. Rabbitt, Effectiveness of collaborative problem solving in affectively dysregulated youth with oppositional defiant disorder: Initial findings. Journal of Consulting and Clinical Psychology **72**, 1157–1164 (2004)

R.W. Greene, J. Biederman, S. Zerwas, M. Monuteaux, J.C. Goring, S.V. Faraone, Psychiatric comorbidity, family dysfunction, and social impairment in referred youth with oppositional defiant disorder. American Journal of Psychiatry **159**, 1214–1224 (2002)

R.W. Greene, A.E. Doyle, Toward a transactional conceptualization of oppositional defiant disorder: Implications for assessment and treatment. Clinical and Family Psychology Review **2**(3), 129–147 (1999)

R.W. Greene, T.H. Ollendick, Behavioral assessment of children, in *Handbook of psychological assessment*, ed. by G. Goldstein, M. Hersen, 3rd edn. (Elsevier Science (Pergamon), Oxford, 2000), pp. 453–470

J.D. Harnish, K.A. Dodge, E. Valente, Mother-child interaction quality as a partial mediator of the roles of maternal depressive symptomatology and socioeconomic status in the development of child conduct problems. Child Development **66**, 739–753 (1995)

S.C. Hayes, R.O. Nelson, B.B. Jerrett, The treatment utility of assessment: A functional approach to evaluating assessment quality. American Psychologist **42**, 963–974 (1987)

S.P. Hinshaw, B.B. Lahey, E.L. Hart, Issues of taxonomy and comorbidity in the development of conduct disorder. Development and Psychopathology **5**, 31–49 (1993)

A.E. Kazdin, Treatment of conduct disorder: Progress and directions in psychotherapy research. Development and Psychopathology **5**, 277–310 (1993)

A.E. Kazdin, Parent management training: Evidence, outcomes, and issues. Journal of the American Academy of Child and Adolescent Psychiatry **36**(10), 1349–1356 (1997)

A.E. Kazdin, K. Esveldt-Dawson, N.H. French, A.S. Unis, Problem-solving skills training and relationship therapy in the treatment of antisocial child behavior. Journal of Consulting and Clinical Psychology **55**, 76–85 (1987)

A.E. Kazdin, T.C. Siegel, D. Bass, Cognitive problem-solving skills training and parent management training in the treatment of antisocial behavior in children. Journal of Consulting and Clinical Psychology **60**(5), 733–747 (1992)

P.C. Kendall, Toward a cognitive-behavioral model of child psychopathology and a critique of related interventions. Journal of Abnormal Psychology **13**, 357–372 (1985)

P.C. Kendall, Guiding theory for therapy with children and adolescents, in *Child and adolescent therapy: Cognitive-behavioral procedures*, ed. by P.C. Kendall (Guilford Press, New York, 1991), pp. 3–22

P.C. Kendall, J.P. MacDonald, Cognition in the psychopathology of youth and implications for treatment, in *Psychopathology and cognition*, ed. by K.S. Dobson, P.C. Kendall (Academic Press, San Diego, CA, 1993), pp. 387–426

C.B. Kopp, Regulation of distress and negative emotions: A developmental view. Developmental Psychology **25**(3), 343–354 (1989)

B.B. Lahey, R. Loeber, Framework for a developmental model of oppositional defiant disorder and conduct disorder, in *Disruptive behavior disorders in childhood*, ed. by D.K. Routh (Plenum, New York, 1994)

J.E. Lochman, Cognitive-behavioral interventions with aggressive boys. Child Psychiatry and Human Development **16**, 45–56 (1992)

J.E. Lochman, P.R. Burch, J.F. Curry, L.B. Lampron, Treatment and generalization effects of cognitive-behavioral and goal-setting interventions with aggressive boys. Journal of Consulting and Clinical Psychology **52**, 915–916 (1984)

J.E. Lochman, L.B. Lampron, T.C. Gemmer, S.R. Harris, Anger coping intervention with aggressive children: A guide to implementation in school settings, in *Innovations in clinical practice: A source book*, ed. by P.A. Keller, S.R. Heyman, vol. 6 (Professional Resource Exchange, Sarasota, FL, 1987), pp. 339–356

A. Martin, H. Krieg, F. Esposito, D. Stubbe, L. Cardona, Reduction of restraint and seclusion through Collaborative Problem Solving: A five-year, prospective inpatient study. ***Psychiatric Services* 59**(12), 1406–1412 (2008)

R.J. McMahon, K.C. Wells, Conduct problems, in *Treatment of childhood disorders*, ed. by E.J. Mash, R.A. Barkley, 2nd edn. (Guilford, New York, 1998), pp. 111–210

B. Milner, Aspects of human frontal lobe function, in *Epilepsy and the functional autonomy of the frontal lobe*, ed. by H.H. Jasper, S. Riggio, P.S. Goldman-Rakic (Raven Press, New York, 1995), pp. 67–81

W. Mischel, Delay of gratification as process and as person variable in development, in *Interactions in human development*, ed. by D. Magnusson, V.P. Allen (Academic Press, New York, 1983), pp. 149–165

T.E. Moffitt, D. Lynam, The neuropsychology of conduct disorder and delinquency: Implications for understanding antisocial behavior, in *Experimental personality and psychopathology research 1994*, ed. by D.C. Fowles, P. Sutker, S.H. Goodman (Springer, New York, 1994), pp. 233–262

G.R. Patterson, P. Chamberlain, A functional analysis of resistance during parent training therapy. Clinical Psychology: Science and Practice **1**(1), 53–70 (1994)

G.R. Patterson, M.E. Gullion, *Living with children: New methods for parents and teachers* (Research Press, Champaign, IL, 1968)

G.R. Patterson, J.B. Reid, T.J. Dishion, *Antisocial boys* (Castalia, Patterson, OR, 1992)

B.F. Pennington, S. Ozonoff, Executive functions and developmental psychopathology. Journal of Child Psychology and Psychiatry **37**, 51–87 (1996)

R.J. Prinz, G.E. Miller, Family-based treatment for childhood antisocial behavior: Experimental influences on dropout and engagement. Journal of Consulting & Clinical Psychology **62**, 645–650 (1994)

A. Sameroff, Early influences on development: Fact or fancy? Merrill-Palmer Quarterly **21**, 263–294 (1975)

A. Sameroff, General systems theory and developmental psychopathology, in *Developmental psychopathology (Vol. 1): Theory and methods*, ed. by D. Cicchetti, D.J. Cohen (Wiley, New York, 1995), pp. 659–695

C.A. Stifter, T.L. Spinrad, J.M. Braungart-Rieker, Toward a developmental model of child compliance: The role of emotion regulation in infancy. Child Development **70**(1), 21–32 (1999)

T.K. Taylor, A. Biglan, Behavioral family interventions for improving child rearing: A review of the literature for clinicians and policy makers. Clinical Child and Family Psychology Review **1**(1), 41–60 (1998)

C. Webster-Stratton, Enhancing the effectiveness of self-administered videotape parent training for families with conduct-problem children. Journal of Abnormal Child Psychology **18**, 479–492 (1990)

D. Zillman, Cognition-excitation interdependencies in aggressive behavior. Aggressive Behavior **14**, 51–64 (1988)

9

Cognitive Behavior Therapy for the Group-Based Treatment of Oppositional Youth

JOHN E. LOCHMAN, CAROLINE BOXMEYER, NICOLE P. POWELL and KAREN C. WELLS

Aggression is one of the most stable problem behaviors in childhood (Lochman, Barry, Powell, Boxmeyer, & Holmes, 2008), and may escalate over time to include a wide range of severe antisocial behaviors in adolescence (Loeber, 1990). The negative developmental trajectory for aggressive children can lead to poor adjustment in the middle school years (Coie, Lochman, Terry, & Hyman, 1992) and to negative outcomes in adolescence such as drug and alcohol use, truancy and dropout, delinquency, and violence (e.g., Lochman & Wayland, 1994). The negative trajectory continues into adulthood for a portion of these children, with higher rates of criminal convictions and antisocial behavior (Cernkovich & Giordano, 2001). Because of the serious negative outcomes that can occur for aggressive children, intervention is critically important. Two related evidence-based interventions that will be discussed in this chapter are the group-based Anger Coping Program and the Coping Power Program. The Coping Power program is a multicomponent intervention that has 34 child sessions and 16 parent sessions (Lochman & Wells, 1996). The Coping Power child component evolved from the earlier 18-session Anger Coping program (Lochman, Nelson & Sims, 1981).

JOHN E. LOCHMAN • The University of Alabama
CAROLINE BOXMEYER • The University of Alabama
NICOLE P. POWELL • The University of Alabama
KAREN C. WELLS • Duke University Medical Center

R.C. Murrihy et al. (eds.), *Clinical Handbook of Assessing and Treating Conduct Problems in Youth*, DOI 10.1007/978-1-4419-6297-3_9,

ANGER COPING AND COPING POWER PROGRAM MODELS

Contextual Social-Cognitive Model for Aggressive Behavior

The contextual social-cognitive model which serves as the basis of our Anger Coping (Lochman, Nelson, & Sims, 1981) and Coping Power programs (Lochman & Wells, 2002a) has been based on empirically identified risk factors which predict children's antisocial behavior (Lochman & Gresham, 2008). As children develop, they can experience an accumulation of risk factors, increasing the probability that they will eventually display serious antisocial behavior (Loeber, 1990). Malleable risk factors that are incorporated into the intervention include risks in the family context, in the peer context, and in social cognitive processes and emotional regulation.

Family Factors. There is a wide array of factors in the family that can affect child aggression, ranging from poverty to more general stress and discord within the family (e.g., Loeber and Stouthamer-Loeber, 1998). Children's aggression has been linked to family background factors such as parent criminality, substance use and depression, poverty, stressful life events, single and teenage parenthood, and insecure, disorganized attachment. All of these family risk factors inter-relate with one another and build upon one another, and, in turn, can influence child behavior through their effect on parenting processes. For example, marital conflict during the preschool years can cause parents to become harsher and less consistent in their discipline and increased harsh, inconsistent discipline contribute to children's high levels of stress and consequent aggression.

Parenting processes linked to children's aggression (e.g., Patterson, Reid, & Dishion, 1992) include: (a) nonresponsive parenting at age 1, with pacing and consistency of parent responses not meeting children's needs; (b) coercive, escalating cycles of harsh parental demands and child noncompliance, starting in the toddler years, especially for children with difficult temperaments; (c) harsh, inconsistent discipline; (d) unclear directions and commands; (e) lack of warmth and involvement; and (f) lack of parental supervision and monitoring as children approach adolescence. The relations between parenting factors and childhood aggression are bi-directional, as child temperament and behavior also affect parenting behavior (Fite et al., 2006).

Peer Factors. Children with disruptive behaviors are at risk of being rejected by their peers. Aggressive children who are also socially rejected exhibit more severe antisocial behavior than children who are either aggressive only or rejected only (Lochman & Wayland, 1994). The match between the race of students and their peers in a classroom influences the degree of social rejection that students experience (Jackson, Barth, Powell, & Lochman, 2006), and race and gender appear to moderate the relation between peer rejection and negative adolescent outcomes. For example, Lochman and Wayland (1994) found that peer rejection ratings of African-American children within a mixed-race classroom did not predict subsequent externalizing problems in adolescence, whereas peer rejection ratings of Caucasian children were associated with future disruptive behaviors. Similarly, while peer rejection can predict serious delinquency in boys, it can fail to do so with girls (Miller-Johnson, Coie, Maumary-Gremaud, Lochman, & Terry, 1999).

As children with conduct problems enter adolescence they tend to associate with deviant peers. Adolescents who have been continually rejected from more prosocial peer groups because they lack appropriate social skills turn to antisocial cliques for social support (Miller-Johnson et al., 1999). The tendency for aggressive children to associate with one another increases the probability that the seriousness of their antisocial behavior will be escalated (e.g., Fite, Colder, Lochman, & Wells, 2007).

Social Cognition. On the basis of children's temperament and biological dispositions, and on children's contextual experiences from their family, peers, and community, they begin to form stable patterns of processing social information and regulating their emotions. The contextual social–cognitive model (Lochman & Wells, 2002a) stresses the reciprocal interactive relationships between children's initial cognitive appraisal of problem situations, their efforts to think about solutions to the perceived problems, children's physiological arousal, and their behavioral response. The level of physiological arousal will depend on the individual's biological predisposition to become aroused, and will vary depending on the interpretation of the event (Williams, Lochman, Phillips, & Barry, 2003). The level of arousal will further influence social problem solving, operating to intensify the fight or flight response, and interfere with the generation of solutions. Because of the ongoing and reciprocal nature of interactions, it may be difficult for children to extricate themselves from aggressive behavior patterns.

Aggressive children have cognitive distortions at the appraisal phases of social–cognitive processing because of difficulties in encoding incoming social information, and in accurately interpreting social events and others' intentions. In the appraisal phases of information processing, aggressive children have been found to recall fewer relevant nonhostile cues about events (Lochman & Dodge, 1994), and reactively aggressive children have a hostile attributional bias, as they excessively infer that others are acting toward them in a provocative and hostile manner (Dodge et al., 1997; Lochman, & Dodge, 1994).

Aggressive children also have cognitive deficiencies at the problem solution phases of social–cognitive processing. They tend to have dominance and revenge-oriented social goals, (Lochman, Wayland, & White, 1993) which guide the maladaptive action-oriented and nonverbal solutions they generate for perceived problems (Dunn, Lochman, & Colder, 1997; Lochman & Dodge, 1994). Aggressive children frequently have low verbal skills, and this contributes to their difficulty in accessing and using competent verbal assertion and compromise solutions. When aggressive children consider possible solutions to socially challenging situations, they evaluate aggressive behavior in a positive way at the next processing step (Crick & Werner, 1998) and expect it will lead to positive outcomes for them (Lochman & Dodge, 1994). Deficient beliefs at this stage of information processing are especially characteristic for children with proactive aggressive behavior patterns (Dodge et al., 1997) and for youth who have callous-unemotional traits consistent with early phases of psychopathy (Pardini, Lochman, & Frick, 2003). Indeed, children's schematic beliefs and expectations affect each of these information processing steps (Lochman & Dodge, 1998; Zelli, Dodge, Lochman, Laird & The Conduct Problems Prevention Research Group, 1999).

The Coping Power Model: Procedures, Content, and Structure

The Coping Power program includes separate child and parent components which are designed to run concurrently. The child and parent components differ in content, but both seek to address the main goal of reducing aggression and other disruptive behaviors in school-aged children. Toward this end, children and parents attend sessions in small groups across a period of approximately 16–18 months. The structure, content, and procedures used within each of these components will be described in the following sections.

Coping Power Child Component

The Coping Power child component (Lochman, Wells, & Lenhart, 2008) is an extension of the earlier Anger Coping program (Larson & Lochman, 2002), and consists of 34 weekly sessions, typically delivered to groups of five to seven children in the fourth through sixth grades (ages 9–12 years). Group meetings are designed to last 45 min to 1 h and are led by two clinicians, one of whom takes primary responsibility for delivering the content of the session while the other maintains primary responsibility for behavior management. Originally designed for implementation in the school setting, Coping Power can also be used in other venues such as clinics and community centers. With modifications, the program can also be delivered to individual students and to children who are slightly younger or older than the original target age group.

Sessions are highly structured and are organized around the teaching of targeted cognitive behavioral skills. Each group meeting follows a consistent format including standard opening and closing activities. During the main part of the sessions, active teaching methods including discussions, games, and role plays are used to deliver the specific material for each session (examples of procedures used to teach the program content are provided below). In addition to the group meetings, participants are seen individually on a monthly basis to increase leader–student rapport and to individualize the program as needed.

A behavior management system is built into the program, employing positive reinforcement for appropriate and prosocial behaviors as well as consequences for negative and/or disruptive behaviors. Students have the opportunity to earn "points" during each group meeting for their positive participation in activities and for following group rules, which are clearly established during the first meeting and posted for all subsequent sessions. Up to five additional points may be earned each week as part of the program's goal-setting system, described below. Several sessions also offer the opportunity to earn points for completing homework assignments or for demonstrating knowledge of program concepts on quizzes. Students may spend accumulated points each week on tangible rewards that range from small, inexpensive items (e.g., stickers, pencils) to larger prizes (e.g., basketballs, video games), which are included to encourage children to delay gratification and work toward the goal of a desired object.

Given that the majority of children referred for participation in Coping Power demonstrate oppositional and disruptive conduct problems, the program also includes a standard plan for delivering consequences. When appropriate, strategies such as differential reinforcement of appropriate behaviors and selective ignoring are employed to address negative behaviors that occur during group meetings. However, when problems continue, group leaders deliver warnings or "strikes" verbally (e.g., "James, you earned a strike for calling Michael a name") and/or visually on a white board or strike poster. Strikes are used because of the analogy with American baseball, in which the batter has three strikes before he or she is "out." Students can receive up to three strikes during each meeting, after which they fail to earn their point for following the rules. Students who have difficulty handling this consequence may be asked to leave the group to process what has occurred with one of the group leaders, or may be required to return to class. In such instances, the group is led by the remaining clinician.

A main feature of the program involves the use of weekly "goal sheets" to set, monitor, and reward students' progress toward individualized goals. With assistance from group leaders and input from parents and teachers, students set an operationally defined behavioral goal each week (e.g., "I will complete and turn in math homework," "I will use respectful words with teachers and peers"), which is recorded on a standard goal sheet. Each student is responsible for keeping track of the goal sheet throughout the week and for asking his or her teacher to provide feedback on the sheet each day. Students may earn one point for each day that the goal is met. The goal sheet system is particularly helpful in promoting the generalization of treatment effects outside of the group sessions.

Opening Activities. Each group meeting begins with a review of students' goal sheets. Each child discusses contributing factors to their successes and difficulties toward meeting their goals, and goals are modified or new goals are set for the following week. Next, the previous session's content is reviewed. Students are asked to recall one thing they learned during the previous week's meeting, allowing leaders to assess the students' retention and comprehension and to provide additional instruction as needed.

Closing Activities. Each Coping Power child component session ends with three activities. First, students provide positive feedback to each other about appropriate or prosocial behaviors demonstrated either during the group meeting or prior to the meeting in the classroom or on the playground. Each student gives and receives such feedback, which serves to reinforce positive behaviors and enhance feelings of self-esteem and self-efficacy. Next, leaders inform students of their point totals and allow them to redeem their points for prizes. Finally, if time permits, students who have demonstrated appropriate in-session behavior by earning at least one of the "following rules" or "positive participation" points are rewarded with 5–10 min of free time during which they may play games or visit with one another. The free time period operates not only as a reinforcer, but also as an opportunity for leaders to observe and evaluate students' social skills and their abilities to negotiate any conflicts that arise. Students who do not earn free time will spend this period processing their behavior with leaders. If leaders determine that a child is too upset to productively engage in such a conversation, the leaders can meet with him or her individually prior to the next meeting.

Coping Power Child Component Content. The Coping Power child component consists of seven main foci including goal setting, organization and study skills, emotional awareness, anger management, perspective taking, social problem-solving, and handling peer pressure. The goal setting unit comprises activities designed to assist students in identifying long-term goals that are personally meaningful (e.g., "I will improve my grades so that I can play on the basketball team"), and to break their long-term goals down into more readily accomplished short-term goals (e.g., "I will read for 30 min each evening."). A staircase analogy is often used in helping students comprehend the "steps" they need to take to reach their long-term goals. Short-term goals identified during these early sessions can then be used on the students' weekly goal sheets.

A unit on organization and study skills is included in the Coping Power program because problems in these areas frequently accompany disruptive behaviors in the school setting, and because difficulties in these areas are frequent sources of conflict between students and their teachers and parents. Organization and study skills are addressed through several games and activities. Though designed to be competitive in nature, the games may be modified if leaders are concerned that students will react negatively. For example, students can participate in the activities individually and compete against their own times, rather than against one another. In one such activity, students compete against each other to find a common object (e.g., pencil, assignment sheet) in their book bags. They are then given the opportunity to reorganize their book bags and the activity is repeated. Another activity requires students to organize a set of cards with the names of objects printed on them, after which they compete to find a given word in the least amount of time. Students who have organized the cards most effectively are the "winners" and are asked to explain their strategies to the rest of the group. In addition to session-specific activities, the development of good organization skills is encouraged in the Coping Power program by requiring students to be responsible for their goal sheets each week.

In the emotional awareness unit, students develop abilities to identify their feelings and how to verbalize them in constructive ways. Key to this set of skills is the use of a thermometer analogy in which words describing low levels of emotion (e.g., "irritated," "down") are placed at the bottom of the scale and more intense levels (e.g., "enraged," "depressed") are placed higher up. In this way, the idea that emotions occur in varying degrees of intensity is illustrated, an important concept for children who often conceptualize their feelings in an "on–off" manner. Other activities are designed to help children recognize the thoughts, physiological sensations, and behaviors that accompany various emotions, as well as the "triggers" that lead to these feelings.

The anger management unit builds on skills taught in the emotional awareness sessions. Particularly important to the goal of anger management is students' ability to recognize their anger at its earliest, lowest levels when anger management strategies are most likely to be successful. Anger management skills taught in the program include distraction techniques, relaxation exercises, and self-statements. Students are taught to use distraction through exercises in which they engage in a memorization task or a construction task while being taunted by their peers. These exercises are designed to illustrate that by directing one's focus elsewhere, emerging feelings of anger can be diminished and controlled. Another set of activities center on the use of coping self-statements (e.g., "Stay calm," "What he says doesn't matter") in response to peer teasing. In initial activities, students use puppets to practice adaptive self-talk. After mastering this skill with puppets, students engage in a more real-to-life scenario in which other children in the group tease them directly. The student being teased uses coping self-statements to manage resulting feelings of anger.

The next series of sessions addresses deficits in perspective taking commonly experienced by children with conduct behavior problems. Several activities are designed to challenge students' tendencies to make hostile attributions and to encourage them to consider alternate explanations for others' actions. Role-plays of hypothetical and actual situations frequently occur in these sessions, as they tend to be engaging for the students and effective in illustrating the key points. Given the frequency of student–teacher conflicts experienced by Coping Power children, other perspective-taking activities are specifically designed to improve the understanding of teachers' viewpoints. For example, students participate in a "family feud" style game in which they guess the top 10 things teachers expect from their students in the classroom. Students also conduct an interview with one of their teachers, including questions that allow opportunities for teachers to explain their reasons for disciplinary procedures and to express things they enjoy about teaching.

Given that children with disruptive conduct problems frequently demonstrate deficiencies in their ability to solve social problems, 12 of the program's 34 sessions are devoted to social problem-solving training. Central to the social problem-solving unit is the PICC model, which involves three main steps: (1) **P**roblem **I**dentification, (2) **C**hoices that are possible in response to the problem situation, and (3) **C**onsequences that might occur for each of the potential choices. First, students are taught to accurately define a social problem in a solvable manner. For example, a problem initially stated as "my mom isn't fair" could be restated as "my mom wants me to clean my room but I want to go to the movies with my friend." Next, students practice generating multiple solutions for social problem situations, including choices that are both "good" (e.g., having a calm discussion) and "bad" (e.g., whining and complaining). Identifying a range of choices is important for the next step in the PICC model, identifying consequences for solutions. Students identify potential consequences for each of the solutions generated, and evaluate each of the consequences as "good," "bad," or "okay." The process of evaluating consequences includes a discussion of whether the consequence helps the person to reach important goals. In the above example, a "good" consequence would involve the child going to the movies and not getting into trouble with his or her mother.

A favorite activity from the problem-solving unit offers the opportunity for students to write a script, act out, and videotape a skit illustrating the PICC model's use. In an active and engaging way, the video-making exercise serves to reinforce the students' understanding of and ability to use the PICC model. In addition, the videotape-making sessions are, by design, less structured than typical Coping Power sessions, which introduces the potential for real-life problem situations to develop during the meetings. Such problems offer opportunities for leaders to assist students in applying the PICC model, furthering the main goal of students' internalization of the problem-solving process.

The problem-solving component is expanded on by introducing the importance of deliberate versus automatic responding in social problem situations. To illustrate this concept, students are asked to quickly list choices for a hypothetical problem situation in one session; in the following session, the activity is repeated, but students are instructed to reflect upon the potential consequences of their choices before volunteering them. The exercise demonstrates that by stopping to think, students are likely to come up with better solutions for their problems and are more likely to achieve their desired outcomes. Other concepts addressed in the problem-solving component involve identifying good times to approach another person to solve a problem, the importance of being persistent when working on solving a problem, and applying social problem-solving to potential conflicts with teachers, siblings, and peers.

The final unit in the Coping Power child component involves responding adaptively to peer pressure and promoting prosocial peer relationships. Students are taught a variety of skills to handle peer pressure (e.g., make a joke, leave the situation) and are given opportunities to practice the skills in role-plays. Other activities encourage students to identify positive peer groups with which to associate. Students also learn to recognize their personal strengths and the positive leadership qualities that they have to offer in friendships.

The Coping Power program concludes with a review session in which students demonstrate their knowledge of key program content through a board game activity. Leaders also often hold a party for their students with snacks and fun activities to promote closure and to end the program on a positive note.

Coping Power Parent Component

The Coping Power parent component (Wells, Lochman, & Lenhart, 2008) consists of 16 sessions, offered to groups of parents whose children are participating in child groups. To support children's mastery of skills taught in the child component and to promote generalization of these skills to the home setting, parents are instructed in the content covered in the Coping Power child component and are encouraged to reinforce their children's use of the skills at home. In addition, the parent component is designed to enhance parenting skills, addressing parent involvement in academics, management of parents' own stress, behavior management, family communication, and parent–child relationship building.

The content of the Coping Power parent component is delivered mainly through didactic presentation of material by leaders. Parents are encouraged to participate in discussions and to share personal experiences relevant to the sessions' content. In addition, role-plays are frequently included to provide opportunities for modeling and practice of parenting skills.

Activities designed to encourage parent involvement in academics include an exercise in which parents develop a structure (e.g., setting routine homework times) to support their children's completion of homework. Parents are instructed to review the plan with their children and to implement the system on a daily basis. Another activity involves discussion and role-play of effective practices for parent–teacher conferences (e.g., being prepared with questions, demonstrating a willingness to work cooperatively with the teacher). Sessions on parent stress management are included to support parents' emotional functioning and to improve their abilities to remain calm during stressful interactions with their children. These sessions tend to be very well-received and include discussions on the importance of taking care of oneself through scheduling of positive events and practice in progressive muscle relaxation.

The behavior management component covers a variety of parenting techniques for promoting children's positive behaviors and managing their inappropriate behaviors. Parents discuss and practice skills including praise for desired behaviors, ignoring minor disruptive behaviors, delivering effective instructions, and establishing consistent rules and expectations at home. Several sessions are devoted to the use of effective disciplinary practices, including privilege removal, time out, and work chores.

The importance of family communication and relationship building is emphasized throughout the program and parents are encouraged to set aside a period for uninterrupted positive interaction with their child each day toward this goal. Parents also learn the PICC model that is taught in the child component and work through examples of how the model can be applied to conflicts among family members. Finally, parents develop a structure for family communication (e.g., family meetings) around topics such as children's activities away from parental supervision and negotiating changes to family rules. The family communication skills are presented in the context of children's approaching adolescence, and parents are encouraged to have a communication system in place to effectively work through the important issues likely to arise as their children become older and wish to become more independent.

In the last session of the program, parents review material covered in the curriculum and leaders provide referral information for community resources in the event that they are needed in the future. Positive activities are also often planned for the final session, including a viewing of children's PICC videos, special snacks, and a review of positive changes observed by leaders in both parents and children during the course of the program.

EVIDENCE FOR EFFICACY

Anger Coping Outcome Effects

The Anger Coping program, unlike the Coping Power program, has sessions only for children, and was the predecessor for the Coping Power program. An initial within-group pilot study indicated that second and third grade children had reduced aggression following involvement in an Anger Control program (Lochman, Nelson, & Sims, 1981), indicating the promise of cognitive-behavioral interventions with these young children. However, to focus on less concrete and more advanced social cognitive skills subsequent research has focused on somewhat older children. In a randomized control trial, 76 aggressive boys were randomly assigned to Anger Coping (AC), goal setting (GS), Anger Coping plus goal setting (AC+GS), or untreated control (UC) (Lochman et al., 1984). The two to three most aggressive children in each of the classrooms were identified as participants based on teachers' behavior checklist ratings. The boys were in fourth through sixth grades, and 53% were African-American and 47% were Caucasian. They participated in 12 weekly school-based Anger Coping group sessions. In comparison to the UC and GS conditions, aggressive boys in the Anger Coping cells (AC, AC+GS) at the end of training displayed less parent-reported aggressive behavior, and had lower rates of disruptive classroom behavior as observed by independent raters. The addition of a goal-setting component in the AC+GS cell tended to enhance the treatment effects of the program (Lochman et al., 1984).

The Anger Coping program effects have been found to be augmented by the use of an 18-session version of the program, in comparison to the earlier 12-session version (Lochman, 1985). In this quasi-experimental study, 22 teacher-identified aggressive boys in the fourth and fifth grades (55% African-American; 45% Caucasian); received an 18-session version of the Anger Coping program (with more emphasis on perspective taking, role playing, and more problem solving about anger-provoking situations) and were compared to the boys who had received the 12-session program in the Lochman et al. study (1984). With the longer 18-session program, aggressive boys displayed significantly greater improvement in on-task behavior according to independent observers time-sampled ratings, and greater reduction in passive off-task behavior, illustrating the need for longer intervention periods for children with chronic acting-out behavior problems. Using the 18-session version of the program, Lochman et al. (1989) randomly assigned 32 boys in the fourth, fifth and sixth grades (31% African-American; 69% Caucasian) to Anger Coping, Anger Coping plus Teacher Consultation, or to an Untreated Control condition. In comparison to the boys in the control condition, Anger Coping boys displayed reductions in teacher-rated aggression, improvements in perceived social competence and in self-esteem, and reductions in off-task classroom behavior, although teacher consultation did not appear to augment the intervention effects (Lochman et al., 1989).

In a study of inner-city African-American children who had been rejected by their peer group, Lochman and colleagues (1993) found that a social relations program which included the Anger Coping components addressing anger management and social problem-solving skills along with additional social skill training components had significant impact at post-intervention and at a 1-year-follow-up with aggressive-rejected fourth grade children, but not with rejected-only children. Relative to control conditions, the intervention aggressive-rejected children had reductions in peer-rated and teacher-rated aggressive behavior.

At a 3-year follow-up, when boys were 15-years old on average, boys who received the Anger Coping program ($N = 31$) exhibited lower levels of marijuana and drug involvement, lower rates of alcohol use, and maintained their increases in self-esteem and problem-solving skills in comparison to an untreated control condition ($N = 52$; Lochman, 1992). These results indicate the Anger Coping program delivers both long-term maintenance of social–cognitive gains and important preventive effects for adolescent substance use.

The Anger Coping boys' functioning in these domains was within the range of a nonaggressive comparison group ($N = 62$) at the end of training, indicating the clinical significance of these positive effects. However, the Anger Coping boys did not have significant reductions in delinquent behavior at follow-up, and their reductions in independently observed off-task behavior and parent-rated aggression were maintained only for a subset of Anger Coping boys who had received a brief six-session booster intervention for themselves and their parents a year later.

Thus, across multiple-controlled intervention studies, this child-centered cognitive-behavioral intervention reduced children's conduct problems immediately after treatment and provided important preventive effects on adolescent substance use.

Coping Power Program Outcome Effects

Several studies have also examined the efficacy and effectiveness of the Coping Power program, as well as factors affecting program dissemination. In an initial efficacy study, (Lochman & Wells, 2004), 183 boys (61% African-American; 39% Caucasian) who had high rates of teacher-rated aggression in fourth or fifth grades were randomly assigned to either a school-based Coping Power child component, to a combination of Coping Power child and parent components, or to an untreated control condition. Outcome analyses indicated that Coping Power produced lower rates of self-reported delinquent behavior and parent-rated substance use at a 1-year follow-up than did the control cell, and these intervention effects were most apparent for the combined child and parent Coping Power program. Boys also displayed teacher-rated behavioral improvements in school during the follow-up year, and these effects were evident in both intervention conditions and appeared to be primarily influenced by the Coping Power child component. Normative comparison analyses with a non-risk sample of 63 boys from the same schools indicate that the intervention moved at-risk boys into normative ranges for substance use, delinquency and school behavior, in contrast to at-risk control boys who significantly differed from the normative group on the latter two outcomes.

Path analyses indicate that the intervention effects were at least partly mediated by changes in boys' social–cognitive processes, schemas, and parenting processes (Lochman & Wells, 2002a). Intervention-produced changes in both social–cognitive appraisal processes, involving boys' hostile attributions and resulting anger, and decision-making processes, involving reductions in the boys' expectations that aggressive behavior would lead to good outcomes for them, reduced the risk for antisocial behavior. Similarly, changes in boys' schemas regarding their beliefs about their degree of internal control over successful outcomes and the complexity of their internal representations of others, and changes in the consistency of their parents' discipline efforts led to lower levels of delinquency, substance use, and school behavioral problems.

A series of effectiveness studies have subsequently examined the effects of the program in school or clinic settings with conditions more typical of regular clinical care (e.g., higher case loads; using regular clinicians from the intervention setting). In a first effectiveness study, the Coping Power (Lochman & Wells, 2002b, 2003) intervention began in the fall of the fifth grade year and continued midway through the sixth grade year. The sample consisted of 245 male (66%) and female (34%) aggressive fourth grade students (78% African-American; 20% Caucasian) who were randomly assigned to one of four conditions: Coping Power plus a universal intervention, Coping Power alone, the universal intervention alone, and a control condition. The universal intervention consisted of five workshops with teachers and six school-wide parent meetings about behavior management and about the social–cognitive skills children were learning in the targeted Coping Power intervention. Analyses of post-intervention effects (Lochman et al., 2002b), comparing intervention to control conditions, indicate that the combined Coping Power program plus a universal intervention produced lower rates of self-reported substance use, lower teacher-rated aggression, higher perceived social competence, and greater teacher-rated behavioral improvement, indicating the value of nesting the Coping Power program within a universal prevention program in producing immediate intervention effects. However, Coping Power had positive outcome effects at a 1-year follow-up regardless of whether children had also received the universal intervention or not (Lochman & Wells, 2003). In this follow-up study, Coping Power produced reductions in substance use, delinquency, and school behavior problems in comparison to the control condition, replicating the pattern of findings from the earlier efficacy study (Lochman & Wells, 2004).

To examine outcomes of an abbreviated version of Coping Power that can be implemented in one school year (with 24 child sessions and 10 parent sessions), 240 at-risk aggressive fifth graders were randomly assigned to abbreviated Coping Power or control conditions. The program produced significant reductions in teacher-rated externalizing behavior for children in analyses that controlled dosage of parent attendance (Lochman, Boxmeyer, Powell, Roth, & Windle, 2006). In another effectiveness study, the Coping Power program was adapted for use with deaf children (Lochman et al., 2001). Deaf children in a residential school were screened for aggressive behavior ($N = 49$), using teacher ratings, and were randomly assigned by classroom to the Coping Power program or to a wait-list control condition. The children in the multicomponent Coping Power program attended group sessions, and their teachers and dormitory staff received behavioral management training. Because of the residential nature of this program, the Coping Power parent component was not used in this study. The Coping Power program was adapted to meet the unique needs of deaf and hard of hearing children. According to teacher ratings, Coping Power children displayed behavioral improvement, and an increase in social problem solving and communication skills across the intervention year in comparison to control children.

Coping Power has also been adapted for use with clinic populations. A Dutch version of Coping Power with 18 parent and child sessions was evaluated in a study in which children with disruptive behavior disorders ($N = 77$) were randomly assigned to Coping Power or to clinic Care-as-Usual (CAU). Therapists in the CAU condition primarily used cognitive–behavioral and family therapy strategies. Both conditions improved significantly on disruptiveness post-treatment and at a 6-month follow-up, but only the Coping Power group had a significantly greater reduction in overt aggression by post-treatment (van de Wiel et al., 2007). Coping Power clinicians had significantly less experience than CAU therapists, indicating Coping Power's cost-effectiveness (van de Wiel et al., 2003). At a 4-year follow-up, Coping Power children had significantly lower marijuana and tobacco use than did CAU children indicating long-lasting and preventive effects of the intervention (Zonnevylle-Bender et al., 2007).

A dissemination study of the Coping Power program was recently conducted in 57 schools in five school systems in Alabama. School counselors were trained to implement Coping Power with high-risk aggressive fourth and fifth grade students ($N = 531$). The intensity of training provided to counselors had a notable impact on child outcomes. Significant improvements in child externalizing behavior occurred only when a more intensive form of training was provided, that is when counselors received immediate supervisory feedback based on recorded sessions (Lochman, Boxmeyer, Powell, Qu, Wells, & Windle, 2009). School-level factors and counselor traits were associated with quality of program implementation with agreeable and conscientious counselors demonstrating the best program implementation. Counselors who were high on cynicism and who were in schools with low levels of staff autonomy and high levels of managerial control had a particularly poor quality of implementation and child and parent engagement (Lochman, Powell, Boxmeyer, Qu, Wells, & Windle, 2009).

Overall Evaluation of Anger Coping and Coping Power Programs

This series of studies indicate that a cognitive–behavioral intervention can have immediate effects at post-intervention on children's aggressive behavior at home and at school, according to parent, teacher, and independent observer ratings. The effect sizes are typically in the moderate range. The Anger Coping program, which included only a child component, had lasting preventive effects on children's later substance use, up to 3 years following intervention completion, but it appeared necessary to include an adjunctive parent intervention component to have longer-term effects on children's delinquency. As a result, the Coping Power program was developed with both child and parent components. In a series of studies, the Coping Power program has produced significant effects on delinquency, substance use, and aggression in school settings at 1-year follow-up, and has produced long-term effects on marijuana use at a 4-year follow-up. Mediational analyses have indicated that Coping Power follow-up effects are due to intervention-produced changes in children's social–cognitive skills and in parental consistency. A universal intervention with teachers has strengthened Coping Power's immediate post-intervention effects. Altogether, the results emphasize that this form of cognitive behavioral intervention can be useful not only for short-term treatment purposes, but also for longer-term prevention purposes and that the program can be effectively delivered in school and clinic settings.

CASE EXAMPLE FOR COPING POWER CHILD COMPONENT

After providing individual therapy to a number of clients with oppositional defiant disorder and conduct disorder, two licensed clinical social workers at the Valley View Youth and Family Services clinic, Mrs. Sewell and Mr. Munoz, decided to start a therapy group. They felt that providing group-based intervention would allow them to better assess their clients' interpersonal needs by observing their peer interactions directly. They also felt that group-based intervention would provide valuable opportunities for the clients to practice emotional coping and social problem solving skills with their peers and to be reinforced for behavioral improvements. The clinic had recently sponsored a training workshop in the Coping Power program, so Mrs. Sewell and Mr. Munoz decided to use this curriculum for their small group.

Mrs. Sewell and Mr. Munoz identified five clients for the Coping Power group, including three clients from their existing caseloads and two clients from the list of new intakes. In forming the group, they sought to include clients who were similar in age and who appeared to be functioning well enough cognitively and interpersonally to contribute to group discussions and activities. The group included: Jesse, a 10-year-old-Caucasian boy who had been treated off and on at the clinic since age 5 for explosive anger outbursts and attention problems; La'Quesha, an 11-year-old African–American girl who had recently been referred to the clinic for talking back to her teacher and parents; Jamal, an 11-year-old African–American boy who was at risk of being removed from his foster placement due to noncompliant and aggressive behavior; Ricardo, a 10-year-old Hispanic boy who refused to do his schoolwork and had few friends; and Jessica, a 10-year-old girl of mixed race/ethnicity, whose mother indicated that she had coddled Jessica for a number of years following her husband's sudden death and was now concerned about Jessica's lack of respect for her mother and other authority figures.

Coping Power Child Group Session 1: Getting Acquainted and Goal Setting

During the first session, Mrs. Sewell and Mr. Munoz welcomed the children and informed them that the purpose of the group was to help them cope with strong feelings and handle difficult situations so that they could reach the goals they set for themselves. Mrs. Sewell led the group in a get-acquainted activity in which the group members took turns passing a ball, repeating the name of the person who passed the ball and stating one thing that they had in common. The leaders then encouraged the members to generate a name for their group. Jamal and Jessica began to argue, as they each wanted a different name for the group. Mr. Munoz intervened, suggesting that they fuse their ideas and the group agreed upon the name "Valley View Power All-Stars." Next, the members generated a list of rules for the group (e.g., take turns talking; keep your hands and feet to yourself; what we say here stays here). Mrs. Sewell showed the group the "prize box" containing toys and prizes that the members could purchase with points earned for participating positively and following the rules during each session. She informed them that they could also earn additional points for meeting weekly behavioral goals, for participating in games during sessions, and for completing periodic intervention homework assignments.

The group was excited to see the prizes, but Mr. Munoz had to assign warning "strikes" to La'Quesha and Ricardo after they began shoving each other to get a better look at the prize box. He informed the group members that anyone who receives three "strikes" will not earn a point for following the group rules for that session. Mrs. Sewell suggested that the group members look at the prize box one at a time instead. Mr. Munoz then led a discussion about personal goals and showed the group members a handout they would be using to set weekly behavior goals for themselves throughout the program. He asked the group members to think about what kinds of goals they would each like to work toward as a homework assignment for the next session.

To end the session, each group member was asked to share something that he or she had learned that day and also to provide a compliment to another group member. The children had great difficulty with this, so Mr. Munoz modeled the process first. He told Jamal and Jessica that he was proud of them for reaching a compromise about the group name. He told La'Quesha and Ricardo that he was proud of them for settling down and taking turns at the prize box. Finally, he complimented Jesse for being able to describe what a personal goal is and for sharing with the group that he would like to bring his grades up so that he can play on the school's baseball team. With additional coaching from the leaders, the group members provided similar positive feedback to each other.

Coping Power Child Group Session 10: Practice Using Coping Statements for Anger Coping

Mrs. Sewell began the session by welcoming the members and asking them to report on their behavior goals for the week. Jesse proudly stated that he met his goal of not getting his name on the board in class 4 out of 5 days this week. Mrs. Sewell praised Jesse for his big improvement from previous weeks and asked him what he had done differently. He said that when he felt like getting out of his seat or talking back to the teacher, he looked at the baseball sticker on his desk to remind himself that he was trying to make the baseball team. He said that the day he got his name on the board, he had gotten into an argument with another student in Physical Education where he did not have the sticker to remind him of his goal. Mrs. Sewell reiterated that getting his name on the board only one time was a big improvement for Jesse and said that they could role play the situation that happened in Physical Education later in group to practice how Jesse might have handled the situation differently. Ricardo and Jamal had both forgotten to have their goal sheets signed by teachers so Mr. Munoz led the group in brainstorming ways to help them remember to have it signed in the future. Ricardo and Jamal said they would try clipping the goal sheet to their daily assignment sheet, which had worked for Jesse. Jessica had only had her goal sheet signed on 2 days, but on both days the teacher indicated that Jessica had talked to her respectfully. La'Quesha had not attended the group for several weeks and was absent again. Mrs. Sewell planned to call La'Quesha's mother after group to check on her.

Next, Mrs. Sewell asked the group members to recall one main point discussed during last week's session. They each gave answers indicating that they recalled practicing ways to cope with rising levels of anger on their "anger thermometers." Jamal recalled learning about deep breathing; Jessica recalled learning about using coping self-statements; and Jesse recalled using distraction to cope with low levels of anger. Mrs. Sewell praised them for remembering these positive coping techniques and awarded two points to each group member who completed the homework assignment of recording an anger-arousing event, using their favorite coping technique, and recording the effect on their anger level. She informed the children that they were going to continue to practice using coping self-statements in group today.

In preparation for the group self-control activity, Mr. Munoz asked each child to take out the list they made last week of their three favorite coping statements. Jesse was the first to find his list, which included: (a) "Grow up, don't blow up"; (b) "Stay calm, just relax"; and (c) "It's not worth fighting." While the other children were searching for their lists, Mrs. Sewell placed a large laminated thermometer on the floor. Once he had the group's attention, Mr. Munoz informed them that they were going to practice using self-control while being provoked by peers, as they had in the three previous sessions. This time, the group members were going to practice using coping statements while being teased by their peers and they would walk up and down the thermometer to show how angry they feel inside. Prior to beginning the activity, Mr. Munoz reminded the group members of the rules they must follow during the activity (e.g., no cursing, no racial comments, no physical contact).

Jesse was selected to go first so that the group could reenact the incident that he had encountered in Physical Education. Jesse told the other group members that his classmate had called him a "wuss" and said that he didn't want Jesse on his kickball team. Jesse agreed to let the group members tease him about his athletic skills while he tried to stay calm using coping statements. Jesse took his place on the thermometer while the other group members gathered around him. "You're so weak, you couldn't even hurt a fly," Jessica shouted. "It's no wonder your team always loses, you're a wuss," Jamal piped in. "You stink at kickball – and every other sport – you're a joke," Ricardo chimed in. Jesse walked up the thermometer as the teasing made him angry. "Grow up, don't blow up," he recited loudly, "grow up don't blow up ... it's not worth fighting, don't let them bother you ... they don't mean it, they're probably just having a bad day." Gradually, Jesse started to walk down the thermometer as the use of coping statements helped calm his anger. Eventually, the teasing died down as the children ran out of ideas and saw that the teasing no longer had the desired effect of making Jesse angry. Mr. Munoz gave each group member a turn to practice using self-statements to cope with teasing from the group. One of Jamal's taunts made Ricardo extremely angry and Ricardo nearly lashed out in anger at Jamal. Mr. Munoz paused the activity, discussed what had happened, and stood next to Ricardo, whispering coping statements in his ear. Ricardo was able to stay calmer with this direct coaching.

Each group member was given two turns to practice using coping statements; first stating them aloud for the group to hear, and the second time reciting them internally. After each member had two turns, Mrs. Sewell led a discussion of what the children learned from the activity (e.g., "How did you feel when you were teased? What did you say to yourself when you first noticed you were getting angry? Did these thoughts help you cope with your anger? How? What happened to your anger level when you used your coping statements? What happened to the teasing when the group members noticed they weren't getting a reaction from you?"). With 10 min remaining, Mr. Munoz began the session closing activities. He led the group in the positive feedback activity, informed each group member how many new points he/she had earned, and let the group members decide whether they wanted to purchase a prize or save their points. He informed the group that they had earned 5 min of free play time since they had each earned their points for positive participation and following the rules. The leaders used the free play time to reinforce the children for prosocial behaviors, such as taking turns, sharing, and solving problems successfully.

Coping Power Child Group Session 21: Social Problem Solving

After reviewing the children's goals sheets, Mrs. Sewell asked the children what they recalled learning about during the last session. Jessica shouted, "Oh, oh, I know! We talked about the PICC model!" Mrs. Sewell said, "That's right, can anyone tell me what the letters P-I-C-C stand for?" "Problem Identification, Choices, and Consequences," shouted La'Quesha, who had returned to the group after her family saved enough money to fix their car. "That's right, now who can remember when we can use the PICC model?" Mr. Munoz asked. "When something makes us angry or we have a problem to solve," offered Ricardo. Mr. Munoz praised Ricardo for speaking up, and was pleased that Ricardo continued to be more engaged in the group. Mrs. Sewell told the group, “now that you have gotten good at using the PICC model to think of different choices when you have a problem and picking the choice that will lead to the best consequence, there is one more thing we would like to practice.” She told the children that “sometimes things don’t go the way you expect them to, even when you take the time to think ahead and pick the best choice, so today we are going to practice overcoming barriers and not giving up when things don’t work out the way you hoped.”

Mr. Munoz told the group that they were going to play a “Blockers” and “Solvers” game. He assigned Ricardo, Jessica, and Jamal to start out as the “Solvers.” Their job was to help a child named Brian come up with a solution to the following problem: he wants to go to a friend’s house and play, but his mom said he had to stay home and do his chores. Jessica suggested that Brian could offer to do the chores first and then go to the friend’s house. Her teammates agreed to select this solution. Jesse and La’Quesha were the “Blockers” and they said that this would not work because Brian’s friend was going to basketball practice in an hour so there would not be enough time for Brian to play with him after he finished his chores. The “Solvers” had 1 min to think of a new solution. They said Brian could try to make a deal with his mom that if he straightened up his room first, he could go play and then do the other chores when he came back. The “Blockers” said this would not work because Brian’s mother said he had to do all of his chores first. The “Solvers” had another minute to come up with a new solution and they said Brian could play with his friend later in the day when he returned from practice instead. The “Blockers” said this would not work because Brian wanted to play now. The “Solvers” said Brian’s mother usually gave him a special treat after he finished his chores, so this would help him wait to play until his friend came home. The “Blockers” could not come up with a reason this would not work, so the “Solvers” won the game. The teams then switched roles so that Jesse and La’Quesha also had a turn to practice overcoming barriers to solving social problems.

Mrs. Sewell asked the group what they had learned from this activity. They said that you shouldn’t give up or get mad when things don’t work out the way you want them to the first time because you might still be able to figure out a way to solve the problem and reach your goal. Mrs. Sewell said she was proud of the group members for learning this lesson and told them that she would ask each of them to tell her one time that they used this skill at the next session. The leaders then ended the group with positive feedback, the point box transactions, and 5 min of free play time.

Coping Power Child Group: Concluding Sessions

Midway through the group process, Mrs. Sewell and Mr. Munoz learned that they would only be able to hold 24 of the 34 possible Coping Power child group sessions because of insurance restrictions. They reviewed the remaining curriculum and decided to devote two of the remaining sessions to social skills training and affiliating with positive peers, with the final session devoted to reviewing the skills learned throughout the program and to celebrating the behavioral gains made by each participant. During the final session, Mr. Munoz asked each child to describe the improvements he or she had made. Jesse said he was proud of himself for making the baseball team. Mrs. Sewell praised Jesse for reaching this goal and asked the group what they thought Jesse had done differently to accomplish this. Jessica said that Jesse was much better at keeping his cool and not letting things get to him when they didn't go his way. Mr. Munoz agreed with Jessica's comment and then asked her what changes she had made in her own life while in Coping Power. Jessica said that she was getting along much better with her mother now. She said that whenever her mother told her she wasn't allowed to do something, she tried to remind herself that her mother just wanted what was best for her. Mrs. Sewell said that this was a good example of a coping statement and that she had also seen Jamal make a big improvement in using coping statements while in Coping Power. Jamal said that he was glad that he was getting along better with his foster parents and proudly announced that they were considering adopting him. Ricardo said that he was glad that he had found some friends to hang out with but that he was still getting really bad grades at school. Mr. Munoz praised Ricardo for his efforts to connect to others, both in the group and at school. He acknowledged that it is difficult to end the group knowing that they had not been able to improve in every area, such as Ricardo's grades, but that hopefully Ricardo and the other group members could apply the skills they learned to continue to make progress in the future. La'Quesha appeared sullen that the group was ending and the leaders shared that they would miss the group members too. La'Quesha said that her teacher had complimented her that week for improving her attitude. Mrs. Sewell said that the biggest change seemed to occur when La'Quesha became friends with a classmate who did well in school and stopped spending as much time with several classmates who frequently got into trouble. Mrs. Sewell reminded the whole group that who we spend time with affects our behavior and that the transition to middle school would be an important opportunity to find friends who will be a good influence and help you meet your goals.

Mrs. Sewell and Mr. Munoz ended the group by sharing their regards with the group members; informing the group members that they would be meeting with their parents individually to discuss their progress and to provide needed referral information; distributing certificates of completion; and then saying goodbye.

CONCLUSIONS AND SUMMARY

When implementing group interventions with angry and aggressive youth, there are a set of potential obstacles that can interfere with the optimal functioning of the group and which can detract from the effectiveness of the intervention (Lochman, Powell, Barry, Deming & Young, 2007). Two primary issues involve children's reactive behavior in the group, and deviancy training and deviant norms. These issues will be briefly described, and then relevant methods for overcoming these obstacles will be discussed (Lochman & Wells, 1996; Lochman et al, 2007).

Obstacles

Reactive Behavior in Groups. Children who are chosen for a CBT group because of their aggressive behavior with peers can be noncompliant and challenging with adult group leaders and they can readily respond to perceived provocations from other children in the group with quick bursts of reactive, angry aggression. Reactive aggressive children have difficulty regulating their anger and arousal, causing their "hot" angry cognitions to interfere with their information processing. Children's emotional reactions to each other in these situations can be highly contagious, and can lead to bursts of aversive, conflictual interpersonal behavior between group members.

Deviancy Training and Deviant Norms. In addition to being exposed to a number of children with high levels of aggressive behavior in a deviant peer group, the members of the deviant peer group may directly reinforce each other for their antisocial attitudes and behaviors (Dishion & Andrews, 1995). Delinquent adolescent dyads have been found to provide high rates of positive reinforcement for their partners' deviant talk, while nondeviant dyads provide reinforcement for each others' normative, nondeviant discussions (Patterson, Dishion, & Yoerger, 2000). This pattern of reinforcement of rule-breaking talk among deviant dyads directly affects these youths' subsequent substance use and delinquency (Dishion, Eddy, Haas, Li, & Spracklen, 1997). Dishion and Andrews (1995) found that deviancy training led young adolescents who were in a group intervention program to have higher rates of tobacco use and more delinquent behaviors at a 1-year follow-up than did control children. These iatrogenic effects remained even at later 3-year follow-ups, especially for youth with more moderate levels of antisocial behavior at baseline (Poulin et al, 2001). These deviant group effects can also be apparent in children's power struggles with group leaders. If a group member is often involved in challenging group leaders, and if that child is relatively well accepted by his or her peers in the group, this can stimulate broad oppositional power struggles between the group and the leaders, and can reduce children's group involvement and motivation for change.

Ways to Overcome These Obstacles

Intervention Structure. The two primary ways to address problems with children's reactive aggressive behavior and with deviancy training effects are to closely address certain structural issues in the intervention and to provide enhanced behavioral management strategies, as needed. An initial planning issue has to do with the age of the youth in the group. Iatrogenic deviancy training effects seem to be more evident in adolescent-age groups than in preadolescent groups. The inclusion of two group leaders can increase the likelihood that leaders can scan children's behavior continually in the group, and be alert to subtle signs of peers' reinforcement of deviant behaviors.

Once the group is formed, it is useful to carefully follow aspects of the intervention that involve monitoring and providing consequences for children's behavior. Thus, in our Coping Power groups, we place emphasis on having clear Group Rules, starting in the first session, and on providing points for children's adherence to these rules and for their positive participation in group sessions. Other program elements which alert children to how their behavior can lead to consistent consequences include the use of weekly goal setting procedures for each group member, having group contingent rewards for the entire group successfully attaining a certain number of points over several months, and working with the parents in the parent group sessions on their ability to provide clearer instructions to the children and to provide consistent consequences for children's positive and negative behaviors. Ongoing contact by the group leaders with the teachers can be critically important in facilitating teachers' abilities to monitor children's social behavior and to provide logical consequences within the school setting.

Group Behavioral Management Strategies. Minor structural changes in the group can be helpful in providing stimulus control to prevent behavioral escalation in the group. Such minor structural changes include changing seating arrangements so that a group leader is between two particularly reactive children. Group leaders' use of nonverbal cues (e.g., eye contact, physical proximity, animated voice tone) can also be an important means for gaining children's optimal attention. Effective group leaders also are able to assist children with making smooth transitions from one group activity to another or from the group back to the class or the waiting room by verbally preparing them several minutes prior to the change of activity, and guiding them through the transition. If some group members are demonstrating high levels of positive involvement in the group, they can also be used to serve as a "buddy" for reactive peers, reminding the peer of group rules.

Major structural changes can also be implemented in the relatively rare occasions when these minor structural changes and usual program structural elements are insufficient to reduce individual children's serious problem behaviors in the group. When a central concern is intense rivalry between two children, leading them to frequently initiate conflict with each other, or when two children are actively involved in deviancy training with each other, the group can be temporarily split into two subgroups. If there were two group leaders, each leader can then work with a subgroup in a more contained way until group members' functioning improves and the subgroups can be reintegrated again. In cases with a severely and chronically disruptive individual in the group, the individual can be seen individually rather than in the group for a period of time. If this child begins to demonstrate a stronger therapeutic alliance after several individual sessions, then he or she may be carefully reintegrated into the group.

Summary

In this series of research studies on the Anger Coping program (with a child component only) and the Coping Power program (with child and parent components) cognitive–behavioral group intervention with aggressive children produced significant effects on youths' aggressive behavior and substance use. However, intervention effects on delinquency were only evident with the Coping Power program, with its combination of parent and child components. The long-term effects on children's behaviors have been found to be mediated by intervention-produced changes in children's attributions and outcome expectations and in parents' consistency in their use of discipline. Because of the difficulties in conducting group interventions with aggressive children, it is important for clinicians to use clear behavioral management and to structure sessions well so that problems related to youths' reactive behavior and deviancy training can be minimized.

REFERENCES

Cernkovich, S. A., & Giordano, P. C. (2001). Stability and change in antisocial behaviour: The transition from adolescence to early adulthood. *Criminology, 39*, 371–410.

Coie, J. D., Lochman, J. E., Terry, R., & Hyman, C. (1992). Predicting early adolescent disorders from childhood aggression and peer rejection. *Journal of Consulting and Clinical Psychology, 60*, 783–792.

Crick, N. R., & Werner, N. E. (1998). Response decision processes in relational and overt aggression. *Child Development, 69*, 1630–1639.

Dishion, T. J., & Andrews, D. W. (1995). Preventing escalation in problem behaviors with high-risk young adolescents: Immediate and 1 year outcomes. *Journal of Consulting and Clinical Psychology, 63*, 538–548.

Dishion, T. J., Eddy, J. M., Haas, E., Li, F., & Spracklen, K. (1997). Friendships and violent behavior during adolescence. *Social Development, 6*, 207–223.

Dodge, K. A., Lochman, J. E., Harnish, J. D., Bates, J. E., & Pettit, G. S. (1997). Reactive and proactive aggression in school children and psychiatrically impaired chronically assaultive youth. *Journal of Abnormal Psychology, 106*, 37–51.

Dunn, S. E., Lochman, J. E., & Colder, C. R. (1997). Social problem-solving skills in boys with conduct and oppositional disorders. *Aggressive Behavior, 23*, 457–469.

Fite, P. J., Colder, C. R., Lochman, J. E., & Wells, K. C. (2006). The mutual influence of parenting and boys' externalizing behavior problems. *Journal of Applied Developmental Psychology, 27*, 151–164.

Fite, P. J., Colder, C. R., Lochman, J. E., & Wells, K. C. (2007). Pathways from proactive and reactive aggression to substance use. *Psychology of Addictive Behaviors, 21*, 355–364.

Jackson, M. F., Barth, J. M., Powell, N., & Lochman, J. E. (2006). Classroom contextual effects of race on children's peer nominations. *Child Development, 77*, 1325–1337.

Larson, J., & Lochman, J. E. (2002). *Helping school children cope with anger: A cognitive-behavioral intervention.* New York: Guilford.

Lavallee, K.L., Bierman, K.L., Nix, R.L. & the Conduct Problems Prevention Research Group. (2005). The impact of first-grade "Friendship Group" experiences on child social outcomes in the fast track program. *Journal of Abnormal Child Psychology, 33*, 307–324.

Lochman, J. E. (1985). Effects of different treatment lengths in cognitive behavioral interventions with aggressive boys. *Child Psychiatry and Human Development, 16*, 45–56.

Lochman, J. E. (1992). Cognitive-behavioral interventions with aggressive boys: Three-year follow-up and preventive effects. *Journal of Consulting and Clinical Psychology, 60*, 426–432.

Lochman, J. E., Barry, T. D., Powell, N., Boxmeyer, C., & Holmes, K. (2008). Externalizing conditions. In M. L. Wolraich, D. D. Drotar, P. H. Dworkin, & E. C. Perrin (Eds.), *Developmental and behavioral pediatrics* (pp. 603–626). Philadelphia, PA: Elsevier.

Lochman, J. E., Boxmeyer, C., Powell, N., Qu, L., Wells, K., & Windle, M. (2009). Dissemination of the Coping Power Program: Importance of Intensity of Counselor Training. *Journal of Consulting and Clinical Psychology, 77*(3), 397–409.

Lochman, J. E., Boxmeyer, C. L., Powell, N. P., Roth, D., & Windle, M. (2006). Masked intervention effects: Analytic methods for addressing low dosage of intervention. *New Directions for Evaluation, 110*, 19–32.

Lochman, J. E., Burch, P. P., Curry, J. F., & Lampron, L. B. (1984). Treatment and generalization effects of cognitive-behavioral and goal setting interventions with aggressive boys. *Journal of Consulting and Clinical Psychology, 52*, 915–916.

Lochman, J. E., Coie, J. D., Underwood, M., & Terry, R. (1993). Effectiveness of a social relations intervention program for aggressive and nonaggressive rejected children. *Journal of Consulting and Clinical Psychology, 61*, 1053–1058.

Lochman, J. E., & Dodge, K. A. (1994). Social-cognitive processes of severely violent, moderately aggressive, and nonaggressive boys. *Journal of Consulting & Clinical Psychology, 62*, 366–374.

Lochman, J. E., & Dodge, K. A. (1998). Distorted perceptions in dyadic interactions of aggressive and nonaggressive boys: Effects of prior expectations, context, and boys' age. *Development & Psychopathology, 10*, 495–512.

Lochman, J. E., FitzGerald, D. P., Gage, S. M., Kannaly, M. K., Whidby, J. M., Barry, T. D., et al. (2001). Effects of social-cognitive intervention for aggressive deaf children: The coping power program. *Journal of the American Deafness and Rehabilitation Association, 35*, 39–61.

Lochman, J. E., & Gresham, F. M. (2008). Intervention development, assessment, planning and adaptation: Importance of developmental models. In M. J. Mayer, R. Van Acker, J. E. Lochman, & F. M. Gresham (Eds.), *Cognitive behavioral interventions for emotional and behavioral disorders: School-based practice* (pp. 29–57). New York: Guilford.

Lochman, J. E., Lampron, L. B., Gemmer, T. C., Harris, S. R., & Wyckoff, G. M. (1989). Teacher consultation and cognitive-behavioral interventions with aggressive boys. *Psychology in the Schools, 26*, 179–188.

Lochman, J. E., Nelson, W. M., III, & Sims, J. P. (1981). A cognitive behavioral program for use with aggressive children. *Journal of Clinical Child Psychology, 10*, 146–148.

Lochman, J. E., Powell, N., Boxmeyer, C., Qu, L., Wells, K., & Windle, M. (2009). Implementation of a school-based prevention program: Effects of counselor and school characteristics. *Professional Psychology: Research and Practice, 40*(5), 476–482.

Lochman, J. E., & Wayland, K. K. (1994). Aggression, social acceptance, and race as predictors of negative adolescent outcomes. *Journal of the American Academy of Child and Adolescent Psychiatry, 33*, 1026–1035.

Lochman, J. E., Wayland, K. K., & White, K. J. (1993). Social goals: Relationship to adolescent adjustment and to social problem solving. *Journal of Abnormal Child Psychology, 21*, 135–151.

Lochman, J. E., & Wells, K. (1996). A social-cognitive intervention with aggressive children: Prevention effects and contextual implementation issues. In R. Dev Peters & R. J. McMahon (Eds.), *Prevention and early intervention: Childhood disorders, substance use, and delinquency* (pp. 111–143). Newbury Park, CA: Sage.

Lochman, J. E., & Wells, K. C. (2002a). Contextual social-cognitive mediators and child outcome: A test of the theoretical model in the Coping Power Program. *Development and Psychopathology, 14*, 971–993.

Lochman, J. E., & Wells, K. C. (2002b). The coping power program at the middle school transition: Universal and indicated prevention effects. *Psychology of Addictive Behaviors, 16*, S40–S54.

Lochman, J. E., & Wells, K. C. (2003). Effectiveness study of coping power and classroom intervention with aggressive children: Outcomes at a one-year follow-up. *Behavior Therapy, 34*, 493–515.

Lochman, J. E., & Wells, K. C. (2004). The coping power program for preadolescent aggressive boys and their parents: Outcome effects at the one-year follow-up. *Journal of Consulting and Clinical Psychology, 72*, 571–578.

Lochman, J. E., Wells, K. C., & Lenhart, L. A. (2008). *Coping Power child group program: Facilitator guide*. New York: Oxford.

Loeber, R. (1990). Development and risk factors of juvenile antisocial behavior and delinquency. *Clinical Psychology Review, 10*, 1–41.

Loeber, R., & Stouthamer-Loeber, M. (1998). Development of juvenile aggression and violence: Some common misconceptions and controversies. *American Psychologist, 53*, 242–259.

Miller-Johnson, S., Coie, J. D., Maumary-Gremaud, A., Lochman, J. E., & Terry, R. (1999). Relationship between childhood peer rejection and aggression and adolescent delinquency severity and type among African American youth. *Journal of Emotional and Behavioral Disorders, 7*, 137–146.

Pardini, D. A., Lochman, J. E., & Frick, P. J. (2003). Callous/unemotional traits and social cognitive processes in adjudicated youth. *Journal of the American Academy of Child and Adolescent Psychiatry, 42*, 364–371.

Patterson, G. R., Dishion, T. J., & Yoerger, K. (2000). Adolescent growth in new forms of problem behavior: Macro- and micro-peer dynamics. *Prevention Science, 1*, 3–13.

Patterson, G. R., Reid, J. B., & Dishion, T. J. (1992). *Antisocial boys*. Eugene, OR: Castalia.

Poulin, F., Dishion, T. J., & Burraston, B. (2001). 3-year iatrogenic effects associated with aggregating high-risk adolescents in cognitive-behavioral interventions. *Applied Developmental Science, 5*, 214–224.

van de Wiel, N. M. H., Matthys, W., Cohen-Kettenis, P. T., Maassen, G. H., Lochman, J. E., & van Engeland, H. (2007). The effectiveness of an experimental treatment when compared with care as usual depends on the type of care as usual. *Behavior Modification, 31*, 298–312.

van de Wiel, N. M. H., Matthys, W., Cohen-Kettenis, P. T., & van Engeland, H. (2003). Application of the Utrecht coping power program and care as usual to children with disruptive behavior disorders in outpatient clinics: A comparative study of cost and course of treatment. *Behavior Therapy, 34*, 421–436.

Wells, K. C., Lochman, J. E., & Lenhart, L. A. (2008). *Coping Power parent group program: Facilitator guide*. New York: Oxford.

Williams, S. C., Lochman, J. E., Phillips, N. C., & Barry, T. D. (2003). Aggressive and nonaggressive boys' physiological and cognitive processes in response to peer provocations. *Journal of Clinical Child & Adolescent Psychology, 32*, 568–576.

Wright, J. C., Giammarino, M., & Parad, H. W. (1986). Social status in small groups: Individual-group similarity and the social "misfit". *Journal of Personality and Social Psychology, 50*, 523–536.

Zelli, A., Dodge, K. A., Lochman, J. E., Laird, R. D., & Conduct Problems Prevention Research Group. (1999). The distinction between beliefs legitimizing aggression and deviant processing of social cues: Testing measurement validity and the hypothesis that biased processing mediates the effects of beliefs on aggression. *Journal of Personality and Social Psychology, 77*, 150–166.

Zonnevylle-Bender, M. J. S., Matthys, W., van de Wiel, N. M. H., & Lochman, J. (2007). Preventive effects of treatment of DBD in middle childhood on substance use and delinquent behavior. *Journal of the American Academy of Child and Adolescent Psychiatry, 46*, 33–39.

10

Functional Family Therapy

A Phase-Based and Multi-Component Approach to Change

JAMES F. ALEXANDER and MICHAEL S. ROBBINS

Functional Family Therapy (FFT) is all about helping youth and families who are in trouble. Central to FFT is the belief this can be accomplished by changing family interactions and improving relationship functioning as the primary vehicle for changing dysfunctional individual behaviors. FFT shares many similarities with other systems approaches; however, FFT offers a comprehensive framework for understanding adolescent behavior problems that is quite unique. This framework provides the context for integrating and linking behavioral and cognitive intervention strategies to the specific familial and ecological characteristics of each family. As such, FFT is also about therapists, about training and supervision, and about treatment and other (educational, judicial, religious, cultural, political, economic, marketing) systems that surround families, therapists, and agencies.

Like all coherent models of change, FFT is phasic and developmental. Every system, ranging from human beings (and all animal life) to all created products (cars, symphonies, clay figures and so on) begins in a different form than what it later becomes. Physical systems and most conceptual systems undergo phases which build upon each other, and this development usually follows a specific pattern. So too do families and therapists as they undertake and complete their journey together toward positive family change. For over 3 decades, FFT itself has evolved from the experiences and results of clinical research, critical review, and

JAMES F. ALEXANDER • University of Utah
MICHAEL S. ROBBINS • Oregon Research Institute

R.C. Murrihy et al. (eds.), *Clinical Handbook of Assessing and Treating Conduct Problems in Youth*, DOI 10.1007/978-1-4419-6297-3_10,

dissemination across populations, cultures, and treatment contexts. Not surprisingly, across multiple contexts, research teams, and clinical providers there is a core philosophy or value about the critical importance of research and evaluation and accountability. This value epitomizes our ultimate focus on providing the highest quality of care possible to youth and families by monitoring and studying all aspects of training, supervision, and implementation.

The purpose of this chapter is to help readers understand the essential philosophy and components of FFT. In doing so, we describe how FFT systematically matches interventions to the unique and special qualities of each youth, family, culture, and treatment system. In addition, we describe how findings from research studies have led to evolutions in the clinical model.

BRIEF HISTORY OF THE DEVELOPMENT OF FFT AS AN EVIDENCE-BASED INTERVENTION

FFT is viewed as an empirically supported model for adolescent drug use and behavior problems (Barton, Alexander, & Sanders, 1985; Waldron & Turner, 2008). However, the emergence of FFT as an empirically based intervention did not occur suddenly, nor is it complete. Since the early 1970s, the conceptual development of FFT and research on FFT has been inextricably linked. Moreover, this dynamic and reciprocal process persists today as FFT is currently being implemented and evaluated in numerous contexts. These processes continue to shape the clinical model by providing new results and experiences that enhance our ability to understand and communicate about the essential components of successful implementation. From examining moment to moment experiences of therapists in the room with families, to working with state agencies to support community treatment centers and clinical teams, these experiences continue to shape FFT.

The first published articles on FFT established the efficacy of the approach, compared to alternative treatments, for adolescents with delinquent behavior problems (Alexander, Barton, Schiavo, & Parsons, 1976; Alexander & Parsons, 1973). Over time, the efficacy of FFT for adolescent delinquency has been replicated across sites and settings (cf. Barton, Alexander, Waldron, Turner, & Warburton, 1985). FFT has also been established as an efficacious treatment for adolescent substance use disorders (Waldron & Turner, 2008). Moreover, evidence has been found for the preventive effects of FFT for siblings of problem youth (Klein, Alexander, & Parsons, 1977) and for the long-term effectiveness of the intervention into early adulthood (Gordon, Graves, & Arbuthnot, 1995). Research has shown that FFT is associated with improvements in family communication patterns and relationships (Parsons & Alexander, 1973; Waldron, Slesnick, Brody, Turner, & Peterson, 2001). Finally, one of the advantages of FFT, relative to other family based models, is that it has been shown to be effective when implemented by professionals with diverse backgrounds and training and that effectiveness has been demonstrated across cultural groups (Alexander, Pugh, & Parsons, 1998; Waldron et al., 2001).

As evident in the references above, FFT has been profoundly influenced by many individuals. The model was first fully described by Alexander and Parsons (1982). However, the clinical experiences and research findings of numerous individuals and research teams have continued to shape and refine FFT. With respect to research, for example, the independent replications of the efficacy of FFT by numerous research teams in the United States (Waldron, Gordon) and Sweden (Hansson), has led to FFT receiving numerous designations such as "Level 1 Model Program" (Youth Violence: A Report of the Surgeon General, 2001), "Best Practice" (Thornton, Craft, Dahlberg, Lynch, & Bear, 2000 – Centers for Disease Control), "Evidence-Based Effective program" (OJJDP Juvenile Justice Bulletin; December, 2000), and "Promising Strategies to Reduce Substance Abuse" (U.S. Department of Justice, Office of Justice Programs, 2000). FFT was also designated by the Center for The Study and Prevention of Violence (CSPV) as one of 12 Blueprint Programs for treating adolescent delinquency, substance use, and violence. The Blueprints initiative (Elliott, 1998; Elliott & Mihalic, 1997) involved a thorough and rigorous review of the research literature to identify effective programs for helping troubled youth. This initiative has had a profound influence on the treatment of adolescents with behavioral problems by influencing state and local policy and funding, requiring the development of user-friendly treatment manuals and training and supervision programs, and by providing a context for providers, model developers, and policy makers to work together to bridge the gap between research and practice and provide research proven services to youth in need.

In 1998, FFT was included in the Blueprints series (Alexander, Pugh, & Parsons, 1998). Since that time, numerous FFT replications have been supported and guided by the Blueprints initiative. To maintain pace with training and dissemination demands, an independent company was formed, Functional Family Therapy LLC (FFT-LLC). FFT-LLC has trained more than 270 local, state, national, and international organizations to implement FFT. In this work, FFT-LLC has supported over thousands of therapists who have served over 60,000 adolescents/families across the globe. At present, large-scale projects (10 plus sites) are ongoing in California, Washington, Pennsylvania, New York, Florida, and the Netherlands.

In response to the needs of community providers, several variations of FFT have been developed to facilitate the implementation of FFT-informed interventions with diverse clinical providers and populations. For example, Functional Family Probation (FFP) was developed and has been adopted as case management model for Juvenile Justice Systems statewide in Utah and Washington. In this variation, probation officers receive specialized training in FFT Engagement, Motivation, and Relational Assessment principles to facilitate their ability to engage adolescents, work with the youth's family, and effectively plan and implement case management strategies to address the multiple needs of youth. Also, in our current efforts to sustain and extend FFT to new populations and challenges, FFT-LLC is involved in programs working with youth and parents in the Child Welfare system (FFT-CW) as youth are being reunified or reintegrated with their families (FFT-Reunification Services).

CLINICAL MODEL OVERVIEW

FFT consists of five major components in addition to pre-treatment and post-treatment activities (see Fig. 10.1): (1) Engagement in change; (2) Motivation to change; (3) Relational/interpersonal assessment and change planning; (4) Behavior change; and (5) Generalization across behavioral domains and multiple systems (Alexander, Waldron, Barton, & Mas, 1983; Alexander et. al., 1998; Barton et. al., 1985).

Pre-treatment Preparation

Prior to seeing or contacting the family, therapists engage in linking with referral sources, gathering information about the youth and family, and preparing/planning for the initial contact. The therapist, upon receipt of a referral, first contacts the referral source(s) to acknowledge the referral and to solicit all information (including impressionistic as well as formal assessments) available. In the case of formal legal involvement (e.g., Juvenile Justice System), the therapist also clarifies system expectations and requirements, as well as issues of confidentiality. In situations where the therapist might not have experience with the culture or other characteristics of the referral, s/he will contact additional resources within or outside of the treatment system to become better informed. The ultimate goal of these activities is to be fully ready to assist the youth and family, and to anticipate potential barriers and utilize strengths to create a positive initial impression and experience for family members.

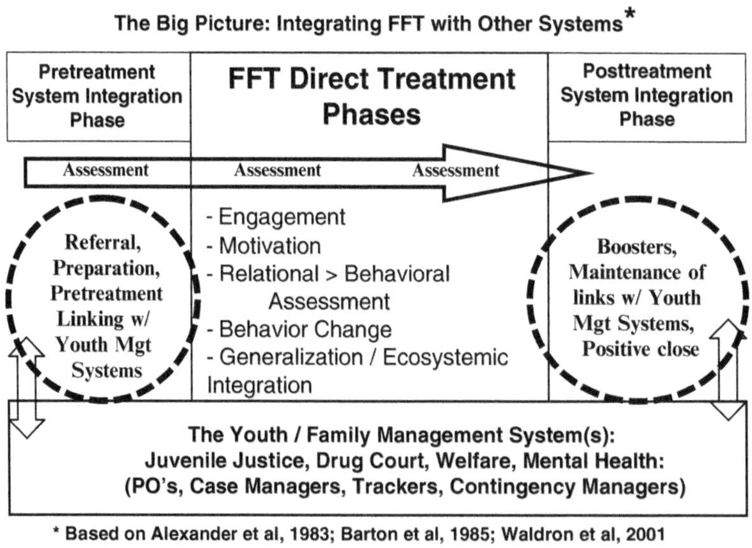

Fig. 10.1. The phases of FFT within treatment and community systems.

The First Phase: Engagement in Change

The Engagement Phase begins prior to first contact, and quickly blends into the Motivation Phase. Engagement refers to any activity that can facilitate the family's willingness to attend early sessions (or allow an interventionist into their home). Engagement also involves creating an initial positive reaction to the therapist. These activities can include "superficial" but important activities such as wearing clothes that seem appropriate for family members and "matching" therapists to families with regards to ethnicity and gender. If a desired match is not available, therapists must be as culturally competent and work to help family members feel comfortable and respected. FFT therapists also make their own initial appointments via telephone so therapists can listen for potential problems such as transportation difficulties, distrust of and resistance to treatment, and confusion about the referral and/or treatment goals. Thus, the Engagement Phase is less characterized by a formal set of therapeutic techniques than it is of an attitude on the part of FFT therapists that families should be shown as much respect as possible and be made to feel comfortable during the initiation of the process of intervention.

Pre-intervention Information and Assessment. Referral information is generally already available about youth and families. Sometimes this information consists only of a name and a reason for referral (e.g., runaway; found in possession of drugs at school; parent called expressing concern that youth is becoming uncommunicative; social services receives referral regarding possible neglect). At the other extreme are cases involving youth with extensive diagnostic test information and perhaps even behavioral records in institutions, and families with a history of many social service contacts. FFT therapists review such information, along with as much demographic information as is available, to understand as much as possible about the context in which intervention is to occur. For example: "Is there information available that might facilitate cultural sensitivity, enlighten about multisystem pressures (e.g., poverty) and resources, and that might suggest individual constraints (e.g., learning disability, illiteracy) which must be considered?"

The Second Phase: Motivation for Change

The Engagement Phase consists primarily of transitory activities that are designed to get the process of intervention "off on the right foot." As direct contact is initiated in the first session, FFT therapists quickly move to more powerful motivational interventions. The primary objective of the Motivation Phase of intervention is to create a motivational context within which change can occur; the family members are helped to experience a reduction in change-interfering negativity (anger, blaming, and hopelessness), coupled with an increase in change-enhancing hopefulness. Decreasing negativity is essential in this early phase of intervention prior to initiating formal behavior change techniques because family members' intense negative emotions can preclude them from making a realistic commitment to change. Often family members have developed a rigid defensive schema through which all information is filtered, and their interactions are characterized by cycles of coercive and defensive interchanges that reinforce their automatic negative processing patterns.

FFT addresses the early session (Engagement and Motivation) risk factors for drop out by engaging in two major domains of activity: Changing Focus and Changing Meaning. *Change Focus* techniques include (a) Divert and Interrupt, (b) Point Process, (c) Sequencing, and (d) Strength-based Relational Statements. *Change Meaning* techniques include (a) Relabeling, (b) Reframing, (c) Creating Themes, and (d) Offering Theme Hints.

Change Focus Techniques

Change focus interventions are intended to disrupt negativity and unproductive family interactions by shifting, stopping, or redirecting communications. Change focus interventions are relatively simple interventions to implement, and are often used when the therapist is still getting a sense of how to effectively intervene with the family, but recognizes the need to attempt to address negative behaviors in the session.

Divert and Interrupt. The most basic change focus techniques are divert and interrupt. Although simple, disrupting family members' negative interactional sequences through divert/interrupt represents a major interpersonal maneuver, which helps families deescalate their toxic negativity. Therapists *divert* family negativity when they intercept a negative speech act made by a family member instead of allowing the family member to whom it was directed to answer. Therapists *interrupt* family negativity when they do not allow a family member who is making a negative or defensive speech act to complete a blaming diatribe. In our prior research, we have found that if a therapist simply diverts or interrupts a family member's negative speech acts, then the subsequent family member's speech act is almost twice as likely to be positive than if the therapist allowed another family member to respond to the negative statement (Robbins, Alexander, & Turner, 2000). In FFT, divert and interrupt interventions require an active and involved therapist that is highly attuned to the meaning and nature of interactions in the family. As such, these interventions are used in a manner that is sensitive to the current interactions, and – although they involve interfering or speaking over family members – they are delivered in a manner that is respectful and accepting of the family.

Pointing Process. Another change focus technique is pointing process. As therapists observe and attend to each family members' perception of within-family and extra-family interactions, they can comment on the process of how family members relate to each other. This is especially important with respect to those interactions that are characterized by negativity and blaming. By pointing process, especially in a non-blaming (and if possible strength-based) manner, therapists are able to make explicit the interrelatedness of family members' feelings, thoughts, and behaviors. These interventions often serve to defuse negativity by shifting the focus from the specific content being discussed to the underlying relational aspects that underlie, but are hidden from family members in the current moment.

Sequencing. The third change focus technique, sequencing behavior or circular questioning, is a method used to assess what happens and who does what within a family with regards to the specifics of a presenting problem. Because information is drawn out in a sequence and in a circular fashion, it is visually easier to see the context in which behavior occurs. Sequencing interventions create depth of knowledge about all the family members involved in a presenting problem, including the action each took, and the meaning of each participant's behavior in relation to one another. When a sequence is completed to include what occurs before, during, and after an event, there is often an identifiable outcome that can be tied to a theme or function of the participants (see Reframes and Themes below). When used in a relationally focused and non-blaming way, the focus of sequencing is not on the presenting problem or other problems, but on family members' interactions. That is, the focus is not on the content or problem that occurred, but rather on family relationships and the meaning of relationships and behaviors to individual family members. For instance, when a father steps into harshly punish his son after he has talked back to his mother, a problem focus would be to understand why the son's behavior was disrespectful. In contrast, a relationally focused sequencing intervention would focus on framing the father's actions as a way of protecting and supporting the values of the family. When used in the Motivation Phase of treatment the goal of this sequencing is for the father to feel acknowledged for having a positive intent – even if his "way of doing it" might have been harsh and non-productive. Sequencing reveals family patterns, which lead to either positive or negative familial outcomes. Sometimes the sequence when drawn (e.g., on paper) and shown to the family can in itself act as a reframe (see below), particularly when the sequencing is accompanied with non-blaming, contextual description. Sequencing also occurs when therapists focus on adding depth to sequences that result in positive behavioral outcomes. Systematically focusing on positive sequences creates a working climate in the session in which family members gain a new perspective about themselves and each other. In many respects, the lens is shifted from the negative behaviors and problems, which they enter treatment with to the positive aspects of relationships that have been overwhelmed by the negativity. This shift in focus helps family members to begin to see what they do "through different eyes."

Strength-Based Relational Statements. Strength-based relational statements include interventions that ascribe a positive (even noble) attribution about one person's efforts toward another person. This includes seeing the positive side of apparently negative relational patterns: For example (to parent and child who are beginning to argue loudly with each other), "*OK – I'm going to jump in here for a second. You both are angry right now, and pretty much yelling. I'm sure that at times you or someone else wants you to stop yelling. But for now, I want to note that you seem to be at least on the same page ... no one seems to be holding back much, and both of you are honest in expressing your anger. Lots of families tend to go underground with their anger ... but with you two, I can trust that you will bring it out and deal with it directly. That gives me something to work with that often I don't have. Now, I wonder ...*" This strength-based relational focus pervades

FFT interventions. Even simple reflections or acknowledgements of family members are expected to convey a strength-based relational focus. For example, instead of acknowledging a mother's anger about her daughter's truancy by simply stating "*I can hear how angry you are*," therapists may rather state "*Your exasperation is even more difficult for you because you have such high expectations and ideas for how she can excel in school.*" Both interventions serve to acknowledge the mother's anger, but the latter goes further by highlighting the strength-based aspects evident in the mother's anger.

Change Meaning Techniques

Like change focus interventions, change meaning techniques are intended to disrupt negativity and unproductive family interactions. However, change meaning techniques involve attempts to change the meaning of how family members understand themselves and each other. The goal of change meaning techniques is not cognitive change, but rather is to create the opportunity (or possibility) of a different frame. Thus, these techniques are not intended to challenge "maladaptive" cognitions or provide an interpretation for a family member's behavior. Rather, the focus is on providing a non-blaming, even positive perspective about behaviors that creates an opportunity in the session for family members to experience one another in a new way.

Relabeling. The therapist relabels by reflecting to family members a similar, but less harmful explanation for a behavior, for the purpose of shifting some of the negative intensity in the meaning of that behavior. Consider a teenage son's complaint about his mother arising in an early (Engagement and Motivation Phase) session, "*As soon as I walked in the door she just went off on me!*" and the therapist's response of, "*So she let you know right off the bat that she had an issue with you.*" While these statements may seem quite similar, "*she just went off*" conjures up a more intense image than "she *let you know right off that she had an issue with you.*" This relabel also added a "softer" relational component ("*she* ... <u>with</u> *you.*") rather than the more "attacker – victim" tone of "*she* ... <u>on</u> *you.*" Relabels set a tone that is less negative and provide the therapist more positive avenues to pursue. They also represent an intervention style that families generally experience in more positive ways than therapist interventions that amplify the negativity with which they already struggle. In addition, they do not involve any element of blaming or suggestion that the behaviors will need to change.

Reframing. Reframing is generally described as a "technique," and although its elements may differ across therapy models, the process of reframing seems to transcend most family-based intervention models. Many in fact consider it a "core technique" for all family therapy approaches. As defined by Paul Watzlawick and colleagues, a reframe is a change of "... *the conceptual and/or setting or viewpoint in relation to which a situation is experienced and to place it in another frame ... and thereby change its entire meaning*" (Watzlawick et al., 1974). As an evidence-based model, FFT has worked to describe precisely the process of reframing as we have used it in our clinical trials and multiple replications. Research on reframing has further helped to articulate the immediate effectiveness of reframing in the session (Robbins, Alexander, Newell, & Turner, 1996; Robbins et al., 2000). This in-depth knowledge has helped us to develop consistency in the training and supervision process across agencies, therapists, and treatment populations. In the process of doing so we have realized that reframing is not only a technique; it is also an attitude, a perspective, and a belief system that helps FFT therapists facilitate positive change even when all of the technical elements of a reframe cannot be presented.

Reframes, as defined in FFT, add two components to the change meaning process (a) acknowledgment of the negative, and (b) proposal of a possible alternative (and perhaps benign or even "noble but misguided") motive. These components add significantly to the therapist's ability to impact upon family negativity while maintaining an overall non-blaming relationship with all family members. Reframes include a clear acknowledgement of the negative aspects of a behavior (thereby supporting those that are negatively impacted by the behaviors in question). This acknowledgement does not include an agreement with the family member. Rather, the focus of the acknowledgement is to establish that the therapist is attuned to and understanding of the relevance of the negative behavior or problem to the family member. After the acknowledgement, therapists then offer an alternative and possibly more benign *motive* for the behavior.

In our experience, the most powerful reframes acknowledge negative behavior, but rather than offering an alternative neutral or benign *motive* for the behavior (e.g., mom's frustration) the hypothesized motive is labeled as "noble" in its intent. Usually the noble intentions are seen as "misguided" but they are nonetheless well intended. As we move from relabeling reframes with noble intent, the complexity and level of inference increases. We are not concerned that we do not "know" if family members' motives are "truly" positive or noble in order to suggest they might be. In fact, hopeless families often are surprised and feel more supported when therapists seem willing to "see the strength and possible nobility" in them even when it is not apparent.

Creating Themes. To generate *behavioral* themes, therapists identify sequences of several problem family member interactions in which all of the negative elements are identified but reframed (or at least relabeled). This focus has the advantage of helping create a family (versus individual) focus, and because all members are subject to reframing the therapist can identify negative interactions and yet still "come across" as seeing the possible benign intent of each member. In this way, the therapist avoids taking sides with family members, and prevents defensiveness that typically occurs when only an individual's negative behavior is the focus. *Relational* themes are so called because they switch the focus to relationships rather than behaviors. Of course, specific behaviors may be noted, but often they are not. Instead, relational patterns, and how they have been *experienced*, become the major focus. And while relational themes maintain the basic elements of reframes (acknowledge negative, reframe intent or meaning in more benign if not noble terms), they often seem more like "stories" and even "myths" than specific sequences of negative behaviors.

Coupled with our core generic principles of matching and respectfulness, our powerful change meaning techniques help families move quickly to being open and responsive to techniques that change behavior (in both the short and long term).

Assessment in Early Phases (Engagement and Motivation): Relational Functions

By the time FFT receives referrals for dysfunctional behaviors, the relational functions expressed in important relationships are usually well established and easy to recognize; rarely do adolescent disruptive behaviors or parenting "styles," nor "challenges" emerge "all of a sudden." As a result, FFT therapists look for stable patterns, first assessing the relational functions. These "relational functions" represent *inferred* internal motivations of family members based on overtly expressed (behaviorally, verbally, emotionally, physiologically) patterns within the family. This notion has had diverse articulations and controversies within our field for decades (and centuries if one considers the early philosophers), but for us it is fairly straightforward and is illustrated nicely in an analogy about motivations for eating. We reflect a pattern of eating food when we experience hunger, anxiety or loneliness. While the exact dynamic factor may take a while to detect (usually through understanding *the pattern*) it is usually straight forward; and yet still an inference based upon the *pattern*. Of course, where the sense of "hunger" (or whatever it is we infer as a motivation) comes from may be arguable, but most theorists (and people) do not have too much of a problem with the explanation that we eat because we are hungry. In the same way, family members relate to one another based on their own inferred internal motivations. In the assessment process of FFT, the focus is not on the inferred internal process, but rather on the resultant patterns that emerge from family interactions.

The assessment process in FFT also examines the functional relationships and problem behavior patterns outside the family (especially with peers). FFT does not attempt to change the relational function itself, but we do change the *cognitive, physiological, emotional, and behavioral strategies* in which the youth or parent engages to meet relational functions. If a child acts out to "get attention" FFT does not work hard to eliminate children's need for attention! Instead, we change the *means* through which this attention is elicited. This of course usually requires dealing with the rest of the system(s) involved with the youth, because "comfort" or "attention" may only be (or at least seem to be) available through maladaptive behavioral patterns.

Relational Connection: Contact/Closeness Versus Distance /Autonomy / Independence. The first and most salient category for determining *Relational Function* is the degree of interpersonal *connectivity* that is expressed in the behavior patterns that directly or indirectly impacts another person (or persons) in the family (and other systems). The degree of connection can range from "close" and highly interconnected to "distant" and quite independent or autonomous. These dimensional anchors are not considered to be fixed and invariant points on a dimension; they are instead the central tendency (or apparent "default mode," or "average") behavioral pattern that best characterizes the ongoing relationship. Imagine a couple in an ongoing relationship: They are not *always* close or *always* distant or *always* a mixture of both. In general; however, couples can be distinguished in terms of whether their pattern is generally close and connected, generally distant and autonomous, or generally variable. Whatever the behavioral pattern is over time, FFT's intervention philosophy, that is, "the *respectful acceptance of the diversity that all family members bring,*" is what we identify as Relational Functions. All three of the aforementioned relational states can be adaptive, and all three can be maladaptive. The problem is not what the relational function is, but how it is expressed and met.

The Second Dimension: Relational ("Relative Power") Hierarchy. Relational Hierarchy reflects the pattern of relative influence parents and youth have over each other in terms of "controlling" each others' behavior. With adolescent conduct problems, it is common to use such phrases as "S/he's out of control." However, FFT examines more than the behavior patterns of one individual. Instead, we examine the relative balance of control and power rather than simply isolating our focus on whether or not the parent can control the youth. When we broaden our focus to look at the relative balance of power, it is not uncommon to find that sometimes a youth is able to exert more "control" over a parent's behavior than vice versa. In other families, the youth, although "acting out," is not able to control the parental behavior any more than the parent can control the youth! Thus the power differential is more one of balance than of one or the other "in control." Interventions that fail to examine the relative balance of the interpersonal "control" in these relationships often fail repeatedly if all they attempt to do is to increase the "control" the parent has over the youth.

Of course, in many ways parents experience the "power" issue as the most salient in raising adolescents. However, FFT asserts that primarily what parents want is a sense of being able to control (if not help) their youth. As a result, when therapists provide alternative ways to influence youth, hierarchy itself becomes less salient. In fact, many parents are quite pleased when their kids begin to comply because the relationship with the youth has been repaired and the youth now wants to maintain a positive and less blaming relational pattern with the parent(s). Power and consequences are important and have their role, but often are more difficult to change and certainly less positive than relational changes that motivate youth to comply and develop positive behaviors.

Unlike the concept of personality, which presumes a core underlying motivational structure, FFT assessment of functions often identifies important differences in motivation within one person. The FFT therapist understands, for example, that the motivational needs of a parent with different children can be markedly different. As a result, child behaviors that would be comfortable for the parent with respect to the "close" child could be quite unacceptable with respect to the "distanced" child (or vice versa). Thus, prescriptions for good parenting cannot be homogeneous, because the behaviors through which effective parenting is carried out will differ depending on the child in question.

Finally, the assessment of relational functions is essential if therapists want to ensure rapid compliance with change interventions. Prescribing tasks or change strategies for one family member with respect to another member will elicit considerable resistance if the prescriptions are implicitly or explicitly inconsistent with the family members' functions. Simply put, the more divergent the techniques are from the relational functions, the more resistance (e.g., poor participation and dropout) the therapist will face, and the more external forces will be needed to facilitate and maintain change. As an empowerment model, FFT offers a more relational and less oppositional belief system and intervention philosophy.

Transitioning between Engagement & Motivation into Behavior Change

Over the years, FFT has utilized two broad classes of techniques for Behavior Change. The first class is represented by *general skill-building* processes such as communication training, problem solving, and conflict management techniques. We use these techniques in almost all families, and they represent skill development, which is useful to family members when they interact, but also generalize nicely to other extra-family systems (school, work, friendships). The second class of techniques represents problem-specific techniques, which may apply to some people and families but not others including: (a) "internal" coping techniques for people with anger impulse problems, and cravings; (b) techniques for overcoming challenges unique to some families, such as a single parent with a physical disability which precludes the use of many parenting strategies; and (c) techniques specific to youth with developmental disorders. Special techniques or unique configurations of Behavior Change approaches also may be utilized, for example, when severe trauma has been experienced by a youth (or parent, or both), or when youth spend time with two active parent figures who live separately and who may have their own new family relationships.

Specific Elements of Behavior Change

Communication Training. Communication training is commonly used in FFT. In some families, the training represents a focus on a true skill deficit; family members do not know the basics of interpersonal communication. In many other families; however, family members know how to communicate (e.g., some have been effective teachers, professors, clergy, Girl Scout leaders, etc.), but in the current context are unwilling or unable to communicate in the effective ways they can demonstrate in other contexts. With family members who truly are characterized by skill deficits, emphasis is on explaining and practicing the positive elements of communication listed below. When the problem is one of performance rather than ability, emphasis is placed on reattribution (e.g., reframing) interventions, and providing constant reminders of the rationale behind effective communication.

The most common examples of communication training in FFT are not unique to the model but rather are core elements of effective communication that are described in many behavioral intervention programs. A common feature of communication training in FFT is to enhance *Source Responsibility*. Individual family members are encouraged or coached to express their needs and reactions in "I" statements which facilitate the centering of responsibility on the speaker. Family members are helped to avoid "non- I" statements such as, "*In this house* ...," "*Kids shouldn't* ...," "*It's not right for you to* ...," and "*It would be nice if* ...." Instead, family members are taught to say, "*I want* ...," and "*When (this particular) thing isn't done, I feel* ..." Keeping statements at a personal level reduces blaming and defensive communications. In addition, family members are guided to be direct and specific in their communications. *Source Directness* complements source responsibility and involves the specific identification of "you" in expressions. This helps avoid third-person comments, innuendo, and inappropriate generalizations. To be avoided are such "non-you" expressions as, "*No one around here* ...," and a wife in front of her husband, "*He never* ...." In place of this third-person invisible process, families are encouraged to directly say, "*I don't want you to* ...," and the like. In either circumstance, brevity is encouraged. Communications must be short to avoid overloading and facilitate listening. Family members are often literally asked to state their needs or reactions in 10 words or fewer. By requiring family members to do this, it reduces unnecessary statements and the opportunity to blame others or make provocative accusations. Statements such as, "*I want you to help around the house*," instead of "*You never do anything around here, except come home and read the paper, and if you think the lawn stops growing just because you're at work, you're crazy*," reduce defensiveness and increase the opportunity for change. An effective therapist will quickly seize on the idea that mowing the lawn and doing some evening chores will provide the husband with distance and private time while giving his wife the necessary help, thus providing desired change without disrupting functions which regulate intimacy levels.

Abstractions such as "being responsible" must be translated into specific behaviors to be performed at specific times. When trust is only emerging, or still not present, an ambiguous situation provides too many opportunities for failure. *Concreteness and Behavioral Specificity* helps family members translate their feelings and demands into specifics to facilitate negotiation, contracting, and presenting alternatives. Family members are helped to present messages that are *Congruent*, or consistent, at the verbal, non-verbal, behavioral, and contextual levels. For example, an assertion from a husband that he wants his wife to spend more time with him should be spoken in a friendly manner, and he must make it contextually possible by being available. Family members are assisted by the therapist to provide congruent verbal and non-verbal cues, and then taught how to help each other do this in the absence of the therapist.

Family members are also taught how to *Present Alternatives* when making requests, and moving away from rigid non-negotiable demands. Presenting Alternatives creates flexible and open problem-solving focus in the session. For example, the statement "*I want you home every night at 8:30, or if you'd prefer coming home four nights at 8:00 and staying out one night until 10:00*" presents a message of flexibility and openness. In this way, the presenter is able to retain a sense of control, yet also provide the recipient with a sense of having options.

Therapists help family members to be more effective *Active Listeners* by providing guidance about how to use cues during and after the time someone else communicates. These cues reflect accurate listening and include eye contact, nodding, leaning forward, and restating or rephrasing what was communicated, in content as well as in the feelings expressed. Good listening and expressiveness is not an innate skill, however, and must be practiced. At the beginning of training active listening is practiced one sentence at a time. In addition, therapists guide family members to provide *Impact Statements* in response to someone else's communication. Impact statements provide feedback about one's personal reaction that requires no justification from either party. By training family members to be specific in their reactions, therapists help to break the established links between feelings and behavior that characterize relationships. This is particularly important because the standard, automatic emotional reactions are often negative or hostile, which leads to maintaining high conflict in the interaction. By breaking this link, therapists are able to reduce negativity, increase the accuracy and specificity of communication, and facilitate the emergence of new behavioral sequences that are not charged with the same emotional negativity. Examples of impact statements include: "*When you do _____, the effect on me is ______*"; "*The impact on me when ______, is that I feel _______*."

Basic Parenting Principles/Techniques

Forehand et al. (1979), Patterson (1974), Patterson and Reid (1973), Webster-Stratton (1992), Chamberlain and Mihalic (1998) and many others provide technical descriptions of numerous basic behavior change techniques and concepts. Positive reinforcement/praise, negative reinforcement, ignoring, distracting, clear limit-setting with consistent follow-through and a reasonable number of limits, parent–child special time, and parental monitoring of activities are applied when deemed appropriate during the Behavior Change Phase of FFT. On their own, parent management techniques appear to be more effective with younger rather than older adolescents. Because FFT is a systemic model and all family members are included in therapy, choosing and relaying these techniques to family members must be done in a sensitive and flexible way. The educational descriptions of reinforcement principles that are sometimes used in parent training are likely to come across as manipulative to an adolescent who is in the session, and should be rethought/rephrased by the therapist prior to presentation in the family setting. In general, the use of these basic parenting principles is encouraged in FFT through incorporation into the more systemic and collaborative techniques of response-cost and contracting. Therapists should keep these principles in mind, but their application is more commonly conducted through more systemic means than classic parent training.

Contracting. Contracting involves having family members identify specific things they would like other family members to do in exchange for interactions/behaviors or tangible rewards. This procedure is especially important with adolescents (as opposed to children). In fact, other than basic communication training, contracting is the parent–youth interaction/

influence technique that is most commonly used by FFT therapists because it is systemic (e.g., involves considering the idea of reinforcement/reward for all members of a system or subsystem), it can be initiated inside the therapeutic environment, and it can be adapted for use with youth at almost all developmental levels. Contracting should initially be conducted within the therapy session since therapists need to do a number of things to make early contracting as positive an experience as possible.

Therapists also need to monitor contracts to make certain they are attainable based on the functional relationship needs of each participant. Finally, therapists need to monitor the in-session contracting process to maintain the decreased negativity attained during the Motivation Phase. To this end, therapists often refer back to specific reframes and themes that were particularly helpful in creating positive attributions in family members during the Motivation Phase. If communication training was conducted earlier in the Behavior Change Phase, the therapist will also model and remind the family to use communication techniques during their in-session contracting discussions.

Response Cost Techniques. Especially effective with children and pre-adolescents, the specific approach to reward and punishment identified by Webster-Stratton and Herbert (1994) as *Response-Cost Techniques* provide a framework that helps a parent or parents learn how to set clear penalties (typically loss of privileges/current rewards) for inappropriate child behaviors or failures to perform. Expected behaviors and penalties should be fair and clearly stated, and augmented by visual aids whenever possible.

Additional Intervention Strategies. In addition to providing communication and additional skill training, FFT interventionists prescribe specific activities and behaviors that will enhance the family's experience of positive change. In particular, interventionists utilize as many *technical aids* as possible. These technical aids include such simple items as sticky-type notes that can be put on mirrors to remind family members about a particular behavior, audiotape recordings of communication practice sessions that can be taken home for review, commercially available manuals on parenting, a wide range of similar free parenting information provided by social service agencies, training in the use of answering machines and cell phones to leave messages for family members, a schedule of reminder telephone calls made by a volunteer to families who need additional structure to change old behavior patterns, and so on. As programs have replicated FFT formally and informally, the various technical aids and props that have been adopted seem endless, and interventionists can become very creative in developing materials that are consistent with the particular needs, abilities, and resources of the specific population with whom they deal.

Interventionists also are reminded to be very creative and energetic with respect to providing specific and concrete resources for families as they enter the change process. We do not want to send families (many of whom have only limited resources and low motivation for change) out of sessions with little more than suggestions about how to change behavior. Instead, we are in some ways "controlling" (or "educational"), ensuring that the client is given very clear information and directions during

Behavior Change. In fact, FFT agencies often buy sticky-type notes and inexpensive audio cassettes to give to families to consolidate techniques between particular sessions. We also often ask social services and educational agencies to forward pamphlets, and so forth.

The shift in therapist style, during Behavior Change, is to a much more structured, direct, and in some ways more hierarchical style than during Engagement and Motivation. In addition, FFT interventionists prescribe specific *interpersonal tasks* often involving technical aids. As has been discussed throughout, these interpersonal tasks (e.g., setting up a specific plan to supervise homework) must be tailored to the interpersonal needs and abilities of all family members involved.

Using Technical Aids. A number of technical aids are frequently used to facilitate behavior change in FFT. Examples of technical aids include (a) tape recordings of sessions, therapist handouts for family to take home and review, (b) reminder cards, post-it notes, charts, message centers on refrigerators, pictures, "corny sayings," symbols to remind family members about the behavior in question, (c) school-home feedback report sheets with detailed tasks and timelines, and (d) answering machines, beepers, two-way radios, cell phones.

Problem Solving. Behavior Change techniques often follow a very specific sequence for resolving problems. First, therapists help to focus on a specific problem to be addressed. In this process, the therapist helps family members to punctuate the nature of the problem, who it involves, and narrows the focus to a manageable goal that can be accomplished in the session. Second, therapists help family members to utilize the principles of communication described above to help family members clarify desired outcomes and agree/negotiate to accomplish the task. Therapists actively anticipate ways in which problem-solving attempts can be derailed and provide relational based, non-blaming interventions to maintain a positive working context. At the conclusion of problem solving, therapists help family members to review the process of problem solving and to discuss any agreements or plans that were resolved.

The above examples represent the more common techniques used by FFT therapists. However, just about any structured activity can represent a useful technique in FFT Behavior Change, *as long as the behaviors they create and maintain are consistent with Relational Functions.* Over the years FFT therapists have utilized a wide range of techniques (e.g., cognitive-behavioral, trauma-focused and experiential) along with already established cultural practices (e.g., preparing meals together) as contexts for FFT Behavior Change. Once they become comfortable with the core construct of "matching," FFT therapists have found that almost limitless techniques are available during this phase of FFT intervention.

The Generalization Phase of FFT

The FFT Therapist as "Family Case Manager." Families are intertwined in a vast array of social, legal, cultural, economic, community, and other systems. FFT not only recognizes this fact, but also incorporates specific principles which govern the inclusion (as well as exclusion) of these systems in the treatment planning process. Unlike generic treatment planning which sometimes wraps services around families and family members with little consideration of family dynamics, FFT focuses on each individual family's interpersonal and systemic needs when considering adjunctive support services. In addition, before ideas with face validity are implemented to advance a treatment plan, it is necessary for a therapeutic alliance to exist for the family to view these ideas as valid, and the idea must be based on an understanding of the functional aspect of family behavior. For example, job training for a 16-year-old male may be viewed as valuable in that it increases protective factors, supports emancipation, and provides necessary skill building. However, participation in such a program may not be supported by the mother if it replaces the father's role with his son and in doing so enables the father to further disengage from the family. Often, situations like this are associated with low support by key family members (e.g., mother becomes too busy or forgets to drive the son to the job training site on the third day). According to FFT, this noncompliance is predictable if the son's previously disruptive behavior functioned to pull the father into parenting and more importantly into supporting the mother. If for this same mother, however, taking her son to the job training program is coupled with increased support and involvement from the father to the mother, then she will be likely to facilitate the increased system involvement of job training. Again, this paragraph stands as a reminder that the phases of FFT are developmental, synergistic, and dependent upon one another.

Summary of Generalization Phase. FFT extends or exports family functioning into a variety of community systems, which helps the family as well as the community. It is our belief that facilitating and managing appropriate links to adjunctive services often (or usually) must be developed in order for the treatment effects to be generalized outside of the treatment context and sustained over time. In doing so, the FFT therapist helps anchor the family and the family members to a larger supportive community.

We also believe that if this is done without consideration of the family relational functions these efforts will fail. Because of this, successful intervention cannot begin with this phase of intervention. To simply wrap services around a family or family member without considering the impact on family functioning is to risk destabilizing an already precarious family process. Thus, the accomplishments of the Generalization Phase are predicted on successful handling of therapist-family *core therapy processes* described above and again summarized below.

BRIEF SYNOPSIS OF THE IDEAL FFT INTERVENTION

Session 1: Engagement, Intake, and Assessment

1. Further develop relationship with all family members that began during phone contacts, initiate
2. Intake and assessment (if done by the FFT therapist). Otherwise, Session 1 consists of establishing the relationship with the family.
3. Initiate Motivation Phase by using Change Focus and Change Meaning techniques.

4. Begin assessment of Relational Functions and observation of family interaction patterns.
5. End Session with assessment protocol and intake documentation; schedule next session within 3 days.

Between Sessions 1 and 2

1. Review each family member's behavior, feelings, and beliefs and consider additional cultural match issues.
2. Identify unclear relationship dynamics within family and with extended family or other caregivers.
3. Identify resistance patterns of family members/caregivers.
4. Hypothesize Relational Functions for each family member.
5. Plan specific techniques and strategies to complete assessment.
6. Plan specific therapeutic interventions based on the above.
7. Have additional conversations with all systems involved with the family (e.g., child welfare worker, school officials/teachers, probation officers, other treatment providers) to develop relationships and further the therapist's understanding of their perspective and expectations of case.

Sessions 2 and 3

1. Repeat techniques from Session 1 and continue to match and build relationships with family members.
2. Continue to use Change Focus and Change Meaning interventions.
3. Continue assessment.
4. If possible complete Motivation Phase goals.
5. Reschedule next session as needed; high risk families are rescheduled within 3 days.

Between Session 3 and 4

1. Develop intermediate and long-term change goals that will address family relational
2. Pattern deficits (e.g., problem solving skills, communication skills, parenting skills, parent and youth well-being, including specific issues such as PTSD and substance abuse).
3. Establish positive alternatives that provide a rationale and behavioral focus that matches all family members' Relational Functions.
4. Review and develop specific behavior change and educational techniques that will lead to fulfillment of intermediate and long term goals.

Middle Sessions

1. Apply Behavior Change technology consistent with Relational Functions to family members.

2. Resistance is feedback that one or more family member's Relational Functions have not been met – therapist must return to Motivation and Assessment.
3. Develop increased family initiative in behavior change and continue to match Relational Functions.
4. Prompt, look for, and support appropriate family member competence with steadily decreasing assistance from therapist.

Later Sessions

1. Identify relevant systems and specific individual issues (e.g., vocational deficits).
2. Relapse prevention work is initiated.
3. Generalize specific behavior changes to other family situations.
4. Facilitate independence that is consistent with Relational Functions of family members.
5. Maintain and create new links with extra-familial systems to generalize positive intra-family changes.
6. Evaluate quality of life issues and plan for future.

Termination

1. Problem cessation: determined by verbal report and therapist observation.
2. Spontaneous family process: new interaction styles and attributions for all family members are observed.
3. Primary risk factors, including safety issues, reduced or eliminated; protective factors enhanced.

CHANGE MECHANISMS: PROCESS RESEARCH ON THE CLINICAL INTERIOR OF FFT

One hallmark of evidence-based interventions is the clear articulation of the presumed underlying mechanisms of action that are responsible for change, including an understanding of the client processes that need to be addressed and the therapeutic strategies necessary to alter these processes. Treatment manuals provide rich theoretical descriptions and examples for how these clinical processes are manifested within sessions and over the course of treatment. Intensive research on the clinical interior of treatment has been an essential component in the development of FFT. In fact, for over 3 decades, the articulation and understanding of mechanisms of action in FFT has evolved through a systematic program of research and clinical practice. As FFT has matured, the lens for understanding the mechanisms of action has broadened (as the model became more complex and multifaceted), but the focus has become even more sharp and specific (as the targets and treatment strategies became more well defined and understood). In the section below, we describe how observational research, including process research, examining what transpires in therapy sessions, has influenced FFT theory and practice. Specifically, we present a program of process research that has systematically examined the relationship between adaptive (supportive) and maladaptive (defensive/negative) family interactions and clinical outcomes, and therapist characteristics and interventions associated with improvements in these family processes. We conclude this section with a brief description of our most recent research on building therapeutic alliances with family members. This program of research has been critical in the integration of therapeutic strategies for creating a motivational context for change in FFT.

Research on Understanding and Managing Family Conflict

Specific aspects of negativity and high levels of conflict have been shown to predict individual, couple, and family problems in both marital (Gottman & Levenson, 1992; Margolin, Burman, & John, 1989) and family research (Alexander, Waldron, Barton, & Mas, 1989). In our earliest work with families with a delinquent adolescent, Alexander (1973) demonstrated that families with a delinquent adolescent expressed higher rates of system-disintegrating communication (defensive), while families with non-delinquent youth expressed more system-integrating (supportive) communication. Moreover, families with a delinquent adolescent demonstrated higher reciprocity in defensiveness. That is, once defensiveness was present, there was a greater likelihood that other family members would respond in like manner, resulting in an escalation or sequences of strong, pervasive negative interactions. Within the treatment context, these negative interactions have been shown to be associated with negative treatment outcomes. For example, Alexander, Barton, Schiavo, and Parsons (1976) found that the ratio of negative to supportive statements was significantly higher in cases that dropped out of therapy than among cases that completed treatment. In turn, premature termination predicted recidivism in adolescents.

In the field of family therapy; however, research findings suggest that family conflict/negativity is malleable in treatment. For example, Melidonis and Bry (1995) demonstrated that therapists could reduce family members' blaming statements and increase their positive statements by asking questions about exceptions and selectively attending to positive statements. Also, Diamond and Liddle (1996) demonstrated that in successful resolutions of therapy impasses, therapists were able to create an emotional treaty among family members by blocking and working through negative affect, and by amplifying thoughts and feelings that promoted constructive dialogue.

Within FFT, research has not only shown that family negativity is common among families with behavior problem youth, but also that systematic interventions aimed at altering the cognitive and affective context can be highly influential in reducing this negativity. For example, Barton, Alexander, and Turner (1988) provided evidence about the critical relevance of the current context on family interactions in a basic (non-therapy) study with delinquent adolescents. This study investigated the effect of attribution sets on the behaviors of 16 families with a delinquent youth and 16 families with a non-delinquent youth. Families were audio-taped during competitive and cooperative experimental situations. As predicted, families with a delinquent youth expressed significantly lower rates of adaptive communication in the cooperative set than families with a non-delinquent adolescent. However, families with a delinquent adolescent expressed significantly lower rates of negativity in the cooperative set condition than in the competitive set condition.

Alexander, Waldron, Barton, and Mas (1989) further evaluated parents' data in three studies of families with a delinquent adolescent. Families were provided with different forms of a positive versus negative interactional (attributional) context. Study 1 demonstrated that the families exposed to a negative attributional context demonstrated more negative behaviors than did families exposed to the positive context when parents interacted with each other and with their delinquent adolescent. Study 2 demonstrated that the dispositional attributions of parents were influenced by the manipulation of set, with a dissatisfied set producing negative blaming attributions and a satisfied set producing non-blaming, positive attributions. Study 3 demonstrated that parents' negative sets regarding their adolescent's negative behaviors, once established and discussed by the family for 5 min, were unresponsive to a subsequent positive reattribution regarding those behaviors.

Taken together, the data provide some support for reattribution techniques, which are explicitly focused on expanding the families frame to include a more workable frame where family members are willing to try out new behaviors. These observational studies have been critical in influencing the development (subsequent evolution) of specific intervention strategies, such as relabeling and reframing, and for creating a motivational context conducive to adaptive and supportive family behaviors. For example, the results of Study 3, demonstrating the stability of defensive interactions, was a precursor to our adoption of a relentless focus on opening new frames for family members (e.g., systematically attending to strength-based relational aspects of interactions, reframing, creating relational themes, particularly during early sessions where interactions are typically devoid of positive sentiments and affective connections between family members).

Applying this knowledge to therapy sessions, Robbins et al. (1996) examined the impact of specific types of therapist intervention (e.g., reframing, reflection, and structuring) on family members' negative attitude during the initial session of FFT with a delinquent adolescent. Therapist interventions and family member behaviors were coded at the speech act level. Family members' immediate responses to therapist interventions were compared. The results revealed that (a) across all therapist's interventions, adolescents demonstrated significantly more negative attitude than mothers following therapist behaviors, but (b) adolescents' attitudes improved from negative to neutral following therapist reframes. Thus, reframing may be used as a tool for decreasing adolescents' negativity in therapy.

In a subsequent investigation, Robbins, Alexander, and Turner (2000) further examined the impact of therapist interventions on family processes. Similar to the previous study, the immediate effects of therapist reframing, reflection, and structuring interventions on family member behaviors were compared; however, to control for previous family member status, only those therapist interventions that followed family member defensive statements were included in the analysis. Results demonstrate that reframing is more effective than reflection and structuring statements in reducing family members' negative behaviors. In addition, the results not only replicated the previous finding that adolescents respond more favorably to reframes than do mothers and fathers, but also provide evidence of the effectiveness of reframing for all family members.

Within the treatment context, we have also conducted a series of studies examining the complex relationships between therapist gender and family support/negativity in therapy sessions. For example Warburton, Alexander, and Barton (1980) demonstrated that mothers expressed significantly higher rates of supportive behaviors to female therapists and that this gender-linked pattern was not evident with fathers and male therapists. However, fathers displayed significantly higher rates of negative behaviors to female therapists. Female therapists likewise showed elevated rates of negativity to fathers.

Building on this research, Newberry, Alexander, & Turner (1991) examined the effects of therapist and client sex roles on the behaviors of 34, two-parent families with a delinquent adolescent that received FFT. In this study, therapist and client behaviors during the first phase of therapy were transcribed and divided into thought units. Each thought unit was classified as supportive, structuring (relational command or demand), pejorative (defensive), or non-therapy related. While molar rates of coded behaviors did not differentiate effects of therapist or parent gender, microsequential analyses (contingency analysis – Z statistic) detected different gender-linked sequential dependencies of therapist and client behaviors. In particular, results indicated that family members responded differently to male and female therapist behaviors. For example, both mothers and fathers were significantly more likely to respond supportively to female therapist supportive statements than to male therapist supportive statements. Also, fathers were more likely to respond supportively to therapist structuring than were mothers. Interestingly, the results suggested that female and male therapists also responded differently to client behaviors. Specifically, female therapists were more likely than male therapists to respond to client supportive statements with structuring statements.

In a recent process study, we examined the relationship between family members' alliance with therapists and dropout (Robbins, Turner, Alexander, & Perez, 2003). In this study, we found that the balance (parent–therapist alliance minus adolescent–therapist alliance) was a better predictor of engagement/retention in treatment than the overall level of alliance. In fact, the overall level of alliance with therapist was actually misleading, with the highest levels of alliance observed among parents in the families that dropped out of treatment. Therapists that were able to achieve a more balanced or similar level of alliance with parents and adolescents were more likely to keep the families engaged in treatment.

How therapists negotiate early sessions in FFT to build balanced alliances with family members and manage family negativity is currently being examined in our most recent evaluation of the clinical interior of treatment. For example, Robbins, Turner, Alexander, Liddle and Szapocznik (2010, in preparation) demonstrate that families that engage in treatment have a significantly higher level of balance in therapist support to family members (support to parents minus support to adolescent) than families that dropout of treatment. And, perhaps more importantly, therapists in the dropout cases appear to have a higher rate of support to parents than therapists in the families that are successfully retained in treatment. In addition, the results indicated that family negativity was significantly higher for the dropout families than the families that completed treatment. Taken together, these findings suggest that therapists who successfully engage families into treatment are able to effectively achieve balanced alliances with family members by engaging in higher rates of supportive interventions to adolescents (compared to parents) than are therapists of cases that dropout of treatment. Support to parents *and* adolescents is still critical; however, in that the overall level is more balanced in the completer families than the dropout families. Given that adolescents are frequently the target of much of the negativity that is expressed in therapy sessions (Robbins et al., 2003), it is not surprising that a systematic attempt to support their perspective is associated with positive outcomes, such as engagement in FFT.

SUMMARY OF THE FFT MODEL AND CORE ELEMENTS

FFT is a relational, family-based, ecosystemic, communication theory, and cognitive–behavioral-based model, with consideration of intrapsychic (or at least intra-individual) factors and biogenic influences. FFT produces change through a phase-based process (Engagement, Motivation, Relational Assessment, Behavior Change, Generalization/Ecosystemic focus). These phases are wrapped in, and informed by core concepts of matching, non-blaming relational focus, balanced alliance and respectfulness with all family members. Various theoretical models have informed the development of FFT but none has been adopted in its entirety. Instead, FFT recognizes that each perspective, and the processes they assume to be relevant to successful treatment, may be more or less influential or appropriate in any given family. FFT is an "integrative" model which allows us to conceptualize families and problem behaviors, as well as family strengths, from various perspectives depending on a number of contextual variables. However, these perspectives must not be mutually exclusive nor represent paradigm shifts or clashes with respect to FFT core principles.

FFT therapist are trained and supervised to be clear about the overall principles and perspective that guides the integrative process. Our "default mode" is relational and respectful, but it is accommodating enough to utilize other perspectives as long as they are consistent with the core FFT model and they help the therapist understand and intervene with *this particular family, effectively, at this particular time.*

And finally, FFT represents a motivational and a systems model; that is, the behaviors we address clinically are assumed to be "internally" motivated by the people evincing them, yet also "co-influenced" by others in the environment. As such, FFT is both an individual *and* a relational model. This fact, in reality, makes FFT a complex and rich intervention, and places demands for accountability and thoughtful behavior on therapists, trainers, dissemination vehicles, and treatment programs. If families were simple, so too should be a treatment program. If families are complex and challenged on multiple levels and domains, successful treatment requires that our intervention models match those levels and domains. At the same time, this reality best fits the realities of troubled families, in which the whole is indeed more than the sum of the parts, but the parts each contribute their unique variance to the functioning of the whole.

REFERENCES

Waldron, H. B., & Alexander, J. F. (Draft). *Integrated Functional Family Therapy and contingency management program (FFTCM) for adolescent substance use and dependence.* Eugene, OR: Oregon Research Institute.

Alexander, J. F. (1973). Defensive and supportive communications in normal and deviant families. *Journal of Consulting and Clinical Psychology, 40*(2), 223–231.

Alexander, J. F. (2008). *Functional family therapy (FFT) clinical training manual.* Salt Lake City, UT: FFC INC.

Alexander, J. F., & Barton, C. (1995). Family therapy research. In R. H. Mikesell, D. D. Lusterman, & S. McDaniel (Eds.), *Integrating family therapy: Handbook of family psychology and systems therapy* (pp. 199–215). Washington, DC: American Psychological Association.

Alexander, J. F., Barton, C., Schiavo, R. S., & Parsons, B. V. (1976). Behavioral intervention with families of delinquents: Therapist characteristics and outcome. *Journal of Consulting and Clinical Psychology, 44*(4), 656–664.

Alexander, J. F., & Parsons, B. V. (1973). Short term behavioral intervention with delinquent families: Impact on family process and recidivism. *Journal of Abnormal Psychology, 81*(3), 219–225.

Alexander, J. F., & Parsons, B. V. (1982). *Functional family therapy: Principles and procedures.* Carmel, CA: Brooks & Cole.

Alexander, J. F., & Pugh, C. (1996). Adolescent oppositional and conduct disorders. In F. Kaslow (Ed.), *Handbook of relational diagnosis* (pp. 210–224). New York: Wiley.

Alexander, J. F., Pugh, C., & Parsons, B. V. (1998). *Functional Family Therapy.* In D. S. Elliott (Series Ed.), *Blueprints for violence prevention* (Book 3). Boulder, CO: Center for the Study and Prevention of Violence, Institute of Behavioral Science, University of Colorado.

Alexander, J. F., Waldron, H. B., Barton, C., & Mas, C. H. (1983). Beyond the technology of family therapy: The anatomy of intervention model. In K. D. Craig & J. McMahon (Eds.), *Advances in clinical behavior therapy* (pp. 48–73). New York: Brunner/Mazel.

Alexander, J. F., Waldron, H. B., Barton, C., & Mas, C. H. (1989). Minimizing blaming attributions and behaviors in delinquent families. *Special series on marital and family disorders. Journal of Consulting and Clinical Psychology, 57*(1), 19–24.

Bandura, A. (1977). *Social learning theory.* New York: General Learning Press.

Bandura, A. (1986). *Social foundations of thought and action.* Englewood Cliffs, NJ: Prentice-Hall.

Barnoski, R. (2002). Washington State's implementation of Functional Family Therapy for juvenile offenders. Preliminary findings. *Washington State Institute for Public Policy*, www.swipp.wa.gov.

Barton, C., Alexander, J. F., & Sanders, J. D. (1985). Research in family therapy. In L. L'Abate (Ed.), *The handbook of family psychology and therapy*. Homewood, IL: The Dorsey Press.

Barton, C., Alexander, J. F., & Turner, C. W. (1988). Defensive communications in normal and delinquent families – the impact of context and family role. *Journal of Family Psychology, 1*(4), 390–405.

Barton, C., Alexander, J. F., Waldron, H., Turner, C. W., & Warburton, J. (1985). Generalizing the treatment effects of Functional Family Therapy: Three replications. *American Journal of Family Therapy, 13*(3), 16–26.

Brofenbrenner, U. (1979). *The ecology of human development: Experiments by nature and design.* Cambridge, MA: Harvard University Press.

Chamberlain, P., & Mihalic, S. F. (1998). *Blueprints for violence prevention: multidimensional treatment foster care.* Boulder, CO: University of Colorado at Boulder, Center for the Study and Prevention of Violence.

Diamond, G., & Liddle, H. A. (1996). Resolving a therapeutic impasse between parents and adolescents in multidimensional family therapy. *Journal of Consulting and Clinical Psychology, 64*(3), 481–488.

Centers for Disease Control, Thornton, T. N., Craft, C. A., Dahlberg, L. L., Lynch, B. S., & Baer, K. (2000). *Best practice of youth violence prevention: a sourcebook for community action.* Atlanta: Centers for Disease Control and Prevention. National Center for Injury Prevention and Control.

Elliott, D. S. (1998). (Series Ed.) *Blueprints for violence prevention.* Boulder, CO: Blueprints Publications. University of Colorado, Center for the Study and Prevention of Violence.

Elliott, D. S., & Mihalic, S. (1997). *Blueprints for violence prevention and reduction: The identification and documentation of successful programs.* Boulder, CO: Center for the Study and Prevention of Violence.

Forehand, R., Sturgis, E. T., McMahon, R. J., Aguar, D., Green, K., Wells, K., et al. (1979). Parent behavioral training to modify child noncompliance: Treatment generalization across time and from home to school. *Behavior Modification, 3*, 3–25.

Gordon, D. A., Graves, K., & Arbuthnot, J. (1995). The effect of Functional Family Therapy for delinquents on adult criminal behavior. *Criminal Justice and Behavior, 22*, 60–73.

Gottman, J. M., & Levenson, R. W. (1992). Marital processes predictive of later dissolution: Behavior, physiology, and health. *Journal of Personality and Social Psychology, 63*, 221–233.

Grover, P. L. (1998). *Preventing substance abuse among children and adolescents: Family-centered approaches: Prevention enhancement protocols system reference guide.* Rockville, MD: Center for Substance Abuse Prevention.

Haley, J. (1963). *Strategies of psychotherapy.* New York: Grune & Stratton.

Hansson, K. (1998). *Functional family therapy replication in Sweden: Treatment outcomes with juvenile delinquents..* Santa Fe, NM: Paper presented to the Eighth International Conference on Treating Addictive Behaviors. February.

Klein, N., Alexander, J. F., & Parsons, B. V. (1977). Impact of family systems intervention on recidivism and sibling delinquency: A model of primary prevention and program evaluation. *Journal of Consulting and Clinical Psychology, 45*, 469–474.

Loeber, R., & Farrington, D. P. (2001). *Child delinquents: Development, intervention, and service needs.* Thousand Oaks, CA: Sage Publications.

Margolin, G., Burman, B., & John, R. S. (1989). Home observations of married couples reenacting naturalistic conflicts. *Behavioral Assessment, 11*(1), 101–118.

Maslow, A. (1943). A theory of human motivation. *Psychological Review, 50*, 370–396.

Melidonis, G. G., & Bry, B. H. (1995). Effects of therapist exceptions questions on blaming and positive statements in families with adolescent behavior problems. *Journal of Family Psychology, 9*(4), 451–457.

Mihalic, S. W., & Elliott, D. S. (1997). Short- and long-term consequences of adolescent work. *Youth & Society, 28*(4), 464–498.

Morris, S. M., Alexander, J. F., & Turner, C. W. (1991). Do reattributions reduce blame? *Journal of Family Psychology, 5*(2), 192–203.

Morton, T. L., Alexander, J. F., & Altman, I. (1976). Communication and relationship definition. In G. R. Miller (Ed.), *Annual reviews of communication research, Volume V: Interpersonal communication.* Beverly Hills, CA: Sage Publications.

Newberry, A. M., Alexander, J. F., & Turner, C. W. (1991). Gender as a process variable in family therapy. *Journal of Family Psychology, 5*(2), 158–175.

OJJDP Juvenile Justice Bulletin (December, 2000). Office of Juvenile Justice and Delinquency Prevention, U.S. Department of Justice, Office of Justice Programs

Parsons, B. V., & Alexander, J. F. (1973). Short term family intervention: A therapy outcome study. *Journal of Consulting and Clinical Psychology, 41*(2), 195–201.

Patterson, G. R. (1974). Interventions for boys with conduct problems: Multiple settings, treatments, and criteria. *Journal of Consulting & Clinical Psychology., 42*(4), 471–481.

Patterson, G. R., & Reid, J. B. (1973). Intervention for families of aggressive boys: A replication study. *Behavior research and therapy, 11*, 383–394.

Reid, J. B., Patterson, G. R., & Snyder, J. (2002). *Antisocial behavior in children and adolescents: A developmental analysis and model for intervention.* Washington, DC: American Psychological Association.

Robbins, M. S., Alexander, J. F., Newell, R. M., & Turner, C. W. (1996). The immediate effect of reframing on client attitude in family therapy. *Journal of Family Psychology, 10*(1), 28–34.

Robbins, M. S., Alexander, J. F., & Turner, C. W. (2000). Disrupting defensive interactions in family therapy with delinquent adolescents. *Journal of Family Psychology, 14*, 688–701.

Robbins, M. S., Turner, C. W., Alexander, J. F., & Perez, G. A. (2003). Alliance and dropout in family therapy with drug using adolescents: Individual and systemic effects. *Journal of Family Psychology, 17*(4), 534–544.

Sale, E., Springer, F., Sambrano, S., & Turner, C. W. (2003). Evaluation of the high risk youth intervention project. *Journal of Drug Education, 33*, 91–105.

Substance Abuse and Mental Health Services Administration (SAMSHA). (2001). *Summary of findings from the 2000 National Household Survey on Drug Abuse.* Rockville, MD: Substance Abuse and Mental Health Services Administration (SAMSHA).

Thornton, T. N., Craft, C. A., Dahlberg, L. L., Lynch, B. S., & Baer, K. (2000). *Best practice of youth violence prevention: A sourcebook for community action.* Atlanta, GA: Centers for Disease Control and Prevention. National Center for Injury Prevention and Control.

U.S. Department of Justice, Office of Justice Programs (2000). *Promising Strategies to Reduce Substance Abuse.* www.ojp.usdoj.gov

Waldron, H. B. (1997). Adolescent substance abuse and family therapy outcome: A review of randomized trials. In T. H. Ollendick & R. J. Prinz (Eds.), *Advances in clinical child psychology* (Vol. 19, pp. 199–234). New York: Plenum.

Waldron, H. B., Brody, J. L., & Slesnick, N. (2001). Integrative behavioral and family therapy for adolescent substance abuse. In P. M. Monti, W. M. Colby, & T. A. O'Leary (Eds.), *Adolescents, alcohol, and substance abuse: Reaching teens through brief interventions.* New York: Guilford Press.

Waldron, H. B., Slesnick, N., Brody, J. L., Turner, C. W., & Peterson, T. R. (2001). Treatment outcomes for adolescent substance abuse at 4- and 7-month assessments. *Journal of Consulting and Clinical Psychology, 69*, 802–813.

Waldron, H. B., & Turner, C. W. (2008). Evidence-based psychosocial treatments for adolescent substance abuse. *Journal of Clinical Child & Adolescent Psychology, 37*, 238–261.

Waldron, H. B., Turner, C. W., Barton, C., Alexander, J. F., & Cline, V. B. (1997). Therapist defensiveness and marital therapy process and outcome. *American Journal of Family Therapy, 25*(3), 233–243.

Warburton, J. R., & Alexander, J. F. (1983). Treatment of female delinquency: Perspectives and techniques. In E. A. Blechman (Ed.), *Behavior modification with women.* New York: Guilford Press.

Warburton, J. R., & Alexander, J. F. (1985). The family therapist: What does one do? In L. L'Abate (Ed.), *The handbook of family psychology and therapy*. Homewood, IL: The Dorsey Press.

Warburton, J., Alexander, J. F., & Barton, C. (1980, August). *Sex of client and sex of therapist: Variables in family process study*. Montreal: Paper presented at the Annual Convention of the American Psychological Association.

Watzlawick, P., Beavin, J., & Jackson, D. D. (1967). *Pragmatics of human communication*. New York: W. W. Norton.

Watzlawick, P., Weakland, J., & Fisch, R. (1974). *Change: Principles of problem formation and problem resolution*. New York: Norton.

Webster-Stratton, C. (1992). *The incredible years: A trouble-shooting guide for parents of children ages 3-8 years*. Toronto, Canada: Umbrella Press.

Webster-Stratton, C., & Herbert, M. (1994). *Troubled families – problem children: Working with parents: A collaborative process*. Chichester: Wiley.

Youth violence: A report of the surgeon general (2001). Department of Health and Human Services, U.S. Public Health Service, Rockville, MD.

11

Multisystemic Therapy for Conduct Problems in Youth*

CINDY M. SCHAEFFER, MICHAEL R. McCART, SCOTT W. HENGGELER, and PHILLIPPE B. CUNNINGHAM

Multisystemic Therapy (MST; Henggeler, Schoenwald, Borduin, Rowland, & Cunningham, 1998, 2009) is a comprehensive family- and community-based treatment for youth with serious conduct problems who are at imminent risk of out-of-home placement (e.g., detention, incarceration, residential treatment). The effectiveness of MST has been established with chronic and violent juvenile delinquents and substance abusing youth. Adapted versions of the MST model have also been successfully applied to youth with other clinical problems, such as problem sexual behavior, psychiatric disturbance, and pediatric chronic illness. This chapter outlines the theoretical and empirical foundations of MST and provides a brief overview of the MST treatment model. A case example is used to illustrate the clinical aspects of the MST approach. The remainder of the chapter summarizes the growing evidence base for MST established through efficacy, effectiveness, and transportability trials.

*Portions of this chapter were published previously in *Evidence-Based Psychotheropies for Children and Adolescents, Second Edition*, edited by J.R. Weisz and A.E. Kazdin (2010), New york: Guilford Press. We greatly appreciate the permission from Guilford Press to reprint this material.

CINDY M. SCHAEFFER • Medical University of South Carolina
MICHAEL R. McCART • Medical University of South Carolina
SCOTT W. HENGGELER • Medical University of South Carolina
PHILLIPPE B. CUNNINGHAM • Medical University of South Carolina

R.C. Murrihy et al. (eds.), *Clinical Handbook of Assessing and Treating Conduct Problems in Youth*, DOI 10.1007/978-1-4419-6297-3_11,

CHARACTERISTICS OF THE MST MODEL

Theoretical and Empirical Foundations

MST is designed to address the array of risk factors commonly associated with conduct problems among youth. Decades of cross-sectional and longitudinal research has shown that risk factors for conduct problems involve influences at multiple individual and environmental levels (Deater-Deckard, Dodge, Bates, & Pettit, 1998; Elliott 1994; Loeber, Farrington, Stouthamer-Loeber, & Van Kammen, 1998; Thornberry & Krohn, 2003). At the individual level, for example, conduct problems are associated with low IQ, cognitive biases about the advantages of aggression, and social skill deficits. Environmental influences are present in the contexts of the family, peer network, school, and neighborhood. For example, high levels of parental substance use, low parental supervision, and inconsistent family discipline are linked with elevated risk for behavior problems among youth, and association with deviant peers is a consistently strong predictor of adolescent conduct problems. School-level influences include low academic achievement, low commitment to education, and an overly authoritarian teaching style. Further, neighborhoods characterized by high levels of poverty, residential mobility, and drug availability predict high rates of adolescent involvement in antisocial behavior.

Given that risk factors for conduct problems exist within and across multiple domains of a person's life, Bronfenbrenner's (1979) social ecological model provides a useful organizing framework for MST. According to this model, youth behavior is largely determined by the functioning of the systems (i.e., family, peer, school, and neighborhood) in which the youth is embedded and the reciprocal interplay between these systems. Consistent with this view, MST contends that for treatment to be effective, interventions must have the capacity to target risk factors in multiple domains and between systemic levels (e.g., caregiver interactions with school). Factors in the broader ecology (e.g., caregiver work hours, lack of prosocial activities in neighborhood) that create barriers to the effective functioning of proximal systems also must be addressed for positive change to occur.

According to the social ecological perspective, behavior must be considered within its naturally occurring context. This view has direct implications for the design of MST interventions. MST uses a home-based model of service delivery that emphasizes ecological validity in the assessment of behavior and delivery of interventions. Assessments are considered ecologically valid when they solicit information from multiple sources (e.g., caregivers, siblings, extended family, teachers) and gauge the youth's functioning in a variety of real world settings (e.g., at home, in school, during neighborhood activities). Similarly, MST interventions are provided where problems occur (homes, schools, community locations) and, whenever possible, are delivered to the youth by key members of the ecology.

MST Theory of Change

A central assumption of MST is that caregivers are the key to achieving and sustaining positive long-term outcomes. Thus, interventions focus intensely on empowering caregivers to obtain the resources and skills needed to more effectively parent and manage their children. As caregiver competencies (e.g., ability to provide consistent monitoring and supervision) increase, the therapist guides caregiver efforts to address other factors that might be contributing to a youth's problem behavior, such as associations with deviant peers and poor school performance. The ultimate goal is to create a context that supports adaptive youth behavior (e.g., relationships with prosocial peers, effective parenting), rather than a context that encourages antisocial behavior. Treatment also aims to surround caregivers with support from family, friends, and members of the community to help sustain the changes achieved during treatment. Importantly, the central emphases of MST on improved parenting and decreased youth association with deviant peers as central vehicles for change have been supported in several studies (e.g., Henggeler et al., 2009; Huey, Henggeler, Brondino, & Pickrel, 2000).

CHARACTERISTICS OF MST CLINICAL IMPLEMENTATION

Treatment Delivery

MST teams consist of two to four full-time Master's level therapists, an advanced Master's level or doctoral level supervisor who devotes at least 50% of his or her professional time to supervisory activities on the team, and administrative support. Therapists carry caseloads of four to six families each. Members of an MST team usually work for private service provider organizations contracted by public juvenile justice, child welfare, and mental health authorities. Therapists provide 24 h/day and 7 day/week availability, which allows them to work with families at times the family finds convenient and to respond to clinical crises wherever and whenever they emerge. The duration of MST treatment is relatively brief, ranging from 3 to 5 months. However, the intervention process is intensive and often involves a total of 60 or more hours of direct contact with the family and other members of the ecology. As noted previously, there is a strong emphasis on the delivery of MST services in home- and community-based settings, which enhances the ecological validity of assessments and interventions, helps overcome barriers to service access, and facilitates family engagement in the treatment process.

Clinical Procedures

MST is highly individualized and does not follow a rigid manualized plan for treatment. Instead, nine treatment principles provide the underlying structure and framework upon which therapists build their interventions (see Table 11.1). The second treatment principle, for example,

Table 11.1. MST treatment principles

1. The primary purpose of assessment is to understand the "fit" between the identified problems and their broader systemic context
2. Therapeutic contacts should emphasize the positive and use systemic strengths as levers for change
3. Interventions should be designed to promote responsible behavior and decrease irresponsible behavior among family members
4. Interventions should be present-focused and action-oriented, targeting specific and well-defined problems
5. Interventions should target sequences of behavior within and between multiple systems
6. Interventions should be developmentally appropriate and fit the developmental needs of the youth
7. Interventions should be designed to require daily or weekly effort by family members
8. Intervention efficacy should be evaluated continuously from multiple perspectives
9. Interventions should be designed to promote treatment generalization and long-term maintenance of therapeutic change

emphasizes that all aspects of MST must be strength-based. Therapists communicate an optimistic perspective to the family and other members of the youth's ecology throughout the assessment and treatment process. Therapists look for potential strengths within the contexts of the child (e.g., hobbies and interests, academic skills), family (e.g., problem-solving ability, affective bonds), peers (e.g., prosocial activities, achievement orientation), school (e.g., management practices, prosocial after-school activities), and the neighborhood/community (e.g., concerned and involved neighbors, voluntary associations such as Boys and Girls clubs). Identified strengths then are leveraged in interventions. For example, a neighbor or extended family member might be enlisted to assist with monitoring the youth after school until a caregiver gets home from work.

Importantly, the nine treatment principles are applied using an analytical/decision-making process that structures the treatment plan, its implementation, and the evaluation of its effectiveness. Specific goals for treatment are set at individual, family, peer, and social network levels. Moreover, as noted previously, the adolescent's caregivers are viewed as key to achieving desired outcomes and as crucial for the generalizability and sustainability of treatment gains.

Early in the treatment process, the problem behaviors to be targeted are specified clearly from the perspectives of key stakeholders (e.g., family members, teachers, juvenile justice authorities), and ecological strengths are identified. Then, based on multiple perspectives, the ecological factors that seem to be driving each problem are organized into a coherent conceptual framework (e.g., the youth's marijuana use seems to be associated with a lack of caregiver monitoring, association with substance using peers, and poor school performance). Next, the MST therapist, with support from other team members (other therapists, supervisor, consultant), designs specific intervention strategies to target those "drivers." Strategies incorporate interventions from empirically supported, pragmatic, problem-focused treatments such as structural/strategic and behavioral family therapies, behavioral parent training, cognitive behavioral therapy, and motivational interviewing. Psychopharmacological interventions might also be incorporated into treatment when evidence indicates biological contributors to identified problems. Importantly, these empirically supported interventions are highly integrated and are delivered in conjunction with interventions that address other pertinent ecological drivers of the identified problems (e.g., supporting caregivers in advocating for more appropriate school services, connecting caregivers with the parents of the youth's peers).

Intervention effectiveness is monitored continuously from multiple perspectives. When interventions are ineffective, identified drivers are reconceptualized, and modifications are made until an effective strategy is developed. This reiterative process reinforces two important features of the MST model. First, MST teams strive to never give up on youth and families, doing "whatever it takes" to help families reach treatment goals. Second, when interventions are not successful, the failure is the team's, not the family's. In other words, when the team develops accurate hypotheses of the drivers, identifies barriers to implementation success, and delivers corresponding interventions appropriately, families tend to achieve their goals, and conduct problems among youth usually diminish. In the next section, a case example is presented to illustrate the clinical implementation of MST.

Case Example

Deon, a 15-year old African-American male, was referred to MST by the juvenile court after he obtained his third assault charge in a year. In the most recent incident, Deon assaulted another neighborhood boy with a baseball bat late one weeknight a few blocks from Deon's house. Deon alleged that he was riding his bike in his neighborhood when several boys "jumped" him in an attempt to steal his bike, and that the assault was an attempt to defend himself. The probation officer confirmed that Deon's charges all involved youth from a particular crowd of same-age and older youth in Deon's neighborhood who were no longer in school and who were known for their involvement in drug and gang activity.

Deon lived with his biological father (Mr. Henry) and paternal grandmother in his grandmother's home, which was in a high crime neighborhood. Deon's mother had died of a heroin overdose when he was 8 years old. Since then his father had not allowed Deon to see his maternal side of the family, stating that "they're all drug addicts." The father had been laid off from his factory job for 4 months and was unemployed. He spent most nights at his girlfriend's (Ms. Smith's) house a few miles away, leaving Deon alone with his grandmother, who was frail and did not discipline him. At school, Deon was reported to be well-liked by staff, but his attendance was sporadic (2–3 days/week) and he was two grades behind (in eighth grade instead of 10th), with a sixth grade achievement level.

In line with structured MST clinical procedures, the initial assessment was multifaceted, and strove to identify systemic strengths, treatment outcomes desired by all stakeholders, and the fit between identified problems and their broader systemic context (MST Treatment Principle 1; Table 11.1). Through initial conversations with Deon, his father, and his grandmother, as well as a meeting with the vice principal at Deon's school, the therapist identified many strengths and needs across Deon's key ecological systems (see Table 11.2). Key systemic strengths included Deon's

Table 11.2. Strengths and needs: Deon's ecology

System	Strengths	Needs
Youth	• Attractive – tall and slim, looks older than 15 • Athletic • Polite to adults • Prosocial interests: freestyle biking, connecting to mother's family	• Untreated ADHD (unfocused and restless at school) • Low verbal skills • Gets angry quickly when provoked • Positive view of aggressive retaliation • Poor organizational and study skills
Family	• Strong father–son bond • Strong work ethic (father, girlfriend, father's sisters) • Relatively most affluent family in neighborhood (father has worked and has a car, etc.) • Large extended network on father's side, all positive – father has two sisters; Deon has several same-age cousins • Father's girlfriend cares, has positive relationship with father and Deon • Maternal grandmother has a desire to reconnect with Deon	• Poor parental monitoring (father gone most nights, grandmother too frail) • Few consequences for misbehavior • Volatile arguments between Deon and father • Father and paternal grandmother both drink heavily • Paternal grandmother declining health/extensive medical needs • Mother's side – little contact with Deon and conflict with Mr. Henry; history of drug use.
Peer	• Likeable, pleasant • Several prosocial cousins close in age	• No friends (prefers to be alone) • Limited verbal abilities • Immature/low social skills • Older and bigger than classmates • Neighborhood peers mostly drug and gang involved; one particular group harasses him
School	• Bonded to the Vice Principal, who is concerned and wants Deon to do well • Teachers like him • Attends most days	• Two or more grade levels behind • Struggles to understand material • Poor work habits (e.g., no structure for homework) • Encounters deviant peers while walking home from school (one assault occurred then)
Community	• Church within walking distance; grandmother active there • Home is close to father's work (when not laid off)	• No recreational facilities/places for adolescents to hang out • Alcohol and drugs easily available • Gang presence; difficult to avoid the crowd that harasses Deon • Few other job opportunities other than factory

politeness and prosocial interests, affection among family members, and a large paternal family social network. Some key ecological needs included family problems with alcohol use, high family conflict, and limited opportunities for prosocial activities in the neighborhood. Deon's desired treatment outcomes were to "see his mother's family" and to "do more freestyle 'trick' biking." Mr. Henry's desired outcomes were for Deon to "do well in school" and to "stay in the house and out of trouble in the neighborhood." His grandmother wanted for "Deon and his father to fight less" and for Deon to "not roam the streets." Deon's probation officer wanted him to "complete an anger management group," "attend school every day," and "comply with all house rules." Ms. Smith (Mr. Henry's girlfriend), whom Deon liked and saw often, shared the family's concerns for Deon, and privately expressed to the therapist a desire for Mr. Henry to "drink less" and "start working again."

With these strengths, needs, and desired outcomes in mind, the MST therapist gained a consensus among all stakeholders on several overarching treatment goals, including (a) no new criminal charges for Deon and compliance with probation officer requests, (b) compliance with all house rules, (c) demonstration of success in school (i.e., no unexcused absences or suspensions/expulsions, completion of assignments), (d) improved relations between Deon and his father, as evidenced by fewer arguments reported by family members and therapist observation, and (e) increased contact with prosocial peers. Consistent with MST Principles, overarching goals used strength-based language (Principle 2) and set forth explicit criteria for judging when goals had been met (Principle 8).

The MST therapist combined information across sources and identified the most likely drivers for Deon's assault incidents and poor school performance. As illustrated in Fig. 11.1, the drivers of many problems were shared (e.g., low parental monitoring was a factor in Deon being out on the streets late at night and of his poor school attendance) or mediated by other problems (e.g., father's alcohol use decreased his ability to monitor and led to conflicts with his son, both of which increased the likelihood that Deon would be out late at night). Prioritized drivers were then targeted in treatment sessions occurring several times each week. Initially, the therapist addressed a few straightforward drivers that would give the family some early successes, such as having Mr. Henry recontact Deon's former psychiatrist for an appointment to address ADHD medication issues and enrolling Deon in an after school homework club to improve his core academic skills. To ensure that Deon could attend the after school program and to prevent him from spending time with other adjudicated youth, the MST therapist requested that she be allowed to provide anger management skills training to Deon individually, rather than have him attend a court-sponsored group, and the probation officer agreed. This treatment component was accomplished through individual sessions with Deon with Mr. Henry's occasional involvement (i.e., he was given skills for how to coach Deon on when to use the skills and to praise him for doing so) using a structured empirically supported protocol.

Two prioritized drivers of Deon's behavior problems were Mr. Henry's low monitoring and ineffective discipline and the fact that Deon had few

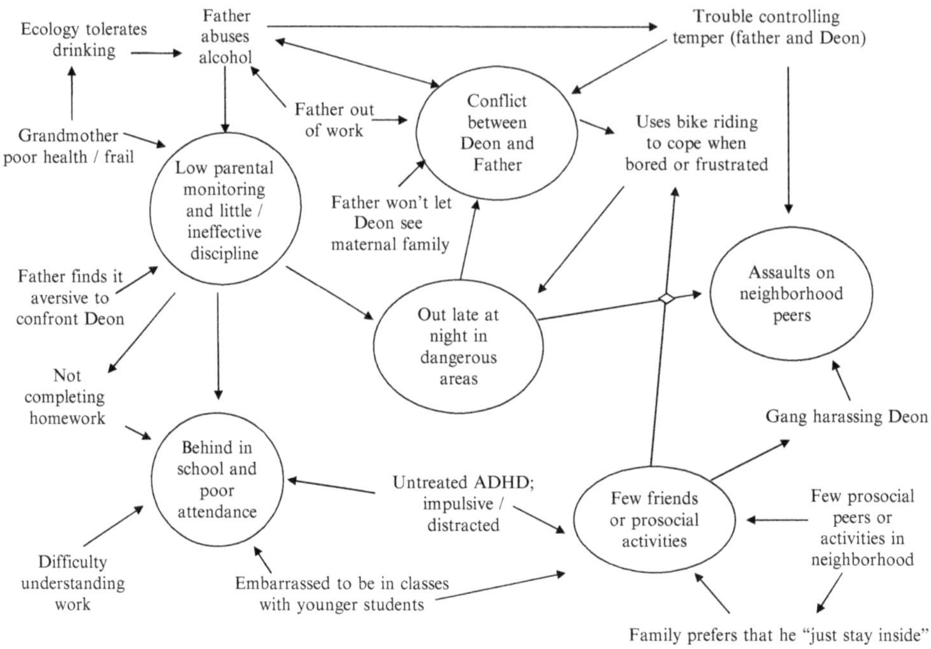

Fig. 11.1. Drivers of Deon's criminal offenses and poor school functioning.

friends or prosocial activities. In addressing these drivers, the therapist began by challenging some of Mr. Henry's misconceptions about parenting an adolescent, such as his belief that the grandmother's mere presence in the home was sufficient to monitor Deon's whereabouts (even though she was in bed by 9 pm every night), or that contact with peers only during the school day was enough to meet Deon's developmental need for friendships and peer support. Maintaining a strength-focus (Principle 2), the therapist framed Mr. Henry's rigid and ineffective attempts to control Deon's behavior (e.g., yelling at him to "just stay home or else") as caring efforts to prevent his son from engaging in deviant behavior that could be built upon. Consistent with the MST belief that intervention generalizability and maintenance of positive changes is enhanced when multiple ecology members are involved (Principle 9), the therapist included Ms. Smith in some sessions with Mr. Henry. Ms. Smith became an ally in the therapist's efforts, helping to persuade Mr. Henry that Deon needed more supervision and positive peer connections. With the help of the MST therapist, Ms. Smith was able to express her concerns to Mr. Henry about his drinking and its adverse effects on his temper, health, and job seeking activities. With her encouragement, Mr. Henry agreed to take a break from drinking for awhile until "this mess with Deon is straightened out" and to resume looking for work. Mr. Henry also agreed to spend more nights at home monitoring Deon, ensuring that he went to school in the morning, and implementing a behavior plan that involved rewards (allowance, time playing videogames) and consequences (taking his bike away) for school attendance, homework completion, and staying home through the night. These interventions encouraged more responsible behavior from both Deon and Mr. Henry (Principle 3) and required consistent daily effort (Principle 7).

As Mr. Henry became more active and effective in disciplining Deon, their conflicts increased, and the therapist became concerned about the potential for physical violence between them. Ms. Smith was enlisted to assist in a safety plan to be implemented at the first sign of conflict escalation (yelling, etc.) identified by the grandmother. The grandmother agreed to call Ms. Smith, who would come over and help Deon and his father calm down, either by taking Deon out for a drive or supervising him while Mr. Henry took a jog. The family implemented this present-focused and action-oriented plan (Principle 4) successfully on two occasions.

As Mr. Henry implemented Deon's behavior plan consistently over several weeks, it became apparent that new, more varied rewards were needed to sustain Deon's motivation to comply. One of Deon's strengths, his desire to do more "trick biking," was leveraged to gain better compliance (Principle 2). Although there were no safe places for him to ride in his neighborhood, some investigation revealed that a skate park was located about 10 mi away near Mr. Henry's sister's house. The therapist accompanied Mr. Henry to verify that the park was an appropriate place for Deon to be with minimal supervision. A plan was set up for Deon's aunt to pick him up each Saturday after she got off work and take him to the park, contingent upon his adherence with the behavior plan during the week. Either Mr. Henry or Ms. Smith would pick Deon up and drive him home 2 h later, and Deon had to use allowance money to pay for admission. Deon's behavior improved greatly with this extra incentive, and he began making friends who shared his interest in freestyle biking, thereby helping to meet Deon's developmental need for appropriate peer contacts (Principle 6).

To address another driver of Deon's behavior problems, the high degree of conflict between he and his father, the therapist held dyadic sessions regularly with Mr. Henry and Deon to help them with their communication and problem-solving skills. Although Deon frequently protested the increased demands made on his behavior in these sessions, he also expressed his appreciation that his father had reduced his drinking, began looking for jobs, and facilitated Deon's access to the skate park. In addition, Deon learned to calmly communicate his reasons for wanting to see his maternal family, and Mr. Henry discussed the reasons for his hesitation to allow it (i.e., his fear that they would expose Deon to illicit activities) without resorting to criticisms of that side of Deon's family. Using a problem-solving approach, Deon and his father identified a maternal family member who did not use drugs (maternal grandmother) who Mr. Henry felt more comfortable allowing Deon to see and set rules for their contact (e.g., Mr. Henry would be present for initial visits). The therapist then held a dyadic session with Mr. Henry and the maternal grandmother to discuss these visits and to help them start to resolve past issues (e.g., Mr. Henry felt she had enabled his wife's drug use; she was hurt that he had denied her access to Deon for years). These focused family sessions were critical for addressing the maladaptive behavioral sequences that had become entrenched between Deon and his father (i.e., volatile arguments) and between Mr. Henry and his former mother-in-law (i.e., a refusal to talk to one another; Principle 5).

Throughout the course of treatment, the MST therapist solicited opinions from all stakeholders regarding whether or not interventions were helping the family meet their overarching goals (Principle 8) and made adjustments accordingly. By the end of treatment, both Mr. Henry and Deon reported fewer and less severe arguments, an appraisal supported by Ms. Smith and Deon's grandmother. School stakeholders confirmed that Deon's attendance had increased and that his academic skills had improved. To facilitate the maintenance of Deon's school improvements (Principle 9), Mr. Henry advocated that the school promote Deon to ninth grade and place him in an accelerated dropout prevention curriculum that would provide him with smaller classes, a supportive community of peers and teachers, and the possibility of graduating with his agemates. Deon had no additional arrests and began spending larger parts of his weekend biking and visiting new skate park friends at his aunt's house. At the time MST ended, Mr. Henry had several leads on jobs, and he and his girlfriend were looking for a larger house in a safer neighborhood where they, Deon, and his grandmother could live together.

As with drivers for problem behaviors, MST therapists also identify drivers for improved behaviors. Hypothesized drivers for Deon's improved behaviors included (a) increased and consistent supervision by his father, (b) strictly enforced rules by Mr. Henry regarding school and whereabouts, (c) improved communication, decreased conflict, and increased warmth between Deon and his father, and (d) Deon's involvement in prosocial age-appropriate activities with nondeviant peers.

Training, Supervision, and Ongoing Quality Assurance

Training and supervision in the MST model are provided in several ways. First, new therapists participate in a 5-day orientation training that provides initial grounding in MST. The training includes both didactic (instruction in social learning theory, review of research on correlates of conduct problems) and experiential (role plays on engagement, assessment, and intervention strategies) components. Second, as therapists gain experience delivering MST to families, quarterly booster trainings are conducted on site. Third, the Master's or doctoral level clinical supervisor meets with therapists weekly to review cases, problem-solve barriers to successful family engagement, and ensure the multisystemic focus of therapeutic interventions. Fourth, the clinical team discusses cases with an MST expert consultant once a week to obtain additional feedback and direction as needed. This consultant also helps facilitate adherence to the MST model.

Training, supervision, and consultation take place within a comprehensive quality assurance/quality improvement (QA/QI) system designed to enhance fidelity to the MST treatment model. Considerable resources are devoted to this system because research supports a strong relationship between therapist adherence to MST and positive outcomes, including improved family relations, decreased affiliation with delinquent peers, and reduced long-term rates of arrest and incarceration (Henggeler, Melton, Brondino, Scherer, & Hanley, 1997; Henggeler, Pickrel, & Brondino, 1999; Huey et al., 2000; Schoenwald, Carter, Chapman, & Sheidow, 2008; Schoenwald, Ward, Henggeler, & Rowland, 2000). The process underlying the QA/QI system has been worked out through more than 15 years of experience assisting community-based agencies in developing and maintaining sustainable MST teams. In addition to the well-specified initial and ongoing training, supervision, and consultation protocols, key components of the QA/QI system include validated measures of implementation adherence at all levels (therapists, supervisors, and consultants) and a web-based implementation tracking system to provide teams and provider organizations with ongoing specific feedback about adherence and youth outcomes.

In addition to providing weekly consultation to the clinical team, MST consultants offer support to provider agencies who are interested in establishing MST programs. This support initially involves (a) community assessments to determine whether the needs that prompted stakeholder interest in MST are likely to be met by an MST program, (b) determination of whether an MST program is viable in a specific practice context (e.g., mechanisms are in place to reimburse therapists for mileage used to travel to families' homes), and (c) cultivation of stakeholder buy-in and commitment to the success of the program. After an MST program has been implemented in a community, consultants provide ongoing organizational support in the form of semi-annual program reviews, problem solving of organizational and stakeholder barriers to implementation, and support for program directors.

EMPIRICAL SUPPORT FOR MST

More than 20 independent reviewers, including researchers (e.g., Eyberg, Nelson, & Boggs, 2008; Waldron & Turner, 2008), entities charged with evaluating research (e.g., Margo, 2008; National Institute on Drug Abuse, 1999; U.S. Public Health Service, 2001), and consumer advocates (e.g., National Alliance on Mental Illness, 2008) have concluded that MST is either promising or effective in treating conduct problems in youth. MST has been evaluated in 15 published randomized clinical trials and two published quasi-experimental trials, most of which have examined outcomes with adolescents presenting with serious conduct problems. An overview of the samples, design, and outcomes of these trials is presented in Table 11.3. The following text summarizes these results.

Efficacy Trials

Early MST outcome studies were conducted in ways to maximize the probability that the new treatment would achieve favorable outcomes, assuming that it was actually efficacious. Henggeler and Borduin provided close supervision to therapists (highly trained graduate students), and the MST program, implemented in a university setting, was sheltered from the many challenges of implementation in real world (i.e., community-based clinics) settings. These studies (i.e., Borduin et al., 1995; Borduin, Henggeler,

Table 11.3. Published MST outcome studies

Study	Population	Comparison	Follow-up	MST Outcomes
Henggeler et al. (1986) $N = 57$[a]	Delinquents	Diversion services	Post treatment	Improved family relations; decreased behavior problems; decreased association with deviant peers
Brunk, Henggeler, & Whelan (1987) $N = 33$	Maltreating families	Behavioral parent training	Post treatment	Improved parent–child interactions
Borduin, Henggeler, Blaske, & Stein (1990) $N = 16$	Adolescent sexual offenders	Individual counseling	3 years	Reduced sexual offending; reduced other criminal offending
Henggeler et al. (1991)[b]	Serious juvenile offenders	Individual counseling usual community services	3 years	Reduced alcohol and marijuana use; decreased drug-related arrests
Henggeler, Melton, & Smith (1992) $N = 84$	Violent and chronic juvenile offenders	Usual community services – high rates of incarceration	59 weeks	Improved family relations; improved peer relations; decreased recidivism (43%); decreased out-of-home placement (64%)
Henggeler, Melton, Smith, Schoenwald, & Hanley (1993)	Same sample		2.4 years	Decreased recidivism (doubled survival rate)
Borduin et al. (1995) $N = 176$	Violent and chronic juvenile offenders	Individual counseling	4 years	Improved family relations; decreased psychiatric symptomatology; decreased recidivism (69%)
Schaeffer & Borduin (2005)	Same sample		13.7 years	Decreased re-arrests (54%); decreased days incarcerated (57%)
Henggeler, Melton, Brondino, Scherer, & Hanley (1997) $N = 155$	Violent and chronic juvenile offenders	Juvenile probation services – high rates of incarceration	1.7 years	Decreased psychiatric symptomatology; decreased days in out-of-home placement (50%); decreased recidivism (26%, nonsignificant); treatment adherence linked with long-term outcomes

Henggeler, Rowland et al. (1999) *N* = 116 (Final sample = 156)	Youth presenting psychiatric emergencies	Psychiatric hospitalization	4 months post recruitment	Decreased externalizing problems (CBCL); improved family relations; increased school attendance; higher consumer satisfaction; reduction in days hospitalized (75%)
Schoenwald, Henggeler, Brondino, & Rowland (2000)	Same sample		4 months post recruitment	Reduction in days in other out-of-home placements (50%)
Huey et al. (2004)	Same sample		16 months post recruitment	Decreased rates of attempted suicide
Henggeler, Rowland et al., (2003)	Same sample		16 months post recruitment	Favorable 4-month outcomes, noted above, dissipated
Sheidow et al. (2004)	Same sample		16 months post recruitment	MST cost benefits at 4 months, but equivalent costs at 16 months
Henggeler, Pickrel, & Brondino (1999) (*N* = 118)	Substance abusing and dependent delinquents	Usual community services	1 year	Decreased drug use at post treatment; decreased days in out-of-home placement (50%); decreased recidivism (26%, nonsignificant); treatment adherence linked with decreased drug use
Henggeler, Pickrel, Brondino, & Crouch (1996)	Same sample			98% rate of treatment completion
Schoenwald, Ward, Henggeler, Pickrel, & Patel (1996)	Same sample		1 year	Incremental cost of MST nearly offset by higher rate of costly out-of-home placement in control condition
Brown, Henggeler, Schoenwald, Brondino, & Pickrel (1999)	Same sample		6 months	Increased attendance in regular school settings
Henggeler, Clingempeel, Brondino, & Pickrel (2002)	Same sample		4 years	Decreased violent crime; increased marijuana abstinence
Borduin & Schaeffer (2001) – preliminary report (*N* = 48)	Juvenile sexual offenders	Usual community services	9 years	Decreased behavior problems and symptoms; improved family relations, peer relations, and academic performance
Borduin, Schaeffer, & Heiblum (2009) – full report				Decreased caregiver distress; decreased sex offender recidivism (83%); decreased recidivism for other crimes (50%); decreased days incarcerated (80%)
Ogden & Halliday-Boykins (2004) (*N* = 100)	Norwegian youth with serious antisocial behavior	Usual child welfare services	6 months post recruitment	Decreased externalizing and internalizing symptoms; decreased out-of-home placements; increased social competence; increased consumer satisfaction
Ogden & Hagen (2006)	Same sample		24 months post recruitment	Decreased externalizing and internalizing symptoms; decreased out-of-home placements

(continued)

Table 11.3. (continued)

Study	Population	Comparison	Follow-up	MST Outcomes
Ellis, Frey et al. (2005a) (N = 127)	Inner-city adolescents with chronically poorly controlled type 1 diabetes	Standard diabetes care	7 months post recruitment	Increased blood glucose testing; decreased inpatient admissions; improved metabolic control
Ellis, Naar-King et al. (2005)	Same sample		7 months post recruitment	Decreased medical charges and direct care costs
Ellis, Frey et al. (2005b)	Same sample		7 months post recruitment	Decreased diabetes stress
Ellis, Templin et al. (2007)	Same sample		13 months post recruitment	Decreased inpatient admissions sustained; favorable metabolic control outcomes dissipated
Rowland et al. (2005) (N = 31)	Youth with serious emotional disturbance	Hawaii's intensive Continuum of Care	6 months post recruitment	Decreased symptoms; decreased minor crimes; decreased days in out-of-home placement (68%)
Timmons-Mitchell, Bender, Kishna, & Mitchell (2006) (N = 93)	Juvenile offenders (felons) at imminent risk of placement	Usual community services	18-month follow-up	Improved youth functioning; decreased substance use problems; decreased re-arrests (37%)
Henggeler et al., (2006) (N = 161)	Substance abusing and dependent juvenile offenders in drug court	Four treatment conditions, including Family Court with usual services and Drug Court with usual services	12 months post recruitment	MST reduced substance use; drug court was more effective than Family Court at decreasing self-reported substance use and criminal activity
Rowland, Chapman, & Henggeler (2008) (N = 70)	Nearest age siblings		18 months post recruitment	Evidence-based treatment decreased sibling substance use
Stambaugh et al. (2007)[a] (N = 267)	Youth with serious emotional disturbance at risk for out-of-home placement	Wraparound	18-month follow-up	Decreased symptoms; decreased out-of-home placements (54%)
Sundell et al. (2008) (N = 156)	Swedish youth met diagnostic criteria for conduct disorder	Usual child welfare services in Sweden	7 months post recruitment	No outcomes favoring either treatment condition; low treatment fidelity
Letourneau et al. (2009) (N = 127)	Juvenile sexual offenders	Usual sex offender-specific treatment	12 months post-recruitment	Decreased sexual behavior problems; decreased delinquency, substance use, and externalizing symptoms; reduced out-of-home placements

[a]Quasi-experimental design (groups matched on demographic characteristics), all other studies are randomized
[b]Based on participants in Henggeler et al. (1992) and Borduin et al. (1995)

Blaske, & Stein, 1990; Brunk, Henggeler, & Whelan, 1987; Henggeler et al., 1986) demonstrated favorable effects for MST with juvenile offenders and their families (e.g., reduced rearrest and incarceration, reduced substance use, improved family functioning), some of which have been sustained for 14 years post-treatment (Schaeffer & Borduin, 2005).

Effectiveness Trials

Building off the favorable results in the efficacy trials, studies of MST were conducted in collaboration with community mental health centers using public sector practitioners. Results from these studies (i.e., Henggeler et al., 1997; Henggeler, Melton, & Smith, 1992; Letourneau et al., 2009) further supported the capacity of MST to improve family functioning and decrease the rearrest and incarceration rates of serious juvenile offenders. Importantly, this work also highlighted the critical role that treatment fidelity plays in achieving favorable outcomes.

Trials for Juvenile Offenders with Substance Use Disorders

In light of favorable reductions in substance use achieved in early trials of MST with juvenile offenders (Henggeler et al., 1991), two subsequent trials of MST were conducted with juvenile offenders meeting diagnostic criteria for substance abuse or dependence. The first study (Henggeler, Pickrel, & Brondino, 1999; Henggeler, Clingempeel, Brondino, & Pickrel, 2002) demonstrated favorable MST effects in several areas, including the reduction of substance use. The second study (Henggeler et al., 2006) showed that MST enhanced the favorable effects of juvenile drug court, a court-based program that provides specialized services for drug-involved youth and their families, in reducing substance use and criminal behavior. Sheidow and Henggeler (2008) provide a detailed overview of substance-related MST outcome research.

Independent Transportability Trials

With the transport of MST programs to many states within the United States and nations around the world, several independent groups of researchers have published rigorous evaluations of MST for youth with conduct problems. For example, in a randomized trial conducted in Norway, Ogden and colleagues (Ogden & Hagen, 2006; Ogden & Halliday-Boykins, 2004) replicated the favorable outcomes of MST found in earlier studies (e.g., decreased youth symptoms and out-of-home placement, high consumer satisfaction). Similarly, Timmons-Mitchell and colleagues (Timmons-Mitchell, Bender, Kishna, & Mitchell, 2006) provided the first independent replication with serious juvenile offenders in the United States. MST improved youth functioning and decreased both recidivism and substance use problems.

On the other hand, in Sweden, Sundell et al. (2008) failed to support the greater effectiveness of MST in treating youth with conduct disorder. This failure might have been due to the low therapist adherence observed in this study or the relatively high quality of services provided in the comparison condition. Nevertheless, across the 12 efficacy, effectiveness, and transportability trials of MST with youth presenting with serious conduct problems and their families, MST has achieved relatively consistent outcomes, including (a) reduced short- and long-term (up to 14 years) rates of criminal offending, (b) reduced rates of out-of-home placements, (c) decreased substance use, (d) decreased behavioral and mental health problems, (e) improved family functioning, and (f) cost savings in comparison with usual mental health and juvenile justice services.

Adaptations to the Basic MST Model

Several groups of investigators have adapted the basic MST model (i.e., focus on serious clinical problems with multi-determined causation, intervention design guided by treatment principles, home-based model of service delivery, strong quality assurance system, integration of evidence-based treatment techniques, and view that caregivers are the key to long-term outcomes) to address other types of serious clinical problems presented by youth and their families and have evaluated the effectiveness of these adaptations.. For example, three randomized trials of MST with juvenile sexual offenders have been published (Borduin et al., 1990; Borduin, Schaeffer, & Heiblum, 2009; Letourneau et al., 2009), and these studies provide strong evidence of the short- and long-term effectiveness of MST with this population. MST for youth with Problem Sexual Behavior (MST-PSB) goes beyond standard MST by focusing on aspects of the youth's ecology that are functionally related to the youth's sexual delinquency. Specific adaptations include creating a safety plan to minimize the youth's access to potential victims, addressing youth and caregiver denial about the severity of the offense, and improving youth's peer relations so that more age-appropriate and normative sexual experiences can occur with peers (for more information about MST-PSB, go to www.mstpsb.com).

Other clinical problems for which MST has been adapted and demonstrated to be effective include youth with serious emotional disturbance/psychiatric crises (Henggeler, Rowland et al., 1999; Rowland et al., 2005; Stambaugh et al., 2007), chronic pediatric health care conditions (e.g., diabetes, HIV-positive youth; Cunningham, Naar-King, Ellis, Pejuan, & Secord, 2006; Ellis, Naar-King, Cunningham, & Secord, 2006; Ellis, Frey, et al., 2005; Ellis, Frey, et al., 2005; Ellis, Naar-King, et al., 2005), and child maltreatment (Swenson et al., 2005, in press). Studies of other adaptations of MST, such as for families experiencing co-occurring child maltreatment and caregiver substance abuse are underway.

CONCLUSIONS

In conclusion, MST is a well-validated, evidence-based intervention for conduct problems in youth. The MST model has been widely disseminated, with more than 17,000 youth and families treated annually through MST programs in more than 30 states in the United States and 10 nations worldwide. A key feature of MST is its emphasis on addressing known risk factors for conduct problems comprehensively, with caregivers viewed as critical to achieving sustainable outcomes. Further, services are provided in community-based settings and incorporate pragmatic, behaviorally oriented intervention techniques. Another defining feature of MST is its use of a well-conceived quality assurance/quality improvement protocol to support fidelity to the treatment model. Future research is needed to examine therapy process variables (e.g., therapist–client interactions) that are linked with favorable youth and family outcomes. Other key areas for research include an examination of the most effective and efficient strategies for recruiting, training, and retaining therapists, supervisors, and consultants, and the exploration of organizational (e.g., agency structure and mission) and service system (e.g., financing methods, interagency working relationships) factors that are critical for the sustainability of high-quality MST programs.

REFERENCES

Borduin, C. M., & Schaeffer, C. M. (2001). Multisystemic treatment of juvenile sexual offenders: A progress report. *Journal of Psychology & Human Sexuality, 13*, 25–42.

Borduin, C. M., Henggeler, S. W., Blaske, D. M., & Stein, R. (1990). Multisystemic treatment of adolescent sexual offenders. *International Journal of Offender Therapy and Comparative Criminology, 35*, 105–114.

Borduin, C. M., Mann, B. J., Cone, L. T., Henggeler, S. W., Fucci, B. R., Blaske, D. M., et al. (1995). Multisystemic treatment of serious juvenile offenders: Long-term prevention of criminality and violence. *Journal of Consulting and Clinical Psychology, 63*, 569–578.

Borduin, C. M., Schaeffer, C. M., & Heiblum, N. (2009). A randomized clinical trial of multisystemic therapy with juvenile sexual offenders: Effects on youth social ecology and criminal activity. *Journal of Consulting and Clinical Psychology, 77*, 26–37.

Bronfenbrenner, U. (1979). *The ecology of human development: Experiments by design and nature.* Cambridge, MA: Harvard University Press.

Brown, T. L., Henggeler, S. W., Schoenwald, S. K., Brondino, M. J., & Pickrel, S. G. (1999). Multisystemic treatment of substance abusing and dependent juvenile delinquents: Effects on school attendance at posttreatment and 6-month follow-up. *Children's Services: Social Policy, Research, and Practice, 2*, 81–93.

Brunk, M., Henggeler, S. W., & Whelan, J. P. (1987). A comparison of multisystemic therapy and parent training in the brief treatment of child abuse and neglect. *Journal of Consulting and Clinical Psychology, 55*, 311–318.

Cunningham, P. B., Naar-King, S., Ellis, D. A., Pejuan, S., & Secord, E. (2006). Achieving adherence to antiretroviral medications for pediatric HIV disease using an empirically supported treatment: A case report. *Journal of Developmental and Behavioral Pediatric, 27*, 44–50.

Deater-Deckard, K., Dodge, K. A., Bates, J. E., & Pettit, G. S. (1998). Multiple risk factors in the development of externalizing behavior problems: Group and individual differences. *Development and Psychopathology, 10*, 469–493.

Elliott, D. S. (1994). Serious violent offenders: Onset, developmental course, and termination. The American Society of Criminology 1993, presidential address. *Criminology, 32*, 1–21.

Ellis, D. A., Frey, M. A., Naar-King, S., Templin, T., Cunningham, P. B., & Cakan, N. (2005a). Use of multisystemic therapy to improve regimen adherence among adolescents with type 1 diabetes in chronic poor metabolic control: A randomized controlled trial. *Diabetes Care, 28*, 1604–1610.

Ellis, D. A., Frey, M. A., Naar-King, S., Templin, T., Cunningham, P. B., & Cakan, N. (2005b). The effects of multisystemic therapy on diabetes stress in adolescents with chronically poorly controlled type 1 diabetes: Findings from a randomized controlled trial. *Pediatrics, 116*, e826–e832.

Ellis, D. A., Naar-King, S., Frey, M. A., Templin, T., Rowland, M., & Cakan, N. (2005c). Multisystemic treatment of poorly controlled type 1 diabetes: Effects on medical resource utilization. *Journal of Pediatric Psychology, 30*, 656–666.

Ellis, D. A., Naar-King, S., Cunningham, P. B., & Secord, E. (2006). Use of multisystemic therapy to improve antiretroviral adherence and health outcomes in HIV-infected pediatric patients: Evaluation of a pilot program. *AIDS, Patient Care, and STD's, 20*, 112–121.

Ellis, D. A., Templin, T., Naar-King, S., Frey, M. A., Cunningham, P. B., Podolski, C., et al. (2007). Multisystemic therapy for adolescents with poorly controlled type I diabetes: Stability of treatment effects in a randomized controlled trial. *Journal of Consulting and Clinical Psychology, 75*, 168–174.

Eyberg, S. M., Nelson, M. M., & Boggs, S. R. (2008). Evidence-based psychosocial treatments for children and adolescents with disruptive behavior. *Journal of Clinical Child & Adolescent Psychology, 37*, 215–237.

Henggeler, S. W., Rodick, J. D., Borduin, C. M., Hanson, C. L., Watson, S. M., & Urey, J. R. (1986). Multisystemic treatment of juvenile offenders: Effects on adolescent behavior and family interactions. *Developmental Psychology, 22*, 132–141.

Henggeler, S. W., Borduin, C. M., Melton, G. B., Mann, B. J., Smith, L., Hall, J. A., et al. (1991). Effects of multisystemic therapy on drug use and abuse in serious juvenile offenders: A progress report from two outcome studies. *Family Dynamics of Addiction Quarterly, 1*, 40–51.

Henggeler, S. W., Melton, G. B., & Smith, L. A. (1992). Family preservation using multisystemic therapy: An effective alternative to incarcerating serious juvenile offenders. *Journal of Consulting and Clinical Psychology, 60*, 953–961.

Henggeler, S. W., Melton, G. B., Smith, L. A., Schoenwald, S. K., & Hanley, J. H. (1993). Family preservation using multisystemic treatment: Long-term follow-up to a clinical trial with serious juvenile offenders. *Journal of Child and Family Studies, 2*, 283–293.

Henggeler, S. W., Pickrel, S. G., Brondino, M. J., & Crouch, J. L. (1996). Eliminating (almost) treatment dropout of substance abusing or dependent delinquents through home-based multisystemic therapy. *American Journal of Psychiatry, 153*, 427–428.

Henggeler, S. W., Melton, G. B., Brondino, M. J., Scherer, D. G., & Hanley, J. H. (1997). Multisystemic therapy with violent and chronic juvenile offenders and their families: The role of treatment fidelity in successful dissemination. *Journal of Consulting and Clinical Psychology, 65*, 821–833.

Henggeler, S. W., Schoenwald, S. K., Borduin, C. M., Rowland, M. D., & Cunningham, P. B. (1998). *Multisystemic treatment of antisocial behavior in children and adolescents*. New York: Guilford.

Henggeler, S. W., Pickrel, S. G., & Brondino, M. J. (1999). Multisystemic treatment of substance abusing and dependent delinquents: Outcomes, treatment fidelity, and transportability. *Mental Health Services Research, 1*, 171–184.

Henggeler, S. W., Rowland, M. R., Randall, J., Ward, D., Pickrel, S. G., Cunningham, P. B., et al. (1999). Home-based multisystemic therapy as an alternative to the hospitalization of youth in psychiatric crisis: Clinical outcomes. *Journal of the American Academy of Child & Adolescent Psychiatry, 38*, 1331–1339.

Henggeler, S. W., Clingempeel, W. G., Brondino, M. J., & Pickrel, S. G. (2002). Four-year follow-up of multisystemic therapy with substance abusing and dependent juvenile offenders. *Journal of the American Academy of Child & Adolescent Psychiatry, 41*, 868–874.

Henggeler, S. W., Rowland, M. D., Halliday-Boykins, C., Sheidow, A. J., Ward, D. M., Randall, J., et al. (2003). One-year follow-up of multisystemic therapy as an alternative to the hospitalization of youths in psychiatric crisis. *Journal of the American Academy of Child & Adolescent Psychiatry, 42*, 543–551.

Henggeler, S. W., Halliday-Boykins, C. A., Cunningham, P. B., Randall, J., Shapiro, S. B., & Chapman, J. E. (2006). Juvenile drug court: Enhancing outcomes by integrating vidence-based treatments. *Journal of Consulting and Clinical Psychology, 74*, 42–54.

Henggeler, S. W., Letourneau, E. J., Chapman, J. E., Borduin, C. M., Schewe, P. A., & McCart, M. R. (2009). Mediators of change for multisystemic therapy with juvenile offenders. *Journal of Consulting and Clinical Psychology, 77*, 451–462. doi: 10.1037/a0013971.

Henggeler, S. W., Schoenwald, S. K., Borduin, C. M., Rowland, M. D., & Cunningham, P. B. (2009). *Multisystemic therapy for antisocial behavior in children and adolescents* (2nd ed.). New York: Guilford.

Huey, S. J., Henggeler, S. W., Brondino, M. J., & Pickrel, S. G. (2000). Mechanisms of change in multisystemic therapy: Reducing delinquent behavior through therapist adherence and improved family and peer functioning. *Journal of Consulting and Clinical Psychology, 68*, 451–467.

Huey, S. J., Jr., Henggeler, S. W., Rowland, M. D., Halliday-Boykins, C. A., Cunningham, P. B., Pickrel, S. G., et al. (2004). Multisystemic therapy effects on attempted suicide by youth presenting psychiatric emergencies. *Journal of the American Academy of Child & Adolescent Psychiatry, 43*, 183–190.

Letourneau, E. J., Henggeler, S. W., Borduin, C. M., Schewe, P. A., McCart, M. R., Chapman, J. E., et al. (2009). Multisystemic therapy for juvenile sexual offenders: 1-year results from a randomized effectiveness trial. *Journal of Family Psychology, 23*, 89–102.

Loeber, R., Farrington, D. P., Stouthamer-Loeber, M., & Van Kammen, W. B. (1998). *Antisocial behavior and mental health problems: Explanatory factors in childhood and adolescence.* Mahwah, NJ: Lawrence Erlbaum Associates.

Margo, J. (2008). *Make me a criminal: Preventing youth crime.* London: Institute for Public Policy Research.

National Alliance on Mental Illness. (Winter, 2008). *Medicaid coverage of multisystemic therapy. NAMI Beginnings.* Arlington, VA: National Alliance on Mental Illness.

National Institute on Drug Abuse. (1999). *Principles of drug addiction treatment: A research-based guide.* NIH Publication No. 99-4180.

Ogden, T., & Hagen, K. A. (2006). Multisystemic therapy of serious behaviour problems in youth: Sustainability of therapy effectiveness two years after intake. *Journal of Child and Adolescent Mental Health, 11*, 142–149.

Ogden, T., & Halliday-Boykins, C. A. (2004). Multisystemic treatment of antisocial adolescents in Norway: Replication of clinical outcomes outside of the US. *Child & Adolescent Mental Health, 9*, 77–83.

Rowland, M. R., Halliday-Boykins, C. A., Henggeler, S. W., Cunningham, P. B., Lee, T. G., Kruesi, M. J. P., et al. (2005). A randomized trial of multisystemic therapy with Hawaii's Felix Class youths. *Journal of Emotional and Behavioral Disorders, 13*, 13–23.

Rowland, M. R., Chapman, J. E., & Henggeler, S. W. (2008). Sibling outcomes from a randomized trial of evidence-based treatments with substance abusing juvenile offenders. *Journal of Child & Adolescent Substance Abuse, 17*, 11–26.

Schaeffer, C. M., & Borduin, C. M. (2005). Long-term follow-up to a randomized clinical trial of multisystemic therapy with serious and violent juvenile offenders. *Journal of Consulting and Clinical Psychology, 73*, 445–453.

Schoenwald, S. K., Ward, D. M., Henggeler, S. W., Pickrel, S. G., & Patel, H. (1996). MST treatment of substance abusing or dependent adolescent offenders: Costs of reducing incarceration, inpatient, and residential placement. *Journal of Child and Family Studies, 5*, 431–444.

Schoenwald, S. K., Henggeler, S. W., Brondino, M. J., & Rowland, M. D. (2000). Multisystemic therapy: Monitoring treatment fidelity. *Family Process, 39*, 83–103.

Schoenwald, S. K., Ward, D. M., Henggeler, S. W., & Rowland, M. D. (2000). MST vs. hospitalization for crisis stabilization of youth: Placement outcomes 4 months post-referral. *Mental Health Services Research, 2*, 3–12.

Schoenwald, S. K., Carter, R. E., Chapman, J. E., & Sheidow, A. J. (2008). Therapist adherence and organizational effects on change in youth behavior problems one year after multisystemic therapy. *Administration and Policy in Mental Health and Mental Health Services Research, 35*, 379–394.

Sheidow, A. J., & Henggeler, S. W. (2008). Multisystemic therapy with substance using adolescents: A synthesis of research. In A. Stevens (Ed.), *Crossing frontiers: Inter-*

national developments in the treatment of drug dependence (pp. 11–33). Brighton, England: Pavilion Publishing.

Sheidow, A. J., Bradford, W. D., Henggeler, S. W., Rowland, M. D., Halliday-Boykins, C., Schoenwald, S. K., et al. (2004). Treatment costs for youths in psychiatric crisis: Multisystemic therapy versus hospitalization. *Psychiatric Services, 55*, 548–554.

Stambaugh, L. F., Mustillo, S. A., Burns, B. J., Stephens, R. L., Baxter, B., Edwards, D., et al. (2007). Outcomes from wraparound and multisystemic therapy in a center for mental health services system-of-care demonstration site. *Journal of Emotional and Behavioral Disorders, 15*, 143–155.

Sundell, K., Hansson, K., Lofholm, C. A., Olsson, T., Gustle, L. H., & Kadesjo, C. (2008). The transportability of MST to Sweden: Short-term results from a randomized trial of conduct disordered youth. *Journal of Family Psychology, 22*, 550–560.

Swenson, C. C., Saldana, L., Joyner, C. D., Caldwell, E., Henggeler, S. W., & Rowland, M. D. (2005). *Multisystemic therapy for child abuse and neglect.* Charleston, SC: Family Services Research Center, Medical University of South Carolina.

Swenson, C. C., Schaeffer, C. M., Henggeler, S. W., Faldowski, R., & Mayhew, A. M. (in press). Multisystemic therapy for child abuse and neglect: A randomized effectiveness trial. *Journal of Family Psychology*

Thornberry, T. P., & Krohn, M. D. (Eds.). (2003). *Taking stock of delinquency: An overview of findings from contemporary longitudinal studies.* New York: Kluwer/Plenum.

Timmons-Mitchell, J., Bender, M. B., Kishna, M. A., & Mitchell, C. C. (2006). An independent effectiveness trial of multisystemic therapy with juvenile justice youth. *Journal of Clinical Child and Adolescent Psychology, 35*, 227–236.

U.S. Public Health Service. (2001). *Youth violence: A report of the Surgeon General.* Washington, DC: U.S. Public Health Service.

Waldron, H. B., & Turner, C. W. (2008). Evidence-based psychosocial treatments for adolescent substance abuse. *Journal of Clinical Child and Adolescent Psychology, 37*, 238–261.

Section III

Evidence-based Treatment of Youth with Conduct Problems in Diverse Settings

12

Social Competency CBT-Based Group Training for Youth in Alternative School Settings

RACHAEL C. MURRIHY

The need for alternative educational places for at-risk youth has increased dramatically in the United States with enrolments quadrupling in the last 15 years, and demand exceeding available placements (Kleiner, Porch, & Farris, 2002). Kleiner and colleagues have estimated, based on a nationally representative sample, that alternative schools serve 613,000 or 1.3% of all public school students in the United States. Even so, this figure is likely an underestimation of the true need for alternative education, not only because it excludes students who already attend alternative programs located within mainstream schools but also because many students who seek to enroll in alternative programs are unable to do so. It is estimated by Kleiner et al. that in the 3 years preceding their survey, over half (54%) of the school districts had faced a time when demand exceeded capacity and further enrolments could not be accepted. The United States is not alone in this predicament. Students from other western countries have a similar need for alternative school placements. Australia, Canada, England, Scotland, and Wales all report behavioral problems and their consequences, expulsion and transfer to alternative programs, as growing challenges for their educational system (Elliot, 2009; Gendron, Royer, Bertrand, & Potvin, 2004; Gulchak & Lopes, 2007; Head, Kane, & Cogan, 2003; Hemphill, 2009; Humphrey & Brooks, 2006).

RACHAEL C. MURRIHY • University of Technology, Sydney

R.C. Murrihy et al. (eds.), *Clinical Handbook of Assessing and Treating Conduct Problems in Youth*, DOI 10.1007/978-1-4419-6297-3_12,

This dramatic rise in the need for alternative school placements is thought to be due, at least in part, to the "default" strategy traditionally adopted by mainstream schools for dealing with students who evince serious conduct problems (Skiba & Peterson, 2000). The *punitive approach* stipulates that aggressive students are segregated from others, either through suspension or through expulsion, and eventually, if problems are severe enough, these students are transferred to alternative education programs and schools. This system exists mainly for the protection of mainstream school students who are thought to benefit from the removal of disruptive influences from the classroom (van Acker, 2007). "Zero tolerance" policies, widely adopted after the Columbine High School mass shootings in the United States, take the punitive approach to a new extreme, whereby students receive the highest possible consequence for transgressions such as verbal and physical aggression or the carrying of weapons (van Acker, 2007). Rather than achieving the goal of decreasing school aggression, however, zero tolerance is believed to be responsible for the massive skyrocketing of suspensions and expulsion rates in schools in the United States that has, in turn, resulted in a greater need for alternative school placements (Kingery, 2000; Skiba, 2000).

The transfer of students with conduct problems to alternative programs or schools attracts considerable controversy amongst educators. Supporters assert that in addition to providing a separate setting for disruptive students to learn, thereby protecting the learning of mainstream school students, alternative schooling provides a personalized, flexible approach for students who do not respond in the traditional setting. Furthermore, supporters assert that it prevents students from being sent out into society, emotionally and vocationally unprepared or ill-prepared to prematurely assume adult responsibilities. Detractors, on the other hand, refer to comments made by former alternative school students (taken from a 5-year evaluation of students in North Carolina) who have severed ties to their former school referring to it as a "dumping ground," or "junior jail" (Cobb et al., 1997, p. 7). Critics argue that the major goal of these schools, to eventually return students to mainstream schooling, is unrealistic as poor resourcing means facilities and opportunities are inequitable (e.g., alternative schools may not have a fully equipped science laboratory, adequate computers, or full access to athletic and enriched academic opportunities) (Cobb et al., 1997; Editorial, 2006; Lehr & Lange, 2003). These substandard educational opportunities mean students are more likely to fall further behind their mainstream peers the longer they remain in alternative schooling. Furthermore, alternative schools tend to "... target behavioral change, but place less emphasis on academic achievement" (Center for Effective Collaboration and Practice, 1999, p. 252). Thus, lowered academic expectations may further disadvantage these students (Fitzsimons Hughes & Adera, 2006). Finally, the opportunity to interact with prosocial peers is also removed and contact with deviant peers increased in alternative programs (Dodge, Lansford, & Dishion, 2006). Ultimately, those opposed to alternative schools contend there is no evidence to suggest removal to alternative school settings, with the associated disruption, stigma, and deviant exposure, is any more effective than less severe remedial practices that could take place within mainstream schools (Cortez & Montecel, 1999).

In response to these criticisms, government policy makers ratified legislation aimed at improving the effectiveness of alternative schooling (and schooling in general) through the adoption of evidence-based practices (U.S. Department of Education, 1998, 2002a). To achieve this, the President's Commission on Excellence in Special Education recommended that research in this field would need "enhanced rigor ... and the current system does not always embrace or implement evidence-based practices once established" (U.S. Department of Education, 2002b, p. 2). Prompted by the push for research-backed practices, a number of researchers have since put forward recommendations for evidence-based practice in alternative schooling programs (Fitzsimons Hughes & Adera, 2006; Fitzsimons-Lovett, 2001; Tobin & Sprague, 1999; Unruh, Bullis, Todis, Waintrup, & Atkins, 2007; van Acker, 2007). Evidence-based practices were recommended for adoption within alternative education curricula, instructional practices, and, relevant to this chapter, therapeutic interventions.

Most educators agree that whether alternative programs or schools "empower or entrap" students depends upon the adoption of evidence-based practice in both academic and therapeutic interventions (Fitzsimons-Lovett, 2001, p. 40). Therapeutic treatment and the effectiveness of these treatments constitute the focus of this chapter. To provide a context for this discussion, an overview of the historical background of alternative schooling programs will be undertaken, followed by a summary on how these schools operate today including: program settings, curricula, inclusion criteria, demographic profiles of students, and uniformity amongst alternative education programs. As will be shown, therapeutic groups such as anger management and social skills training are widely used in alternative programs. They are commonly accepted as effective treatments for the treatment of youth with conduct problems, yet no empirical reviews have been undertaken in this domain. Given the large number of students serviced by alternative schools, it is critical that students are offered effective remediation (Fitzsimons Hughes & Adera, 2006). In light of this, published studies will be reviewed to (a) ascertain the effectiveness of skills-based group therapy programs (e.g., anger management training) and (b) consider current knowledge with regard to the risk associated with aggregating groups of youth with conduct problems (i.e., deviancy training).

ALTERNATIVE EDUCATION: A HISTORICAL BACKGROUND

Emerging in the early nineteenth century in various forms, alternative schooling grew at a steady but slow rate until the 1960s and 1970s when the social justice movement prompted a rapid proliferation of alternative programs and schools for students unsuccessful in traditional educational settings and at risk of dropping out of school (Fitzsimons-Lovett, 2001). At that time, alternative schools could typically be found in urbanized areas and their students were from low socioeconomic and primarily minority backgrounds (Unruh et al., 2007). Later, alternative schools spread from urban areas to suburban and even rural areas (Kleiner et al., 2002), yet students largely remained from poor African American and Hispanic backgrounds (Cortez & Montecel, 1999).

Definitions of Alternative Education

Whilst it is widely acknowledged that alternative schools (also known as learning centers and behavioral schools) were developed for youth with conduct problems who were at risk of dropping out, there is no commonly agreed upon definition for alternative schooling in the field (van Acker, 2007). The United States Department of Education defines alternative schools as a "public elementary/secondary school that addresses the needs of students that typically cannot be met in regular school" (Kleiner et al., 2002, p. 55). The state government in Oregon elucidates further: "(alternative schooling is) a school or separate class group designed to assist students to achieve the goals of the curriculum in a manner consistent with their learning styles and needs ... (in) learning situations that are flexible with regard to environment, time, structure and pedagogy" (Oregon Department of Education, 2007).

Students referred to alternative schooling may receive a placement in various settings. An alternative school may exist as an independent site separate from a mainstream school or students may remain at the mainstream campus either within a separate wing or between special and mainstream classes (Tobin & Sprague, 1999). The majority of students (59%) attend alternative school in a separate facility (Kleiner et al., 2002). Most districts offer programs for grades 9–12, and 46–67% of districts offer programs for grades 6–8. Although student numbers are on the increase, only 10–21% offer services to grades 1–5 (Kleiner et al., 2002). The average duration of enrolment in Oregon State was 7 months (Unruh et al., 2007).

Philosophies and Goals of Alternative Education Programs

Although philosophies, structures, and goals of alternative educational programs for at-risk youth differ markedly (Quinn, Poirier, Faller, Gable, & Tonelson, 2006), their broad purpose is typically aligned: to provide an individualized academic program to students, prevent drop-out, reduce antisocial and aggressive behavior and delinquency, and to attain a high school diploma or certificate. Most programs endeavor to teach the student skills that will enable them to reenter mainstream school requiring an improvement in both academic work (most students are significantly behind their peers; Atkins, Allen, & Meredith, 2001) and conduct behavior problems. Alternatively, students are prepared to enter the workforce or further vocational/educational training.

Similar approaches apply to teaching practices. Compared to mainstream public schools, teachers in (exemplary) alternative schools are less authoritarian, more flexible, demonstrate more caring, emphasize fair rules (and take care in enforcing these), and are more collaborative in their decision-making (Quinn & Poirier, 2006; Quinn et al., 2006). The aim is to create personalized environments in smaller classrooms for students who, working towards their high school diploma, need intensive remedial support (Lange & Sletten, 2002). Studies proceed at the student's pace and are delivered in an engaging style where "real life" examples are frequently employed. Research has shown that alternative school students benefit from a personalized environment, one in which they perceive that teachers genuinely care for them (Castleberry & Enger, 1998; Quinn & Poirier, 2006). Behavior modification systems that provide contingencies for both prosocial and antisocial behaviors are also commonly used within alternative programs.

Clinical Profile of Alternative School Students

A national survey of 49 state directors of special education in the United States by Lehr and Lange (2003) found that alternative schools, instead of representing an innovative educational alternative of choice, are typically "last chance" placements for students who have been threatened with (or undergone) suspension or expulsion. According to the state directors, students who attend alternative schools typically exhibit behavior and/or academic problems and are at risk of dropping out (Lehr & Lange, 2003). Although minimal data were kept on disabilities in this population, they indicated that the primary disability experienced by these students is emotional and behavioral disorders. Emotional and behavioral disorders (EBD) is an umbrella term used to describe youth experiencing internalizing or externalizing disorders or a comorbid presentation of both (Atkins et al., 2001).

This being said, most referrals to alternative schools are for conduct problems rather than primary anxiety or depression. In a large-scale study of teachers from 156 alternative schools in the United Kingdom, Cole, Visser, and Upton (1998) found that placements were typically a result of overt conduct problems as opposed to internalizing emotional needs. Consistent with this research, in a survey of 767 public school districts, Kleiner and colleagues confirmed that the following actions are sufficient for admission to alternative programs or schools in the United States: selling, using or possessing drugs and/or alcohol (52%); physical assaults (52%); chronic truancy (51%); academic failure (50%); possession or use of a weapon other than a firearm (50%); disruptive verbal behavior (45%); possession or use of a firearm (44%); and arrest or involvement with the juvenile justice system (38%). Interestingly, mental health problems were the least likely reason for referral from mainstream school (22%; Kleiner et al., 2002).

Given the entrance criteria above, a number of studies have confirmed a high rate of externalizing disorders in the mainly male (80%) alternative school population. Comorbidity has also been identified as a common feature (Cassidy, James, & Wiggs, 2001; Place, Wilson, Martin, & Hulsmeier, 2000; Wheatley et al, 2009). Cassidy et al. (2001) studied the psychological profile of students enrolled in alternative education. They conducted semistructured diagnostic interviews (Kiddie-Schedule for Affective Disorders and Schizophrenia – Present and Lifetime Version, K-SADS-PL), based on Diagnostic and Statistical Manual of Mental Disorders criteria (DSM-IV), to determine the psychological profile of students aged 11–16 years attending a secondary alternative education school. After interviewing 28 students (25 boys, three girls) and 26 parents, they showed that 89% of students received a psychological diagnosis; 78% had Conduct Disorder (CD) and 32% met the criteria for Attention Deficit Hyperactivity Disorder (ADHD). Internalizing disorders were present in smaller numbers, but not as independent diagnoses (with the exception of one case). In all, 14% of the sample had depression or anxiety in addition to comorbid externalizing disorders. Indeed, cormorbity was generally high with one-quarter (seven of the 28 students) meeting diagnostic criteria for both CD and ADHD.

Rates of comorbidity and externalizing disorders were found to be even higher in an Australian study of two alternative schools by Murrihy et al. (*N* = 25; 2007). As in the Cassidy et al. study, students were interviewed using the K-SADS-PL to assess psychological diagnoses. The full parent interview was substituted for the background K-SADS-PL interview only (Murrihy et al., 2007; Wheatley et al., 2009). Parent and adolescent interviews, in combination with parent, teacher, and student self-report questionnaires, were used to determine clinical diagnoses. All students met DSM-IV criteria for either CD (76%) or Oppositional Defiant Disorder (ODD; 24%). Three-quarters met criteria for ADHD, half had anxiety-related disorders, 40% had depression, and 33% were diagnosed with a substance abuse disorder. Students on average met criteria for three comorbid diagnoses. The psychological profile of students in alternative programs such as these indicates that most students possess CD and at least one or two other comorbid disorders, especially ADHD. At any rate, these studies reflect a student psychological profile that is severe and complex in nature, perhaps more so than commonly thought.

Does Alternative Education Work?

Alternative schooling represents a crucial component of the public education system for students who cannot be traditionally schooled, but is it effective in improving educational and psychosocial outcomes? Despite some positive effects in the literature (Cox, Davidson, & Bynum, 1995; Groth, 1998; Munoz, 2002; Yearwood, Abdum-Muhaymin, & Jordan, 2002), overall there is insufficient research at this time to draw firm conclusions about the effects of alternative schooling on students' outcomes (Kleiner et al., 2002; Quinn et al., 2006; Unruh et al., 2007; van Acker, 2007). Differing alternative school philosophies and goals have led to diverse curricula. Hence, "the nature and quality of these educational programs is still unclear" (Fitzsimons Hughes & Adera, 2006, p. 26) making it difficult to reach conclusions about the general effectiveness of alternative school programs (Unruh et al., 2007). Another criticism is the overreliance on anecdotal and survey methodologies, at the expense of controlled, comparison studies (van Acker, 2007).

In the absence of firm conclusions about the effectiveness of alternative schooling in general, recommendations have been made by researchers for the use of certain "empirically validated" components within alternative school programs (Quinn, Rutherford, & Osher, 1999; Tobin & Sprague, 1999). These recommendations range from general educational strategies, such as instructional techniques and curricula changes, to therapeutic interventions. Narrowing the focus to therapeutic interventions, a number of prominent authors in this field have recommended the use of Cognitive Behavior Therapy (CBT)-based anger management/social skills/conflict resolution groups for students in alternative schooling, claiming they are evidence-based (Fitzsimons-Lovett, 2001; Tobin & Sprague, 1999). But are they in actuality? Lochman (see Chap. 9) has demonstrated positive effects at postintervention for students with conduct problems attending group anger control training in mainstream schools, but it is unclear if these effects translate to students in alternative education programs and schools. The next section of this chapter will consider these questions in more depth.

CBT ANGER MANAGEMENT GROUP INTERVENTIONS

Aggression is a defining characteristic of many students attending alternative schools. Moreover, aggression management is of critical importance to healthy adult adjustment, as aggression can create significant barriers to educational, vocational, and relational success (Kim-Cohen et al., 2003; Zoccolillo, Pickles, Quinton, & Rutter, 1992). Therefore, most therapeutic programs (whether they are labeled anger management, social skills, or conflict resolution programs) are primarily focused on helping the student manage anger and communicate more effectively. Anger management, conflict resolution, and social skills training programs are generic terms, often used interchangeably, to describe CBT-based group therapy programs that draw on an assortment of therapeutic strategies including psychoeducation, social problem solving, goal setting, anger management skills/assertiveness training, social skills training, conflict resolution, moral reasoning and perspective taking, self-instruction, cognitive restructuring, self-monitoring, and relaxation techniques (Olatunji & Lohr, 2004). Common among these approaches are the underlying assumptions that aggressive students have skills deficits which prevent them from establishing healthy relationships and that direct skills-based instruction will allow them to learn and use more adaptive response patterns (Robinson et al., 2002).

Although recommended in the literature, it is unclear how many schools are actually implementing groups of this nature. One study offering some insight was a state-wide survey of alternative programs and schools conducted by the University of Oregon in 2002–2003 (Unruh et al., 2007). This survey revealed that 75% of alternative programs and schools offered social skills training and/or individual or group counseling. No information was given regarding the breakdown of figures within each group. Similarly, in a national study of 105 model alternative education programs in the United States, Tyler (1997) reported that 66% offered conflict resolution or peer mediation training.

Social Cognitive Model

Most anger management programs[1] conducted in alternative schools (and mainstream schools) are informed by the social cognitive model, a model based on empirical research, which evolved from Novaco's (1975) early work on the cognitive behavioral conceptualization of anger and Dodge's social information processing model (Crick & Dodge, 1994; for an in-depth discussion of these models, see Lochman, Barry, & Pardini, 2003; see Chap. 9 in this book for a case study illustrating the use of an anger management program by Lochman and colleagues). The fundamental assumption underlying the social cognitive model is that it is not the event itself, but the individual's perception of that event that influences their subsequent behavior (Lochman et al., 2003). Deficiencies in two major areas that perpetuate ongoing social problems have been identified in students with conduct problems. First, they appraise social situations in a problematic fashion, and second, their social problem-solving skills are ineffective (Lochman et al., 2003). From the perspective of the social cognitive model, aggressive students' appraisal of situations are typically distorted by unhelpful core beliefs or schemas held about the world around them (e.g., other people are not trustworthy), prompting selective attention to cues consistent with those core beliefs, and a failure to notice cues that are not consistent with the distorted beliefs (Crick & Dodge, 1994; Lochman, Whidby, & FitzGerald, 2000). Because of these ingrained core beliefs, aggressive youth are more likely to have difficulties perceiving and interpreting social situations accurately and, often as a result, attribute hostile intent to ambiguous cues (Dodge, 1980).

With regard to the second major deficit area, social problem solving, the first component in the response search process is the ability to generate solutions to social problems. Studies have revealed mixed findings as to whether aggressive adolescents generate fewer solutions than nonaggressive adolescents (Lochman & Dodge, 1994; Slabby & Guerra, 1988). That said, the number of solutions generated to social problems appears to be of secondary importance to the quality of the solutions offered. Consistently, studies have found that, alongside more direct actions, aggressive children use verbal assertion solutions less than nonaggressive children (Lochman & Dodge, 1994; Lochman & Lampron, 1986). Moreover, goals of dominance and revenge in this population are common. These youths expect that aggressive actions will accomplish successful outcomes by reducing aversive behavior from others and helping them gain tangible awards. They also believe that their victims do not suffer (Lochman & Dodge, 1994; Slabby & Guerra, 1988). In essence, they value aggressive actions over prosocial solutions.

Social Cognitive Model: Treatment Overview

Treatment, according to the social cognitive model, is first targeted at the appraisal stage of social interactions (Lochman et al., 2000). Distorted cognitions are challenged and students are taught to interpret situations

[1]The term "anger management training" will be used henceforth to denote all skills-based therapy groups used to treat anger and aggression including social skills and conflict resolution training.

and the motives of others more accurately (e.g., perspective taking). The second phase of treatment addresses deficient social problem solving skills. Students are asked to identify short- and long-term goals for their future and then are given the task of considering their responses to perceived provocation in light of these goals.

Social problem solving is broken down into a number of steps and the student is coached in the execution of each step using techniques such as instruction, modeling, role play, direct observation, and feedback (Lochman et al., 2003). Initially, the student learns to brainstorm solutions to social conflict (particularly prosocial solutions), before being encouraged to weigh the pros and cons of each alternative action, essentially performing a cost–benefit analysis to inform the choice of a solution (i.e., do their actions help them achieve their short- and long-terms goals?). As skill deficiencies become apparent throughout this process, students are engaged in CBT skills training, to "replace" ineffective skills with more adaptive ones (e.g., managing affect – relaxation training and self-instruction). The final stage of the social problem-solving process oversees the generalization of new skills from the classroom to the student's life through the practice of homework tasks.

Whilst most anger management groups incorporate various cognitive behavioral (CB) techniques (in line with the social cognitive model), the actual CB components used, and the order in which they are used, differs substantially across groups. Indeed it is not always possible to say how much they vary, given the sometimes scant details provided in program outlines in published papers. This variation needs to be kept in mind in reviewing outcome research associated with CBT-based group therapy in alternative education.

OUTCOME RESEARCH

Brief, Intensive Outcome Studies Conducted in Alternative Schools

The first group of studies to be considered in this review focuses on the effectiveness of CBT anger management group therapy for adolescents in alternative schools when training is delivered in an intensive, short-term format (see Table 12.1 for a full list of outcome studies including those in the current section). First, Etscheidt (1991) investigated the effects of group therapy for 12- to 18-year-old youth attending a school for behaviorally disturbed adolescents (N=30). As with most studies in this field, the real-world approach to treating students in classrooms precluded random assignment of students. Instead, a cluster sampling procedure was used to assign six preexisting classrooms to one of three conditions. Students in two classrooms received a teacher facilitated CB intervention adapted from Lochman's Anger Control program; another two classrooms received the same intervention in addition to positive reinforcement for using skills (e.g., listening to music for 10 min); and the remaining two classrooms served as control groups. Each group consisted of five students who, over a 3-week period, attended 12 sessions.

Table 12.1. Review of the effectiveness of anger management training programs for students in alternative school settings

Research study	Conditions	Assignment sample size attrition	Sessions	Measures	Posttraining outcomes	Follow-up
Amish, Gesten, Smith, Clark, & Stark, 1988 Two alternative schools	I Social problem-solving group II Control group	Quasiexperimental Established classrooms One school experimental group and one control group N=40 (started with 50) Male=44 (based on pretest N) 7–12 Years	3–4 Months (15 sessions)	Interview Role play Simulated problem situation Adjustment measures – Classroom rating scale Human resources inventory Sociometric rating (peer)	Group I (compared to control): Generated more antisocial solutions to problem situations Decrease in average solution effectiveness No differences in adjustment were found	
Etscheidt, 1991 Alternative school	I CBT training program (modified from Lochman's anger control program) II CBT+positive consequence for using skills III Control groups	Cluster sampling Established classrooms assigned randomly N=30 Male = 24 38% Latino, 31% African American 12–18 Years	3 Weeks 12 Sessions 30–40 min/session	Aggressive behavior observed daily by independent rater (40 min/day in 3-week pretraining and posttraining period) Self-control rating scale (SCRS – teacher)	Groups I and II (compared to control): Reductions in observer-rated aggressive behavior Increases in teacher-rated self-control No additional benefit from adding rewards for using skills	1 Month No differences maintained in aggressive behavior (teacher ratings not collected)
Feindler, Marriott, & Iwata, 1984 Specialized program for multisuspended adolescents in a mainstream school	I Anger control training II No-contact control	Random assignment N=36 12–15 Years	7 Weeks (10 biweekly sessions in total)	Means–ends problem-solving inventory (student rated) Locus of control scale for children (LOCS-C) Matching familiar figures test (MFFT) SCRS (teacher rated) School records of fines Continuous measures of single fines and double (result in school expulsion) fines during program	Group I (compared to control): Improvement in social problem solving and self-control No differences on MFFT or LOCS-C Reduction in double fines	5 Weeks Reduction in double fines No other measure use at f/up

Hovell et al., 2001 Alternative schools (from four sites)	I Anger prevention social skills training II AIDS education (control)	Quasiexperimental *N* = 29 (started with *N*=40) 62% Male 13–18 Years	4 Weeks 12 Sessions 1.2–2 h session	Videotaped role plays to assess anger management skills – blind coding Student interviews anger management attitudes and skills (pretest and follow-up only)	Group I (compared to control): Significantly reduced negative reactions to provocation and aggressive behavior Increase in assertion and positive reactions	6 Months No differences maintained
Kellner, & Bry, 1999 Alternative school	I CBT anger management training	Quasiexperimental *N*=7 Males=6 14–18 Years	10 Weekly sessions(30 min)	Conner's parent and teacher rating scale revised-short form (CPRS-R-S & CTRS-R-S) Incidents of physical aggression	Improvement in behavior (parent and teacher rated) No student received a worse score after completing program Trend toward fewer incidents of physical aggression	Maintained at 6 months
Kellner, Salvador, & Bry, 2001 Alternative school	I Anger management training II Control (anger logs only)	Established classrooms *N*=46 (20 students in intervention group) 74% Male 12–16 years	10 Weeks+3 monthly booster sessions	Behavioral observation (independent observers) of behavior in classroom and recess (not at f/up) Incident reports Anger logs completion child behavior checklist (CBCL) – teacher rated Knowledge quiz Monthly teacher and interdisciplinary team reports	Group I (compared to Group II): During program, observed improvements in prosocial behavior toward teachers in class time and less antisocial verbal and nonverbal behavior toward classmates in break time CBCL (teacher), knowledge quiz, team reports – no differences found	3 Months Group I (compared to Group II): Increase in anger logs, fewer aggressive incidents

(continued)

Table 12.1. (continued)

Research study	Conditions	Assignment sample size attrition	Sessions	Measures	Posttraining outcomes	Follow-up
Kellner, Bry, & Colletti, 2002 Alternative school	I Anger management training II Control (anger logs only) Boosters given to two classrooms (n = 19) compared to third classroom	Established classrooms (slightly larger groups than norm – nine students each) N=46 (27 in intervention group) 76% Male 62% Caucasian American 28% African American 12–16 Years	10 Weeks+4 monthly booster sessions	School records Anger logs completion Consulting with school counselor	Group I (compared to Group II): Fewer peer fights, more anger logs, more frequently consulting with school counselor Students who received boosters (two intervention classrooms) used more anger logs than the one classroom that did not	4 Months Increase in anger logs main-tained only, especially for booster students Fighting with peers and talking with school coun-selor were not main-tained
Mandel, 1991 Alternative school	I Anger control training (ACT) II ACT+parent training III Untreated attention control group (sexual ed class)	Group was divided into two groups (not randomly assigned) N = 16 (started with 30) All male 60% African American 40% Hispanic 16–18 Years	12 Weeks Parents – four sessions	Videotaped role plays of provocation Satisfaction questionnaire STAXI	Groups I and II (compared to control) :Improvement in use of anger control techniques No differences between groups on anger feelings or expression Parent group did not have superior outcomes (group attendance by parents was poor – eight attended sporadically)	4 Weeks Students found pro-gram useful and recom-mended it for others No other follow-up conducted

McWhirter & Page, 1999 Alternative school	I Psychoeducational anger management group II Psychoeducational goal-setting group III Control	Established classrooms were designated to each condition $N=57$ (started with 85) Males = 53 (outset) Caucasian American 16–19 Years	5 Weeks Once or twice a week (AM – nine 1-h sessions, GS – six 1-h sessions)	State trait anger expression inventory (STAXI) Self-efficacy scale for anger management, goal setting, and interpersonal communication Demographic questionnaire	Group I: No reduction in state anger levels, anger expression, and self-efficacy using anger management skills Teachers informally commented some students showed improved behaviors in classroom and breaks, and better problem-solving skills
Petit, 1998 Two mainstream schools – students had previous assignment to alternative education centers	I Anger management group II Placebo group (educational videos) III Control group	Random assignment $N=55$ (started with 90; half dropped out of exptal group, one-third dropped out of other two groups) Males = 26 87% African American 13% Caucasian American 15–18 Years	9 Weeks (two sessions/week)	STAXI Teacher-rated CBCL Positive behavior survey (teacher rated)	No differences between three groups; however, trends in expected direction Group I (compared to Groups II & III) more inhibited, greater reduction in expressed anger Teachers reported two-thirds of group positively impacted by program

(continued)

Table 12.1. (continued)

Research study	Conditions	Assignment sample size attrition	Sessions	Measures	Posttraining outcomes	Follow-up
Robinson, Smith, & Miller, 2002 Alternative school + self-contained programs in two mainstream schools	I Anger control curriculum II Control group	Cluster sampling procedure to assign randomly one established classroom to treatment or control N=41 All male 58.5% African American, 33.5% Caucasian American Sixth to eighth grade students	10 Weeks (two sessions/week over first 5 weeks, weekly thereafter)	STAXI Teacher interview perceptions of ACC (4 teachers) Teacher-rated CBCL – aggression scale Recall tests Satisfaction interview (9 students)	Group I (compared to control): Reduced internal feelings of anger, expressed anger less frequently, better anger control (both physical and verbal) Improvements on the CBCL aggression scale Students found program beneficial and teachers reported improvements in class (less impulsivity)	4 WeeksAnger control maintained on STAXI – not state anger, angry temperament, angry reaction, or anger-out CBCL – no differences
Wheatley, Murrihy, van Kessel, Wuthrich, Remond, Tuqiri, Dadds, & Kidman, 2009 Alternative school	I Anger management training (outcomes compared to equivalent control period prior to training)	Quasiexperimental study Established classrooms N=8 (started with 15) Males=7 13–15 years	16 Weeks, two sessions per week	School records Parent and student interview: Kiddie-schedule for affective disorders and schizophrenia Parent- and teacher-rated strengths and difficulties questionnaire combined with antisocial process screening device CPRS-R-S & CTRS-R-S Focus groups	Of five students with CD, four had improved at posttraining (two moved from clinical to nonclinical significance). Three students with ODD improved at posttraining Three parents and two teachers reported clinically significant improvement in ext behavior Five of eight students received fewer withdrawals and suspensions during training compared to that in control period Attendance rates did not differ significantly	No follow-up Focus groups with teachers revealed that students had increased their repertoire of problem-solving strategies. An increase in empathy and understanding was also observed

Wignall, 2006 Four alternative schools	I Modified – adolescents coping with emotions for students with comorbid behavioral and depressive symptoms (content to address anger management, cognitive distortions, and interpersonal problems)	Quasiexperimental study (pre–post design) *N* = 17 (from 19 at outset) Males = 13 Mean = 14.25 years	11 Weekly sessions	Symptom measures – Center for epidemiological studies' depression scale for children & youth self-report Social problem-solving inventory (self-report) Children's automatic thoughts scale (self-report) Bryant empathy scale (self-report) SDQ parent and teacher report Satisfaction questionnaires	Significant improvements in depressive symptoms (scores dropped from clinical to nonclinical range) and externalizing behaviors between pre- and posttest (self-report measures) Significant improvements in empathy and negative problem orientation (dysfunctional orientation toward solving life problems) (self-report) Parent and teacher reports not analyzed as response rate was too low	1–2 Weeks posttraining, students indicated via satisfaction survey that the program was useful and appropriate. Anger management and problem solving were nominated as skills that were most practiced

Analysis of postintervention effects, comparing the intervention conditions to the control condition, indicated that the program produced (a) significant reductions in observer-rated aggressive behaviors and (b) significant increases in teacher-rated self-control. Interestingly, no additional benefit was derived from adding the positive consequences or rewards for using skills learnt in the group. The authors suggested that the reinforcer selected may not have been salient enough to act as an incentive or alternatively an existing behavior modification program in the classrooms may have diminished the impact of this additional reinforcer. At 1-month follow-up, the differences between intervention and control groups were no longer observed.

Hovell et al. (2001) conducted a quasi-experimental study in which students, aged 13–18 years, from four alternative schools, received either anger prevention social skills training or Acquired Immune Deficiency Syndrome (AIDS) education in an intensive format. The AIDS group was intended to serve as an attention control for the anger prevention group. Group interventions were run over a 4-week period with students attending 12 sessions in total. Attrition was high in this sample and a starting sample of 40 decreased to 29 by the end of the three measurement periods. Compared to the control condition, anger management group training resulted in significantly reduced negative reactions to provocation and aggressive behavior, and an increase in assertion and positive reactions (according to videotaped role plays and student interviews). Unfortunately, as was the case in Etscheidt's study, none of these differences were maintained at 6-month follow-up.

Another intensive short-term intervention was undertaken by McWhirter and Page (1999) who compared 57 adolescents (16–19 years) from an alternative school, assigned to one of three groups: a psychoeducational anger management group, a psychoeducational goal-setting group, and a control group. Although labeled as psychoeducation, the anger management curriculum included many components common to standard CB anger management programs (e.g., anger logs, self-statements, role playing, goal setting). A total of 28 students dropped out and attrition was equivalent across groups. Remaining in their regular classrooms, students were given the option of attending the group designated for that class (either anger management or goal setting) or continue on with their regular class work. Groups ran for 5 weeks with sessions held once or twice a week. The hypothesized expectation that students in the anger management training group would show a reduction in state anger levels, anger expression, and an improvement in self-efficacy in using anger management skills (measured by the State Trait Anger Expression Inventory (STAXI) and a Self-Efficacy Scale for anger management) was not supported. It is possible that the sole reliance on self-report data did not afford a sufficiently comprehensive assessment into progress made by students. Students may be motivated to overreport anger (to show off) or to underreport (to avoid punishment). Regardless, the measures used in this study were less robust than the multimethod approach employed in most studies in this field, limiting confidence in the findings.

Research drawn from the above three studies (Etscheidt, Hovell et al., and McWhirter & Page) suggests that the less than impressive follow-up outcomes (and posttraining results in the case of McWhirter & Page) may be a result of temporal factors. Brief, intensive interventions may not have sufficient power to effect ongoing change in students from a high-risk population with chronic and severe problems. It is well recognized that establishing therapeutic rapport with students with conduct problems, who tend to reject authority, can be a challenging task requiring persistence over time, particularly if students perceive they are being pressured to participate in training (Howells & Day, 2003). Treatment readiness varies greatly in this population (see discussion in the penultimate section of this chapter), and the limited time available to establish a working alliance in these brief studies may influence group participation, drop-out rates, and ultimately treatment outcomes.

To address some of these shortcomings, Kellner and colleagues (Kellner & Bry, 1999; Kellner, Bry, & Colletti, 2002; Kellner, Salvador, & Bry, 2001) have conducted a series of studies over a longer time period (incorporating the use of booster sessions) comparing anger management training to the completion of anger management logs (a self-reflection instrument allowing students to address real-life concerns). Following on from the success of pilot trials (see Table 12.1), Kellner and colleagues evaluated the effectiveness of anger management training compared to the completion of anger logs only in a sample of 46 alternative school students (Kellner et al., 2002). Based on established classrooms, 27 students were assigned to the anger management condition and 19 to the anger log condition. Training was conducted over 10 weeks, followed by monthly booster sessions over 4 months for two of the three intervention classrooms. At postintervention, students in the anger management group (according to school records) were in significantly fewer fights with peers than the control (anger log only) group. They were also using more anger logs and were "talking things out" more frequently with a school counselor when angry (p. 400). At 4-month follow-up, only the increase in completion of anger logs was maintained. No differences were found with regard to peer fights and visits to the school counselor.

The impact of booster sessions was investigated in this study by offering four booster sessions to two of the three intervention classrooms only and comparing these results to those of the classroom that did not receive a booster session. Results indicated that students in the classrooms who received boosters were more likely to continue to use anger logs than students in the classroom who did not receive the booster sessions. The continued use of anger logs is desirable because they "represent purposeful training for generalization" (Robinson, Smith, & Miller, 2002, p. 268). In other words, anger logs assist the maintenance of learnt skills by reinforcing these skills through real-life situations.

These positive findings were partially replicated in another study by Kellner and colleagues using additional measures with the same age cohort (Kellner et al., 2001). Forty-six students from a therapeutic day school were recruited after teachers agreed to participate. The sample consisted of 20 students attending anger management training in three established classrooms and 26 students who did not receive the program, but were instructed in the use of anger logs (control group). Training was conducted for 10 weekly sessions followed by monthly booster sessions over 3 months for the students in the program group. During the program, significant improvements were observed in students in the intervention condition in prosocial behavior toward teachers (in classroom time) and students (in unstructured time) as measured by independent observers. At 3-month follow-up, school records reflected significantly fewer aggressive incidents in the anger management group compared to students in the control group. Moreover, students in the intervention group completed significantly more anger logs than the control group – evidence that they continue to use skills learnt in group. However, improvements on other dependent variables were not maintained at follow-up (see Table 12.1 for details). Thus, although the findings are limited, the series of studies by Kellner and colleagues lend weight to the argument that anger management programs that include booster sessions can lead to a reduction in aggression in alternative school students both at posttraining and up to 3–4 months later.

Outcome Studies Conducted in Self-Contained Units Within Mainstream Schools

Positive results have also been evident for anger management training conducted across different alternative education settings. This study, by Robinson et al. (2002), represents one of two that, in addition to investigating students in a stand-alone alternative school, also examined students attending self-contained programs within two mainstream schools. The effectiveness of 10-week anger control training was evaluated in a controlled trial of 41 students, aged 11–15 years which examined pre- and postintervention measures of internal and expressed anger (Robinson et al., 2002). At the alternative school (n = 13), two classrooms were randomly assigned to intervention and control group. The same process took place for students enrolled in four self-contained programs in the two general education schools (School 2, n = 15; School 3, n = 13). The anger control intervention included two lessons over the first 5 weeks of the program and one lesson per week for the remainder of the program (10 weeks in total).

Results indicated that, compared to controls, students in the anger control group had significantly reduced internal feelings of anger at postintervention. They expressed anger less frequently and were better able to control their aggressive behavior (physical and verbal; measured by STAXI and teacher-rated Child Behavior Checklist (CBCL) and an interview). At 4-week follow-up, students in the intervention group still differed significantly in terms of anger control, but not on the other two dependent variables (angry feelings, anger expression) found at postintervention. This suggests that angry feelings had returned at 4 weeks; however, students attending the program were still more successful in controlling their anger compared to controls. After group completion, interviews conducted with students revealed that they had found the training beneficial in managing their anger, and cited instances where they had used skills outside of school. In contrast, teachers (group leaders) reported that although student behavior, in particular impulsivity, had improved in class, they did not expect skills to generalize to other settings.

It is noteworthy that the intervention group scores in this study were pooled across all intervention settings (including both stand-alone schooling and self-contained schooling on a mainstream site; Robinson et al., 2002). No breakdown in the figures was offered between the intervention groups in stand-alone schools and those in self-contained programs within mainstream schools. Therefore, it can be surmised that the intervention was effective across settings, but this cannot be stated with certainty.

A further study investigating 12- to 15-year-old students with conduct problems assigned to a specialized behavior modification program for frequently suspended delinquents in a mainstream education setting was conducted by Feindler and her colleagues (Feindler, Marriott, & Iwata, 1984). A total of 36 students were selected from a pool of 100 attending a specialized program for disruptive students because they had the highest rates of problematic behavior. Next, this select group was randomly assigned to an intervention group or a no-contact control condition. Anger control training was conducted over 7 weeks with 20 sessions in total. Analysis of postintervention effects, comparing the intervention to the control condition, revealed that student self-control and social problem solving had significantly improved (measured by the student-rated Means-Ends Problem-Solving Inventory and teacher-rated SCRS). School records of "double fines" (fines for severe aggressive behavior such as physical fights, property damage, and severe verbal abuse), administered daily in class, reflected substantial change for the experimental group between pretreatment and a 5-week follow-up.

Outcome Studies Conducted in Mainstream Schools with Students Previously Assigned to Alternative Education Centers

In the only study to randomly select and assign students to experimental conditions, Petit (1998) recruited 55 students from a list of students who had previously been assigned to alternative education centers for chronically disruptive adolescents. Students aged 15–18 years were assigned to one of three conditions: (a) a 9-week anger management group ($n = 15$), (b) a placebo group who watched educational videos ($n = 20$), and (c) a control group ($n = 20$). Again, attrition was high in this study. Although 90 students were assigned at the outset, only 55 completed the interventions. Results reflected no statistically significant differences (measured by the STAXI and the teacher-rated CBCL) between the three groups at posttreatment. However, it is noteworthy that trends in the expected direction were observed. Compared to students assigned to the placebo and control groups, students in the anger management group were more inhibited and showed a greater reduction in expressed anger towards others or objects at posttraining. Teachers concurred that two-thirds of the treatment group were positively impacted by the program.

Anger Management Training in an Elementary/Primary School Cohort

Although alternative schools do increasingly accept elementary school-aged children, all studies in this review up to now have been conducted with adolescents only. The one study to investigate an elementary school cohort (7- to 12-year olds) conducted a controlled trial of 40 students (started with 50) which compared a social problem solving condition located in a Severely Emotionally Disturbed (SED) center (n = 18) to a control condition in another SED school (n = 22) (Amish, Gesten, Smith, Clark, & Stark, 1988). The program, run by classroom teachers, extended over 3–4 months for a total of 15 sessions. Students were matched for sex, age, ethnicity, and intelligence. Results indicated that children in the social problem solving condition generated significantly more solutions to problem situations compared to a matched control group (measured by interview and role play), but upon further investigation it was apparent that these solutions were antisocial in nature. Teachers reported that children were "perseverating on aggressive themes especially during brainstorming exercises (p. 183)." It is not surprising then, given these observations, that improvements in student adjustment did not eventuate.

Parent Involvement in Anger Management Training

Despite considerable support in the literature for family involvement in the treatment of youth with conduct problems (see Chap. 11, Multisystemic Therapy), only one study has specifically included parents in the treatment program. Mandel (1991) examined the effectiveness of anger control training with students only compared to the addition of parent training to improve anger control amongst conduct disordered youth aged 16–18 years attending a government school for conduct disordered males. The intervention groups comprised 30 students chosen because they demonstrated interest, and had a regular attendance history. They were assigned either to a cognitive behavioral anger control group (n = 15) or a cognitive behavioral anger control group and parent training (n = 15, an abbreviated form of the training program aimed at reinforcing techniques taught in the student program). The size of an untreated attention control group (sex education class) was not given. Attrition, common to many of these reviewed studies, saw almost half of these students drop out due to lack of attendance, disruption, and aggression in group, leaving a final N of 16. The authors emphasized that no students were "kicked out" of the study. The student program ran over a 12-week period and it was intended that parents would participate in four school-based sessions.

Consistent with an earlier study by Robinson et al. (2002), postintervention results revealed that the use of anger control techniques (measured by videotaped role plays) was significantly improved in both treatment groups compared to the control group. No differences were found between the groups on anger feelings or expression. At 4-week follow-up, results (N = 14) from a satisfaction questionnaire revealed that the majority of students had found the training useful and would recommend it for other students.

The anger control training group with parent involvement, expected to have better outcomes than anger control training group alone, did not, although there were small effects for anger experience and expression compared to the control group. Group attendance by parents was extremely poor and had to be supplemented with phone meetings. According to the authors, these meetings were generally "less than satisfactory ... parents were often rushed and harried, seemingly overwhelmed by financial, employment and family obligations (p. 32)."

This difficulty in engaging parents is a commonly observed phenomenon within this population (Lochman & Wells, 2002; Wheatley et al., 2009) and is believed to be due to reasons such as defensiveness and learned helplessness, disillusionment with psychological care, poverty and the associated need to work, lack of social supports, mental health problems (e.g., substance abuse), chaotic lifestyles, and marital discord (Mandel, 1991). Thus, engagement and commitment difficulties represent significant barriers to the successful implementation of systemic treatment approaches. Mandel (1991) concluded that parent participation might have yielded better results had the parents been convinced to invest more effort.

Summary of Research Outcomes

Taken together, the practical implications that can be drawn from these studies is that anger management skills can be taught to conduct disordered adolescents attending alternative programs and schools, and that these skills do translate, at least *in the short term*, to better anger control and less observed aggression *within school*. Whether these positive outcomes translate from the school setting to the external environment cannot be said. Compared to control and comparison groups, the majority of studies (10 out of 13) found favorable results at posttraining for a small group training format, extending over a 2- to 6-month period. In particular, the series of studies by Kellner and colleagues and Robinson et al. with robust designs and respectable samples represent the most convincing evidence of program effectiveness. Furthermore, the multimethod approach to assessment employed in the majority of these studies (self-report, teacher report, independent behavioral observation, social problem-solving role play, and school records) increased methodological rigor, lending weight to the strength of these conclusions. And while it is likely that training works (at least in the short term in the school setting), effect sizes have not been given; thus, the magnitude of the effect is not clear, nor is the clinical significance of outcomes (with the exception of Wheatley et al., 2009). Future research would do well to consider issues of clinical significance, given the severity of conduct problems in this population. For *children* in alternative education programs, there is currently insufficient evidence to comment on program effectiveness.

Social Validity. The social validity of these training programs, important for determining whether students will use strategies learnt in training (Wolf, 1978), has also been formally investigated in three studies (Mandel, 1991; Robinson et al., 2002; Wignall, 2006). According to interview and satisfaction questionnaire data, students found anger management training acceptable, preferred shorter classes (40–50 min) to circumvent boredom, believed that anger management should be taught to more students, and used anger management skills both inside and outside of the school environment. Teachers in one study, despite giving generally positive feedback about the effectiveness of the program, were concerned about the generalizability of skills from the classroom to outside of school (Robinson et al., 2002).

Questions raised by teachers about generalizability cannot be answered by the research conducted to date. Whether positive results occur outside school or after group completion is not entirely clear as few studies have used measures (e.g., parent reports) that capture behavioral improvement outside of school. Although many studies reported positive follow-up data, this must be interpreted with caution, as results often diminished substantially compared to postintervention (Kellner et al., 2002; Robinson et al., 2002), and fewer dependent variables were used (three studies used one outcome variable only; see Table 12.1, Etscheidt, 1991; Feindler et al., 1984; Mandel, 1991; Wignall, 2006). Follow-up outcomes in future studies need to be collected over a longer time period (follow-up has been short – 4 weeks to 6 months) using more rigorous methods that extend beyond the classroom.

Having reached these conclusions, it is important to note the limitations of this anger management research, related to the benefits and confounds of real-life effectiveness studies. Such limitations make recommendations about the use of anger management training difficult to make. These research limitations will be considered in the next section.

RESEARCH LIMITATIONS AND CONSIDERATIONS FOR FUTURE RESEARCH

Lack of Random Assignment. Although there are many advantages of research set in a real-world natural environment, one threat to internal validity present in effectiveness studies is a lack of random assignment of subjects to experimental and control conditions (many studies left subjects in their established classrooms and randomly assigned classroom to conditions, not individual students; see Table 12.1). Without such, it is unclear whether groups are equivalent in terms of individual differences before training starts. Differences between groups may lead to systematic variability and confound the true effects of treatment. That said, the majority of studies did attempt to address this issue by testing for group differences at the start of the training program. Results from these comparisons revealed, for the most part, that the experimental groups were equivalent at pretreatment (except for Amish et al. who were matched on all but one interview and role-play variable), and therefore, it is unlikely that systematic differences accounted for observed differences between groups.

Pretraining Diagnostic Status. To be eligible for placement in alternative schools adolescents have to "move beyond the tolerance level of classrooms" (Quinn & Poirier, 2006, p. 1). Each school jurisdiction has different inclusion criteria (Lehr & Lange, 2003), but generally students must have risk factors that place them at risk of drop-out including academic failure, suspension, truancy, and disruptive conduct (Kleiner et al., 2002). Students are not admitted by psychiatric diagnosis. As a result, minimal information is available about the diagnostic profile of students in these schools, making generalizability of results across alternative schools difficult (e.g., one alternative education program may have students that as a group are more emotionally and/or behaviorally disturbed than students in another program). In the absence of clinical diagnoses (e.g., CD or ODD) at pretraining, it is often difficult to ascertain how severe the conduct problems experienced were and whether comorbidity was present. Singh and colleagues warn that "it behooves the field to settle this issue before any meaningful research with this population can be undertaken (Singh, Deitz, Epstein, & Singh, 1991, p. 85)."

Identifying Salient Ingredients in Multi-Component Programs. Authors vary as to how comprehensively they describe their treatment programs, but from what information is able to be gleaned from published studies, it appears they include a similar array of CB components (social problem solving, anger management training, etc.), adopted in an idiosyncratic fashion. Because programs have not typically followed manuals or identical formats, however, it is difficult to pinpoint with certainty the salient ingredients associated with change and the maintenance of change (Robinson et al., 2002). Feindler et al. (1984) argue that component analyses should be conducted in future studies to ascertain which techniques are most effective.

Other interventions already in place in alternative programs and schools, such as behavioral modification systems, functional behavior assessments, and individual counseling also confound the outcomes in these studies. It is unclear how these factors might impact upon the success of group therapy programs. The school climate is another important contributor to treatment success that is generally overlooked in this research. A positive school climate is one wherein (a) anger management training is supported, (b) change is supported, (c) teachers possess desired personal qualities (e.g., warmth and positive regard) and employ appropriate instructional techniques, (d) training and resources are provided, and (e) general curricula is challenging (Fitzsimons-Lovett, 2001; Quinn et al., 1999; Tobin & Sprague, 1999). It is also important to know if students are involved in wraparound services in which school and staff collaborate with family and external agencies to develop individually tailored support services, for example, Multisystemic Therapy (Schaeffer, McCart, Henggeler, Cunningham, see Chap. 11). Future research also needs to be more process oriented to ensure a better understanding of the many factors that impact upon the success of these training programs.

Generalization of Skills to the Student's External Environment. Programs of this nature have been criticized for modifying aggressive behavior in the immediate classroom only and not ensuring skills transfer to the youth's wider environment (Gresham, 1985). It is thought that skills learnt in class fail to consolidate because of a lack of practice outside of school, mainly due to an absence of support for these skills by significant others in the student's environment who may continue to model aggressive behaviors

(Kellner & Bry, 1999). Few studies, with the exception of Wheatley et al. (2009) and Mandel (1991), have included parent reports regarding the student's progress away from school perhaps because of the difficulties discussed earlier in ascertaining parental cooperation. Thus, conclusions about the generalizability of the program are difficult to make. We can say that the program is probably effective in reducing aggression and other conduct problems inside school, but outside the school is unclear. External assessment by researchers needs consideration if this research is to answer the question of how these programs generalize to the student's external environment (e.g., parent interview, legal offenses).

Generalization of Skills to the Wider Alternative School Population. Another issue relating to generalization is how relevant these outcomes are to the wider alternative school population (Gresham, 1985). Rather than accessing random samples, convenience samples have been drawn upon when teachers have volunteered their classrooms as a whole, when researchers have accepted interested students with good attendance, or when the most highly disturbed students have been recruited. These convenience samples potentially consist of a subsample of the population and therefore results may not be generalizable to other alternative school populations (e.g., less severe presentations). Only a few studies have collected samples across a number of schools avoiding any location-related biases that may exist (e.g., lower socioeconomic status).

Maintenance of Gains. Studies have not adequately addressed the issue of maintenance of gains after program completion (Gresham, 1985; Robinson et al., 2002). Many studies have simply not collected follow-up data and it is not clear why this is the case – perhaps the transitory nature of the population makes follow-up difficult. Commonly, when follow-up data has been collected, fewer dependent variables have been employed than at postintervention (sometimes only one), and follow-up has been too short (up to 6 months) to establish maintenance of gains and properly screen for iatrogenic effects. A number of strategies promote maintenance of gains – teachers and parents are trained to reinforce skills outside of the group program, students are taught to use anger logs, skills are practiced on real-life situations, homework tasks aim to generalize skills from the classroom to the outside world (Robinson et al., 2002) – but none have been specifically tested, with the exception of Kellner et al. (2002) who illustrated the importance of booster sessions. Research should focus on what techniques best maintain gains (Robinson et al., 2002). It would also be useful to understand the potential value of parent involvement in training; however, it is noteworthy that researchers have experienced difficulty in engaging parents to attend group or telephone meetings (Mandel, 1991; Wheatley et al., 2009).

Facilitator Role. Studies have also varied in terms of the facilitation role, ranging from the use of regular classroom teachers to school counselors (less commonly) to trained counselors, and because of this, it is difficult to know if the choice of facilitator influences program outcome. Furthermore, in conducting future studies, it is important to consider whether the facilitators chosen for training (e.g., mental health professionals) are available in numbers to run groups on a larger scale. There is already controversy as to whether teachers have the time to assume roles as mental health treatment providers, given their already substantial workloads (Lashley & Boscardin, 2003; Mayer, Lochman, & van Acker, 2005). Logistical issues faced by teachers include the time required for training, and whether they receive adequate emotional support and sufficient resources from their school (Fitzsimons-Lovett, 2001). Teachers must undergo a significant change in role if they are to assume the position of mental health facilitator. The challenge they face in switching roles is summarized nicely by an alternative school principal who, after a 16-week program in her school, stated "It is much easier for an external psychologist to come into the school and maintain a non-judgmental stance. If a teacher has had a blow up with a student the period before and they have had to be the disciplinarian, it can make it difficult to be non-judgmental" (Wheatley et al., 2009, p. 33). On the contrary, Durlak (1982) contends that there are simply not enough school-based mental health professionals to meet demand, especially given the small amount of time school counselors are able to apportion to therapeutic client contact.

Attrition Rates and Small Sample Sizes. This is another major problem within this population and most studies reported high attrition rates, ranging from 20% to 50%, between the commencement and completion of training (see Table 12.1). Very few studies have included detailed information about the students who drop-out, yet this information is critical for determining if a certain group of students is not responding to the program. It is possible that students with the most severe conduct problems are dropping out of the program, rendering the program ineffective for this subsample of clients. For example, in a comparison of program completers (n = 29) and noncompleters (n = 13), Hovell et al. (2001) identified four behaviors had occurred more often in noncompleters over the previous 6 months, including marijuana usage, friends encouraging them to fight, damaging property, and physically injuring others. This prompted Hovell and colleagues to conclude that the program may have only been effective for students with a less extreme risk profile. Another byproduct of high attrition is small sample sizes, and associated problems such as less power in statistical calculations (effects may be missed) and a decreased ability to generalize results to other alternative school populations.

Lack of Studies at the Elementary School Level. Although research provides some support for the use of anger management programs in adolescents, inadequate evidence exists for the use of these programs with younger students. Further research is needed before anger management training can be recommended in the elementary school setting.

In sum, future research would benefit from (a) the random assignment of students to ensure groups are equivalent at the outset of treatment, (b) psychiatric assessment of students (including severity) conducted at the outset of training to aid generalization across settings, (c) component analyses to delineate the salient components of treatment and treatment maintenance, (d) identification of strategies that will aid skill transfer to the student's external environment, (e) addressing attrition problems by collecting information on drop-outs with the aim of overcoming barriers to program engagement (and thus increasing sample size), and (f) conducting more research on skills-based group treatment with elementary school students. Lastly, and most importantly, is the collection of long-term (1–2 years) follow-up data. Over the last decade, concern has been voiced in the literature, with increasing volume, about the possibility of iatrogenic effects resulting from the aggregation of deviant peers (Dishion, McCord, & Poulin, 1999). More research is needed urgently in this area before groups of this kind can be recommended with confidence. Indeed, an understanding of the literature concerning potential iatrogenic effects of group treatment of deviant youth is an important requirement for a discussion on group therapy effectiveness, and thus is included in the following section.

FIRST, DO NO HARM (*PRIMUM NON NOCERE*): AGGREGATING HIGH-RISK YOUTH

Anger management programs are commonly delivered in group format, first because they provide a social environment where students can interactively practice prosocial skills through the use of modeling, role playing, and reinforcement of appropriate behavior, and second because they constitute a cost-effective way of providing therapeutic skills to greater numbers. However, the emergence of research in the 1990s prompted Dishion and colleagues to argue that the aggregation of high-risk youth with conduct problems into homogenous groups should be avoided under some circumstances because it can cause deleterious effects (Dishion et al., 1999). Indeed, their argument extends further than aggregating at-risk youth in mental health groups, to the larger system of alternative programs and schooling. They suggest that the current default system of removing students from mainstream classes to segregate them into self-contained settings with other deviant peers may exacerbate problems rather than reduce them (Dishion, Dodge, & Lansford, 2008). (This discussion is outside the scope of this chapter but an overview is provided by Dodge et al. (2006) and Dishion, Dodge, & Lansford (2006).

Dishion and colleagues maintain that increasing the amount of contact between deviant youth encourages *deviancy training* to take place. Deviancy training occurs when a young person receives positive verbal and nonverbal reinforcement for delinquent or rule-breaking dialogue with peers (Dishion et al., 1999). In a series of studies by Dishion and colleagues associations were found between deviancy training observed at 13–14 years of age (25-min videotaped discussion of a natural conversation between a youth dyad) and conduct problems in subsequent adolescent years including an increase in delinquency (self-reported), violent behavior (self-reported and police reported), and use of tobacco and marijuana (Dishion, Capaldi, Spracklen, & Li, 1995; Dishion, Eddy, Haas, Li, & Spracklen, 1997; Dishion, Spracklen, Andrews, & Patterson, 1996). Thus, the authors conclude that deviant peer exposure can influence and reinforce undesirable behaviors creating a "deviant peer contagion." Peer contagion contributes to an escalation in conduct problems most likely through the processes of modeling, reinforcement, identity formation (wanting group acceptance), and by creating more opportunities for deviance (Dishion et al., 2006). Dodge et al. summarized "when the reason that deviant youth are placed with each other is because they are deviant, their identity and common ground become deviance" (Dodge et al., 2006, p. 4).

To further support their argument that aggregation of at-risk youth can be iatrogenic, Dishion et al. (1999) assert that deviancy training and peer contagion, shown to exist in naturally occurring friendships in the above studies, also occur when youth have been grouped for skills-based therapeutic treatment (Adolescent Transitions Program, Dishion & Andrews, 1995). One hundred and nineteen self-referred families with high-risk adolescents (11–14 years) were randomly assigned to one of five 12-week group training conditions. These included (a) parent focus training, a combination of parent management skills and strategies for strengthening peer support; (b) teen focus, improving prosocial behavior with family and peers; (c) both parent and teen focus; (d) self-directed change (materials only); and (e) a quasiexperimental control group. Measures of family interactions, problem behavior and smoking were assessed via structured interview, CBCL, Family Events Checklist, and videotaped family interaction collected at pre- and posttraining and at 1-year follow-up.

Results showed that although observed and parent-rated family conflict decreased by the end of training in both the teen and parent group compared to families in the inactive intervention conditions, at 1-year follow-up iatrogenic effects in the teen group had become evident. At follow-up, adolescents in the teen group and teen group combined with parent intervention reported higher levels of teacher-rated externalizing behavior problems and smoking compared to other conditions (Dishion & Andrews, 1995). Poulin and colleagues revealed that both the teacher-reported delinquency and increase in smoking continued to be evident at 3-year follow-up (Poulin, Dishion, & Burraston, 2001).

One would expect based on Dishion's deviancy training hypothesis that a dose–response relationship would exist; that is, the greater the exposure to deviant youth, the higher the level of deviancy training and associated negative outcomes (Dishion et al., 2008). However, this has not always been the case. The literature has shown the association between deviant youth, levels of deviancy training, and negative outcomes to be more complex. For example, a study by Mager et al. investigated the effects of problem solving skills training (9–12 weeks) in 139 sixth and seventh grade students (mean age = 12) assigned to either "pure" CD groups or a "mixed" CD and non-CD group (Mager, Milich, Harris, & Howard, 2005). Participants were asked to complete questionnaires including the CBCL, Attitudes towards Delinquency and Alcohol and Drugs, Social Skills Rating System, and information about peer associations. School records provided information about adjustment and behavioral observation was also undertaken. Contrary to expectations that the pure CD group would fare worse, the study showed that students in the pure CD group actually did better than the mixed group in terms of teacher- and parent-rated externalizing behavior. The mixed group condition did improve in their problem behaviors compared to pretraining, but not as much as the pure group condition. Of interest, more deviancy training was observed in the mixed group, consistent with Dishion et al.'s hypothesis that deviancy training is correlated with poorer outcomes.

Whilst the strength of these outcomes may have been affected by treatment groups of unequal sizes (mixed groups were larger than pure CD groups) and a relatively short follow-up that may not have fully captured iatrogenic effects (Mager et al., 2005), these outcomes highlight that results can vary depending upon specific circumstances. The nature of exchanges that take place within groups is complex; exchanges are moderated by both the individual's characteristics and group characteristics. With regard to the former, individual characteristics of relevance include gender, personality characteristics (impulsivity), and age. Young adolescents are particularly vulnerable to peer contagion especially from associating with older youth. Initial levels of delinquency are also important as moderately deviant youth, not yet committed to a delinquent lifestyle, are most at risk (Dishion et al., 2008). In terms of group characteristics, a number of variables are of interest including gender (or masculine and feminine group norms; Hartup, 1983), competitiveness, group cohesiveness, and group size. The skill level of the facilitator and session format (structured vs. unstructured) may also moderate outcomes (Dishion et al., 2008; Hartup, 2005). Susceptibility to peer exposure is an important concept as some youth with conduct problems are less likely to be influenced than others; they may differ in their inclination to attend to delinquent models, and how much they enjoy the delinquent model's attention (Hartup, 1999, 2005). Dishion et al. summarize that the "evidential landscape is underdeveloped" and research, although growing rapidly, has a long way to go in identifying the conditions that contribute to deviant peer contagion (Dishion et al., 2006, p. 371).

Recommendations for Avoiding Deviancy Training in Groups. Dodge and colleagues assert that presently the "... challenge is to understand how group treatments and interventions might be structured so that deviant peer influence is minimized" (Dodge et al., 2006, p. 13). In 2002, a commission of 27 scholars from the fields of psychology, sociology, law, media, business, and education formed to investigate the influences of peer contagion in youth (Dishion et al., 2006). Over 3 years this team conducted a metaanalysis, literature review, interviews with program officials, and focus groups with practitioners and youth. The team reported that one of the strongest factors leading to deviant peer influence is interaction with deviant peers in settings which are unsupervised and structurally lacking. In line with Lochman and colleagues' recommendations (see Chap. 9), the team recommended that facilitators of anger management training groups be alert to signs of deviancy training and minimize these through group structure (e.g., group rules and use of reward points) as well as enhanced behavioral management strategies (see Lochman et al.). Facilitators must be skilled – or at least closely supervised – and should work arduously at the outset of group to influence the establishment of a prosocial culture among students.

GROUP TREATMENT CONSIDERATIONS FOR CLINICIANS AND RESEARCHERS: FACILITATING ENGAGEMENT AND MINIMIZING DROP-OUT

Treatment Readiness. "Low (treatment) readiness refers...to the presence of characteristics...within either the client or the therapeutic situation, which are likely to impede engagement in therapy and which, thereby, are likely to diminish therapeutic change" (Howells & Day, 2003, p. 320). The success of skills-based training programs for students in alternative education programs can be compromised if the facilitator fails to appreciate the unique aspects of anger and aggression that make treatment readiness and group engagement more important in this population than perhaps is the case for other disorders (Howells & Day, 2003). Without a focus on treatment readiness and group engagement, group members are likely to drop-out through disinterest or stay and disrupt other students.

Howells and Day (2003) argued that low treatment readiness in externalizing students can result from a number of factors. First, the student's personal goals can conflict with those of the therapist. Depression and anxiety, unlike anger, are emotions that typically create distress for the person, motivating them to attend and fully engage in treatment. Anger, on the other hand, is often ego-syntonic, and can have social benefits for the aggressor (as least in the short term through intimidation and obtained outcomes); thus, students are not always personally motivated to receive treatment. Typically, it is left to parents and school staff to instigate treatment.

Further to this, students with anger problems often hold firm beliefs about the value of anger that can interfere with treatment readiness. DiGuiseppe (1995) identified a number of these beliefs, including (a) anger is appropriate, (b) self-righteousness ("my reaction is just"), (c) anger is effective and helps me to meet my needs, (d) blaming others for their aggression (low personal responsibility), and (e) the belief that if therapists try to change their aggressive behavior, this means the therapists do not believe that the other party is responsible. Beliefs such as these make it unlikely that the therapist and student will agree on therapeutic goals. Moreover, voluntary participation in group does not equate to treatment readiness. Even if the students decide of their own free will to attend group, they may not see the value in pursuing the therapeutic goals and thus resist treatment. Affiliative goals need to replace dominance goals for the students to become more treatment ready.

The high comorbidity in the alternative school population may also present a barrier to treatment readiness. Substance abuse, personality disorders, ADHD, and family dysfunction are commonly experienced and can interfere with the success of therapy (e.g., an ADHD diagnoses may make sitting and attending challenging; Howells & Day, 2003). Furthermore, youths with "callous–unemotional traits," characterized by callousness and pursuit of one's own needs at the expense of others, represent a subsample of this population that may have particularly low treatment readiness.

According to the training outlines provided in the studies reviewed, it appears these anger management programs tend to commence skills-based instruction early with little time devoted to the issue of treatment readiness and the development of intrinsic motivation to participate in group. Perhaps these students have less severe presentations and are treatment ready or, alternatively, perhaps this speediness in commencing skills training may account for some of the high attrition rates evidenced. Change strategies may be undertaken in these groups (e.g., assertiveness training) before the students perceive a need to alter their communication style. The author's experience in alternative schools in Australia has highlighted the need to focus on treatment readiness, by expanding the rapport building and motivational components of the program, for anger management training to successfully engage alternative school students who have chronic and severe comorbid presentations and are unlikely to be treatment ready at group commencement.

Anecdotally, based on clinical experience, many strategies are useful in increasing treatment readiness and motivation to participate in alternative school students:

1. Students are invited to attend a "social skills" group (or another generic term) to distance the group from stigma attached to mental health treatment and to reduce the possibility that the group is viewed as a punishment for bad behavior.
2. The facilitator can be removed from the role of disciplinarian. A school staff member[2] typically sits at the back of the classroom (as is legally required in Australia), just within earshot but physically removed (e.g., marking papers), and steps in to enact behavior modification procedures when behavior escalates to the point where warnings for time out are required (minor behavior modification strategies are also used by the facilitators). By divorcing oneself from the disciplinary role, the therapist avoids being drawn into time depleting power struggles with students (e.g., the therapist instructs a student to go to time out and they refuse to recognize the facilitator's authority, creating a standoff), and they are able to maintain a warm supportive stance, one that increases the likelihood that therapeutic rapport will be established, and then maintained. The stronger the therapeutic alliance, the more likely the student will be motivated to please the facilitator and participate in group (and discourage the disruptions of others).
3. The student's goals and that of the therapist need to be aligned for therapy to be successful (Howells & Day, 2003). A relatively large section of the curricula is dedicated to exploring personal goals and raising student awareness of their own strengths and weaknesses and the need for change (moving students from precontemplation

[2] The choice of teacher, teacher's aide, and school counselor here is clearly important. They must be well respected, capable of disciplining students, and cognizant of the importance of confidentiality.

to contemplation and action as per DiClemente and Prochaska's Stages of Change model; Prochaska, DiClemente, & Norcross, 1992). Thus, Miller and Rollnick's motivational interviewing strategies are woven throughout activities to raise cognitive dissonance (e.g., goal setting) for at least five to six sessions, before action strategies are embraced (Miller & Rollnick, 1991). When students begin to understand that achieving their goals is dependent on choices, they have the power to make (e.g., learning skills in group) intrinsic motivation to participate in group builds. The therapist also works to bridge the gap between their goals for therapy and those of the students. For example, a student may have the goal of joining the army and to achieve this goal they need to satisfactorily pass at least grade 10. The therapist's goal of getting the student to pass school in the short term is enabled by the student's longer term goal of joining the army.

4. Instructional strategies used by facilitators need to be highly engaging and appropriate to students with learning and attention difficulties for motivation to be maintained. Preferred activities tend to be short and active, and engaging methods employed. Multimedia strategies, recommended in pedagogical research (R. Mayer, 2003), were observed to be particularly effective. For example, psychoeducation about anger, depression, and anxiety was conducted through the medium of movies. Excerpts were screened from well-known movies (e.g., Meet the Parents) of characters exhibiting these emotions. Students then discuss what cognitions, behaviors, and physiological reactions are associated with each emotion, whether consequences are desirable or undesirable, and what other alternative courses of action might have been taken. By focusing on a character, students are able to discuss emotions in a less threatening way. Video recording exercises (e.g., asking students to write and act in short movies) was a simple but effective strategy that could be used repeatedly for motivating students to engage in social problem solving activities. These multimedia strategies are thought to be effective because students learn more deeply from words matched with pictures than words by themselves. Mayer also notes the benefits of a "personalization effect" whereby students learn more effectively when words are delivered in a conversational rather than a formal style (p. 125).
5. Participation needs to be linked to both immediate end-of-session and longer term rewards (see Lochman et al., Chap. 9).
6. Having two facilitators increases the likelihood that students will find a facilitator they can develop a good working alliance with. A good working alliance can motivate the student to participate in group.
7. Prior to commencing group, group suitability assessments should be conducted by the facilitators to ensure (as much as possible) that members of the group are likely to cooperate with each other (e.g., putting dyads who have experienced high conflict in the same group should be avoided).

As noted, these observations represent suggestions at this stage and need to be trialed and examined empirically using process-oriented research.

SUMMARY AND CONCLUSIONS

As the number of students being schooled through alternative education grows rapidly, the United States government, concerned about the quality of educational services, has encouraged the adoption of school-wide evidence-based practices. Against this background, this chapter considered the effectiveness of one of those recommended practices: anger management group therapy, a therapy widely practiced in the alternative school system for the alleviation of conduct problems in students with moderate to severe presentations. A review of 13 studies of anger management group training in alternative school settings revealed that adolescents participating in training groups typically demonstrated fewer conduct problems in school at posttraining than those in comparison or control groups. It is not known if these results generalized to the student's external environment. Specifically, outcomes included less verbal and physical fights with peers, more self-control, less suspensions, and fewer aggressive incidents. These findings were consistently demonstrated through multimethod approaches, and provide early evidence for the effectiveness of skills-based group training. Still, the magnitude of training effects have not been determined and future studies, given the initial severity of these presentations, would benefit from including effect sizes and measures of clinical significance in outcome data.

Findings were not as clear cut, however, with regard to maintenance of group gains over short-term follow-up (4 weeks to 6 months). Even though many studies reported positive follow-up results, compared to posttraining, outcomes were often significantly diminished. Moreover, fewer assessment measures were drawn upon compared to posttreatment assessment with some studies employing one measure only. Thus, outcomes derived from short-term follow-up assessments appear promising, but to be fully satisfied, gains are being maintained over time, and further research is necessary.

There is a possibility that generalizing skills to outside of the school setting and maintaining gains over the long term may require support from the adolescent's wider environment. A transactional perspective would warn against any treatment interventions that did not take into account the influence of parents/caregivers on treatment outcomes. Researchers need to consider how parents might be engaged in treatment, and once engaged, comparisons between training programs that include parents, and adolescent-only groups need to be conducted.

Follow-up periods also need to be longer than 6 months to ensure iatrogenic effects do not emerge at a later stage. Iatrogenic effects are a significant concern with groups that aggregate high-risk youth and facilitators need to be continually alert to the possibility of deviancy training and deviant peer contagion in research trials. Amish et al. (1988) findings that children left to brainstorm tend to perseverate on aggressive themes stand as a warning about the importance of keeping therapist vigilance on the agenda and maintaining highly structured environments. That said, the research into peer contagion is still in its infancy. Research revealing poorer training outcomes in mixed groups (internalizing and externalizing disorders) of students compared with pure CD groups highlights the complexity of this issue. Clearly, susceptibility to peer contagion is influenced by many factors and more remains to be discovered about what increases vulnerability.

Future studies will need to overcome a number of important methodological shortcomings identified in the literature if the quality of research in this domain is to be improved:

1. Assessment of a student's clinical diagnoses (including severity) prior to training would enable conclusions to be reached about which clinical presentations benefit most from training (e.g., perhaps training is more effective in less severe presentations). This knowledge can also help in determining whether results from one setting are generalizable to other alternative school settings.
2. A detailed overview of the training program should be included in published research, and if possible researchers should aim to conduct studies using a common program so that dissemination of evidence-based manuals may be possible.
3. Process-oriented research should be conducted to determine which components of anger management training are the most successful for enhancing group engagement, generating change, and maintaining that change over time.
4. A better understanding is needed about the generalization of skills from the classroom to the external environment, both during training and over the long-term. It is difficult to determine from the literature whether generalization from the classroom to the external environment is taking place because behavioral measures (with the exception of self-report) are typically used in school only. Whether students are successful in transferring skills from the classroom to outside school can be evaluated using parent/carer reports and police records of legal offenses (in combination with student self-report). Mechanisms that facilitate the transfer of skills across settings (e.g., parent reinforcement, homework exercises) also warrant further exploration.
5. Attrition rates are unacceptably high in this population and researchers need to capture information about causes of drop-out for two reasons. First, to investigate if there is a certain population (e.g., students with high comorbidy) who are less likely to benefit from this group training, and second, to help facilitators in determining how they might overcome attrition as they prepare for group. If high rates of drop-out can be curtailed, problems associated with small sample sizes can be minimized as much as possible.

Based on findings from this literature review, it can be concluded that although results thus far are encouraging, educators should proceed with caution in continuing to use anger management group training in alternative education programs until further long-term research is conducted. At present, it can only be concluded that there are positive effects at the completion of group treatment *within* the school setting. Researchers urgently need to conduct more methodologically rigorous studies with follow-up assessed over a 1–2-year period, to establish maintenance of program gains and ensure iatrogenic effects are not present. If iatrogenic effects are present, researchers need to shift focus to consider how group treatments might be delivered or structured to minimize peer contagion or consider other treatment modalities for these students (Dodge et al., 2006). In the meantime, facilitators continuing to run training programs need to ensure that groups are highly structured skill-building interventions, and that they are monitored with deviancy training in mind. Moreover, facilitators need to address engagement and motivational barriers to treatment as well as consider how they will ensure skills are transferred from the classroom to the home environment. Finally, given the rise in alternative schooling at the elementary level, more research is needed to determine whether similar outcomes occur in children.

REFERENCES

Amish, P. L., Gesten, E. L., Smith, J. K., Clark, H. B., & Stark, C. (1988). Social problem solving training for severely emotionally and behaviorally disturbed training. *Behavioral Disorders, 13*(3), 175–186.

Atkins, T., Allen, J., & Meredith. M. (2001). *Alternative schools information for families.* Washington, DC: Center for Effective Collaboration and Practice. Retrieved September 10, 2003, from http://cecp.air.org/familybriefs/docs/AltSch.pdf

Cassidy, E., James, A., & Wiggs, L. (2001). The prevalence of psychiatric disorder in children attending a school for pupils with emotional and behavioral difficulties. *British Journal of Special Education, 28*(4), 167–173.

Castleberry, S., & Enger, J. (1998). Alternative school students' concepts of success. [Electronic version] *NASSP Bulletin,* 105–111.

Center for Effective Collaboration and Practice. (1999). Emphasizing achievement [electronic version]. *Reclaiming Children and Youth, 7,* 252–254.

Cobb, C., Brewer, D., Bauman, A., Groves, P., Rayle, J., & Noblit, G. (1997). Alternative learning programs evaluation: Part 3 report. *Case studies of alternative schools and programs* [Electronic source]. Raleigh, NC: North Carolina State Department of Public Instruction.

Cole, T., Visser, J., & Upton, G. (1988). *Effective schooling for children with emotional and behavioral difficulties.* London: David Fulton.

Cortez, A., & Montecel, M. R. (1999). *Disciplinary alternative education programs in Texas – What is known: What is needed.* [Electronic version]. San Antonio: Intercultural Development Research Association. (ERIC Document Reproduction Service No. ED434963)

Cox, S. M., Davidson, W. S., & Bynum, T. S. (1995). A meta-analytic assessment of delinquency-related outcomes of alternative education programs. *Crime and Delinquency, 41*(2), 219–234.

Crick, N. R., & Dodge, K. A. (1994). A review and reformulation of social information-processing mechanisms in children's social adjustment. *Psychological Bulletin, 115,* 74–101.

DiGuiseppe, R. (1995). Developing the therapeutic alliance with angry clients. In H. Kassinove (Ed.), *Anger disorders: definition, diagnosis and treatment* (pp. 131–150). Philadelphia, PA: Taylor and Francis.

Dishion, T. J., & Andrews, D. W. (1995). Preventing escalation in problem behaviors with high-risk adolescents: Immediate and 1-year outcomes. *Journal of Consulting and Clinical Psychology, 63*, 538–548.
Dishion, T. J., Capaldi, D. M., Spracklen, K. M., & Li, F. (1995). Peer ecology of male adolescent drug use. *Development and Psychopathology, 7*, 803–824.
Dishion, T. J, Dodge, K. A., & Lansford, J. E. (2006). Findings and recommendations: A blueprint to minimise deviant peer influence in youth interventions and programs. In K. A Dodge, T. J. Dishion, & J. E. Lansford, J. E (Ed.), *Deviant peer influences in programs for youth* (pp. 366–394). NY: Guilford Press.
Dishion, T. J., Dodge, K. A., & Lansford, J. E. (2008). Deviant by design: Risks associated With aggregating deviant peers into group prevention and treatment programs. *The Prevention Researcher, 15*(1), 8–11.
Dishion, T. J., Eddy, J. M., Haas, E., Li, F., & Spracklen, K. (1997). Friendships and violent behavior during adolescence. *Social Development, 6*, 207–223.
Dishion, T. J., McCord, J., & Poulin, F. (1999). When interventions harm: Peer groups and problem behaviors. *American Psychologist, 54*(9), 755–764.
Dishion, T. J., Spracklen, K. M., Andrews, D. W., & Patterson, G. R. (1996). Deviancy training in male adolescent friendships. *Behavior Therapy, 27*, 373–390.
Dodge, K. A. (1980). Social cognition and children's aggressive behavior. *Child Development, 51*(1), 162–170.
Dodge, K. A., Lanford, J. E. & Dishion, T. J. (2006). The problem of deviant peer influences in intervention programs. In K. A. Dodge, T. J. Dishion, & J. E. Lansford, J. E (Ed.), *Deviant peer influences in programs for youth* (pp. 366–394). NY: Guilford Press.
Durlak, J. A. (1982). Use of cognitive-behavioral interventions by paraprofessionals in the schools. *School Psychology Review, 11*, 64–66.
Editorial (2006, August 16). School's out ... so where do the bad students go? *The Sydney Morning Herald.*
Elliot, A. (2009). Alternatives to school suspensions. *Australian Council for Educational Research eNews, 16*, Retrieved May 1, 2009, from http://www.Acer.edu.au/enews/0403_School_suspension.html.
Etscheidt, S. (1991). Reducing aggressive behavior and improving self-control: A cognitive behavioral training program for behaviorally disordered adolescents. *Behavioral Disorders, 16*(2), 107–115.
Feindler, E. L., Marriott, S. A., & Iwata, M. (1984). Group anger control training for junior high school adolescents. *Cognitive Therapy and Research, 8*(3), 299–311.
Fitzsimons Hughes, A., & Adera, B. (2006). Education and day treatment opportunities in schools: strategies that work. *Preventing School Failure, 51*(1), 26–30.
Fitzsimons-Lovett, A. (2001). Alternative education programs: empowerment or entrapment? *The Council for Children and Behavioral Disorders Monograph* p. 37–41.
Gendron, M., Royer, E., Bertrand, R., & Potvin, P. (2004). Behavior disorders, social competence and the practice of physical activities among adolescents. *Emotional and Behavioral Difficulties, 9*, 249–259.
Gresham, F. M. (1985). Utility of cognitive behavioral procedures for social skills training with children: A critical review. *Journal of Abnormal Child Psychology, 13*, 411–423.
Groth, C. (1998). Dumping ground or effective alternative? *Urban Education, 33*(2), 218–242.
Gulchak, D. J., & Lopes, J. A. (2007). Interventions for students with behavioral disorders: An international literature review. *Behavioral Disorders, 32*(4), 267–281.
Hartup, W. W. (1983). Peer relations. In P. H. Mussen & E. M. Hetherington (Eds.), *Handbook of child psychology* (*Socialization, personality, and social development*, Vol. 4, pp. 103–196). New York: Wiley.
Hartup, W. W. (1999). Constraints on peer socialization: Let me count the ways. *Merrill-Palmer Quarterly [Electronic version], 45*, 172–183.
Hartup, W. W. (2005). Peer interaction: What causes what? *Journal of Abnormal Child Psychology, 33*(3), 387–394.
Head, G., Kane, J., & Cogan, N. (2003). Behavior support in secondary schools. *Emotional and Behavioral Difficulties, 8*, 33–42.

Hemphill, S. (2009, April 27). Suspending students leads to other problems. *The Age newspaper* [Electronic version].

Hovell, M. F., Blumberg, S. L., Powell, L., Morrison, T. C., Duran, G., Sipan, C. L., et al. (2001). Training AIDS and anger prevention social skills in at-risk adolescents. *Journal of Counselling and Development, 79*, 347–355.

Howells, K., & Day, A. (2003). Readiness for anger management: Clinical and theoretical issues. *Clinical Psychology Review, 23*, 319–337.

Humphrey, N., & Brooks, A. G. (2006). An evaluation of a short-term cognitive-behavioral anger management intervention for pupils at risk of exclusion. *Emotional and Behavioral Difficulties, 11*(1), 5–23.

Kellner, M. H., & Bry, B. H. (1999). The effects of anger management groups in a day school for emotionally disturbed adolescents. *Adolescence, 34*(136), 645–651.

Kellner, M. H., Bry, B. H., & Colletti, L. (2002). Teaching anger management skills to students with severe emotional or behavioral disorders. *Behavioral Disorders, 27*(4), 400–408.

Kellner, M. H., Salvador, D. S., & Bry, B. H. (2001, August). *In control: Anger management and the development of prosocial behavior.* CA: Poster session presented at the American Psychological Association Annual Conference.

Kim-Cohen, J., Caspi, A., Moffitt, T., Harrington, H., Milne, B., & Poulton, R. (2003). Prior juvenile diagnoses in adults with mental disorder. *Archives of General Psychiatry, 60*(7), 709–717.

Kingery, P. (2000). *Zero tolerance: The alternative is education.* Washington, DC: Hamilton Fish Institute.

Kleiner, B., Porch, R., and Farris, E. (2002). *Public alternative schools and programs for students at risk of education failure: 2000–01* (NCES 2002–2004). National Center for Education Statistics, U.S. Department of Education. Washington, DC.

Lange, C. M., & Sletten, S. J. (2002). *Alternative education: A brief history and synthesis.* Alexandria: VA. Retrieved May 15, 2009, from, www.nasdse.org.

Lashley, C., & Boscardin, M.L. (2003). *Special education administration at a crossroads: Availability, licensure, and preparation of special education administrators.*[Electronic version] (COPSSE Document No. IB-8). FL: University of Florida, Center on Personnel Studies in Special Education.

Lehr, C. A. & Lange, C. M. (2003). Alternative schools and the students they serve: Perceptions of state directors of special education. *Policy Research Brief* (University of Minnesota: Minneapolis, Institute on Community Integration), *14(1)*, 1–11.

Lochman, J. E., Barry, T. D., & Pardini, D. A. (2003). Anger control training for aggressive youth. In A. E. Kazdin & J. R. Weisz (Eds.), *Evidence-based psychotherapies for children and adolescents* (pp. 263–281). NY: Guilford Press.

Lochman, J. E., & Dodge, K. A. (1994). Social cognitive processes of severely violent, moderately aggressive and non-aggressive boys. *Journal of Consulting and Clinical Psychology, 62*, 366–374.

Lochman, J. E., & Lampron, L. B. (1986). Situational social problem solving skills and Self-esteem of aggressive and non-aggressive boys. *Journal of Abnormal Child Psychology, 14*(4), 605–617.

Lochman, J. E., & Wells, K. C. (2002). The coping power program at the middle-school transition: Universal and indicated prevention effects. *Psychology of Addictive Behaviors, 16(4 S)*, S20–54.

Lochman, J. E., Whidby, J. M., & Fitzgerald, D. P. (2000). Cognitive behavioral assessment and treatment with aggressive children. In P. C. Kendall (Ed.), *Child and adolescent therapy: Cognitive behavioral procedures* (pp. 31–87). NY: Guilford Press.

Mager, W., Millich, R., Haris, M. J., & Howard, A. (2005). Intervention groups for adolescents with conduct problems: Is aggregation harmful or harmful? *Journal of Abnormal and Child Psychology, 33*(3), 349–362.

Mandel, S. (1991). CB anger control training with aggressive adolescent males in a special education high school (Doctoral dissertation, Temple University, 1992). *Dissertation Abstracts International-A, 52/07*, 2471.

Mayer, R. (2003). The promise of multimedia learning: using the same instructional design methods across different media. *Learning and Instruction, 13*(2), 125–139.

Mayer, M., Lochman, J., & van Acker, R. (2005). Introduction to the special issue: Cognitive-behavioral interventions with students with EBD. *Behavioral Disorders, 30*(3), 197–212.

McWhirter, B. T., & Page, G. L. (1999). Effects of anger management and goal setting group interventions on state-trait anger and self-efficacy beliefs among high risk

Miller, W. R., & Rollnick, S. (1991). *Motivational interviewing: Preparing people to change addictive behaviors.* NY: Guilford Press.

Munoz, M. (2002). Alternative schools: Providing a safety net in our high schools to cope with at-risk student challenge [Electronic version]. Lexington: Kentucky State Department of Education. (ERIC Document Reproduction Service No. ED463365)

Murrihy, R., Wheatley, A., Van Kessel, J., Wuthrich, V., Remond, L., Tuqiri, R., Dadds, M., & Kidman, A. (2007, September). *Aggression management training for oppositional adolescents in behavioral schools: Pilot trial of a CBT-based intervention.* Paper presented at the 42nd Annual Conference of the Australian Psychological Society, Brisbane, Australia.

Novaco, R. (1975). *Anger control: The development and evaluation of an experimental treatment.* Lexington, MA: Lexington Books.

Olatunji, B. O., & Lohr, J. M. (2004). Non-specific factors and the efficacy of psychosocial treatments for anger. [Electronic version] *The Scientific Review of Mental Health Practice, 3(2),* 1–26.

Oregon Department of Education. (2007) *Oregon revised statutes: Alternative education.* Retrieved May 15, 2009, from, http://www.leg.state.or.us/ors/336.html

Petit, J. A. (1998). The effects of an anger management program on aggressive adolescents: A cognitive behavioral approach. (Doctoral dissertation, University of New Orleans, 1998). *Dissertation Abstracts International-A,* 59/08, 2871.

Place, M., Wilson, J., Martin, E., & Hulsmeier, J. (2000). The frequency of emotional and behavioral disturbance in an EBD school. *Child Psychology and Psychiatry Review, 5*(2), 76–80.

Poulin, F., Dishion, T. J., & Burraston, B. (2001). Three-year iatrogenic effects associated with aggregating high-risk adolescents in cognitive-behavioral preventive interventions. *Applied Developmental Science, 5*(4), 214–224.

Prochaska, J. O., DiClemente, C. C., & Norcross, J. C. (1992). In search of how people change: Applications to addictive behaviors. *American Psychologist, 47,* 1102–1114.

Quinn, M. M., & Poirier, J. M. (2006). *Study of effective alternative programs: Final grant report.* Washington, DC: American Institutes for Research.

Quinn, M. M., Poirier, J. M., Faller, S. E., Gable, R. A., & Tonelson, S. W. (2006). An examination of school climate in effective alternative programs. *Preventing School Failure, 51*(1), 11–17.

Quinn, M. M., Rutherford, R. B., & Osher, D. M. (1999). Special education in alternative education programs. VA: Eric Clearinghouse on Disabilities and Gifted Education. [Elecronic version]. (ERIC Document Reproduction Service No. ED436054)

Robinson, T. R., Smith, S. W., & Miller, M. D. (2002). Effect of a cognitive behavioral intervention on responses to anger by middle school students with chronic behavior problems. *Behavioral Disorders, 27*(3), 256–271.

Singh, N. N., Deitz, D. E., Epstein, M. H., & Singh, J. (1991). Social behavior of students who are seriously emotionally disturbed. *Behavior Modification, 15*(1), 74–94.

Skiba, R. J. (2000). *Zero tolerance, zero evidence: An analysis of school disciplinary policy.* [Electronic version.] Policy Res. Rep 23. Bloomington, IN: University of Indiana.

Skiba, R. J., & Peterson, R. L. (2000). School discipline at a crossroads: From zero tolerance to early response. *Exceptional Children, 66*(3), 335–346.

Slabby, R. G., & Guerra, N. G. (1988). Cogntive mediators of aggression in adolescent offenders:1. Assessment. *Developmental Psychology, 24*(4), 580–588.

Tobin, T., & Sprague, J. (1999). Alternative education strategies: Reducing violence in school and community. *Journal of Emotional and Behavioral Disorders, 8,* 177–186.

Tyler, J. (1997). *Nine principal components for developing promising alternative education programs for expelled youth.* Washington: U.S. Department of Education.

U.S. Department of Education. (1998). *Twentieth annual report to Congress on the Implementation of the Individuals with Disabilities Education Act.* Washington, DC: U.S. Department of Education.

U.S. Department of Education. (2002a). *No child left behind: Executive summary [Electronic version].* Washington, DC: U.S. Department of Education.

U.S. Department of Education (2002b). *A new era: Revitalising special education for children and their families.* [Electronic version]. Washington, DC.

Unruh, D., Bullis, M., Todis, B., Waintrup, M., & Atkins, T. (2007). Programs and practices for special education students in alternative education settings. *National Center on Secondary Education and Transition.* Retrieved March 13, 2009, from http//:www.ncset.org

van Acker, R. (2007). Antisocial, aggressive and violent behavior in children and adolescents within alternative education settings: prevention and intervention. *Preventing School Failure, 51*(2), 5–12.

Wheatley, A., Murrihy, R., van Kessel, J., Wuthrich, V., Remond, L., Tuqiri, R., et al. (2009). Aggression management training for youth in behavior schools. *Youth Studies Australia, 28*(1), 29–36.

Wignall, A. (2006). Evaluation of a group CBT early intervention program for adolescents with comorbid depression and behavior problems. *Australian Journal of Guidance and Counseling, 16*(1), 119–132.

Wolf, M. M. (1978). Social validity: The case for subjective measurement, or how applied behavior analysis is finding its heart. *Journal of Applied Behavior Analysis, 11,* 203–214.

Yearwood, D. L., Abdum-Muhaymin, J., & Jordan, P. (2002) *Alternative learning programs evaluation: 2000–2001.* [Electronic version]. Raleigh: North Carolina Department of Public Instruction.

Zoccolillo, M., Pickles, A., Quinton, D., & Rutter, M. (1992). The outcome of childhood CD: Implications for defining adult personality disorder and CD. *Psychological Medicine, 22,* 971–986.

13

Residential Treatment Centers for Children and Adolescents with Conduct Disorders

PAUL A. LeBUFFE, SUZANNE ROBISON, and DAVIDA J. CHAMBERLIN-ELLIOTT

Any discussion of residential treatment is complicated by the fact that the term can encompass a variety of program settings and models. Residential treatment has been construed to include acute hospitalization, secure (locked) and open (unlocked) units, group homes, and at times, treatment foster care. This lack of definitional consensus has created considerable confusion and has made it difficult to summarize current research. The use of the term residential treatment center (RTC) in this chapter is based on the definition provided by Butler and McPherson (2007). They define RTCs as requiring a therapeutic milieu, multidisciplinary care, deliberate client supervision, intense staff supervision and training, and consistent clinical/administrative oversight. In addition, as used in this chapter, RTC refers to regulated settings that provide care and support to individuals who present both mental health disorders and significant risk management issues. Residential centers that provide primarily child welfare and

PAUL A. LeBUFFE • Devereux Center for Resilient Children
SUZANNE ROBISON • Psychological Services and Human Development Center
DAVIDA J. CHAMBERLIN-ELLIOTT • Outpatient and Substance Abuse Services Devereux Texas Treatment Network

R.C. Murrihy et al. (eds.), *Clinical Handbook of Assessing and Treating Conduct Problems in Youth*, DOI 10.1007/978-1-4419-6297-3_13,

protective services to individuals removed from their homes due to parental supervision issues are not within the purview of this chapter.

RTCs are a significant component of the child mental health system in the United States, providing services to approximately 8% (change symbol to word throughout text) of children with significant mental health disorders each year (Department of Health and Human Services, DHHS, 1999). At year's end in 2002, there were 35,709 youth receiving services in RTCs for emotionally disturbed children (Substance Abuse and Mental Health Services Administration [SAMHSA], 2004). Although RTCs continue to serve a significant portion of children and adolescents with serious mental health disorders, including those with conduct problems such as oppositional defiant disorder (ODD) and conduct disorder (CD), their effectiveness remains controversial. The landmark Report of the Surgeon General on Mental Health (DHHS, 1999) concluded that residential treatment programs, especially for youth, have "only weak evidence for their effectiveness" (p.170). This assertion represented the consensus at that time that residential treatment was not considered to be an evidence-based intervention. Concerns included: a paucity of outcome research, use of poor research methodology, lack of maintenance of treatment gains postdischarge, and lack of generalization of skills to community settings. The sorry state of research a decade ago led to widespread disparaging of residential treatment, culminating in calls for "sanctions by professional and governmental organizations" on practitioners functioning in noncommunity settings (Burns, 2002, p. 8). It is our position that this view of residential treatment is now outdated and does not reflect more recent approaches and evaluation research, especially in intensive treatment settings, which suggest the positive value of residential treatment for youth, families, and society.

RECENT STUDIES SUPPORTING THE EFFECTIVENESS OF RESIDENTIAL TREATMENT

In the past decade, a variety of studies has demonstrated that residential treatment for youth can have positive effects, which generalize to the community and are often sustained for years. For example, Blackman, Eustace, and Chowdhury (1991) assessed the functioning of 40 clients, 10 of whom had CD or ODD, at admission, discharge, and 1–3 years postdischarge. The treatment program, which was designed for high-risk adolescents with a history of unsuccessful treatment, emphasized the development of coping skills within a multimodal family systems approach. The residential program was also integrated with community-based placements including group homes. The typical length of stay was 4–6 months. This study is noteworthy in that it used independent raters who were not involved in the care of the youth and included follow-up data on more than three quarters of the sample. Outcomes were assessed using the Global Assessment Scale (Endicott, Spitzer, Fleiss, & Cohen, 1974), the Level of Functioning Scale (Newman & Rinkus, 1978), and the Adolescent Functioning Scale (Blackman et al., 1991).

Several findings of this study are worth noting. Clinically significant improvement was reported on all three scales between admission and discharge. Whereas 68% of the sample was rated as demonstrating serious or severe behaviors at admission, only 13% fell in this category at discharge. Similarly, 58% of youth demonstrated serious or severe socialization problems at admission vs. 8% at discharge. Follow-up interviews with parents at 1–3 years postdischarge indicated that all gains were maintained and some areas showed further improvement.

One criticism of residential treatment is the paucity of postdischarge follow-up studies that have been published, making lasting change difficult to document. In response, Frankfort-Howard and Romm (2002) examined the long-term effects of residential treatment on the persistence of antisocial behavior into adulthood. The 42 participants in this study had either a diagnosis of CD or had been found delinquent by the courts. This was a diverse sample of adolescents with an average age at admission of 15 years. All attended a residential treatment program based on an eclectic therapeutic milieu for a minimum of 11, and an average of 18 months. To be included in the study, the youth had to be out of residential treatment for at least 1 year. The average time between discharge and follow-up was 6 years. Adult antisocial behavior was determined by systematic review of police records. The major finding was that only 28.6% of the sample evidenced criminal antisocial behavior as adults. This was viewed as a favorable outcome in comparison to other studies (cited by the authors) reporting a persistence rate of 40–50% for antisocial youth not receiving mental health treatment. Moreover, none of the participants who persisted in antisocial behavior as adults completed the residential treatment program, although the authors did not specify what constituted program completion.

Further evidence of the benefits of residential treatment for youth who have engaged in violent behavior is provided by Lyons and Schaefer (2000). They reviewed the records of a random sample of 392 children and adolescents served in RTCs in Florida. Measures included the Child and Adolescent Strength Assessment (CASA; Lyons Uziel-Miller, Reyes, & Sokol, 2000) and the Childhood Severity of Psychiatric Illness (CSPI; Lyons, 1998). Each child was assessed by agency staff upon admission and at a point at least 60 days into treatment. Based on the CSPI Danger to Others scale, the 392 youths were assigned at the outset to one of three groups: (a) nonviolent, (b) historically dangerous, or (c) currently dangerous. The major findings were that the currently dangerous group had the worst dispositional outcomes (only 52% had positive outcomes), but showed the most positive change during treatment compared to the other two conditions. In contrast, the historically dangerous group had better dispositional outcomes (63% positive outcomes) but showed less positive change during treatment than the currently dangerous group. The nonviolent group had the best dispositional outcomes (74% positive outcomes), but the least amount of change during treatment. The nonviolent and currently dangerous groups also differed significantly on the number of strengths as measured by the CASA, with the nonviolent youth having more Peer strengths and Morality/Spiritual strengths. As noted by the authors, it is to be expected that the most dangerous cases would display the greatest clinical improvement because they had the most room for improvement. In regard to the poorer dispositional outcomes, the authors suggested that the more dangerous cases were more likely to have premature, unplanned discharges due to absent without leave status, or discharge to detention centers or acute hospitals. They concluded that youth are more likely to benefit from an RTC if they remain in placement and complete the treatment program.

Shabat, Lyons, and Martinovich (2008) specifically examined residential outcomes for youth aged 6–20 years with ($n=120$) and without ($n=336$) CD. These youth attended 50 different RTCs and group homes throughout the State of Illinois. Youth with CD showed significant improvement between admission and discharge in overall mental health, depressive symptoms, cognitive performance, interpersonal relationships, and security management needs as measured by the Childhood Functional Assessment Rating Scale (CFARS; Ward et al., 1996). In addition, the CD youth showed greater improvement than non-CD youth on five of the CFARS scales: depression, cognitive performance, traumatic stress, medical/physical needs, and interpersonal relationships. The only comparisons in which the CD youth fared worse than non-CD youth were decrease in school attendance and frequency and type of discharge: CD youth tended to have more negative discharges (52% vs. 42%), with much of the difference being due to discharges to the Department of Corrections. The authors note, however, that this could have been due to events that predated their residential stay. Shabat et al. concluded, "not only do youths with behavior problems improve in RTCs and group homes but they may improve more than other youths" (p. 365).

The largest recent study of the outcomes of residential treatment is the Odyssey Project sponsored by the Child Welfare League of America (Drais-Parillo et al., 2008). This study involved youth admitted to residential group care or therapeutic foster care at 22 agencies, from 1994 to 2000. A total of nearly 2,500 participants, aged 3–20 years were involved in the study. Although the report notes improvement on a number of standardized measures including the Child Behavior Checklist (CBCL; Achenbach, 1991), perhaps the most noteworthy finding was that 71% of the youth in residential group care achieved their permanency planning goals, with 49.8% returned to a biological parent at discharge. The Odyssey Project also reported maintenance of positive outcomes at 2 years post discharge, but the response rate (10% of the sample) makes these data of questionable value. In regard to satisfaction, more than two thirds of the youth reported that the treatment program had been helpful and more than half would recommend it to a friend.

Although brief, this review demonstrates that there are a number of studies documenting the positive effects of residential treatment for youth with CD. In addition, some of these studies indicate that positive treatment results in terms of skills acquisition generalize to the community setting; in some cases for years posttreatment.

CURRENT CHALLENGES IN RESIDENTIAL TREATMENT

The positive findings noted are particularly salient given the challenges presented by conduct problem youth in residential treatment programs. As Spreat and Jampol (1997) observed a decade ago, youth get referred to residential treatment programs primarily because of "barrier behaviors" that pose a threat to the child, the family, and society and "effectively bar the child from meaningful pro-social integration." (p. 106). In this sense, residential programs not only provide treatment, but also serve a critical risk-management function preventing youth from engaging in behaviors that would further jeopardize their future or the safety of others in their communities. Residential treatment also serves as a protective factor for the youth themselves, temporarily providing respite from many risk factors including abuse, neglect, interpersonal violence, the stress of chaotic families, exposure to dangerous neighborhoods, and lack of adult supervision (see Butler & McPherson, 2007).

A review of client demographics at two of our Devereux treatment centers for children and youth with conduct problems indicated that these individuals present with significant comorbid problems. Twenty-two clients at these centers had a primary diagnosis of CD, ODD, or Disruptive Behavior Disorder Not Otherwise Specified. The youths' age at admission to Devereux ranged from 10 to 19 years of age, with a median age at admission of 14. Most of these youth did not live with their biological families. Many of the families of origin had problematic profiles with 45% having a history of substance abuse and more than a third (36%) having a history of mental illness in at least one parent. Because we were unable to obtain information on the biological parents of some of the children in foster care, in adoptive placements, or in custody of the state, the actual figures might be considerably higher than those reported here.

Youth in residential treatment also tend to have histories of abuse and neglect; more than half of the youth (55%) in the Devereux centers had been physically or sexually abused or neglected. Many had experienced multiple episodes and multiple types of abuse and neglect. These youth also had a history of dangerous and illegal behaviors including homicidal threats (32%), fire setting (32%), cruelty to animals (27%), suicide attempts (36%), suicide ideation (50%), and perpetrating sexual abuse on others, usually minors (32%). The three most common problems noted in the histories of these clients were self-injurious behaviors, assault, and property destruction, each reported for 59% of the sample. These Devereux clients are not atypical of youth served in RTCs. The figures cited above are, in many cases, remarkably similar to those reported for over 1,300 youth in the Odyssey Project. These findings lend support to Blackman et al.'s (1991) conclusion that adolescents are often referred to residential treatment because of a multitude of behaviors that pose a threat to themselves and the community.

This was the first episode of care for only one of the Devereux individuals included in this brief review. The range of prior treatment episodes for the remainder of the group was 2–16, with an average of seven prior placements. Similarly, in the Odyssey Project, the youth had an average of five prior living arrangements. Residential treatment continues to be a service that individuals "fail" their way into. With residential treatment often being the last resort before a state hospital or a juvenile facility, youth entering residential programs and their families are, by definition, refractory to many outpatient treatment programs: moreover, they are often jaded, demoralized, and inured to treatment.

Effective residential treatment for youth with conduct problems is a challenge. As noted above, these individuals are often hard to treat, present multiple, complex problems, and often lack families or other significant social supports. However, positive outcomes are possible as the earlier review attests. With increasingly acute clients and decreasing lengths of stay, the need for a targeted, coordinated, effective, multisystems treatment is paramount. The essential elements of such a comprehensive program are included in the Devereux approach and described in the remainder of this chapter.

A MODEL OF CARE FOR CONDUCT PROBLEM YOUTH IN RTCS

As a field, behavioral healthcare has come a long way from operating from a "one size fits all" treatment stance. While common strengths and needs among the population drive a program model as a whole, an individualized approach should drive each person's plan of care. Treating the individual rather than the disorder requires attending to multiple problems through a multimodal approach. One advantage that residential treatment offers is the ability to assess the individual's level of functioning in multiple key life areas, and then to address those areas in a consistent, coordinated and hierarchical fashion.

Within the daily structure, programming may vary quite a bit among facilities and across time. Typically however, a youth's day may include educational programming, group, individual, and family therapy, psychoeducational groups, meetings, or lectures, and recreation and leisure time. Criticisms of residential treatment programs include a lack of opportunity to generalize skills to external environments, a need-driven rather than strength-based focus, and a failure to establish a comprehensive system of care upon discharge. In reality, residential treatment providers are often forced to prioritize safety issues, resulting in secondary or tertiary issues falling by the wayside. Establishing programmatic goals based on common needs of the population enables practitioners to hierarchically prioritize treatment needs among youth with conduct problems. There are four levels within this hierarchy. The Level I goal of practitioners is to establish basic safety and stabilization. Once clients are stable, Level II requires practitioners to develop and enhance their client's skills. As that process begins, and throughout the course of treatment, clinicians assure that these skills are being generalized to the youth's natural environments such as school and home in Level III. Finally, in preparation for and soon after discharge, providers operating within Level IV actively engage in discharge and aftercare planning to foster a system of care that extends beyond the residential setting.

Across each of the above levels, key areas of need or "domains" must also be addressed throughout care. These include (a) psychological and medical conditions, (b) academic and vocational factors, (c) family and social dynamics, and (d) community and legal issues. Multiple deficits in functioning within these areas often present a challenge to clinicians attempting to prioritize the needs of youth and to organize treatment interventions. The model that follows offers a systematic way of addressing common needs of youth and provides professionals with a method for prioritizing program goals effectively. The interventions and approaches presented within this model were developed using both research-based interventions recommended within the field, and practice-based interventions based on clinical judgment and experience, drawing upon Devereux's nationwide treatment network. Furthermore, many of these approaches are recommended by county, state, and national accrediting, funding, and regulatory bodies. Table 13.1 illustrates goals (Levels) to be achieved throughout residential treatment, across multiple areas of need (Domains).

It is important to note that there is no set timeframe in which youth should be expected to transition from one level to the next. Rather, each individual will progress through treatment at his or her own pace, depending on individual factors within the child, his or her family and culture, and the larger community. However, with shorter lengths of stay becoming the norm and not the exception, professionals need to remain cognizant of the fact that youth may potentially be discharged from treatment during any one of these levels of residential care, and should strive to meet as many of the individual's needs as possible throughout the course of treatment.

Level I: Establishing Basic Safety and Stabilization

Level I, establishing basic safety and stabilization, is the primary goal of RTCs and with decreases in funding and shortened treatment episodes, sometimes these are the only interventions facilities are able to offer. In order to reduce youths' risk and the risks to those around them, safety within all domains is crucial. This will enable long-term stabilization, not just simply minimize overt dangerous behaviors. Reducing risk factors within the youth, at home, at school and work, and within the larger community is the overall target of Level I.

Domain A: Psychological and Medical Conditions

There are several issues within the psychological and medical domain that need to be addressed throughout the Level I stage of treatment, including physical illness, high-risk behaviors often accompanying conduct problems, and co-occurring mental health diagnoses such as substance use disorders (SUDs) and posttraumatic stress disorder (PTSD). These problems require early and ongoing evaluation and interventions on the part of the treatment team, in order to thwart the effects these behaviors and co-occurring conditions have on the individual.

Table 13.1. A model of care for CD youth within residential treatment

	Domains			
Levels	A. Psychological and medical conditions	B. Educational and vocational factors	C. Family and social dynamics	D. Community and legal issues
IV. Fostering a system of care	Establish discharge/aftercare planning from admission Establish a relapse prevention plan Arrange post discharge follow up and consultation as needed Arrange outpatient medical/MH care	Assist youth in decision-making processes Enroll in school Apply to trade school/college Secure full-time employment Secure GED/ enroll in tutoring Finalize work skills portfolio	Develop supports Provide aftercare connections Provide support group information Establish steps to access future treatment	Establish clear criteria for resolution for of legal issues Track recidivism rates Provide resources for youth and families within their communities
III. Assuring generalization	Work with third parties to offer increasing off-grounds opportunities Monitor positive and negative progress actively	Teach study skills Provide off-grounds work opportunities Bring in outside individuals to discuss career options Teach life skills	Offer home visits Increase family members responsibility Identify resources for families Increase prosocial peers	Offer opportunities for legal resolution Coordinate increasingly with legal representatives Encourage community involvement
II. Enhancing Skills development	Increase replacement behaviors Develop an early and strong rapport Apply evidence-based/ clinically sound practices	Provide vocational training Provide on-grounds life skills responsibilities Improve school conduct attendance and achievement	Offer parent management training and family therapy Set and maintain healthy boundaries Provide social skills training	Provide BARJ Help youth recognize the impact of criminal behaviors Increase involvement of legal representatives
I. Establishing basic safety and stabilization	Provide a differential diagnosis Reduce/control antisocial behaviors Complete medical/psychiatric evaluations Screen for and manage communicable diseases Address co-occurring diagnoses	Reduce acting out in school Provide educational and vocational assessment Design academics around strengths/need Provide low-risk daily structure Complete a thorough biopsychosocial assessment	Remove youth from dangerous environment Allow family respite Problem solve with third parties to reduce barriers to treatment involvement Provide strong advocacy and clear communication with third parties	Reduce risks to general community and peers within RTC Put in place environmental precautions Begin communication with legal representatives Provide trained, supportive staff within a consistent, structured milieu

Comorbid Medical Conditions

One of the first services provided when a client is referred to a 24-h care setting is a medical and/or psychiatric evaluation, often with the primary focus of assessing psychopharmacological needs. This is a critically important aspect of care. Chronic conditions such as head trauma and seizure disorders are strongly associated with conduct problems in youth (American Academy of Child and Adolescent Psychiatry, 2007), and these youth often have been deprived of healthcare prior to entering treatment for a variety of reasons. The absence of healthcare benefits, substance use among caretakers, or damage resulting from high-risk behaviors are just some factors that put these youth at risk for comorbid medical conditions. In addition, multiple placements such as detention centers, foster care homes, and community shelters put these youth and the individuals residing with them at risk for communicable diseases, which should be screened for and managed throughout care.

A medical plan of care is necessary during Level I, followed by ongoing follow-up care and periodic reassessment of medical needs up to and postdischarge. Furthermore, medical conditions or side effects from psychotropic medications may exacerbate many conduct symptoms, and professionals working in RTCs should be provided training that will increase their awareness of these interactions. Special accommodations may be necessary for youth whose medical or psychiatric conditions are interfering with their ability to follow the daily structure in such programs.

High-Risk Behaviors and Comorbid Mental Health Diagnoses

A diagnosis of a conduct problem is correlated with a number of specific life-threatening behaviors that often lead a youth into residential treatment, such as early-onset sexual behavior, reckless driving, self-injurious behavior, physical aggression, and substance use (Frick & Loney, 2002). The high-risk nature of this population necessitates that RTCs prioritize risk management within all areas of care, and provide early and ongoing risk assessment and corresponding levels of supervision. Areas of behavioral risk to be assessed include, but are not limited, to fire setting, aggression toward others and animals, property destruction, self-injurious behavior, sexual offending and acting out, suicidality, eating disorders, and substance use. It should be noted that some of these high-risk behaviors such as self-injurious behavior may serve an adaptive function for some youth. Clinicians should ensure that alternative coping strategies are in place before these high risk behaviors are eliminated or the youth may be at increased risk. Although skill development is emphasized in Level II, the development of alternative coping strategies for high-risk behaviors is essential to safety and therefore appropriate to Level I as well.

Along with these high-risk behaviors, there is a likelihood of comorbid diagnoses, such as substance use and trauma related diagnoses, that also carry high-risk symptoms with them (AACAP, 2007). In an effort to address these problems, RTCs sometimes add a therapeutic component for youth with these additional symptoms or disorders. However, an "add-on" approach, if not fully integrated with the rest of the treatment program, can be detrimental rather than helpful, leading youth to experience an increase in symptoms. For example, youth with substance use disorders (SUDs) may be placed in a group using a substance use prevention model, as opposed to a treatment group designed toward intervention. Similarly, a traumatized youth engaging in a discussion about his or her trauma with an untrained clinician is more likely to be retraumatized than to appropriately process and resolve that trauma. A discussion of common co-occurring disorders is beyond the scope of this chapter; however, brief strategies for minimizing the effects of two high risk comorbid diagnoses, SUDs and post-traumatic stress disorder, are presented here.

Substance Use Disorders

The presence of SUDs presents obvious risks related to the safety of youth, their loved ones, and society as a whole. Within RTCs, these risks continue to be present, and may manifest themselves in behaviors such as using illegal substances or toxins such as paint or cleaners to get high, or acting out addictive behaviors with food, gambling, and so forth. In the past, mental health providers have been trained to deny admission of clients with suspected SUDs to mental health facilities. In recent years however, many states have been advocating a "no wrong door approach" to client care (Center for Substance Abuse Treatment, 2000, p. 4). This approach is aimed at training service providers in the provision of both mental health and substance use services, in order to avoid either discipline turning clients away.

An integrated approach is driven by the understanding that both SUDs and symptoms of other disorders impact the individual simultaneously, and that it is important to address how each set of symptoms comes together and manifests itself within the individual. As such, this integration is reflected in screening, assessment, and treatment planning, rather than treating one issue as "primary" over another. This requires a strong commitment on the part of the agency and its individual professionals to become educated about the nature of SUDs and the proper way to address these issues in youth.

Post-traumatic Stress Disorder

As noted earlier, youth with conduct problems often have experienced some form of trauma such as abuse or witnessing violence, making the integration of a trauma informed care (TIC) model into RTC programming essential. However, integrating TIC into any program can be challenging. Many models for treating trauma address either a singular aspect of treatment such as clinical interventions (Cohen, Mannarino, Deblinger, 2001), or adopting a culture of TIC within the milieu (Bloom, 2005). In response, RTCs must strive to adopt TIC models at both the individual and the program level.

At the individual level, a thorough assessment must be done with youth to determine how to safely apply restrictive procedures if needed. According to Bloom's (2005) Sanctuary model, client involvement in assessment and treatment helps foster feelings of control and personal investment in the therapeutic process, both of which lead to potentially better treatment outcomes. Evidence-based clinical models for reducing the effects of trauma on the individual should be utilized, such as the Trauma Recovery and Empowerment Model (TREM; Harris, 1998), or other cognitive-behavioral interventions specifically aimed at reducing the effects of trauma.

At a programmatic level, it is important for RTCs to operate from a "universal precautions" model (Hodas, 2006), assuming that all clients have experienced some form of trauma. This will avoid retraumatizing already traumatized youth. In addition, RTCs should strive to keep all employees educated about the impact of trauma on clients, and the importance of utilizing TIC methods and approaches. Like integrating substance use treatment, maintaining a TIC system requires strong organizational commitment, especially for RTCs with high rates of staff turnover. However making such a commitment can greatly reduce risk level for a high-risk population.

Domain B: Educational and Vocational Factors

Much of a young person's time is usually spent in school; however, youth with conduct problems are at high risk for school dropout, learning disabilities, repeated discipline problems, and poor academic achievement (AACAP, 2007). RTCs have the ability to offer consistent and specialized academic programming to youth who may have experienced truancy or who may have dropped out of school altogether.

Communication among clinical and educational staff can be challenging in any setting, and educational needs may be secondary to clinical needs, particularly at Level I care. However, functional academic skills are essential and improving academics and reducing acting out in school is a target met through structured and consistent rewards and consequences, as well as consistent, open communication among disciplines. Within this domain, it is essential to provide thorough educational assessments to determine academic strengths and needs, and to design academic instruction around those findings. Furthermore, learning disabilities should be identified at this level and integrated into the overall treatment plan as well as the individual education plan (IEP), using an interdisciplinary approach.

While vocational needs are typically prioritized in adult RTCs, they are often minimized in RTCs treating younger populations. A thorough biopsychosocial assessment program, however, explores youth's vocational experiences, goals, and strengths, as well as academics. Vocationally, many youth are working illegally, legally, or on a volunteer basis, and often need to work early in life due to their lack of academic opportunities or interest, or their family's economic circumstances. A history of early termination from employment, job abandonment, or being caught stealing from employers is not uncommon, and this information can assist the team in properly conceptualizing the problems and diagnostic profile of youth. Programmatically, RTCs should begin to teach basic adaptive daily living skills in Level I, as a step toward Level II, where more advanced life skills are begun to be taught. This skill development is essential for increasing a sense of competency and helping youth to acquire a work ethic. Fostering in youth a sense of responsibility for themselves, others, and their surroundings is a key aspect of all levels within this model of care. However, during Level I, the focus must be on minimizing risk and maintaining safety while developing this sense of responsibility in youth (e.g., youth with a history of self-mutilation should not be working in a kitchen without constant supervision).

Domain C: Family and Social Dynamics

Many referral agencies seek out RTCs as a means of removing youth from violent, abusive, or neglectful environments. Furthermore, familial issues are an area of need that is often difficult to address due to the considerable amount of time and resources it requires. Many significant others have been involved in family services throughout multiple placements, and may have used all of their resources to help care for and manage these youth. By the time these significant others involve themselves in treatment, they often require a period of respite to rebuild their resources and repair relationships. Because family dysfunction, lack of parental skills and resources, and barriers to involvement in treatment (e.g., complicated work schedules, lack of transportation) can make engaging family members in residential treatment a challenge, Level I is primarily a time to problem-solve around reducing barriers to their treatment involvement.

Another challenge often faced by RTCs is determining the appropriateness and timing of home visits or "passes." This can be problematic when the youth, the family, or the placement agency has requested a home pass but the treatment team is concerned about the youth's readiness for a high-risk environment, or the caretaker's ability to monitor the youth at home. Skills have not yet been developed at this level to resist peer pressure and overcome negative peer involvement such as gang-related activities. In most cases, it is recommended that home visits and most off-grounds visits be delayed until Level II is reached, as the youth has not been stabilized in this level of treatment, and families have not received significant interventions to manage youth in the home. This will likely require strong advocacy for youth and families, and clear and repeated communication and collaboration with third parties.

Domain D: Community and Legal Issues

Perhaps the most obvious benefit of residential placement is the natural reduction in risks to the general community that occurs with 24-h placement. Because youths' interactions with the community at large are greatly reduced, there is less opportunity for them to engage in illegal or reckless behaviors. However, individuals within the RTC community must also be safeguarded against youth acting out within the walls of the RTC, or during off-grounds trips, visits, or medical appointments. Providing appropriate trainings for staff, putting environmental precautions in place to reduce risk (e.g., installing door alarms, reducing access to means of suicide), and providing ongoing risk assessments will increase safety within the RTC. In addition, there must be ongoing communication with legal representatives such as probation officers to work toward resolution of legal issues and to ensure adherence to legal contracts on and off the residential campus.

The consistent structure of the milieu is instrumental in providing a sense of stabilization for youth who often have experienced unstructured, inconsistent limits within their environment. A token economy may be useful in helping youth begin to understand both the positive and negative consequences of their behaviors. A varied yet consistent and full daily schedule provides youth with opportunities to gain a sense of accomplishment, and keeps them actively and productively engaged with peers and staff. Finally, the presence of well trained, supportive staff who are willing to communicate among the team and work collaboratively with youth is vital. These individuals can assist youth in understanding their needs and increasing a sense of safety and stabilization in Level I and subsequent levels.

Level II: Enhancing Skill Development

If treatment were to be terminated after Level I, youth and those around them would be safer, but no skills would have been instilled within the individual or the family to maintain this safety and minimize the likelihood of a subsequent placement. Once safety has been established and the youth is stabilized, RTCs should focus in Level II on skill development, emphasizing psychoeducation and therapeutic interventions for youth and their families. Skills taught must be individualized, targeted, and appropriate to the youth's postdischarge environment. Many evidence-based and promising practices exist that are applicable to residential treatment settings. These should be integrated into this second level of treatment as much as possible. Professionals must focus on using this time to develop functional skills within the individual, in an effort to reduce recidivism and enhance quality of life.

Domain A: Psychological and Medical Conditions

Beyond safety, sobriety, and stabilization, the majority of clinical work focuses on skill development for managing conduct-related problems and comorbid disorders. In many ways this is the most active phase of treatment and, because of that, one important priority for professionals is to ensure that the skills being taught to youth and family members complement rather than contradict each other. For example, while mental health professionals traditionally use more supportive techniques, substance abuse professionals tend to be more confrontational. Although both approaches may be effective at times, the use of both requires coordination and planning among professionals and a close monitoring of individual reactions to interventions. In addition, in order to avoid overburdening clients with multiple problem areas that are being addressed simultaneously, treatment plans should be written in language youth can understand, and should be broken down into manageable and incremental steps with appropriate timeframes. Ultimately, treatment should be happening *with* clients and families, not *to* clients and families.

Several promising training models have been found to have moderate effect sizes (American Psychological Association (APA), 2006) for achieving skill acquisition and, when integrated into well-established therapeutic models, can be important adjunct interventions in the treatment of youth with conduct problems. These interventions include anger management training, social skills training, problem-solving therapy, and various parent training models. All of these interventions have been derived from two broader empirically supported models: Behavioral and Cognitive-Behavioral Therapy (CBT). A description of these interventions can be found in earlier chapters; however, some elements are referred to here as well. It is important to note that within this domain, the opportunity to learn life skills is a large benefit of a residential placement, and learning these skills is essential for youth being discharged into independent living. Incremental life skills training should be integrated into treatment planning from Level II through discharge. Critical life skills to be included are daily living skills such as laundry, cooking, grocery shopping, and cleaning; banking skills such as living within a budget and balancing a checkbook; and health and wellness skills such as nutrition and diet, exercise, and medication management.

The assessment and management of areas of need within this domain has been made easier with the development of functional behavior assessment (FBA). FBA has provided clinicians with a highly effective method for understanding how aberrant behavior is shaped and maintained. It focuses on understanding the underlying function (e.g., attention, escape, avoidance) that the negative behavior serves for the individual. The goal of functional assessment is to lead to the identification and training of replacement behaviors that serve the same function, but are more adaptive and prosocial than the negative behaviors the youth are currently using. FBA is an essential component of contemporary residential care (McCurdy & McIntyre, 2004) and is a key strategy for both identifying critical skills to be acquired and eliminating negative behaviors. When completing FBAs it is important to remember that some of the challenging behaviors exhibited by youth (e.g., aggression) may, in fact, be used as survival skills, and may be functional or appropriate to the individual's environment or culture. Professionals working with youth need to be aware of the nature of the postdischarge environment and ensure that the replacement behaviors are adaptive in that setting.

Domain B: Educational and Vocational Factors

Vocational and educational training, though not considered evidence-based practices as sole interventions, are important components of RTC programming. Within the academic setting, school-wide positive behavioral support (SWPBS; Crone & Horner, 2003) should be implemented. SWPBS is a behavioral approach geared toward providing the supports needed for youth to be both academically and socially successful. Within this model, providing clear expectations for youth, teaching the skills necessary to meet those expectations, ongoing interdisciplinary communication, individualized approaches, and data-based decision making regarding treatment needs are used by all members of the team to reduce problem behaviors and build prosocial skills (Crone & Horner, 2003). Increasingly, positive behavior support approaches are being adopted throughout RTCs. Referred to as program-wide positive behavioral support, this approach is critical in that it provides consistency both in the expectations of the youth and in the behavioral responses of adults.

In addition to academics, vocational training opportunities should be made available at this level, and should extend beyond life skills and those basic living skills targeted in Level I. There should be a hierarchical structure to on-campus employment, resulting in enhanced status that comes with holding these positions (e.g., orientation leader, gardener, clerk). Opportunities for promotions based on displaying solid therapeutic work and positive job performance should be in place and integrated into the behavior modification system. Vocational mastery can be achieved through interviewing for and requesting staff recommendations for on-site jobs, resume writing, and developing a vocational portfolio.

Domain C: Family and Social Dynamics

According to Sholevar and Schwoeri (2003), family interventions for youth with conduct problems should focus on developing the following skills within the family: (a) increase parental figures' involvement with one another; (b) improve appropriate bonding between the parent and youth; (c) improve successful management of youth's behavior; (d) improve family cohesiveness, collaboration, and affect; (e) improve family communication, conflict resolution, and problem-solving skills; (f) establish healthy boundaries; and (g) increase the responsibility of individual family members. The integration of CBT and family therapy models is supported within the literature as an effective treatment approach for achieving many of these goals (see Waldron, Miller, & Tonigan, 2001). In selecting a family therapy model, it is imperative that the treatment team consider the practical (e.g., limited funds, lack of transportation, cultural issues) and emotional (e.g., mental health disorders, exhaustion, or frustration from multiple placements) limitations of the family as a whole, and tailor treatment interventions to meet the needs of each individual family. Multisystemic family therapy (MSFT; Henggeler, Schoenwald, Rowland, & Cunningham, 2002; see Chap. 8) and parent management training (PMT; Chamberlain, 1994; see Chap. 9) are among the methods of family intervention with the most empirical support for helping youth with conduct problems. However, these models are very intensive, and several barriers to treatment involvement may exist for some family members of these youth (e.g., lack of resources, addiction). There are several alternative parent training models discussed within Section II of this handbook that can be used either as adjunct therapies, or as stand-alone interventions.

Along with family relationships, youth with conduct problems experience many challenges with their peers. Associations with deviant peers can make it difficult to avoid peer pressure, and a "street code" makes them reluctant to separate from these peers. Problem-solving and social skills training are important elements in skill building at this level, as exposure to unhealthy peers is to be expected throughout and after care.

Negative outcomes from associating with deviant peers can occur within RTCs as well. There is a risk of "deviancy training" (Dishion, McCord, & Poulin, 1999) in which group sessions with youth can lead to the acquisition and reinforcement of antisocial attitudes and behaviors. Fortunately, the risk of these iatrogenic effects can be minimized by employing several strategies. For instance, using structured skills-oriented groups led by experienced staff reduces risk as compared to unstructured process groups led by less seasoned clinicians. A variety of moderator and mediator variables (e.g., age, attitudes towards delinquency, parental attachment) that influence deviancy training effects have also been identified (Gifford-Smith, Dodge, Dishion, & McCord, 2004).

Domain D: Community and Legal Issues

Youth who are court committed to treatment not only have an additional motivating factor to complete treatment, but have additional resources at their disposal if needed. Similarly, legal involvement increases a clinician's leverage within the program and provides another resource for both funding and assistance with case management. Finally, legal involvement requires the achievement of specific treatment goals, such as those addressed by *Balanced and Restorative Justice (BARJ;* Office of Juvenile Justice Programs, 2006*)*

BARJ, while lacking significant empirical evidence, is considered by many to be a promising practice (Office of Juvenile Justice Programs, 2006), focusing on increasing perpetrator accountability, instilling in youth awareness and empathy for crime victims, and enhancing a sense of safety and protection within communities. Therefore, BARJ reporting by professionals is often an expectation of the court for those youth involved in the criminal justice system, and counties collecting BARJ information maintain extensive data bases from which outcome data can be derived (e.g., recidivism rates, substance use relapse). BARJ includes activities such as empathy training, restitution, and community service. Within Level II, skills should be focused on helping youth understand the impact illegal behavior has on them, their loved ones, and the larger community. Integration of legal goals and objectives, along with ongoing open and regular communication with legal representatives assists youth in actively taking steps toward resolving legal issues.

Level III: Assuring Generalization

While clinicians working within RTCs often report positive outcomes, some youth are unable to transfer learned behaviors to contexts external to the residential placement such as on the street, at home, in school, or in the workplace. To maximize the client's ability to use learned behaviors in everyday living, professionals must collaborate with families, communities, and schools to enhance protective factors and promote generalization.

Domain A: Psychological and Medical Conditions

The effort to generalize learned skills and positive, healthy behaviors can be difficult in RTC environments, mainly due to the nature of the setting itself. Because of the high-risk symptoms, associated conduct problems and the comorbid conditions that resulted in an RTC placement, allowing for off-grounds interactions naturally increases risk to youth and those around them. However, not providing off-campus experiences severely limits the opportunities to practice skills in community settings and may lead to a sense of boredom and frustration for both youth and the treatment team. Level III is an opportunity to partner with families and communities to identify resources and enhance protective factors, incrementally increasing opportunities for skill generalization.

At a programmatic level, this includes expanding external collaborations within the community via marketing strategies (e.g., sending RTC representatives to the local court house to encourage treatment as an alternative to incarceration), maintaining a safe and appropriate environment where outside organizations feel comfortable allowing youth to use their facilities (e.g., providing extra staff to monitor youth while they use a local recreation center to reduce the risk of incidents occurring on their property), and establishing policies and procedures around off-grounds and therapeutic home visits. At the individual level, youth should be afforded opportunities to engage in off-grounds activities and home visits in order to begin to generalize these skills. There are two common problems that serve as barriers to youth gaining experience using skills in community settings. First, it may be difficult for RTCs to find staff to take youth off grounds for appointments or trips. Accompanying a client in the community requires well-trained staff both to manage risk and to take advantage of opportunities for skill rehearsal. Second, staff often have limited time to follow up with youth after off-grounds trips or appointments. It is important to review the client's use of newly acquired skills in naturalistic settings and to problem-solve any challenges the youth may have encountered. Structured home and community pass guidelines and follow-up protocols should be put in place in RTCs, and opportunities for off-grounds activities should be prioritized as critical opportunities to generalize skills.

Symptomatology, although expected to be stabilized by this point, should be monitored throughout care to allow for timely interventions in response to increases in medical or mental health symptoms. If needed, psychopharmacology should be continued throughout this level, with more emphasis placed on psychoeducation, independent medication management, and acceptance of the need for these interventions.

Domain B: Educational and Vocational Factors

Generalizing educational and vocational skills to outside environments is rewarding for both youth and the treatment team. While youth begin to achieve mastery in applying skills to the outside world, members of the treatment team are able to recognize positive changes in their clients and enjoy the natural rewards that come with such changes. Up until this level, youth have been working within the RTC, holding on-campus jobs and fulfilling daily responsibilities, while completing school credits and improving their academics. This level focuses on taking these skills beyond the RTC. Youth are often able to attend school or work at local community organizations, and can thereby begin mainstreaming to such places while still having the security of the RTC in place. It is in this stage of treatment that if youth begin earning money, they can experience some advanced life skill opportunities such as choosing and managing a bank account or learning to shop for healthy foods. Within the RTC, time should be spent on teaching youth independent study skills, assisting them with finding employment in the classifieds or on career websites, and providing them exposure to career counseling with outside representatives.

Domain C: Family and Social Dynamics

Along with gaining more off-grounds experiences, an improvement in positive relationships with family members, peers, and authority figures should occur in Level III. Psychoeducation about medication, mental illness, etcetera; structured monitoring of home visits; and parent training should be offered in an ongoing manner, in order to sustain changes within the family and social system. Finally, the opportunity for family therapy continues in Level III, with deeper issues (e.g., resolving resentments, establishing healthy boundaries) often becoming therapeutic content.

In addition, along with prosocial experiences like work and school, youth should be associating more with prosocial peers (e.g., community youth groups or recreational centers), increasing the chance of dissolving unhealthy relationships and establishing positive relationships with peers. Opportunities for youth to take on leadership roles within the RTC should also be increasingly available, such as allowing youth to serve on advisory boards or as mentors to clients who are new to the program.

Domain D: Community and Legal Issues

Because of the tendency for youth with CD to engage in illegal activities, completion of an RTC episode of care may be a condition of the court for many youth. Therefore, it is important to integrate legal considerations into the treatment plan. In those cases where the legal representative is at a distance from the RTC, maintaining his or her active involvement can be a challenge. Regardless of the extent of this involvement, during RTC placement many legal obligations can be met. Community service hours, restitutions, and fine payments can be arranged while in treatment, often requiring little work on the part of the RTC team, other than active coordination with third parties. Professionals often need to act as advocates and/or liaisons with judges, probation or parole officers, or other legal representatives, working to establish and maintain open communication and cooperation among disciplines.

In addition to resolving legal issues, youth learning to generalize skills to various contexts need to gain a sense that they are part of a larger community, and need to be afforded opportunities to give back to their communities. Volunteer work with animals, the elderly, or organizations of need, as well as less formal activities, such as asking youth to give a tour of the RTC to visitors, are encouraged to instill a sense of community in youth. Finally, discharge and aftercare needs must be assessed carefully at the completion of Level III, in preparation for more active discharge planning throughout the domains in Level IV.

Level IV: Fostering a System of Care

The highest level within residential care, Level IV, requires an active focus on discharge and aftercare planning, in order to foster a system of care postdischarge. This by no means suggests that aftercare planning begins close to discharge. On the contrary, discharge planning should begin preadmission, and continue throughout care. However, this planning becomes more active in the final stages of treatment, requiring more time to be spent on discharge and aftercare planning, and more frequent consultation with ancillary providers. Collaboration with significant others, funding and referral sources, as well as community organizations will establish a wider net of ongoing support for youth to continue to utilize skills acquired for maintaining long-term changes.

Domain A: Psychological and Medical Conditions

The final level of consideration within this domain requires active discharge and aftercare planning related to the youth's psychological and medical needs. Along with planning for discharge, the treatment team must work hard at this stage to provide appropriate closure for youth, an important task due to the high likelihood of these youth experiencing early loss, trauma, or inappropriate closure in other settings. The focus of individual and group sessions during this level of treatment should be on processing feelings related to termination, as well as confronting acting out or regressive behaviors. Finally, establishing a formal relapse prevention plan is crucial at this stage, in order to put strategies into place in the event of exposure to triggers and/or relapse to preadmission behaviors.

Although RTCs are often responsible for aftercare planning, at times professionals wait until discharge is imminent to set up aftercare plans, creating a gap in services that can lead to regression or perceived undoing of positive changes the youth has made. Clear discharge criteria, as well as opportunities for medical and behavioral aftercare programming, should be established before admission to avoid youth and families receiving inappropriate or inadequate postdischarge services. Furthermore, beyond aftercare facilitation, postdischarge follow up can assist in tracking outcomes and the longevity of treatment gains within youth.

Domain B: Educational and Vocational Factors

Within Level IV, youth are most likely enrolled or preparing to enroll in their home-based school, and depending on their age, may be preparing for posthigh school experiences. The treatment team, in concert with third parties such as significant others and agency representatives, will be assisting the youth in making decisions about his or her future, such as whether to graduate from high school or obtain a General Equivalency Diploma (GED); whether to go to college, work, or trade school; and where youth should live, work, or go to school. This decision-making process is extremely important for youth who not only need support in making these choices, but also need to learn how to make these choices for themselves.

Five issues should be considered by the treatment team when helping youth make educational and vocational decisions. First, and most importantly, clinicians, along with the interdisciplinary team, need to recruit the youth's significant others to help determine what type of environments will be most appropriate for sustaining gains made within the RTC program. Second, youth continuing in school need an educational placement that can meet both their academic and social-emotional needs. Third, those who decide to obtain a GED should either have earned it while in placement, or be involved in services that will assist in meeting this goal postdischarge. Fourth, those bound for college or trade school will need help selecting and applying for these schools, as well as exploring funding options and selecting an area of study. Finally, employment opportunities should be increased via skill development and an established portfolio including a resume and letters of reference. Mock interviews for offsite employment can prepare youth to face academic or employment interview processes. Having multiple systems involved with youth can be an advantage at this stage as more resources, assistance, and perspectives are made available. However, this can also be a disadvantage when there are contradictory agendas at work, requiring treatment team members to practice strong advocacy and communication skills.

Domain C: Family and Social Dynamics

As with the youth themselves, discharge from placement can be both an exciting time and a time of great anxiety for significant others. Increasing structured therapeutic home visits is important during this final level of treatment, with methods to track progress put in place to prevent relapses from going unaddressed. While the youth is the identified client in these cases, the family system is an essential part of the youth's recovery, and so establishing aftercare and identifying resources and supports for the family increases the youth's chance of success. Family therapy may be indicated on an outpatient basis, as well as family support groups such as Al-anon or Nar-anon (support groups for family members of individuals with substance use problems), or local parenting groups. In Level IV, significant others and clients often find comfort in the use of telephone consultation or a follow up face-to-face visit with the clinician, even if brief. As part of a comprehensive discharge plan, steps for accessing treatment in the future should be clearly established, including contact names, addresses, and phone numbers of aftercare and RTC team members. Because of the importance of peer relationships with younger individuals, youth who have not established a pro-social peer network by Level IV should be connected with local youth centers and/or recreational activities where positive peer support can be established postdischarge.

Domain D: Community and Legal Issues

The final domain within Level IV involves legal and community issues postdischarge. While legal issues may not be resolved upon discharge, clear criteria for achieving resolution should be in place for the youth and for their significant others. Postdischarge communication with legal representatives should occur to track recidivism rates for the overall program. Finally, quality improvement initiatives can assist programs in continuing to improve future programming for youth, and can help RTCs work to reduce rates of recidivism.

Involvement at local places of worship, places of business, or community centers can instill a larger sense of community in youth postdischarge, and decrease youth's risk of regression by providing structured activities to combat boredom. Youths' ability to "give back" by providing talks or mentoring at-risk youth within the larger community should be encouraged and arranged predischarge as much as possible. Alumni groups can also assist youth in gaining a sense of community by involving them in continuous quality improvement at the RTC. Finally, in addition to postdischarge therapy, support groups within the community are often indicated, such as Alcoholics or Narcotics Anonymous, or groups related to sexuality, gender, or other culture-specific domains.

Summary

The levels and domains described above are not intended to encompass every need with which youth with conduct problems may present. However, professionals working in an RTC setting can use this model to assist with reducing risks commonly associated with these problems, while organizing problems, goals, objectives, and interventions in an incremental way. In implementing this model, certain core elements must be present across all levels. The first is a high level of consistency. This requires the presence of well-trained and supervised professionals who utilize "teachable moments" throughout the day to instill skills and reinforce clinical, educational, and vocational goals. The direct care professional is often viewed as the primary change agent within RTCs and ensures consistency across levels and domains. The second is a consistent, safe, and nurturing environment to provide the context of care, traditionally referred to as a therapeutic milieu. Third is interdisciplinary communication and collaboration that addresses the multiple needs of CD youth in a holistic fashion. The last is a continual focus on the postdischarge environment, which requires advocacy, case management, and inter-agency coordination. The case study that follows offers an example of how the hierarchical approach suggested here assisted one youth in a Devereux RTC to overcome symptoms of conduct problems and related life consequences.

CASE STUDY JOEY: A YOUTH WITH CONDUCT PROBLEMS BENEFITING FROM RTC PLACEMENT

Joey is a 16-year-old African-American male who was born and raised in New Jersey. At the time of this writing he had spent a little over 1 year in one of Devereux's RTCs, and he was considered to be toward the end of Level II in the treatment model presented here. Joey has no significant medical issues other than a history of asthma that required no specific intervention. He reported upon admission that he had been sexually active since he was 13 and up until that time was not practicing safe sex, leaving him at high risk for related complications.

Joey presented with a history of failed outpatient and RTC placements prior to coming to Devereux. He had been placed in acute psychiatric hospitals since the age of 8 for "being out of control" and was in one RTC from age 13 to 14. Joey has a history of hyperactivity and angry outbursts which led to assaultive behaviors. He also had a history of lying when he felt that he would benefit as well as a history of stealing and property destruction.

Upon admission, he was entering his second year of high school and his vocational history consisted only of selling illegal substances to earn money. Joey was referred by his probation officer due to legal issues and expulsion from school. The goal for this placement according to the referral source was to "stabilize Joey's mood and behavior" and he was expected to abstain from drug use and attend a substance abuse program, take mood stabilizing medication compliantly, reduce acting out in school and improve academic achievement, develop a positive relationship with his mother, and develop anger management, problem solving, and social skills.

There were no reported mental or physical health issues in his family history. His mother and father had never been married and Joey's father was reportedly incarcerated at the time of his placement, although at the time of this writing, his father was currently out of prison and requesting a relationship with Joey. He reported that he has never had a "good" relationship with his father, and he was not sure that he really wanted one.

His legal involvement began at age 12 as a result of, according to referral information, "dangerous behaviors." His most recent legal charges resulted in a juvenile detention stay for selling crack cocaine, and subsequently he was placed on probation for charges of possession of illegal substances. He reported that he began using cannabis at age 14 and used heavily at one time. However, he stated that he had not used cannabis since approximately 4 months prior to being placed in juvenile detention. Although he had a history of crack cocaine sales beginning at the age of 15, he denied the use of crack cocaine.

Functional assessment revealed antecedents and consequences of Joey's behaviors, and helped the treatment team identify specific target behaviors needing strengthening or extinguishing. His strengths were assessed to be a willingness to engage in treatment, a desire to improve his physical health, openness to discussing past behaviors, eagerness to improve family relationships, a strong sense of competency related to sports, good listening skills, and a healthy fear of returning to his preadmission environment. Limitations and areas for improvement included difficulty respecting authority, a history of multiple failed placements, a tendency to act out aggressively, and minimization of his drug-related lifestyle. Upon admission, Joey was diagnosed with the following:

Axis I	314.01	ADHD, Combined type
	312.82	Conduct disorder adolescent onset
	296.90	Mood disorder, NOS
	315.0	Learning disorder by history
Axis II	799.9	Deferred
Axis III		History of asthma
Axis IV		Severe: social support, educational, and legal problems
Axis V		GAF: 40 current 45 highest prior year

Level I: Safety and Stabilization

Upon his admission to Devereux, Joey completed a biopsychosocial assessment, risk assessment, psychiatric and medical evaluation, and toxicology screening and was placed on appropriate precautions and levels of supervision to ensure safety. Due to high levels of aggression he remained on the unit and was under close observation throughout the initial assessment phase. Although at the time of this writing Joey was still an active client, a comprehensive aftercare plan and relapse prevention plan are being formulated, and will be in place prior to discharge, including preliminary discharge criteria identified in Level I. These criteria included: demonstrating an ability to maintain stability in his moods, regular use of anger management skills, verbalizing a commitment to ongoing sobriety, and displaying improved behaviors and achievement in an academic setting.

Domain A: Psychological and Medical Conditions

During Level I treatment, triggers to aggressive behavior were identified by Joey and the treatment team as were de-escalation strategies that had been effective in preventing the escalation of anger in the past (identified by Joey and his family). These strategies were implemented to help him remain safe in his environment. The focus up to this point had been placed on what could be done to calm him down after he was already upset with no proactive strategies being employed such as anger management skills or problem resolution techniques. To address his co-occurring substance use, Joey was placed in a weekly substance abuse group aimed at providing psychoeducation and identifying triggers to substance use and related cognitions and behaviors. To address his high-risk sexual behaviors, Joey received psychoeducation about sexually transmitted diseases and safe sex practices.

Domain B: Educational and Vocational Factors

Due to Joey's history of acting out in school and poor academics, his RTC placement has assisted him in maintaining school attendance and receiving academic training appropriate to his strengths and needs. Vocationally, in Level I Joey began taking on daily responsibilities such as doing chores within the RTC, until further vocational training was deemed appropriate by the treatment team.

Domain C: Family and Social Dynamics

Joey's RTC placement served to remove him from unhealthy peer interactions and to give his family respite from assaultive behaviors that had been unmanageable up until this point. However, his mother resided a good distance from his placement, making family therapy and home visits a challenge. The treatment team used the time in Level I to engage Joey's mother and develop plans for telephonic family sessions throughout care. Family and social dynamics were examined via review of records, biopsychosocial assessment, and client and third-party interviews.

Domain D: Community and Legal Issues

There was a natural reduction in risks to Joey's own community resulting from his placement. Involvement with Joey's probation officer began in Level I with the treatment team striving to establish regular, open communication with legal representatives. Programmatically, Joey began interacting with well-trained staff within a secure, therapeutic environment.

Level II: Enhancing Skills Development

After a substantial amount of assessment information had been gathered and basic safety and stabilization had begun, Level II began with a focus on prioritization of treatment goals. Goals were derived from a variety of sources, such as client and third-party interviews, review of past records, biopsychosocial and risk assessment information, and specialized screenings and assessments such as the Devereux Scales of Mental Disorders (DSMD, Naglieri, LeBuffe, & Pfeiffer, 1994) and the Substance Abuse Subtle Screening Inventory-Adolescent Version 2 (SASSI-A-2; Miller, 1990). Joey's identified goals were integrated into his treatment plan, including: (a) development of anger management skills; (b) reduction of substance use; (c) improvement of family relationships; (d) development of social skills; (e) increased academic achievement; and (f) enhanced health and wellness strategies. Throughout the course of treatment, there were notable changes in the way Joey responded to the daily structure inside and outside of the RTC, evidenced by data collection and tracking methods (see Fig. 13.1).

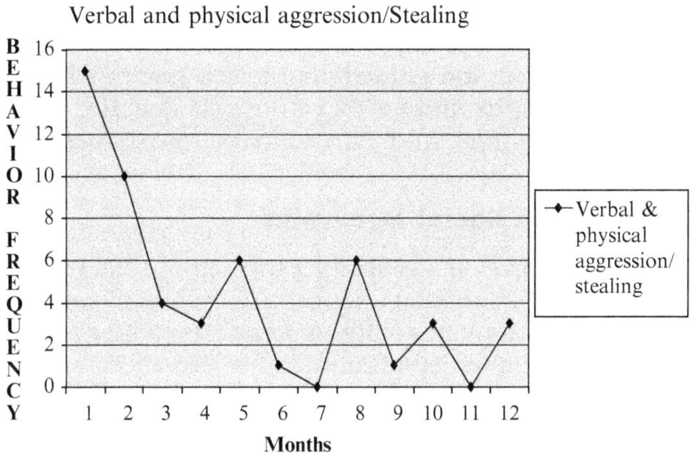

Fig. 13.1. Data analysis across a 12 month span for one youth in residential treatment.

Domain A: Psychological and Medical Conditions

In the area of aggression toward others Joey began exploring his use of aggression, leading to his ability to verbalize the importance of using anger management skills. His therapist utilized the Rational Emotive Behavior Therapy "A-B-C-D-E" method (Ellis & Harper, 1997), allowing him to identify his maladaptive belief system and teaching him specific skills to utilize in lieu of inappropriate expression of his anger. He began participating in substance abuse groups in Level I, and in Level II his participation increased. His verbalizations demonstrated that he had developed an understanding of how substance use impacted his life. He showed insight about his lifestyle as evidenced in discussions with his peers about the effects of his behaviors on his life. In Level III, Joey will begin the intensive substance use group which will help him move beyond psychoeducation and early identification of triggers to substance use. This group will examine more subtle triggers, introduce the 12 Step philosophy, and allow him to identify and address necessary lifestyle changes that must take place after the substance use stops. Postgroup self-report measures will be used to measure the degree to which Joey has internalized these concepts, and to monitor symptomatology related to substance use issues.

Domain B: Educational and Vocational Factors

Academically, Joey has been assessed using Standardized Testing and Reporting (Understanding the STAR, 2008), and although his admission diagnosis included a learning disorder by history, results of these tests and classroom observations led Devereux educational staff to rule this diagnosis out, attributing much of the academic difficulties he has had to symptoms related to ADHD and CD. Overall, he exhibited positive behaviors within the education program, and developed aspirations of attending some type of postsecondary school program, hopefully with a basketball scholarship. Vocationally, he obtained employment as an on-grounds landscaper, and stated that he enjoyed this type of work very much. In Level III, further vocational and educational assessments will take place to better determine strengths and needs within this domain, as well as to assist in formulating vocational and educational aftercare plans.

Domain C: Family and Social Dynamics

Joey has worked to develop social skills throughout his treatment. He began by receiving psychoeducation about the definition of social skills, as he exhibited few and had limited ability to verbalize social skills concepts upon admission. Shortly after admission, he began receiving points for the utilization of proper skills at appropriate times, and at the time of this writing had begun exhibiting more frequent use of specific social skills. He now recognizes and verbalizes impulses to act inappropriately in social situations.

Throughout Level I, Joey's family struggled to find consistent times for family therapy. Once regular interactions over the phone began and rapport had been established between clinic staff and Mrs X, family sessions could commence over the phone. First, this involved psychoeducation to help all parties understand the dynamics of family communication, and second, Joey was able to practice setting limits with his mother. During these sessions both Joey and his mother learned to communicate more effectively. Furthermore, both have openly been discussing Joey's patterns of dishonesty, and have begun at the time of this writing to explore the functions of his dishonesty, as well as the impact it has on their relationship.

Domain D: Community and Legal Issues

Although Joey's probation officer resides quite a distance away from Joey's placement, she has been active in his treatment and regularly involved in team meetings discussing Joey's progress, treatment, and aftercare needs. She has been clear about the status of Joey's legal issues and the steps he needs to take to abide by his probation contract. BARJ principles are being applied with Joey; he and his therapist have begun discussing the impact his drug dealing has had on his life and on the larger community. Further exploration of his juvenile justice involvement and the impact these behaviors have had on him and others will occur in Level III.

Levels III and IV: Assuring Generalization and Fostering a System of Care

At the time of this writing, Joey is just beginning Level III. He is able to recite skills that he uses such as walking away, taking time out, and so forth. He reportedly still gets angry and he can overreact or respond negatively without provocation, but as can be seen in Figure 13.1, this has become the exception rather than the norm. However, he struggles with generalizing these skills to a variety of situations and contexts, reverting to acting out at times. Joey has been proudly able to state that he has had significant periods of time with no incidents; nevertheless, he sometimes expresses hopelessness about his inability to maintain these changes. He often states that he grew up in the streets and he fully expects to go back to the streets when he goes home, where being "good" is viewed by his peers as "bad." In talking with him it is obvious that he is aware that he has learned adaptive skills in a controlled environment in which he is given the opportunity to apply these skills. However, the treatment team will soon need to turn its focus to more actively fostering a system of care to which he can return.

Although Joey has yet to complete Levels III and IV of residential treatment, he has made solid progress. His case is a good illustration of common struggles faced by youth with conduct problems and interventions targeted at these struggles. This case study presents an individualized approach using the key domains and levels within the model of care presented in this chapter. Joey has been in treatment just over a year and has struggled to consistently utilize the prosocial skills developed. His considerable distance from his home makes generalizing the skills learnt to his natural community difficult, but he is beginning to work toward opportunities to generalize skills in a variety of contexts within the nearby community surrounding Devereux. Because of the multiple complex factors and high-risk behaviors that accompany his conduct problems, lengths of stay will vary greatly depending on the needs of the individual and the speed with which each youth progresses in treatment.

SUMMARY AND CONCLUSIONS

Since the publication of Jane Knitzer's book, Unclaimed Children (1982) and Stroul and Friedman's landmark 1986 monograph on systems of care, there have been remarkable developments in community-based, nonresidential programs (Burns & Hoagwood, 2002). The efficacy of some of these programs such as Multisystemic Therapy (Schoenwald & Rowland, 2002), the Wraparound model (Burchard, Bruns, & Burchard, 2002), and Treatment Foster Care (Chamberlain, 2002) led to the expectation that residential treatment would become unnecessary and that all children and youth with serious emotional disorders would be served effectively in their homes, neighborhood schools, and local communities. This expectation has not been realized for at least two reasons. First, many communities still do not have a full continuum of treatment options for youth with conduct problems. Second, even with the most efficacious of community-based treatment programs, it has still been necessary to place at least some youth in psychiatric hospitals and RTCs when their symptoms have become too acute and posed risks that could not be effectively managed in the community (Henggeler et al., 1997).

At the end of the first decade of the twenty-first century, residential treatment remains an important component of a comprehensive system of care for children and youth. There continues to be a cadre of youth whose behavior poses such a threat to their own welfare and the safety of others that residential treatment remains the treatment of choice.

The positive contribution of quality RTCs was recognized by SAMHSA, which in 2006 convened the Building Bridges conference with the explicit goal of better integrating community-based and residential programs (SAMHSA, 2006). The joint resolution that emanated from this conference both affirmed the value of 24-h (i.e., residential) care and called for a commitment to further develop community-based services to decrease the need for 24-h services and facilitate transition back into the community. Importantly, one of the explicit goals of this meeting was to "address the historic tensions between residential and community-based service providers and systems" (p. 2).

Although the overall value of residential services has been reaffirmed by this major organization, it is still the case that much work remains to be done. To facilitate the continued evolution of residential programs as an effective and efficient component of a comprehensive system, we recommend the following steps:

1. Develop a uniform operational definition of residential treatment. As noted in the introduction, the lack of a consistent definition has greatly impeded research, training, and public policy (Butler & McPherson, 2007). We support their definition of residential treatment as requiring a therapeutic milieu, multidisciplinary care, deliberate client supervision, intense staff supervision and training, and consistent clinical/administrative oversight. In addition, in research and policy the distinctions should be made between regulated and unregulated residential care, and RTCs that serve individuals with mental health diagnoses and high-risk behaviors vs. those that serve primarily a child welfare population.
2. Articulate clear program models. A better understanding and the continued evolution of residential treatment is dependent on providers being able to clearly articulate their residential treatment program model. We should emulate the advances in community-based care by clearly describing, to the greatest extent possible, our programs, their components, logic models, and theories of change.
3. Adopt clinical quality improvement models. Residential treatment has long been criticized for its weak research basis, including, among other concerns, the lack of true experimental designs with randomized assignment. True efficacy research is not a possibility in the large majority of residential programs, mainly due to the complex and severe presentation of youth in need of residential treatment. Clearly, random assignment is not ethical, nor is it practical, particularly in publicly funded programs. Neither are some quasi-experimental options such as delayed treatment or wait list controls. Alternatively, it would be far more effective to utilize different research strategies arising from the clinical quality improvement field such as Total Clinical Outcomes Management (Lyons, 2004). These approaches focus on enhancing effectiveness by making successive and incremental improvements over past performance in response to programmatic change. As such, they are far more practical, ethical and contextually valid than more traditional research designs.
4. Redefine the goal of treatment. Historically, residential care was characterized by lengths of stay measured in years and vague and

diffuse treatment goals such as the restructuring of personality or the building of "character." As a result of managed behavioral healthcare, episodes of care are much briefer and the goal of treatment is often the reduction of specific barrier behaviors to a level that can be addressed or at least tolerated in the community. In relation to the model of care presented above, the focus in these cases is squarely on Level 1. However, it is reasonable to think that in many cases, the individual, the family, and society might be better served by a longer length of stay that provides an opportunity to further develop the key competencies and to plan for generalization to the postdischarge environment.

5. Increase involvement with community providers. There is consensus that the probability of postdischarge success is greatly enhanced by detailed, individualized discharge plans and close communication and collaboration with community providers. However, there remain many barriers to this partnership. Some barriers such as distance can be overcome; others, such as agency regulations limiting residential providers' role in postdischarge care, are more challenging. In line with recommendations made at the Building Bridges conference (SAMHSA, 2006), these territorial boundaries must be addressed by RTCs in order to meet their vision of an integrated, comprehensive system of care.

A decade ago, the Surgeon General concluded that there was very weak evidence for residential treatment. This is no longer the case. Although not necessarily compelling, the evidence for the effectiveness of residential treatment, especially for youth with conduct problems, can at least no longer be summarily dismissed. With further elaboration of specific treatment models and the adoption of more appropriate clinical quality improvement methodologies, the unique role of residential care in the comprehensive array of services will continue to evolve.

ACKNOWLEDGMENT

The authors would like to thank the Devereux Professional Psychology Trainees and the Quality Improvement Department's support staff for their diligence and assistance in preparing this chapter.

REFERENCES

Achenbach, T. M. (1991). *Manual for the child behavior checklist/4-18 and 1991 profile.* Burlington, VT: University of Vermont, Department of Psychiatry.

American Academy of Child and Adolescent Psychiatry. (2007). Practice parameter for the assessment and treatment of children and adolescents with attention-deficit/hyperactivity disorder. *Journal of American Academy of Child and Adolescent Psychiatry, 46*(7), 894–921.

American Psychological Association. (2006). Report of the working group on psychotropic medications for children and adolescents: psychopharmacological, psychosocial, and combined interventions for childhood disorders: evidence base, contextual factors, and future directions. http://www.apa.org/releases/PsychotropicMedicationsReport.pdf. Accessed 1 August 2007.

Blackman, M., Eustace, J., & Chowdhury, T. (1991). Adolescent residential treatment: a one to three year follow-up. *Canadian Journal of Psychiatry, 36*, 472–479.

Bloom, S. L. (2005). The sanctuary model of organizational change for children's residential treatment therapeutic community. *The International Journal for Therapeutic and Supportive Organizations, 26*(1), 65–81.

Burchard, J. D., Bruns, E. J., & Burchard, S. N. (2002). The wraparound approach. In B. J. Burns & K. Hoagwood (Eds.), *Community treatment for youth: evidence-based interventions for severe emotional and behavioral disorders*. New York: Oxford University Press.

Burns, B. J. (2002). Reasons for hope for children and families: a perspective and overview. In B. J. Burns & K. Hoagwood (Eds.), *Community treatment for youth: evidence-based interventions for severe emotional and behavioral disorders*. New York: Oxford University Press.

Burns, B. J., & Haogwood K. (Eds.). (2002). Community Treatment for Youth: evidence-based interventions for severe emotional and behavioral disorders. New York: Oxford University Press.

Butler, L. S., & McPherson, P. M. (2007). Is residential treatment misunderstood? *Journal of Child and Family Studies, 16*, 465–472.

Center for Substance Abuse Treatment. (2000). *Changing the conversation: Improving substance abuse treatment. The national treatment improvement plan* (DHHS Publication No. SMA 00-3479). Rockville, MD: Center for Substance Abuse Treatment.

Chamberlain, P. (1994). *Family connections: a treatment foster care model for adolescents with delinquency*. Eugene, OR: Castalia.

Chamberlain, P. (2002). Treatment foster care. In B. J. Burns & K. Hoagwood (Eds.), *Community treatment for youth: evidence-based interventions for severe emotional and behavioral disorders*. New York: Oxford University Press.

Cohen, J. A., Mannarino, A. P., & Deblinger, E. (2001). *Child and parent trauma-focused cognitive behavioral therapy treatment manual*. Philadelphia: Drexel University College of Medicine.

Crone, D. A., & Horner, R. H. (2003). *Building positive behavior support systems in schools: functional behavioral assessment*. New York: Guildford Press.

Department of Health and Human Services (DHHS). (1999). *Mental health: a report of the surgeon general*. Rockville: U.S. Department of Health and Human Services.

Dishion, T. J., McCord, J., & Poulin, F. (1999). When interventions harm: peer groups and problem behavior. *American Psychologist, 54*(9), 755–764.

Drais-Parillo, A.A., Baker, A., Fojas, S., Gunn, S., Kurland, D., & Schnur, E. (2008). *The Odyssey Project: A Descriptive and Prospective Study of children and Youth in Residential Group Care and Therapeutic Foster Care*. Washington, DC: The Child Welfare League of America. http://www.cwla.org/programs/research/odysseyfinalreport.pdf. Accessed 12 November 2008.

Ellis, A., & Harper, R. A. (1997). *A guide to rational living* (3rd ed.). Hollywood: Melvin Powers Wilshire Book Company.

Endicott, J., Spitzer, R., Fleiss, J., & Cohen, J. (1974). *The Global Assessment Scale: a procedure for measuring overall severity of psychiatric disturbance*. New York: New York State Psychiatric Institute.

Frankfort-Howard, R., & Romm, S. (2002). Outcomes of residential treatment of antisocial youth: development of or cessation from adult antisocial behavior. *Residential Treatment for Children and Youth, 19*(3), 53–70.

Frick, P. J., & Loney, B. R. (2002). Understanding the association between parent and child antisocial behavior. In R. J. McMahon & R. D. Peters (Eds.), *The effects of parental dysfunction on children* (pp. 105–126). New York: Kluwer Academic/Plenum.

Gifford-Smith, M., Dodge, K. A., Dishion, T. J., & McCord, J. (2004). Peer influence in children and adolescents: crossing the bridge from developmental to intervention science. *Journal of Abnormal Child Psychology, 33*(3), 255–265.

Harris, M. (1998). *Trauma recovery and empowerment: a clinician's guide for working with women in groups*. New York: The Free Press.

Henggeler, S. W., Rowland, M. D., Pickrel, S. G., Miller, S. L., Cunningham, P. B., Santos, A. B., Schoenwald, S. K., Randall, J. E., (1997). Investigating family-based alternatives to institution-based mental health services for youth: Lessons learned from the pilot study of a randomized field trial. Journal of Clinical Child Psychology, *26*(3), 226–233.

Henggeler, S. W., Schoenwald, S. K., Rowland, M. D., & Cunningham, P. B. (2002). *Serious emotional disturbance in children and adolescents: multisystemic therapy.* New York: The Guilford Press.

Hodas, G. (2006). Responding to childhood trauma: the promise and practice of trauma informed care. http://www.nasmhpd.org/publicationsOTA.cfm. Accessed 1 December 2008.

Knitzer, J. (1982). *Unclaimed children: the failure of public responsibility to children and adolescents in need of mental health services.* Washington, DC: The Children's Defense Fund.

Lyons, J. S. (1998). *Severity of psychiatric illness scale-child and adolescent version.* San Antonio: Psychological Corp.

Lyons, J. S. (2004). *Redressing the emperor: improving our children's public mental health system.* Westport: Praeger.

Lyons, J. S., & Schaefer, K. (2000). Mental health and dangerousness: characteristics and outcomes of children and adolescents in residential placements. *Journal of Child and Family Studies, 9*(1), 67–73.

Lyons, J. S., Uziel-Miller, N. D., Reyes, F., & Sokol, P. T. (2000). The strengths of children and adolescents in residential settings: prevalence and associations with psychopathology and discharge placement. *Journal of the Academy of Child and Adolescent Psychiatry, 39*(2), 176–181.

McCurdy, B. L., & McIntyre, E. K. (2004). "And what about residential...?" Reconceptualizing residential treatment as a stop-gap service for youth with emotional and behavioral disorders. *Behavioral Interventions, 19*, 137–158.

Miller, G. A. (1990). *The adolescent substance abuse subtle screening inventory manual.* Bloomington, IN: The SASSI Institute.

Naglieri, J., LeBuffe, P., & Pfeiffer, S. (1994). *The devereux scales of mental disorders.* San Antonio: The Psychological Corporation.

Newman, F., & Rinkus, A. (1978). Level of functioning, clinical judgment, and mental health service evaluations. *Evaluation and the Health Professional, 1*, 175–194.

Office of Juvenile Justice Programs (2006) Juvenile Offenders and Victims: 2006 National Report. http://www.ojjdp.org. Accessed 1 January 2007.

Shabat, J. C., Lyons, J. S., & Martinovich, Z. (2008). Exploring the relationship between conduct disorder and residential treatment outcomes. *Journal of Child and Family Studies, 17*, 353–371.

Schoenwald, S. K., & Rowland, M. D. (2002). Multisystemic therapy. In B. J. Burns & K. Hoagwood (Eds.), *Community treatment for youth: evidence-based interventions for severe emotional and behavioral disorders.* New York: Oxford University Press.

Sholevar, G. P., & Schwoeri, L. (2003). *Textbook of family and couples therapy: clinical applications.* Washington, DC: American Psychiatric Press.

Spreat, S., & Jampol, R. C. (1997). Residential services for children and adolescents. In R. T. Ammerman & M. Hersen (Eds.), *Handbook of prevention and treatment with children and adolescents.* New York: Wiley.

Stroul, B. A., & Friedman, R. M. (1986). *A system of care for seriously emotionally disturbed children and youth.* Washington, DC: CASSP Technical Assistance Center, Georgetown University Child Development Center.

Substance Abuse and Mental Health Services Administration. (2004). National Mental Health Information Center. http://mentalhealth.samhsa.gov/publications/allpubs/sma06-4195/chp19table5.asp. Accessed 12 November 2008.

Substance Abuse and Mental Health Services Administration. (2006). Building bridges between residential and community based service delivery providers, families and youth. http://www.cwla.org/programs/groupcare/buildingbridgesstatement.pdf. Retrieved 12 November 2008.

"Understanding the STAR." http://www.renlearn.com/products.aspx. Accessed 30 November 2008.

Waldron, H. B., Miller, W. R., & Tonigan, J. S. (2001). Client anger as a predictor of differential response to treatment. In R. Longabaugh & P. W. Wirtz (Eds.). *Project MATCH hypotheses: Results and causal chain analyses* (pp. 134–148). *Project MATCH Monograph Series, Vol. 8.* Bethesda: National Institute of Drug Addiction.

Ward, J., Dow, M., Saunders, T., Halls, S., Musanta, K., Penner, K., Berry, R., et al. (1996, 1997 & 1998). *CFARS: Child or adolescent behavioral health functional assessment.* http://cfars.fmhi.usf.edu. Accessed 8 December 2008.

14

Alternative Treatments for Conduct Problems: Brats, Boot Camps, and Bungee Jumps

GARRY F.A. COVENTRY and LAURA G. SWANSON

> My mum and my step-dad were watching *Brat Camp* the other night and they have told me that if I don't behave they are going to tell the TV people..... (Burnie, 2005).

What to do about troublesome young people or young people with troubles is a perennial problem for governments and the general public. This chapter focuses on boot camps, and to a lesser extent wilderness style programs, from a criminological perspective about the general problem of youth (and young adult) crime and youth crime prevention.

At the time of writing this chapter, the world is facing major economic challenges, which could bring further pressure to bear on detention rates of young people in countries like the United States, the United Kingdom, and others. We contend that juvenile justice correctional jurisdictions are likely to face a new set of challenges with regard to the provision of policies and programs – hopefully, ones that do not use detention as a carte blanche for young people in trouble. One such challenge is whether increasing numbers of young people should be referred to alternative programs (e.g., boot camps), rather than be left out of juvenile detention style programs

GARRY F.A. COVENTRY • James Cook University
LAURA G. SWANSON • James Cook University

R.C. Murrihy et al. (eds.), *Clinical Handbook of Assessing and Treating Conduct Problems in Youth*, DOI 10.1007/978-1-4419-6297-3_14,

altogether. It has been argued by Austin and Krisberg (1981), among others in criminology, that the criminal justice system expands the overall entrapment of offenders through the implementation of various alternative programs, which become grafted onto the main juvenile and adult criminal justice system of police–courts–corrections. This is widely referred to as the process of "net-widening" and we contend that such abatement of these processes is unlikely to occur in the foreseeable future. As long as both adult and juvenile correctional facilities in Western democracies have rising incarceration rates and soaring costs, the considerable pressure on governments to maintain budget surpluses may lead to a greater dependence on "boot camps."

A recent article by Eisler and Schissel (2008) reminds us of the vulnerability of young people in the global market. Their important contribution focuses readers on the interconnectedness between global corporatism, punitive criminal justice system policy, militarism, and disadvantaged Canadian young people. They argue that young people are susceptible to being exploited in the labor market and, being marginal to the political economy, are seen as incorrigible and likely candidates for military service. The authors contend that these young people become a store of labor for the army to be drawn upon when necessary. Indeed, for "bad and idle youth," a military experience is framed by a discourse of character building and discipline. Further, and disturbingly for us, boot camps have become a central point for public debates about creating "better" and more productive young citizens – an approach we consider to be way off the mark. Like Hil (2004), we argue that boot camps and many kinds of wilderness programs for young offenders emphasize a misplaced sense of attempting to enhance individual responsibility and rational choice decision making within a highly regimented and fearful environment.

We are skeptical whether the search for alternatives to reduce imprisonment numbers and correctional costs can be found in the use of military style discipline structuring boot camps or wilderness programs for those young people considered wayward. To understand boot camps and other alternatives to pure detention, we need to reflect on the extent to which these alternative correctional options mirror the correctional or prison warehouse (Irwin, 2005) or truly offer a different approach to dealing with young offenders. While mindful of the fact that most young people should not be in detention, we need to take a considered, evidence-based approach as to what can be offered to rehabilitate young offenders. Do boot camps provide us with a new and defensible alternative to reduce detention numbers and correctional costs? Are these alternatives defensible along moral and ethical lines?

This chapter adopts a critical criminological approach to both understanding and assessing the merits of correctional boot and wilderness camps for juvenile and adult offenders. Critical criminology is described by Stubbs (2008) as an orientation away from mainstream criminology which generally does not question systems of governance and criminal justice systems. Critical criminology is orientated toward issues such as social justice, human rights, and the understanding of social control mechanisms. In part, this approach is defined by what it challenges – traditional criminological definitions, its constructions and its linkages to other disciplines (including clinical psychology), and the broader political, economic, social, and cultural context which shapes human decision making and behavior.

We provide an overview of some of the major criminological traditions and discuss the extent to which these theories are relevant to an assessment of boot camps. Furthermore, we explore the implications of providing sentencing options that are modeled on extreme military style discipline and provide an examination of how alternative sentencing options such as "reintegrative shaming" fit within broader criminal justice frameworks. In addition, we consider whether boot camps are more effective at reducing recidivism and/or reducing the costs of more traditional forms of incarceration or restricted confinement. Ultimately, we argue that the rehabilitation agenda regarding young offenders requires an innovative and progressive conceptual framework that understands the compelling interaction between the structure and agency of offenders, in terms of how people see themselves and how society views them. By structure, we refer to major steering mechanisms of society such as politics and economics (Habermas, 1975), as well as social institutions including education, religion, and recreation which shape the experiences and opportunities for young people. Agency refers to actions of individuals (either on the basis of exercising rational choice or perhaps constrained to render one only capable of irrational decision making). Importantly, Erickson and Murphy (2003) contend that more positive approaches aimed at empowering young people is an essential element of a structure and agency understanding of youth policy.

Overall, this chapter considers the complexities and challenges of boot camps and wilderness programs by offering a critical assessment according to criminological theory and research evidence. What might be a more fruitful programmatic response to the problems faced by young people caught up in the juvenile justice system network is then outlined.

CRIMINOLOGICAL THEORIES

To provide a more comprehensive view of boot camps – and to a lesser extent "wilderness style" programs for young offenders – this chapter requires a brief review of the discipline of criminology in terms of its major theoretical frameworks, as well as divergent assumptions about human nature and the decision-making capabilities of offenders (see also Chap. 2).

Classicism is regarded as the cornerstone theory upon which the United Kingdom, Australian, and American criminal and juvenile justice systems were founded. The early classicists, such as Beccaria in 1764, were a group concerned about the horrific practices of punishment that occurred in European medieval times (see Foucault, 1977, for an account of "The body of the condemned"). This movement posited that criminal acts should be punished equally for all "men" and they should be proportionate to the severity of the offense. They posit that violations of criminal laws were an indication of irrational decision making on the part of offenders (Winfree & Abadinsky, 2003). Women, children, and "impaired" persons were not considered to be capable of rational thought (free will) by the founders of classicism. Neoclassicists revised this theory to include women as capable of rational thought but, even today, our criminal justice and juvenile justice systems have caveats excluding young people under certain ages and the mentally disabled from the full impact of criminal law. The strong and influential remnants of this thinking are still evident when we consider notions of "just deserts" and "mandatory sentencing" guidelines in juvenile justice system jurisdictions across Western democracies.

A shift in thinking away from classicism and neoclassicism occurred in the late nineteenth and early twentieth century in criminology. The rise in positivism as a "science" to explain human behavior led criminologists to search for the root causes of criminality, whether they lay in biological, psychological, or, to a lesser extent, sociological domains (Winfree & Abadinsky, 2003). Positivists, in trying to understand the causes of crime and what to do about it, have human pathology or deficits clearly on the agenda. For positivists, the system needed to be reorientated toward treatment and rehabilitation, rather than punishment per se. The treatment approach, however, took a major blow after a metaanalysis conducted by Lipton, Martinson, and Wilkes (1975) of more than 1,000 studies concluded that rehabilitation programs do not work . It should be noted that this report was seriously challenged with respect to its validity and that rehabilitation has been the adopted framework in many jurisdictions, from time to time.

The agenda for positivist criminologists, many of whom stretch across the criminal justice system, government, nongovernment agencies, academia, and the like, is focused on identification, diagnosis, prognosis, and treatment plans for young offenders. The core issue is one of individual pathology – the "correction" of problematic young people.

SOCIOLOGICAL TRADITIONS

There were some early efforts within the criminology discipline to focus attention onto sociological, nonpositivist approaches to understanding youth crime and justice. Largely, the work of the Chicago School and issues about the nature and structure of social institutions in capitalist societies rose to prominence in the 1940s (Shaw & McKay, 1942). Questions were raised about the extent to which societal structures in urban areas, particularly human services, education, and the labor market, shaped the opportunities of young people who lived in societies marked by the capitalist enterprise. More specifically, hypotheses like Merton's (1938) strain theory posited that the pressure of achieving economic success was a cause of criminal behavior. Some young people were destined for a successful outcome, while others were not, often as a consequence of their original family's socioeconomic status. Social class had crept into criminological debates, as had social institutions – thus, attention had shifted to problems with institutions and away from problem individuals.

This is a critical distinction about how the human condition is interpreted – where we locate the source of the causes of youth crime and whether defensible policy responses are framed in people change or societal change agendas.

MAJOR SHIFTS IN CRIMINOLOGICAL THINKING

The 1960s were marked by other important developments in Western capitalist democracies, including the Anti-Vietnam War and Civil Rights movement, Women's and Gay/Lesbian rights movements – all major challenges to the power and operations of the state. This era represents a fundamental shift in the discipline of criminology. Interest was now directed at the state, its inadequacies, shortcomings, and corruption-related structures (including law) that engendered and promoted the exploitation of particular groups of people. Power became the centerpiece for criminological analysis, beginning with labeling theory, which largely emanated out of research concerned with the use of marijuana (Becker, 1963). Becker raised important matters for consideration such as the notion of who defines rules or criminal statutes that label so-called deviants. His 1963 journal article entitled "Who's side are we on?" challenged the discipline to undertake research with and on behalf of the powerless to bring about change in social structures, particularly law. The foundations for the critical criminological project were largely expanded by reference, for example, in terms of war conflicts, economics, race relations, gender relations, and sexuality relations. The "baby boomers" had delivered a gift to criminology, by getting the focus on people with problems (the relatively powerless in society) because of problems with the state.

This period heralded in the birth of critical criminology. We submit that one of the seminal texts leading the way on these matters was the volume by Taylor, Walton, and Young (1973). At the time, these authors were admitted "socialists," who wrote about criminology in an entirely different way to what had been written previously. For them, capitalism was the central problem which largely created criminal behavior, due to the oppression of the working class. To us, the essence of critical criminology has no substantial steerage, let alone reflection, in boot camp or wilderness style programs for young offenders. Further, Correia (1997) argues that there is little to no theoretical basis for the operation of boot camps to reduce crime. Boot camps are essentially structures based on military style discipline, often buttressed by step programs (akin to Alcoholics Anonymous), designed to "break down" and then "rebuild" people into "conforming" and contributing members of society. These programs are less concerned with power inequities between staff and participants and feasible ways of addressing the enhancement of positive outcomes for young participants.

Quality of life is a vital outcome that needs to be considered. Available evidence suggests that endowing people with a sense of belonging, meaning, competence, usefulness, future, and a sense of psychological security is critical to increase chances of a successful transition into the community for adult prisoners on release (White & Coventry, 2008). Such quality of life notions are derived from the work of Polk and Kobrin (1972) regarding youth crime prevention and community approaches which can foster youth empowerment in local settings. We suggest that all young people, both offenders and nonoffenders alike, should have structures that enhance their quality of life.

UNRAVELING THE KEY ELEMENTS OF BOOT CAMPS

It is important to recognize that boot camps and other "softer" correctional alternatives in juvenile justice were, in part, introduced as ways of controlling state budgets regarding juvenile justice. Often, jurisdictions shift back and forth regarding the fundamental ideology of juvenile/youth corrections – from rehabilitation models to justice models. These shifts are linked to public support for "get tough" election promises on law and order issues.

To understand youth or juvenile justice system practices, it is important to consider the seminal work of Garfinkel (1956). His most important contribution to the discipline of criminology (and to clinical psychology, for that matter) was to introduce the notion of "status degradation" ceremonies that accompany the successive stages of juvenile justice system processing through police, courts, and corrections. A status degradation ceremony is epitomized when "stigma symbols" become the defining factor for a person's identity (Winfree & Abadinsky, 2003). As Garfinkel (1956) stressed, "stigma symbols" are reflected in the significance of the ritualistic nature of court trials and prison intake procedures. Essentially, these "stigma symbols" act as symbolic processes that, in turn, translate as the core criteria for a person's identity, in this case a deviant identity – a negative label by implication.

A central issue is whether boot camps and other alternative correctional diversion programs can alleviate a particular status degradation ceremony, if not transform, an individual's identity. One fundamental step, in this regard, can be drawn from Braithwaite (1989) and his arguments about reintegrative shaming. This alternative approach suggests that it is possible to mitigate against community degradation of young offenders. Braithwaite (1989) defines reintegrative shaming as:

> Shaming which is followed by efforts to reintegrate the offender back into the community of law-abiding or respectable citizens through words or gestures of forgiveness or ceremonies to decertify the offender as a deviant. Shaming and reintegration do not occur simultaneously but sequentially, with reintegration occurring before deviance becomes a master status. It is shaming which labels the act as evil while striving to preserve the identity of the offender as essentially good (p. 100).

Community disapproval can range from lenient warnings at one end of the spectrum through to more formal degradation ceremonies that can have the potential to shape a deviant identity. However, these expressions are followed by gestures of reacceptance into the law-abiding community. The essence of this reintegration argument is that status degradation can be replaced by status enhancement if both shaming and community support structures are adopted. The essential requirements of how to structure community support under an umbrella of quality of life notions are canvassed in this chapter. We need to move much further in this regard.

Moralizing can exert more effectual social control than overtly repressive approaches as it aims for compliance and social integration rather than ostracism or stigmatization (Anleu, 2000). Some boot camps, however, have been described as using shaming and humiliation practices to punish offenders. Humiliation, in combination with the aggressive and confrontational/intimidation military style tactics of boot camp staff, has the potential to result in the emotional abuse of offenders (see Lutze & Brody, 1999; MacKenzie & Souryal, 1995; Morash & Rucker, 1990). Further, Lutze and Brody argue that the use of strict military style discipline in combination with verbal confrontation by those in control (correctional officers) may serve to actually replicate the negative dynamics of previous abusive relationships. In addition, they argue that particularly vulnerable are those who suffer from low self-esteem or have a propensity to behave aggressively. Here, we find no evidence of reintegration along the lines suggested by Braithwaite (1989).

It is important to point out that many boot camp inductees arrive with emotional problems, aggression, and learning difficulties. Further, the use of strict military type discipline in combination with psychological humiliation by boot camp staff leaves little opportunity for a flexible approach for dealing with behavioral transgressions. For some young people, inflexibility on the part of staff can lead to ill health or even death. For example, testimony given before the Committee on Education and Labor described numerous cases of obvious symptoms of serious ill health being mistaken for "faking it" by staff (US Government Accountability Office, 2007).

Reintegrative shaming programs, however, have the potential to structure status enhancement programming for youth justice. In their review of the theoretical underpinnings of reintegrative shaming and some reference to empirical research evidence (see Bazemore & Umbriet, 2001); Winfree & Abadinsky 2003) write that reintegrative shaming alone may not prevent crime, but shaming combined with gestured forgiveness and a ritualistic reinforcement of the offender's status within a group is more likely to reduce the chance of reoffending.

We believe that reintegrative shaming is an important beginning concept to shape both correctional and diversion programs for young offenders. Dignity, human rights, and maximization of possibilities for young offenders to reenter communities are essential. We need to extend the debate around alternative programs with not only a watchful eye on such matters, but importantly policy and program directives about how these can be delivered. Further, we argue that reintegrative shaming, coupled with principles of positive youth development outlined above (cf. Polk & Kobrin, 1972), consistent with the enhancement of the quality of life for young offenders, would be a more progressive and productive juvenile justice system policy than a proliferation of boot camps. Successful reintegration of offenders also requires a reciprocal process involving communities (White & Coventry, 2008) – both acts of offenders giving to communities (e.g., natural disaster recovery and reconstruction efforts) and vice versa (e.g., provision of education and training programs for employability).

KEY GOALS OF BOOT CAMPS AND WILDERNESS PROGRAMS

It is important to distinguish between wilderness style behavioral modification camps (by and large utilized by parents wanting to "deprogram" problem teenagers) and correctional boot camps. Arguably, a major distinction between the two styles of alternative programs is that wilderness programs are about attempts to instill a sense of confidence and responsible decision-making skills associated with "dangerous," if not exhilarating, adventures. On the other hand, boot camps are explicit programs of the administration of adult or institutional power over young people.

The nature, quality, and size of correctional boot camps vary considerably across the United States. Most are based on a military model that encompasses basic training, regimentation, and strict physical discipline. This type of program demands unquestioning compliance, discipline, hard work, and physical toughness and aims to break down the inmate's "individualism" (Atkinson, 1995). Many researchers have questioned how appropriate the military model is to the rehabilitation of offenders (see MacKenzie, Wilson, & Kider, 2001, for an overview of this literature). While drill instructors push inmates to the limits of their emotional and physical capabilities, the support structure associated with a military occupation such as medical, housing, and employment assistance is not a fundamental characteristic of the correctional boot camp.

For Correia (1997) a fundamental aim of the correctional boot camp is to shape inmates into a preconceived "mould" that is premised on an outmoded military model that comprises degradation, harassment, and physical punishment as an enduring feature. Boot camps seek to capitalize on the transformative power of stress to induce behavioral and attitudinal change (Atkinson, 1995). Offenders are usually offered reduced sentences in exchange for their participation in a regimen that demands "unquestioning compliance, discipline, hard work and physical toughness" (Atkinson, p. 2). Most correctional boot camps across the United States are structured in similar ways (MacKenzie & Hebert, 1996). Most programs run, on average, between 90 and 120 days, with the minimum stay being 30 days and the maximum 240 days. MacKenzie and Herbert indicated that the primary element of all programs consisted of physical training, and not all included rehabilitative components such as counseling or educative services. Generally speaking, there are three main objectives for correctional boot camps: to reduce recidivism of offenders; to lessen the financial stressors of running a traditional prison; and to alleviate prison overcrowding (MacKenzie et al., 2001). Only a relatively small number of inmates actually enter boot camps, however, in relation to the entire prison population. Moreover, the numbers of recruits that are siphoned from traditional imprisonment and complete boot camp have only a limited capacity to reduce prison numbers (Atkinson).

There are also "wilderness programs" predominantly for young offenders who are already in detention, and for those perceived as being "at risk" of detention in the future. These programs are intended to be therapeutic in nature and are ostensibly orientated towards building self-esteem and problem-solving skills. It needs to be noted that wilderness programs are different to correctional boot camps and are originally based on the philosophies of the Outward Bound wilderness challenge program. Experiencing the wilderness involves activities that often provide young people with excitement and a dynamic meaningful experience. Whether such activities translate into meaningful attributes in a young person's regular environment is another matter.

Indeed, Reddrop (1997), following a review of 100 US studies, had a number of questions about wilderness style programs and the extent to which they are particularly suited to having a positive impact on youth at risk of criminal behavior. Reddrop argues that with an instructor's guidance, the Outward Bound model could be appropriate for troubled young people, as the excitement of the wilderness may elicit higher levels of motivation. Further, she argues that behavioral and attitudinal changes may occur by presenting young people with a series of unique problem-solving tasks in a natural environment. Reddrop even contends that psychological benefits which can be explicitly measured, such as improved self-confidence, can be attained from successful achievement in outdoor activities. Ultimately, however, despite some short-term success in character building and self-esteem changes, Reddrop, in this review of available empirical studies at the time, notes that the ability of wilderness style programs to achieve long-term success is less clear and remains debatable. There is little evidence to directly link these kinds of programs with a long-term decrease in criminal (or delinquent) behavior among young people.

Most importantly, after conducting a comprehensive review of research evidence, Cuneen and White (2002) argue that nonvoluntary intensive style programs such as boot camps and wilderness programs can fail in rehabilitation and future crime prevention efforts targeted at young offenders. Alternatives to detention, such as wilderness camps, are seen by the authors as an effort to deinstitutionalize young offenders away from secure forms of custody such as prison. This is a laudable objective. They refer to Reddrop's (1997) study and agree that the majority of wilderness programs for young people have only demonstrated limited success in reducing criminal behaviors. As Cunneen and White contend, this failure is due, in part, to the fact that isolating young people in boot camps or wilderness programs is in direct contradiction to the effectiveness of close-knit family and community contact networks.

In the United States between 1990 and 1997, the adult prison population increased by 60% (Austin et al., 2007), while costs of building, maintaining, and staffing facilities have also increased dramatically. Many jurisdictions are looking for less expensive alternatives to overcrowded prisons, yet must also respond to public pressure and expectations of how prisoners should be dealt with. While other options such as home detention and electronic monitoring are perceived as "soft options" for adult and juvenile offenders, many still believe that the correctional boot camp, with its basis in a regime of strict military style physical discipline, is the "golden" solution.

Duwe and Kerschner (2008), for example, write that by the mid-1990s, over 100 boot camps were operated by federal, state, and local agencies in the United States. Nevertheless, while deregulation has made it difficult to effectively calculate the current number of boot camps, there is certainly a decline in the overall number of operational boot camps since the late 1990s. However, there remains strong public enthusiasm for this method of correctional intervention (Duwe & Kerschner).

BOOT CAMP AS ENTERTAINMENT

The populist icon of hard labor as justifiable punishment fits well with the military nature of the boot camp. Instilling core "moral values" into offenders by utilizing strict militarized physical activities has great appeal to the general public and policy-makers alike. Indeed, the concept of the boot camp as an alternative punishment option has become part of the accepted public psyche and is a spectacle that can be viewed on many reality television programs. These programs create a "fly on the wall," voyeuristic experience to view the elaborate "transformation" of people from the unwanted or unlikeable to the desirable. Sending overweight people to a "fitness boot camp" or the unruly girl to a "manners boot camp" is seen, by many, as a perfectly acceptable form of behavioral modification. However, for the correctional boot camp dealing with actual juvenile offenders, there is much more at stake. There are considerable tensions between viewing boot camps as a quick and cheap way to deal with delinquent behavior, and conceptions about boot camps being an inventive and common sense way to rehabilitate offenders through acceptable corporal punishment (Correia, 1997).

The problem with this confused thinking is also evident when we consider wilderness programs. The fun and thrills of adventure in "survival" settings – for example, the television reality show *Survivor* – is not translated into the "real" world of young participants engaging in such activities under the authority of correctional authorities. Consider, for example, a 5-day wilderness adventure trekking across Cape York (Australia). To what extent do "survival skills" learned in that environment translate to "survival" in remote Northern Australian towns where child abuse, alcoholism, poor educational attendance, and chronic unemployment dominate the landscape of such communities? Very little, we suggest.

Disturbingly, there is a relatively new development in the scenarios of boot camps. So-called "well-off" parents seem to be willing to countenance decisions about sending their "uncontrollable" children, even though they have not necessarily committed a criminal offense (and do not suffer from conditions such as ADHD), to wilderness camps. Bratich (2006) notes that reality television programs such as *Brat Camp* become a "mechanism for conducting powers of transformation" (p. 77). These "powers of transformation" are enacted on unruly teenagers who are sent off for "behavior modification" at private military boot camps. Just as reality television can transform ordinary people into pseudocelebrities, can Bratich's "powers of transformation" transform delinquent teens into useful and grateful citizens through shows like *Brat Camp*? At this time, we do not know the answer to this question.

HAVE THE GOALS OF BOOT CAMPS BEEN ACHIEVED?

Although the original purpose of the prison was to reform offenders, it is now widely accepted that prison does not effectively perform this function (e.g., Wrightsman, Nietzel, & Fortune, 1998). Wrightsman et al. contend that when rehabilitation is the primary goal, sentences will usually involve an alternative to incarceration. However, with the advent of boot camps and other "shock incarceration" programs in the 1990s, an ideological shift from the public and policy makers towards the punishment of offenders became apparent. A large body of research over the last 10 years points to an overwhelming finding that, in general, boot camps are no more effective at reducing recidivism than traditional forms of juvenile detention (e.g., Ashcroft, Daniels, & Hart, 2003; Benda, 2001; MacKenzie et al., 2001; Parent, 1994).

The work of MacKenzie et al. (2001) who conducted a systematic metaanalysis of 29 correctional boot camp studies is most informative. It was found, overall, that there were no significant differences in recidivism rates between boot camp participants and comparison samples of offenders who did not participate in such programs. However, it was discovered that recidivism rates varied when examining the impact of specific program characteristics between different boot camps. A key conclusion of this study, therefore, was that correctional boot camps which incorporated after care programming had, overall, significantly lower rates of recidivism amongst offenders than programs that did not include such provisions. While we contend that boot camps, as currently conceived and operated, are not as effective as one would desire, juvenile justice system alternatives which are structured on youth development principles and longer-term community reintegrative programming, beyond the camp, might have greater promise.

With regard to other research evidence, MacKenzie et al. (2001) randomly assigned adult inmates to an adult prison or a correctional boot camp in Maryland for a period of 6 months. This study is thought to be the first experimentally designed study to examine the impact of a correctional boot camp for adult offenders. While those who attended the boot camp program had a slightly lower recidivism rate than those in prison, the results were hardly convincing – certainly, not convincing enough to herald such alternatives as a "silver bullet" approach to stem recidivism rates.

While also investigating recidivism rates, Benda (2001) by contrast adopted a more qualitative research style and individually interviewed 480 boot camp participants to compare recidivists and nonrecidivists after attending correctional boot camps over a 3-year period. Benda examined how factors related to recidivism, personal attributes, sociodemographics, peer association, criminal history, and perceptions of the correctional boot camp environment affected an offender's recidivism rate. He concluded that recidivists were younger when they start unlawful behavior, were incarcerated as a juvenile, had several personality deficits, and viewed boot camp as merely a faster way of being released from incarceration. Nonrecidivists, however, had a sense of self-efficacy, high self-esteem, and were optimistic about their future. Overall, Benda argued that correctional boot camps are no more effective in reducing recidivism than other correctional institutions.

Clearly, key researchers in this field indicate that boot camps are no more effective in reducing recidivism than traditional forms of incarceration (Benda, 2001; MacKenzie et al., 2001). The complexity of reducing recidivism is outlined by Benda who suggests that boot camps will struggle to reduce recidivism because: (a) they are typically made up of a heterogeneous population and therefore the requirements of many participants are not met; (b) the stay in a boot camp is too short to equip youth with needed skills; and (c) staff are typically undertrained to cope with the needs of participants. Further, the lack of postrelease programs after boot camp offering a sufficient amount of vocational, educational, and personal skills development may also contribute to higher recidivism rates.

There is nothing in the findings of this body of research to encourage the proliferation of militarism, confrontations between staff and detainees, and hard labor while detained. These key aspects of boot camps do not appear to unlock the "revolving door" of people moving in and out of the criminal justice system. Furthermore, boot camps are underevaluated and not regulated by governing bodies and can be susceptible to unlicensed operators. Establishing a relationship between theory and delinquency prevention in operational programs is vital. We suggest that youth development approaches, along the lines suggested by Polk and Kobrin (1972), which structure programs for the enhancement of the quality of life for young offenders (discussed earlier in this chapter) are required.

The key questions regarding the reduction of recidivism and alternative interventions for juvenile offenders must be commented upon further. The most useful and effective programs are those that use a comprehensive approach including social competence training, mentoring, and educational and vocational skill development for the enhancement of quality of life. Some argue that individual programming is essential to the success of such programs (Australian Institute of Criminology, 2002), but we point out that the fundamental philosophy of youth development should be applied to all. Today, it is not.

EXCITEMENT WITH DISCIPLINE VERSUS DISCIPLINE WITHOUT EXCITEMENT

For Morash and Rucker (1990), the military model of boot camps has created abuses of power and encouraged aggression by staff and young people. Moreover, images of dehumanizing meaningless labor enacted by a delinquent and "deficient" offender are often celebrated in popular imagery. Importantly, for Morash and Rucker, "The military model has provided a legitimization of severe punishment. It has opened the door for psychological and even physical abuse, that would be rejected as cruel and unusual punishment in other correctional settings" (p. 208).

More recently, reports have surfaced that highlight not only the ineffectual elements of boot camps, but point out the dangerous and in some cases even fatal outcomes for participants. Testimony given before the United States Government Accountability Office in 2007 established that thousands of allegations of abuse were reported between 1990 and 2007 at residential treatment programs, including juvenile boot camps and wilderness programs. Some of these reports included fatalities, and many were instigated by staff who were untrained, unqualified, or in some cases neglectful. This report draws attention to the lack of minimum standardization of operating procedures across the United States and was drawn from hundreds of interviews and obtained documents from closed cases. In addition to the lack of minimum standards, it was also found that there is a deficiency of standard, commonly recognized definitions for boot camps and wilderness programs. For example, one particular pending civil lawsuit alleges that dozens of children were subjected to over 30 types of separate abuse at one facility. In another case cited in the above mentioned report, significant neglect by staff was found to directly contribute to the death of a minor from dehydration on a mountain hike. Taken together, these findings from the United States Government point to lack of regulatory standards in the operation of alternative juvenile/criminal justice system programs and the horrific consequences for individuals, let alone neglect of fundamental underpinnings of life enhancement strategies which might structure more profitable programs for young offenders.

CONCLUDING COMMENTS

Foucault (1977) alerts us to the use of corrections generally, and prison per se, as the institutional framework that metes out the disciplinary regime of regulating or controlling the body, time and space arrangements for offenders. For Foucault, a French philosopher and social scientist, the way to effectively understand disciplinary society is to examine the relationships between power, knowledge, and forms of social control and surveillance. Imprisonment, at the "hard edge" of correctional programming is essentially about the use of discipline. But, so are "softer" forms of sentencing and alternatives to the prison. Correctional programs normalize their inmates through constant surveillance, labor and regulation of time and space (Foucault).

To reflect on this approach in an investigation of correctional boot camps suggests that we need to look at the societal discourses and relationships between government, institution, and prisoner to thoroughly appreciate the wider issues at hand. From a social psychological perspective, the community's support for harsher punishments and penalties relates more to a sense of the dissipation of moral cohesion than to explicit support for the corrective process of dealing with offenders (Anleu, 2000).

For authors such as Welch (1997), an examination of boot camps can be made in relation to Foucault's notion of "normalizing institutions."

In addition, the use of Foucault's notion of the "penal calculus" – that the public will accept shorter sentences for prisoners if sentences can be perceived as much harsher – could explain the popularity of boot camps. Typically, offenders will stay at a boot camp for a shorter period of time and participate in a more rigorous and military-like program compared to traditional forms of incarceration.

Militarization of boot camp systems utilizes dominance through such pervasive regulations. To be clear, military style discipline, the regulation of daily time and space, and obedience to correctional authorities are central organizing themes of boot camp programs. As mentioned above, confrontation, humiliation, and degradation of nonviolent young offenders are a part of the process of attempting to turn young people into law-abiding citizens. These methods are supposed to provide deterrence effects. Other boot camp programs, however, emphasize a welfare model of juvenile justice by including elements such as therapeutic treatment and/or education to enhance the rehabilitative objectives of the intermediate sanction.

Shock incarceration programs or boot camps have come into vogue as an intermediate correctional system sanction against young offenders in particular. The military-style punishment regime, in contrast to extended prison sentences, attracts support from "law and order" politicians who are eager to find ways of "getting tough on crime" and reducing state correctional budgets at the same time. Further, it was hoped that these kinds of interventions would ease the mounting problem of overcrowding in correctional facilities (MacKenzie & Hebert, 1996).

Our review of the literature based on research about boot camps in the United States, Canada, and Australia indicates a number of continuing concerns that require close attention by both policy makers and criminal justice system researchers. These concerns include:

1. The deleterious effects of exposure to the military style "machine" on young people.
2. While there may be short-term desistance effects, with regard to early offending (most likely because they are under surveillance), there is no consensus that boot camps have a long-term impact on recidivism.
3. There is no evidence that prison overcrowding has been eased by alternatives such as boot camps and it appears that some jurisdictions use the sanction as a "net-widening" program, bringing more young people under the control of corrections. Corrections, to be sure, is an industry of massive proportions in the United States and other Western countries.
4. Some studies report that, rather than reducing prison overcrowding, there are patterns of increased use of technical violations for graduates such that they are returned to prison. Technical violations, conditions imposed by courts on people granted probation or parole often include offenders being late to meetings with case workers, failure to submit to drug testing, or not attending counseling sessions.

5. There is no demonstrable evidence that state correctional costs have been eased as a result of introducing boot camp sentencing alternatives.
6. Few programs include a structured aftercare component to monitor, if not maintain, the goals of any rehabilitation services provided.
7. Although a large amount of research has been generated over the last 10 years, there is a paucity of comprehensive process and impact evaluation research related to the effectiveness of boot camps.

It is essential that the matter of preventing young offenders from reoffending is at the center of any new criminal justice legislation. The rehabilitation agenda needs to be revisited through a new conceptual framework that understands the compelling interaction between structure and agency of offenders. In other words, how personal choices and values are made and experienced within the restrictions of circumstances imposed by alternative programs. Institutionalized social interventions in the form of imprisonment or alternatives like boot camps must address the external and internal aspects that shape a person's sense of self. Furthermore, militarized boot camps are less useful methods for preparing juvenile offenders for release into the community.

The challenge is to recognize that a fundamental philosophy is required to work with offenders in ways that encourage them to give back to the community and the community to provide status enhancement opportunities for such people. For example, community service orders that place offenders in not-for-profit agencies are worthy of considered thought. Effective community service orders are described by Cuneen and White (2002) as working in aged homes, hospitals or rehabilitation centers. This is evident at both a theoretical and therapeutic level by those who advocate positive rather than negative interventions (White & Coventry, 2008). Further, the reintegration of offenders needs to be a reciprocal process whereby the community and the offender give to others in a "constructive and active fashion."

The outcome of "doing it on the cheap," particularly with lack of follow up services and support to young participants in remote sites, located far away from family support contacts (and possible cultural insensitivities) can potentially lead to failure. Most importantly, as Hil (2004) points out:

> Perhaps the real story of boot camps begins with the socio-political and economic status of young people, many of whom find themselves increasingly on the margins of contemporary life and are subject to a range of punitive state interventions. This is a story rarely to be found in the glut of empirical studies on boot camps (p. 148).

The persistent push towards punishment rather than rehabilitation in many jurisdictions has meant that, unfortunately, we may not have seen the end of boot camps. With the focus turned away from rehabilitation strategies, there are concerns for how juvenile offenders will integrate in the future. It is inevitable that most prisoners, adult or juvenile will be released eventually. How prepared will we be in dealing with them and they with the broader community? These questions and others remain to be addressed in a more empirical manner.

REFERENCES

Anleu, S. (2000). *Deviance conformity and control* (3rd ed.). Sydney: Addison Wesley Longman.

Ashcroft, J., Daniels, D., & Hart, S. (2003). *Correctional boot camps: lessons from a decade of research.* U.S. Department of Justice Programs, Washington: National Institute of Justice. Publication No. NCJ 197018.

Atkinson, L. (1995). Boot camps and justice: A contradiction in terms? *Trends and Issues in Crime and Criminal Justice* (AIC Publication No. 46). Canberra, Australia.

Austin, J., & Krisberg, B. (1981). Wider, strong and different nets: the dialectics of criminal justice reform. *Journal of Research in Crime and Delinquency, 18,* 165–196.

Austin, J., Clear, T., Duster, T., Greenberg, D., Irwin, J., McCoy, C., et al. (2007). *Unlocking America: why and how to reduce America's prison population.* Washington: The JFA Institute.

Australian Institute of Criminology. (2002). *What works in reducing young people's involvement in crime?* Australian Capital Territory: Australian Government Publishing.

Bazemore, G., & Umbriet, M., (2001). A comparison of four restorative conferencing models. *Juvenile Justice Bulletin,* February. Washington: Office of Juvenile Justice and Delinquency Prevention.

Braithwaite, J. (1989). *Crime, shame and reintegration.* Cambridge: Cambridge University Press.

Bratich, J. (2006). Nothing is left alone for too long: reality programming and control society subjects. *Journal of Communication Inquiry, 30,* 65–82.

Becker, H. S. (1963). *Outsiders: studies in the sociology of deviance.* New York: Free Press.

Benda, B. (2001). Factors that discriminate between recidivists, parole violators, and non-recidivists in a 3-year follow-up of boot camp graduates. *International Journal of Offender Therapy and Comparative Criminology, 45*(6), 711–729.

Burnie, J. (2005). I am threatened with brat camp. Daily Record, March 21.

Correia, M. (1997). Boot camps, exercise and delinquency: an analytical critique of the use of physical exercise to facilitate decreases in delinquent behavior. *Journal of Contemporary Criminal Justice, 13*(2), 94–113.

Cuneen, C., & White, R. (2002). *Juvenile justice: youth and crime in Australia* (3rd ed.). South Melbourne: Oxford University Press.

Duwe, G., & Kerschner, D. (2008). Removing a nail from the boot camp coffin: an outcome evaluation of Minnesota's challenge incarceration program. *Crime and Delinquency, 54*(4), 614–643.

Eisler, L., & Schissel, B. (2008). Globalization, justice and the demonization of youth. *International Journal of Social Inquiry, 1*(1), 167–187.

Erickson, P., & Murphy, L. (2003). *A history of anthropological theory* (2nd ed.). Toronto: Broadview Press.

Foucault, M. (1977). *Discipline and punish: the birth of the prison.* London: Penguin Books.

Garfinkel, H. (1956). Conditions of successful degradation ceremonies. *American Journal of Sociology, 61,* 420–424.

Habermas, J. (1975). *Legitimation crisis.* New York: Beacon Press.

Hil, R. (2004). In pursuit of the responsibilised self. In *Hard lessons: reflections on governance and crime control in late modernity.* Sydney: Ashgate.

Irwin, J. (2005). *The warehouse prison: disposal of the new dangerous class.* Los Angeles: Roxbury.

Lipton, D., Martinson, R., & Wilkes, L. (1975). *The effectiveness of correctional treatment and what works: a survey of treatment evaluation studies.* New York: Praeger.

Lutze, F., & Brody, D. (1999). Mental abuse as cruel and unusual punishment: do boot camp prisons violate the eighth amendment? *Crime and Delinquency, 5*(2), 242–255.

MacKenzie, D., & Hebert, E. (1996). *Preface, correctional boot camps: a tough intermediate sanction.* National Department of Justice, United States: National Criminal Justice Reference Service.

MacKenzie, D., Wilson, D., & Kider, S. (2001). Effects of correctional boot camps on offending. *American Academy of Political and Social Science, 578,* 126–143.

MacKenzie, D., & Souryal, C. (1995). A Machiavellian' perspective on the development of boot camp prisons: a debate. *University of Chicago Law School Roundtable, 2,* 435–453.

Merton, R. (1938). Social structure and anomie. *American Sociological Review, 3,* 672–682.

Morash, M., & Rucker, L. (1990). A critical look at the idea of boot camp as a correctional reform. *Crime and Delinquency, 36*(2), 204–222.

Parent, D. G. (1994). Boot camps failing to achieve goals. *Overcrowded Times, 5,* 8–11.

Polk, K., & Kobrin, S. (1972). *Delinquency prevention through youth development.* Washington: Office of Youth Development. DHEW, Publication No 72-26013.

Reddrop, S. (1997). *Outdoor programs for young offenders in detention: an overview.* Tasmania: National Clearinghouse for Youth Studies.

Shaw, C., & McKay, H. (1942). *Juvenile delinquency and urban areas: a study of rates of delinquency in relation to different characteristics of local communities in American Cities.* Chicago: Chicago University Press.

Stubbs, J. (2008). Critical criminological research. In T. Anthony & C. Cunneen (Eds.), *The critical criminology companion* (pp. 6–18). Sydney: Hawkins Press.

Taylor, R., Walton, P., & Young, J. (1973). *The new criminology: for a social theory of deviance.* New York: Harper and Row.

Welch, M. (1997). A critical interpretation of correctional boot camps as normalizing institutions: discipline, punishment and the military model. *Journal of Contemporary Criminal Justice, 13*(2), 184–205.

White, R., & Coventry, G. (2008). Prisoners, work and reciprocal reintegration. *Proceedings from The Second Australian and New Zealand Sociology Conference.* Sydney, Australia: Crime and Justice Research Network.

Winfree, L. T., & Abadinsky, H. (2003). *Understanding crime, theory and practice* (2nd ed.). Canada: Thomson Wadsworth.

Wrightsman, L., Nietzel, M., & Fortune, W. (1998). *Psychology and the legal system* (4th ed.). California: Brooks/Cole Publishing Company.

United States Government Accountability Office. (2007). Residential treatment programs: concerns regarding abuse and death in certain programs for troubled youth. (GAO Publication No GAO 08-146T). (Testimony given before the Committee on Education and Labor, House of Representatives).

15

Pharmacotherapy for Children and Adolescents with Conduct Problems

HELEN L. SMITH and DAVID R. COGHILL

Conduct problems can be formally classified as "disruptive behavior disorders" which include conduct disorder (CD), oppositional defiant disorder (ODD), and disruptive behavior disorder not otherwise specified (DBD-NOS) in the Diagnostic and Statistical Manual 4th edition (DSM-IV-TR; American Psychiatric Association, 2000). Conduct Disorder is a serious disorder which is characterized by persistent antisocial behavior and can be helpfully divided into early (before the age of 10 years) or late onset. Clinicians are often pessimistic about the effectiveness of treatment options available to manage CD and ODD; in particular, many are skeptical about the value of pharmacological treatments for managing CD and ODD, but is this skepticism justified?

First-line treatments for conduct problems are psychosocial/psychotherapeutic in nature (Findling, 2008; Pappadopulos et al., 2006) and include Multisystemic Therapy and Collaborative Problem Solving approaches (Greene & Ablon, 2003; Henggeler, Schoenwald, Borduin, Rowland, & Cunningham, 1998), among others (see chapters in this book). These first-line interventions are unfortunately not available in all areas, and even where they are accessible, not every child will respond and it may be necessary to consider medication as an alternative.

HELEN L. SMITH • University of Dundee
DAVID R. COGHILL • University of Dundee

R.C. Murrihy et al. (eds.), *Clinical Handbook of Assessing and Treating Conduct Problems in Youth*, DOI 10.1007/978-1-4419-6297-3_15,

In all cases, treatment should follow a detailed assessment, which includes a risk assessment and the clear identification of the aims of and targets for intervention. Most of the medications detailed below have been used with the aim of either (a) generally reducing the core symptoms of conduct problems or (b) specifically targeting and reducing levels of aggression as this is often the most visible symptom of these disorders. One potential benefit of medications over psychosocial interventions is their ability to produce a faster response and therefore result in a quicker reduction in the risk of harm to others (Caldwell, Maltereer, Umstead, & McCormick, 2008). Early intervention is linked to efficacy (Moretti et al., 1997) and the addition of medication can also increase the efficacy of behavior modification programs (Caldwell et al.).

When the clinical team has decided on the targets for intervention, they then need to be clear about how they will be measured and how change will be monitored. Various scales are available, but it is important to remember that whichever scale is used, it should be valid and reliable and be able to accurately measure change and response to treatment. Several of the common scales used in research are listed below.

General scales measuring the symptoms of conduct problems include the aberrant behaviour checklist (ABC; Aman, Singh, Stewart, & Field, 1985) and the Nisonger Child Behaviour Rating Form (Aman, Tasse, Rojahn, & Hammer, 1996). The Clinical Global Impressions-Severity (CGI-S) and Change scale (CGI-C) (Guy, 1976) are useful for measuring general clinical status and change. Specific measures of aggressive behavior include the Modified Overt Aggression Scale (MOAS; Malone, Luebbert, Penea-Areit, Bisecker, & Delaney, 1994) and the Rating of Aggression against People and/or Property scale (RAAPP; Kemph, Devane, Levin, Jarecke, & Millar, 1993). None of these scales have been validated as a core measure for conduct problems or violence, however (Pandina, Aman, & Findling, 2006). See Chap. 4 in this volume for other measures that have been used in various settings.

Each of the medications that have been used in the treatment of conduct problems will be systematically examined to evaluate the evidence supporting their use. The main groups that have been studied are the mood stabilizers, antidepressants, stimulants, selective norepinephrine reuptake inhibitors, and antipsychotics.

MOOD STABILIZERS

Lithium Carbonate

The use of lithium in the treatment of conduct problems was first documented in 1956 when it was used to treat a 17-year-old youth with aggressive and antisocial behavior (Jefferson, 1982). It has since been shown to have antiaggressive properties in several well-controlled studies (Campbell et al., 1991, Campbell et al., 1995; Malone, Delaney, Luebbert, Carter, & Campbell, 2000; Rifkin et al., 1997). The earliest reports compared lithium to haloperidol (an antipsychotic medication; see Campbell et al., 1984).

This study was double blind and included a placebo for the initial 2 weeks to remove placebo responders and thereby reduce the placebo effect. The subjects were inpatients (n=61) and mostly male; there were no females in the lithium treatment group. The children were aged between 5 and 13 years and were of mixed ethnicity with Hispanics making up the largest ethnic group followed by African-Americans. All had a DSM III diagnosis of Conduct Disorder. Haloperidol was started at 1.0 mg/day increasing to 16 mg a day and lithium at 250 mg a day increasing to 2 g a day. Lithium levels were monitored by saliva until the allocation code was broken and it was revealed which medication the patient had been taking after which blood levels were measured. Average daily doses of haloperidol were 0.21 mg/kg/day and for lithium 1,166 mg/day. The length of treatment was 4 weeks. Outcome measures were the CGI, the Children's Psychiatric Rating Scale (CPRS) (Guy, 1976), and the Global Clinical Judgments (Consensus) Scale (GCJCS, Campbell et al.). Lithium and haloperidol both resulted in a significant improvement in hyperactivity, aggression, and hostility on the CPRS as well as a general reduction in the severity of conduct problems as measured by the CGI. However, participants in both conditions also reported adverse drug reactions with the haloperidol group reporting a significantly greater number of side effects than the lithium group. The authors also suggested that haloperidol may have resulted in a degree of cognitive slowing that impacted negatively on the children's daily functioning. This was investigated in more detail in a related paper (Platt, Campbell, Green, & Gregan, 1984) in which formal cognitive testing was conducted on these same patients. Several cognitive tests examining memory and executive functioning were included in the design. While the cognitive effects of both drugs were reported as "mild," the authors concluded that even a slight impairment in these already academically challenged children would be a problem. They therefore advocated the use of lithium over haloperidol due to its effectiveness at reducing conduct problems and producing fewer side effects, cognitive or otherwise.

Campbell et al. (1995) continued investigations into the use of lithium with a second double-blind,placebo-controlled trial. Fifty children aged from 5 to 12 years completed this study. Conduct Disorder diagnoses were made by psychiatrists and all subjects had previously failed to respond to various outpatient psychosocial treatments. This trial had a similar placebo run-in to the previous study to exclude placebo responders from the active treatment phase. No other medications were allowed for the duration of the study. Subjects were treated for 6 weeks only; 25 received placebo and 25 lithium. The doses of lithium were varied, but there did not appear to be any extra clinical benefit with dosages above 1,500 mg a day. There was significant improvement in overall functioning in the lithium group compared to placebo as measured by the CGI. There were also significant reductions in the CPRS measures of aggression, bullying, fighting, and temper outbursts in the lithium group, although these changes were not statistically significant. Conversely, the Profile of Mood States (POM; McNair, Lorr, & Droppleman, 1971) showed that lithium increased self-reported states of confusion and bewilderment and adverse effects were relatively common in the lithium treatment group.

Rifkin et al. (1997) investigated the effects of lithium on aggression in adolescents aged 12–17 years with CD diagnoses (rated via diagnostic interview). Subjects also had three significant episodes of aggression after being hospitalized as measured by the Overt Aggression Scale (OAS; Yudofsky, Silver, Jackson, Endicott, & Williams, 1986). Lithium was administered double blind alongside a placebo group for 2 weeks only. This is the only study that had more female than male participants. Results showed no statistical difference between placebo and lithium on any of the dependent measures. Lithium did, however, have statistically more adverse effects than placebo.

The most recent study (Malone et al., 2000) examined 86 in patients with CD diagnoses between the ages of 10 and 17 years. The sample was mostly male and African–American. The average IQ of the sample was below average, with a median of 80–90. Lithium was given for 4 weeks. Outcome measures included the CGI, the GCJCS, and the OAS. According to the GCJCS, 80% of participants responded to lithium, reducing aggression, compared to 30% of the placebo group. Similarly, the OAS score for the lithium group reduced significantly over 4 weeks. The authors provide an odds ratio (OR) of 9.3, indicating that subjects were nine times more likely to respond to lithium than placebo. It is noteworthy, however, that adverse effects were again an issue for subjects in the lithium condition.

In the above studies (Campbell et al., 1984, 1995; Malone et al., 2000; Rifkin et al., 1997) while no subjects were reported to have stopped lithium treatment due to adverse effects, all authors apart from Rifkin et al. commented on the presence of adverse effects. In Campbell et al. lithium subjects suffered from stomach aches, headaches, weight gain, and hand tremors. Tremor was also common in Campbell et al.'s second study (Campbell et al.). Lastly, in Malone et al.'s (2000) study, the lithium group also reported significantly more adverse effects than the placebo group including nausea, vomiting, and urinary frequency. Further, adverse effects were more prevalent in younger children (Campbell et al., 1991) even when other variables such as weight and dose were taken into account.

In summary, there is evidence to support the use of lithium in CD, but this is limited to inpatients. The effects appear to be greater for children aged less than 12 years than for adolescents, with just one study reporting positive effects in adolescents (Malone et al., 2000). Another adolescent study that reported negative findings was also notable for having included a large number of female subjects and for having given treatment for only 2 weeks (Rifkin et al., 1997). Indeed the length of treatment in all studies was rather short; there are no studies with extensive follow-up. The majority of studies also had a bias towards subjects from Hispanic and African-American ethnicities which limits the generalizability of results. Limitations notwithstanding, a systematic review of these studies confirmed a moderate clinically meaningful effect for mood stabilizers on aggression in children and adolescents with a mean effect size of 0.4 (Pappadopulos et al., 2006).

When prescribing lithium for children and adolescents, monitoring processes identical to those used in adults should be implemented. As children have a higher renal clearance of lithium than adults, higher oral doses may be needed to reach equivalent serum levels (Jefferson, 1982). While it has been suggested that the serum levels required for antiaggressive properties are lower than those required for antimania treatment (Jefferson), this has no empirical support in the literature. From the evidence presented, it does appear, however, that there is no additional clinical benefit associated with dosages above 1,500 mg a day.

Carbamazepine

Carbamazepine is a tricyclic anticonvulsant that has been used for some time in the treatment of behavioral difficulties associated with epilepsy, in particular temporal lobe epilepsy. It has been hypothesized that carbamazepine may have a less negative impact on cognitive performance when compared to drugs like typical antipsychotics, making it a potentially more attractive treatment option (Cueva et al., 1996).

Kafantaris et al. (1992) conducted an open-label trial with carbamazepine in 10 individuals with severe CD. The children, aged between 5 and 10 years old, were all hospitalized because of their behavior. The length of treatment was 3 weeks. Significant improvements were found on the CPRS with significant reductions in fighting with peers, bullying and temper outbursts and improvements in mood lability. Positive results were also evident on the CGI and OAS. There was no direct relationship between serum level of carbamazepine and the clinical response. A number of children in this study reported adverse effects with carbamazepine including headaches, fatigue, blurred vision, and diplopia.

Cueva et al. (1996) examined the use of carbamazepine in children admitted to an inpatient unit. Subjects received active treatment or placebo for 7 weeks. The children entered into the trial were drug free for 4 weeks prior to starting the study medication. The study population was mostly male (20 male, 2 females) and aged between 5 and 12 years. The majorities were Hispanic or African-American with substantial variations in standard measures of intelligence; IQs ranged from 55 to 111. Twenty-two subjects completed the study (11 carbamazepine, 11 placebo). Outcomes for the study were measured using the OAS, CPRS, and CGI. The optimal dose of carbamazepine was 400–800 mg a day. There were no significant improvements in the rating scales for either group. Adverse effects were reported by the carbamazepine group with leucopoenia (decrease in number of white blood cells, placing subject at higher risk of infection) occurring in 45% of subjects and dizziness in 64%. Rashes and headaches were also prevalent.

Currently there is very limited evidence to support the use of carbamazepine for the treatment of CD in children and there are no published studies in adolescents.

Divalproex Sodium

Antiepileptic drugs have been flagged as a treatment for aggression because epileptic-like activity has been observed in the limbic system of those with periodic aggressive behavior problems (Monroe, 1970). Divalproex sodium and its related compounds (sodium valproate) have been used to treat epilepsy with and without behavioral disturbances for many years. It has been speculated that this drug may also have a positive impact on aggressive behaviors due to an effect on γ – aminobutyric acid (GABA) and/or serotonin (5-HT). A limited number of studies have examined the use of divalproex sodium in children and adolescents with conduct problems.

Donovan et al. (1997) reported ten outpatient cases treated with open-label divalproex sodium. Seven of the ten cases were diagnosed with CD; the remaining three had a diagnosis of ODD. Most of the participants were male (80%) and aged between 15 and 18 years. Divalproex sodium was used because it was believed that the participants' temper outbursts were linked to irritable mood. Subjects were given divalproex sodium starting at 250 mg a day increasing to 1 g daily for up to 5 weeks. The mean number of outbursts as rated by a child and adolescent psychiatrist was reduced from 6.5 per week at the start of treatment to 0.1 per week at the end of the study period. Functioning was also assessed with the Global Assessment of Functioning scale (GAF). Subjects improved from 37.8 to 65.7 on the GAF after 5 weeks of treatment. It is worth noting that most of the subjects were also either abusing or dependent on cannabis while in treatment.

Donovan subsequently completed a double-blind placebo-controlled crossover study (Donovan et al., 2000). This study enrolled outpatients who fulfilled diagnostic criteria for CD or ODD. The study had two phases; divalproex for 6 weeks followed by placebo or vice versa. Twenty boys were initially enrolled; 17 completed phase one (the first 6 weeks up to the crossover) and 15 completed both phases. The reduction in numbers from phase one to two was mainly due to withdrawal of consent and subjects being jailed for parole violation. Subjects were younger than in the open label study, aged between 10 and 18 years with a mean age of 13 years. Most were male (80%) and the majority were Hispanic (60%). For this study the researchers utilized a more structured approach to measuring levels of aggressive behavior, using the hostility subscale of the SCL-90 (Derogatis, Lipman, & Covi, 1973). Stimulants and cannabis were being used by most subjects (Donovan et al.). It is not clear, however, whether this drug use continued during the trial or if it was monitored after enrolment. Aggressive behavior in general was measured using the MOAS. The authors reported that 80% of the subjects assigned to the divalproex group responded in 6 weeks, significantly reducing hostility as measured on the SCL-90 compared to placebo. The overall response to divalproex sodium as determined by an independent assessor was significantly better than that for placebo.

The evidence for use of divalproex was further supported by a second randomized controlled dose response trial (Steiner, Petersen, Saxena, Ford, & Matthews, 2003). Sixty-one subjects enrolled into the study. It is possible that the subjects in this sample were more seriously violent than samples in previous studies as a number had been charged with serious offenses including manslaughter, rape, and assault with a deadly weapon. Diagnoses were made by clinicians and as with previous samples there was a high degree of comorbidity; the median number of diagnoses for each subject was three. Subjects were assigned to either high-dose or low-dose divalproex valproate and treated for 7 weeks; there was no placebo arm.

There was no reporting of the randomization process and the study was not blind as all subjects received divalproex. Subjects were, however, blindly assessed with respect to dose level at the end of the trial. Clinical improvement as measured by the CGI severity and improvement scales was noted in both groups. Subjects in the high-dose group were more likely to have shown improvement. Subjects' self-report on the Weinberger Adjustment Inventory also suggested that impulsivity and self-restraint had improved significantly (Weinberger, 1997).

One further naturalistic study that showed a reduction in adolescent aggression with divalproex was primarily aimed at adolescents with Bipolar Affective Disorder (Deltito, Leviton, Damone, Hajal, & Zamberiedetti, 1998). The authors used divalproex sodium in 18% of admissions over a 1-year period. Subjects were aged between 13 and 18 years. Divalproex was not the only intervention as the subjects also received psychotherapy and psychosocial interventions. Additional medications were available for agitation as required including haloperidol, chlorpromazine, diphenylamine, and benzodiazepines. Only one patient had a diagnosis of CD but divalproex was thought to have reduced aggression in subjects with bipolar disorder and psychosis, although no direct measures of aggression were used. This conclusion is tentative, however, given the lack of control group and difficulty in separating out which of the interventions were responsible for change. None of the studies above reported serious adverse effects when using divalproex sodium. The most frequent adverse effects were gastrointestinal upset, increased appetite, and sleepiness. One patient did develop abnormal liver function tests, but these returned to normal when the concurrent chlorpromazine was discontinued (Deltito et al.).

Evidence for the use of divalproex sodium for CD and ODD is limited at present and there is not enough evidence to unequivocally support its use. The results can, however, be seen as promising; clinicians reported global improvement in behavior and few serious adverse effects, but further research is warranted. Studies have not yet extended treatment beyond 7 weeks and there have been no follow-up studies conducted. In future studies it would be of value to use a more structured assessment of violent or aggressive behavior using tools such as the MOAS (Malone et al., 1994) or RAAPP (Kemph et al., 1993). A number of the papers (Donovan et al., 1997, 2000; Steiner et al., 2003) have commented on comorbidity of aggression and substance misuse and abuse, but have not controlled for this or monitored it during the study. This is problematic due to the established link between violence and substance abuse.

ANTIDEPRESSANTS

Serotoxin Reuptake Inhibitors

Only one study has specifically examined the effects of SSRIs on aggression in children. Armenteros and Lewsi (2002) completed an open-label pilot study of citalopram for impulsive aggression. Participants were aged between

7 and 16 years, had been aggressive for over 6 months and had displayed violent behavior at least 3 times in the preceding week with at least two of these acts directed against a person. Eleven of the twelve subjects had CD and comorbidity was extremely common. The study monitored aggression using the MOAS, CGI, and the Child Behavior Checklist (CBCL; Achenbach, 1991). Citalopram was prescribed initially at 10 mg a day, increasing by 10 mg a week (dependent on clinical response) for a total of 6 weeks of treatment to a maximum dose of 40 mg a day. There was a statistically significant reduction in aggression towards objects on the MOAS, but not on any of the other MOAS subscales. There was also a significant reduction in several of the CBCL subscales including aggressive behavior, externalizing problems, attention problems, and total problems subscales. There was also a significant improvement on the CGI severity of illness scale. This study therefore provides some preliminary evidence regarding the potential efficacy of citalopram in the treatment of conduct problems, but more research is needed, including RCTs, before any clear recommendations can be made.

There are concerns that the prescription of SSRI medication in children and adolescents with depression may increase the risk of self harm and suicide (Cipriani, Barbui, & Geddes, 2005). It is not clear if these concerns should be extended to the use of the medications for CD. Although it should be noted that impulsivity increases the risk for harming oneself as well as others. A systematic review (Pappadopulos et al., 2006) of the literature suggested a small effect size for antidepressant use in the treatment of child and adolescent aggression (0.3), but these studies mostly examined children with primary diagnoses of Attention Deficit Hyperactivity Disorder (ADHD) and not CD. Taken together, the evidence suggests that, at this time, SSRI's should not be considered as a first-line medication for the treatment of CD.

Trazodone

Although trazodone is related to the tricyclic antidepressants, its action is thought to be through a modulation of serotoninergic neurotransmission. Zubieta and Alessi (1992) described an open-label trial of trazodone in 22 inpatients. These children, aged between 5 and 12 years, all had impulsive aggressive behaviors that had failed to respond to an average of four medications. The 18 boys and 4 girls were started on 50 mg trazodone at night, which was then increased up to the maximum tolerated dose. The average IQ of the subjects was 80–90. The average length of inpatient treatment with trazodone was 27 days, and the medication was continued as outpatients. Post treatment clinical improvement was noted in both ADHD and ODD symptoms. Improvement was measured using a DSM IV checklist of symptoms for the behavioral disorders, which were completed by clinicians using subjective clinical ratings. Conduct disorder symptoms were also reduced, with cruelty to people and the frequency of physical fights improving to a statistically significant level. Six children did not respond to treatment and three became worse. Fifty percent of subjects developed orthostatic hypotension, but this was not impairing, and 27% reported drowsiness. Subjects were followed up approximately

8 months and all except one patient were still prescribed trazodone. Clinical improvement had been maintained in the opinion of both the clinical team and parents.

No other studies have been reported and we therefore conclude that there is currently insufficient evidence to recommend trazodone as a frontline treatment for CD. Taken together, the evidence suggests that while there have been some encouraging results from a small number of open trials, more research is required and there is insufficient evidence to support the use of antidepressants as frontline treatments for CD or ODD. On the other hand, they have not been ruled out as potential future treatments, and their lower adverse effects profile is positive; however, clinical efficacy and effectiveness need to be more clearly demonstrated.

SELECTIVE NOREPINEPHRINE REUPTAKE INHIBITORS AND ATOMOXETINE

Selective norepinephrine reuptake inhibitors (SNRIs) have been demonstrated to be effective treatments for ADHD. The postulated mechanism of action relates to their impact on ADHD symptoms via their ability to block the noradrenaline transporter and impact on both noradrenergic and dopaminergic neurotransmission. An open-label pilot study of reboxetine in children with hyperkinetic CD has been completed (Mozes, Meiri, Ben-Amity, Sabbagh, & Weizman, 2005). The children in this study were inpatients in Israel, aged between 5 and 14 years and were mostly male (11 of 15 children). They had previously received a broad range of other medications (including stimulants and both typical and atypical antipsychotics) and these continued to be taken during the 12 weeks trial of reboxetine. Aggression was measured by the OAS. Reboxetine was started at 2 mg and increased to 8 mg depending on clinical need. There was a significant reduction in aggression on the OAS measure and a reduction in impulsivity measures. One patient discontinued reboxetine due to the adverse effects of insomnia, hair loss, and weight loss. Almost all of the subjects lost weight. Drowsiness, bed wetting, and reduced appetite were commonly reported as adverse effects. The effect size for reboxetine in the treatment of aggression is very small (0.18; Pappadopulos et al., 2006).

Atomoxetine increases the availability of dopamine and norepinephrine in the prefrontal cortex. It is highly selective for the norepinephrine transporter and therefore does not increase dopamine in the nucleus accumbens and is not associated with an increased risk of substance abuse (Newcorn, Spencer, Biedeman, Milton, & Michelson, 2005). While there are no studies examining atomoxetine in CD it is included here as it is commonly prescribed in ADHD which, as discussed earlier, is closely associated with early-onset CD. Several studies have investigated the effects of atomoxetine on children and adolescents with ADHD and comorbid ODD (Bangs et al., 2008; Kaplan et al., 2004; Newcorn et al.). Kaplan et al. amalgamated the results of two studies examining the safety and efficacy of atomoxetine in the treatment of ADHD with comorbid ODD. The RCT extended over 9 weeks. Ninety-eight subjects were recruited, aged 7–13 years, and structured interviews confirmed that subjects met diagnostic criteria for both ADHD and ODD. Fifty-two subjects were assigned to the atomoxetine condition and 45 to the placebo condition. The only difference between the two groups at baseline was height. The average mean dose was 1.6 mg/kg/day with a maximum dose of 2 mg/kg/day. The Connors Parent Rating scale (Conners, 1998) was used to measure ADHD symptomatology change and the CGI-S. There was a significant reduction in ADHD symptoms on the inattention and hyperactivity subscale of the Connors Scale for the intervention group compared to placebo. These improvements were observed in week 1. Importantly, there was no significant impact of atomoxetine on the oppositional subscale of the Connors Scale. Three subjects in the atomoxetine group discontinued due to adverse events and there was a significant reduction in appetite in the atomoxetine group.

Newcorn et al. (2005) investigated various doses of atomoxetine in a group of children and adolescents aged between 8 and 18 years diagnosed with ADHD and ODD or ADHD alone. Treatment lasted 8 weeks and there were three treatment arms: doses of 0.5, 1.2 and 1.8 mg/kg/day. Three hundred and thirty-three subjects were randomized: 155 subjects with ODD and ADHD, and 178 with ADHD only. Atomoxetine at 1.8 mg/kg/day reduced symptoms of ADHD as measured by the Attention Deficit/Hyperactivity Disorder Rating Scale-IV (ADH-DRS). The ADHD and ODD group, who had more severe ADHD symptoms at baseline, also required higher doses of atomoxetine (1.8 mg/kg/day) to improve their ADHD symptoms. There was also a significant improvement in oppositionality as measured by the Connors oppositionality subscale at the 0.5 and 1.8 mg/kg/day doses, but not at 1.2 mg/kg/day. The improvement in oppositionality was not dependent on the presence of a diagnosis of ODD, but was dependent on there also being a positive response of ADHD symptoms to medication. In other words, oppositional behavior improved only in subjects whose ADHD symptoms improved concurrently.

Bangs et al. (2006) conducted a randomized placebo-controlled trial of atomoxetine at 1.2 mg/kg/day vs. placebo in a group of children recruited from Europe and Australia, aged 6–12 years, with ADHD and ODD. Symptoms of ODD were measured using the Swanson, Nolan and Pelham scale (SNAP IV; Swanson, 1992). Despite a positive response with respect to ADHD symptoms and an initial reduction in ODD symptomatology by week 8, there was no difference in outcomes between the atomoxetine and placebo groups at the end of the study. Adverse events were few, but there was a significant reduction in appetite and weight in the atomoxetine group. Diastolic blood pressure also increased and required monitoring.

There is currently no evidence for the use of atomoxetine in CD. A possibility exists that it may reduce oppositionality in the presence of ADHD, but this needs to be examined further in RCTs as the current evidence is contradictory.

ANXIOLYTIC DRUGS

Only one study has formally examined the use of anxiolytic drugs in children with conduct problems. An open-label pilot study (Petti, Fish, Shapiro, Cohen, & Campbell, 1982) was conducted with nine boys, six of whom were African–American; aged between 7 and 11 years, all in patients with IQs ranging from 71 to 109. After a 3-week placebo period the boys were given chlordiazepoxide starting at 15 mg daily increasing up to a maximum of 120 mg depending on clinical response. The optimal dose range was 15–75 mg a day. Initially, the drug had a stimulating effect on eight of the boys. Six of the boys made clinically significant improvements on the CPRS, but three children demonstrated significantly increased levels of impulsivity. Adverse effects included fatigue and lethargy in almost all of the subjects and slowed or slurred speech. This report is part of a larger study that was a double-blind crossover study comparing chlordiazepoxide, chlorpromazine, trifluoperazine, and placebo. The overall study results suggested that boys with less severe symptoms had a better response to chlordiazepoxide; boys with more severe symptoms had a better response to antipsychotic medications. There is currently no evidence to support the use of anxiolytic drugs for the treatment of CD.

STIMULANTS

Stimulant medications are proposed to be of potential use in the treatment of CD due to the marked comorbidity between CD (in particular early onset CD) and ADHD (Connor, Glatt, Lopez, Jackosn, & Melloni, 2002; Robbins, Tipp, & McEvoy, 1991). ADHD may have long-term effects on the prognosis of CD as children with both disorders have a worse prognosis in terms of continued aggression, substance use, and adult antisocial behaviors than CD alone (Connor et al.). Two studies specifically examined the effects of methylphenidate on the behaviors of adolescents with CD and ADHD (Kaplan, Busner, Kupietz, Wassermen, & Segal, 1990; Klein et al., 1997).

Kaplan et al. (1990) examined the impact of stimulant medication on nine adolescent males aged between 13 and 16 years. In a methodologically mixed study, three participants participated in an open-label trial of methylphenidate while a further six enrolled in a 7-week double-blind randomized controlled crossover trial with methylphenidate and placebo. The Adolescent Antisocial Behaviour Checklist was used (Curtiss et al., 1983) to measure aggression and hyperactivity. Aggressive behaviors significantly improved over the treatment period of the double-blind condition. Physical threats and verbal harm showed the strongest improvements followed by improvements with respect to difficulties with responsibility and rule violation. As expected, levels of hyperactivity significantly reduced in the double blind group ($n=6$). In their concluding comments, Kaplan and colleagues suggested that the subtyping of CD into those with and without ADHD could have implications for treatment.

This idea of using methylphenidate in youth with CD but not ADHD was taken up by Klein et al. (1997). Klein's group conducted an RCT with youth with CD, many of whom did not have ADHD. Subjects were aged between 6 and 15 years and IQs were above 70 with a range of 74–136. Subjects with substance abuse problems were excluded. The youth were assigned to receive either methylphenidate or placebo for a period of 5 weeks. Consistent with the literature, it was noted that the authors had a great deal of difficulty finding "pure" CD subjects. That said, this remains the one study to have documented the impact of methylphenidate on a mainly non-ADHD population. Methylphenidate was not the only intervention used as subjects' parents also received weekly supportive counseling. The study was conducted over a 3-year period with 83 subjects completing the trial. Methylphenidate significantly improved conduct problems, except for socialized aggression, on all measures including the Connors rating scale and an observed classroom rating. On global clinical assessments of impairment the methylphenidate group significantly improved as rated by teachers, parents, and clinicians.

A number of studies of children with ADHD have reported effect sizes for the impact of the stimulant on aggressive behaviors. Kolko, Bukstein, and Barron (1999) examined methylphenidate (low and high dose) and found that the effect size was greater for methylphenidate in combination with a behavior modification than on its own (0.85 vs. 0.59). There were few differences between the high- and low-dose groups, although negative behavior in a social skills group improved more in the low-dose than high-dose group. The combination treatment also had a more positive effect on mood than either treatment alone.

Two meta-analyses (Connor et al., 2002; Pappadopulos et al., 2006) found stimulants to have a significant effect on aggressive behavior independent to the effect on ADHD symptoms. Pappadopulos et al. reported an effect size of 0.78 for stimulants on aggressive behaviors, although they note that this was normally reported as a secondary outcome measure. Connor et al. divided aggression into overt (physical violence) and covert (stealing, etc.) aggression. In a meta-analysis of 683 children with ADHD and CD treated with stimulants the reported effect sizes were impressive. Overt aggression treated with stimulants was associated with a larger effect size (0.86) than covert aggression (0.75). While impressive, it should be noted that these effect sizes are somewhat lower than those that have been reported for the effect of stimulants on ADHD symptoms (around 1.0; Banaschewski et al. 2006)

Adding clonidine may further enhance the effects of methylphenidate (Hazell & Stuart, 2003). Hazell and Stuart conducted a 5-week RCT of 67 subjects aged 6–14 years, all of whom had a diagnosis of ADHD and either ODD or CD. Subjects had clonidine added to their stimulant medication. Subjects in the clonidine and methylphenidate condition showed significantly less aggression than subjects in the methylphenidate-only condition. Significant adverse effects were noted: drowsiness and dizziness and concerns about potentially serious cardiovascular events.

The overall evidence for methylphenidate in children and adolescents with comorbid ADHD and CD is relatively robust with methylphenidate appearing to reduce both sets of symptom clusters. No studies have successfully examined stimulant medication in "pure" CD, however. While Klein et al. (1997) were not able to recruit a pure CD sample, the results of their study do seem to indicate that methylphenidate may be an effective treatment for CD even in the absence of ADHD. It is interesting that this has not been studied further. It is possible that this is a reflection of the rather ambiguous position that CD occupies in respect to whether it is or is not a "psychiatric disorder." One suspects that even if stimulant medications were demonstrated to be an effective treatment for CD there would be a significant debate as to whether they should be used to treat what many see as just "bad behavior."

ANTIPSYCHOTICS

Typical Antipsychotics

Before the introduction of atypical antipsychotics the typical antipsychotics were frequently used to treat aggression and CD. Early studies (Barker & Fraser, 1968; Cunningham, Pillai, & Blachford-Rogers, 1968) reported a significant reduction in aggression with haloperidol in children with behavioral problems. There was a degree of diagnostic fluidity in these studies, but they both employed a double-blind crossover design with placebo. The ages of the children ranged from 4 to 15 years in both studies. Adverse effects included apathy, increased sleepiness, reduced reaction times, impaired hand eye coordination, and muscular pains (Cunningham et al.). In both studies, benzhexol was given to all subjects to reduce the potential for adverse effects and to help maintain the blinding. The study by Cunningham et al. included 12 subjects who had all been admitted to hospital having shown disturbed behavior in the community. Haloperidol was administered up to a dose of 3 mg a day for 4 weeks. The study team devised their own behavior ratings to examine behavior in the ward (completed by nursing staff) and school environments. Haloperidol reduced reported levels of destructiveness and overactivity. Children also bullied and teased less; they were less resentful and dour. There were no significant differences reported for in-school behavior between the treatment and placebo groups.

Barker and Fraser (1968) studied a mixed group of in- and out-patients aged between 4 and 15 years. Haloperidol was prescribed in gradually increasing doses up to a daily dose of 0.05 mg/kg/day. A self-devised rating scale was again used in the study. There appeared to be significant reductions in temper- and attention-seeking behaviors. A more recent study discussed earlier (Campbell et al., 1984, see section on lithium) compared haloperidol to lithium in hospitalized children with CD. While both drugs improved aggression and hostility in subjects, haloperidol was reported to have more adverse effects.

Molindone hydrochloride was compared to thioridazine in a double-blind cross-over study with placebo (Greenhill, Soloman, Pleak, & Ambrosini, 1985). Subjects were inpatients, aged 6–11 years, and had not previously received neuroleptic medication. Children were diagnosed with undersocialized CD, aggressive type. Molindone was given in dose between 2.5 and 10 mg/kg/day for 4 weeks. The treatment phase was both preceded and followed by a placebo phase. Both drugs significantly improved hostile, antisocial, and violence ratings (on the Conner's Parent Ratings scale) compared to placebo, but the molindone group improved significantly more than the thioridazine group across all three subscales. In terms of adverse effects, molindone was associated with more dystonic reactions while thioridazine caused more sedation.

Although effect sizes reported for typical antipsychotics in the treatment of CD are moderate to large (0.7–0.8; Pappadopulos et al., 2006), concerns about dystonic reactions and tardive dyskinesia in children will limit their use. They may, however, continue to have a role as short-term adjunctive medication to psychotherapeutic interventions (Barker & Fraser, 1968).

ATYPICAL ANTIPSYCHOTICS: RISPERIDONE

Risperidone is the medication that has been most thoroughly studied and for which the best evidence exists for use in CD (Findling, 2008). It was initially chosen for study as it was thought to be less likely to result in the adverse effects previously associated with haloperidol, namely sedation and extra-pyramidal side effects (Findling et al., 2000).

Preliminary evidence came from a small double-blind trial (Findling et al., 2000). Ten subjects received risperidone and ten received placebo over a 10-week period. Subjects were aged 5–15 years with a primary diagnosis of CD. The dose of medication was low with a mean dose of 0.028 mg/kg/day. Progress was monitored by the CBCL, CGF, and RAAPP. There was a large attrition rate in this study with four subjects from the risperidone group and seven from the placebo group dropping out. Results from the RAAPP suggested that those receiving risperidone were significantly less aggressive than the placebo group over the final 4 weeks of the study. The CGI-S and CGI-I for the experimental group also improved as the study progressed with significant group by time interactions suggesting that the differences between the risperidone and placebo groups increased over time. Risperidone also resulted in greater reductions in conduct problem subscale in the CPRS than placebo, but there were no group differences on the aggressive behavior subscale of the CBCL. Adverse effects reported included increased appetite, significant weight gain, and sedation. There were no dystonic reactions. The authors stated that although the results were important they should not be inappropriately generalized to other populations.

A larger international study assessed whether risperidone maintained improvement in conduct problems over time (Reyes, Buitelaar, Toran, Augustyns, & Erdekens, 2006). This study recruited over 300 participants in the double-blind period. They were aged from 5 to 17 years and had received CD diagnoses after participation in structured interviews. All subjects had normal IQs, 66% had comorbid ADHD, and the majority were Caucasian (87%). The study commenced with a 6-week open label trial followed by a 6-week single-blind phase and proceeding to a double-blind period of 6 months, during which subjects were randomized to either continued risperidone or placebo. Low doses of risperidone were again used (0.02 mg/kg/day). During the open label phase, response was defined as a greater than 50% reduction in the conduct problem scale of the Nisonger questionnaire. Subjects who continued to receive risperidone maintained their response for longer at the end of 6 months; 29.7% of subjects prescribed risperidone had symptoms of CD re-emerge compared to 47.1% of placebo (Reyes et al.).

Adverse events were more likely in the acute phase of treatment. Dystonias and tardive dyskinesia were very rare. Weight gain was noticeable in the risperidone group but glucose metabolism was not affected. Risperidone did not appear to negatively impact cognitive functioning.

These last two studies (Findling et al., 2000; Reyeset al. 2006) were conducted with children of normal intelligence. While acute RCTs of risperidone have not been conducted in children with normal intelligence, several studies have been conducted in children with “subaverage intelligence” (van Bellinghen & de Troch, 2001; Snyder et al., 2002; Aman, De Smedt, Lyons, Findling R., & Risperidone Disruptive Behavior Study Group, 2002). Van Bellinghen and de Troch (2001) investigated the effects of risperidone on 13 youths (aged 6–14 years), with persistent behavioral disturbances such as hostility, irritability, and aggression. Subjects had IQs between 45 and 85 and were living in residential care. The placebo-controlled double-blind trial extended over 4 weeks. Outcome measures included the ABC, CGI, and a visual analog scale for target symptoms completed by carers. The daily dose was low at 0.05 mg/kg/day and there were no dropouts. Results showed that risperidone led to significantly improved ratings on the ABC subscales of irritability, hyperactivity, and inappropriate speech compared to placebo. The CGI also improved significantly for the risperidone group, as did a visual analog scale that assessed the target symptom severity and was completed by carers. These improvements could be measured in the first week of treatment. Adverse effects were few, but two subjects did increase their body weight by 7%. Van Bellinghen and de Troch (2001) suggested that a slow titration of risperidone can avoid extra-pyramidal side effects.

Two international studies investigating the effects of risperidone on conduct problems in subjects with sub-average intelligence were completed by Snyder et al. (2002) and Aman et al. (2002). Snyder et al. (2002) recruited 110 children, aged 5–12 years with CD, ODD or DBD-NOS. The trial extended over 6 weeks with a 1-week single-blind period to remove placebo responders; co-prescription of methylphenidate was allowed. The Nisonger, ABC, and CGI were used as measures of aggressive behaviors and clinical response. Doses averaged out at 0.03 mg/kg/day. A significant reduction in the conduct problems subscale was evidenced on the Nisonger; symptoms reduced by an average of 47.3% by the end of treatment. All scales of the ABC (i.e., irritability, hyperactivity, and inappropriate speech) also improved significantly. These improvements were maintained when the coprescription of stimulant medication was controlled for. Extra-pyramidal adverse effects were again uncommon. Somnolence affected 41.5% of the risperidone group. The analysis was repeated with those suffering from sedation removed, and the effects remained significant. Weight and Body Mass Index increased significantly in the risperidone group, but blood pressure, electrocardiograms and other biochemical markers remained unchanged.

The Aman et al. (2002) study had an identical design to that of Snyder et al. (2002). The number of subjects in each was also similar; 55 in the risperidone group and 63 in the placebo group. Subjects met criteria for CD, ODD, or DBD-NOS. Unfortunately, a large number of the placebo group withdrew because there were no improvements in symptoms. The results of the study were similar to those of Snyder et al. (2002). The prosocial scale from the Nisonger significantly improved by the completion of treatment compared to placebo. The CGI also significantly improved as did the irritability and lethargy subscales of the ABC. Aman and colleagues' study population did, however, appear to suffer from more adverse events. Ninety-eight percent of the risperidone group had an adverse event as did 70% of the placebo group. Over 50% of the treatment group complained of somnolence, but it was mild and transient. There were no differences in prolactin levels but weight gain was noticeable in the risperidone group.

A number of studies have also examined the use of longer term risperidone to treat behavioral disturbance in low-IQ populations. Reyes, Croonenberghs, Augustyns, and Eerdekens (2006) study followed up subjects who had previously been enrolled in the 1-year study by Croonenberghs et al. (2005). This study was open label. The subjects were aged 6–15 years and met criteria for CD, ODD, or DBD-NOS diagnoses. The diagnoses were assessed during a previous study (Croonenberghs et al., 2005). Subjects were prescribed with a maximum daily dosage of 4 mg of risperidone. Improvements noted in the conduct problems subscale of the Nisonger and ABC continued for 1 year and were maintained for 2 years (Reyes et al.). The number of adverse effects reduced over time, and weight gain was reported to have stabilized after 3–6 months of treatment. Cognitive improvements were maintained through the second year of treatment. Pandina et al. (2007) examined the data from a number of studies and confirmed that risperidone did not affect attention, verbal learning, or memory.

Taken together, these findings suggest that there is evidence to support the use of risperidone in the management of behavioral problems for learning-disabled children and adolescents in both the short and long term. The evidence in a non-learning-disabled population is growing, but rigorous RCTs are required. The effect size reported for atypical antipsychotics is large at around 0.9 (Pappadopulos et al., 2006). There is strong support for the suggestion that risperidone gives a rapid onset of action and reduction in symptoms. Adverse effects are of a concern and need to be studied in larger long-term studies and via increased pharmacovigilance efforts. Somnolence is the most frequent adverse effect, but appears transient and does not affect cognitive functioning. Extra-pyramidal adverse effects are infrequent. Weight gain is more common and needs careful monitoring and early intervention.

Olanzapine

A number of studies have investigated the use of olanzapine in children and young people with CD (Handen & Hardan, 2006; Masi et al., 2006; Soderstrom, Rastam, & Gillberg, 2002). Soderstrom et al. described the use of open-label olanzapine in a case series of six adolescents aged 14–19 years with aggressive behavior. The treatment extended between 2 and 10 months. These young people had previously received behavioral interventions without success. Five subjects had low IQs and other comorbidity including multiple substance abuse, Tourette's Disorder, Bipolar

Disorder, and ADHD. The conduct problems were severe and most of the adolescents had attempted to kill people in the past. Clinicians reported a marked clinical improvement as measured by the CGI, with most subjects responding within a week. The major concern was weight gain. Five of the six subjects gained between 5 and 18 kg. Two subjects were sedated, but there were no problems with extra-pyramidal adverse effects.

Another open-label trial was conducted by Handen and Hardan (2006). Sixteen subjects were recruited to the study. The adolescents were out-patients aged between 13 and 17 years with IQs ranging from 39 to 79. Most subjects were male and had received a generic diagnosis of disruptive behavior disorder; only one patient fulfilled diagnostic criteria for CD. Olanzapine was started at 2.5 mg increasing to 20 mg a day for 8 weeks. The average daily dose was 13.7 mg. Measures included the ABC, Connors, and CGI. Four subjects discontinued the medication due to adverse effects or worsening symptoms. Severity of conduct problems and global impression scores improved significantly in response to olanzapine, as did ratings of irritability on the ABC and hyperactivity subscale of the ABC and Connors hyperactivity index. Weight gain was the major adverse effect, with 10 out of 15 subjects gaining more than 5 kg in 8 weeks. Prolactin blood levels increased over treatment, but this did not cause clinical problems.

Masi et al. (2006) described a retrospective chart review of 23 adolescents with severe CD that had been treated with olanzapine when mood stabilizers had previously failed to produce benefits. Learning-disabled adolescents were excluded from this study. The study population was mixed sex and included both in- and out-patients. The MOAS was used as the main measure of aggression. At the end of 8–12 weeks of treatment the conduct problems of 42% of subjects were said to have clinically significantly improved. Subjects were followed up at 6 months, at which point 61% had improved and were less aggressive. The specific reductions in the MOAS scales were verbal aggression (30%), violence against property (44%), violence against self (78%), and violence against other people (48%). This follow-up period led the authors to conclude that time to respond to treatment can be considerably delayed and may sometimes occur as late as 3 months after initiation of medication (Masi et al.). Subjects were more likely to respond to medication if they had exhibited impulsive/affective aggression. Weight gain was the most common adverse effect with sedation and increased appetite reported.

Evidence supporting the use of olanzapine is limited and all trials have been open label. The populations studied are mostly learning disabled and there have not been any studies conducted in children under the age of 12 years. The major concern with the use of olanzapine is weight gain (Allison et al., 1999) and the possibility of other biochemical abnormalities such as metabolic syndrome.

Quetiapine

It has been suggested that Quetiapine may produce a less serious side effects option among the atypical antipsychotics as it appears to be associated with a lower risk of both extra-pyramidal side effects and weight gain

(Allison et al., 1999). Findling et al. (2006) conducted an open-label trial with quetiapine that extended over 8 weeks. The 17 subjects were children aged 6–12 years with primary diagnoses of CD. A structured diagnostic interview was used to reach diagnoses and comorbid diagnoses, other than ADHD, were excluded. Doses were commenced at 3 mg/kg/day increasing to 6 mg/kg/day at the clinician's discretion. No other medications were allowed at the same time as the trial. Lower doses were needed than those required for antimanic properties. The RAAPPS was used to measure aggression. The CGI and CBCL were also used to measure overall clinical improvements and the CBCL behavior subscale measured aggression. There were significant improvements observed in aggression as measured by the RAAPPS and CGI scores showed significant clinical improvements overall. A large number of subjects had adverse events (88%): these included fatigue, nasal congestion, headache, sedation, increased appetite, vomiting, irritability, and fever. Despite this, all subjects continued to take the medication for the full trial. There was a statistically significant increase in body weight over the trial, but no effects on glucose levels.

CONCLUSIONS

Psychosocial treatment approaches remain the first-line treatment for CD, ODD, and aggression more generally in children and adolescents. It is, however, not uncommon for these initial treatments to be refused or to be only partially effective or completely ineffective. In this chapter, we have reviewed the evidence for pharmacological treatment of conduct problems. A considerable number of medications have been examined; however, there remain, in many ways, more questions than answers. Most studies have been short-term (less than 8 weeks) and although a number were placebo-controlled and double blind there are also many uncontrolled open-label or retrospective chart review studies. The vast majority of subjects were male. Some medications like divalproex sodium and antidepressants show promising results, but require more research. Evidence may be limited, but some general principles can be developed.

On the basis of the available evidence, risperidone should be considered first-line pharmacological treatment of conduct problems, especially in the absence of ADHD. Current evidence for these effects is much stronger for the learning-disabled population than for those children with normal IQs, although this reflects a lack of trials in this second group of children and young people rather than a demonstrated lack of efficacy in this population. Risperidone appears to be associated with a rapid onset of action affecting the general symptoms of conduct disorder and specific measures of aggressive behavior. Monitoring for somnolence, extra-pyramidal adverse effects, and weight gain for the development of metabolic syndrome is essential.

If comorbid ADHD is present with conduct disorder, current evidence points to the use of stimulant medication (methylphenidate) as the first-line pharmacological treatment as this appears to reduce the symptoms of both CD and ADHD. In cases where methylphenidate is not effective at reducing both the ADHD and the CD symptoms, then atomoxetine may be considered. If methylphenidate reduces the ADHD symptoms but does not control conduct symptoms then it may be appropriate to add risperidone. There is some evidence to support the use of lithium in children under 12 years, but this requires regular blood monitoring for serum levels which may severely limit its usefulness. In general, considerably more research is required into the long term efficacy, effectiveness, and safety of these medications in different populations and age ranges.

REFERENCES

Achenbach, T. M. (1991). *Manual for the child behavior checklist/4–18 and 1991 profile.* Burlington: University of Vermont, Department of Psychiatry.

Allison, D. B., Mentore, J. L., Heo, M., et al. (1999). Antipsychotic induced weight gain a comprehensive research synthesis. *American Journal of Psychiatry, 156,* 416–432.

Aman, M., De Smedt, G., Lyons, B., Findling, R., & Risperidone Disruptive Behavior Study Group. (2002). Double –blind, placebo-controlled study of risperidone for the treatment of disruptive behaviours in children with subaverage intelligence. *American Journal of Psychiatry, 159,* 1337–1346.

Aman, M. G., Singh, N., Stewart, A. W., & Field, C. J. (1985). Psychometric characteristics of the Abberrant Behavior Checklist. *American Journal of Mental Deficiency, 89,* 492–502.

Aman, M. G., Tasse, M., Rojahn, J., & Hammer, D. (1996). The Nisonger CBRF: a child behavior rating form for children with developmental disabilities. *Research in Developmental Disability, 17,* 41–57.

American Psychiatric Association. (2000). *Diagnostic and statistical manual of mental disorders (4th ed., text revision).* Washington, DC: American Psychiatric Association.

Armenteros, J. L., & Lewis, J. E. (2002). Citalopram treatment for impulsive aggression in children and adolescents: an open pilot study. *Journal of American Academy of Child and Adolescent Psychiatry, 41*(5), 522–529.

Banaschewski, T., Coghill, D., Santosh, P., et al. (2006). Long-acting medications for the hyperkinetic disorders. A systematic review and European treatment guideline. *European Journal of Child and Adolescent Psychiatry, 15*(8), 476–495.

Bangs, M., Hazell, P., Danckaerts, M., Hoare, P., Coghill, D., Wehmeier, P., et al. (2006). Atomoxetine for the treatment of attention-deficit/hyperactivity disorder and oppositional defiant disorder. *Pediatrics, 121,* e314–e320.

Barker, P., & Fraser, I. (1968). A controlled trial of haloperidol, in children. *British Journal of Psychiatry, 114,* 855–857.

Caldwell, M., Malterer, M., Umstead, D., & McCormick, D. (2008). A retrospective evaluation of adjunctive risperidone treatment in severely behaviourally disordered boys receiving psychosocial treatment. *Journal of Child and Adolescent Psychopharmacology, 18*(1), 34–43.

Campbell, M., Adams, P., Small, A., Kafantaris, V., Silva, R., Shell, S., et al. (1995). Lithium in hospitalized aggressive children with conduct disorder: a double blind and placebo controlled study. *Journal of the American Academy of Child and Adolescent Psychiatry, 34*(4), 445–453.

Campbell, M., Small, A., Green, W., Jennops, S., Perry, R., Bennett, W., et al. (1984). Behavioral efficacy of haloperidol and lithium carbonate. A comparison in hospitalised aggressive children with conduct disorder. *Archives of General Psychiatry, 41,* 650–656.

Campbell, M., Silva, R., Kafantaris, V., Locasio, J., Gonzalez, N., Lee, D., et al. (1991). Predictors of side-effects associated with Lithium administration in children. *Psychopharmacology Bulletin, 27*(3), 373–380.

Cipriani, A., Barbui, C., & Geddes, J. (2005). Suicide, depression and antidepressants. *British Medical Journal, 330,* 373–374.

Conners, C. (1998). *Manual for Conners' Rating Scale.* Toronto: Multi- health care systems.

Connor, D., Glatt, S., Lopez, I., Jackson, D., & Melloni, R. (2002). Psychopharmacology and aggression I: a meta-analysis of stimulant effects on overt/covert aggression-related behaviours in ADHD. *Journal of American Academy of Child and Adolescent Psychiatry, 41*(3), 253–261.

Croonenberghs, J., Fegert, J.M., Findling, R., De Smedt, G., Van Dongen, R., & Risperidone disruptive behaviour study group. (2005). Risperidone in children with disruptive behaviour disorders and subaverage intelligence: a 1 year open label study of 504 patients. *Journal of American Academy of Child and Adolescent Psychiatry, 44*, 67–72.

Cueva, J., Overall, J., Small, A., Armenteros, J., Perry, R., & Campbell, M. (1996). Carbamazepine in aggressive children with Conduct Disorder: a double blind and placebo controlled study. *Journal of American Academy of Child and Adolescent Psychiatry, 35*(4), 480–490.

Cunningham, M. A., Pillai, V., & Blachford-Rogers, W. J. (1968). Haloperidol in the treatment of children with severe behaviour disorders. *British Journal of Psychiatry, 144*, 845–854.

Curtiss, G., Rosenthal, R., Marohn, R., Ostrar, E., Offer, D., & Trujillo, J. (1983). Measuring delinquent behaviour in inpatient treatment settings: revision and validation of the adolescent antisocial behavior checklist. *Journal of American Academy of Child Psychiatry, 22*, 459–466.

Deltito, J. A., Leviton, J., Damone, J., Hajal, F., & Zamberiedetti, M. (1998). Naturalistic experience with the use of divalproex sodium on an inpatient unit for psychiatric patients. *Acta Psychiatrica Scandinavica, 97*(3), 236–240.

Derogatis, L. R., Lipman, R. S., & Covi, L. (1973). SCL-90: an outpatient psychiatric rating scale- preliminary report. *Psychopharmacology Bulletin, 9*, 13–28.

Donovan, S., Stewart, J., Nunes, E., Quitkin, F., Porides, M., Daniel, W., et al. (2000). Divalproex Treatment for youth with explosive temper and mood lability: a double blind, placebo controlled crossover design. *American Journal of Psychiatry, 157*, 812–820.

Donovan, S., Susser, E., Nunes, E., Stewart, J., Quitkin, F., & Klein, D. (1997). Divalproex treatment of disruptive adolescents: a report of 10 cases. *Journal of Clinical Psychiatry, 58*, 12–15.

Findling, R. (2008). Atypical antipsychotic treatment of disruptive behavior disorders in children and adolescents. *Journal of Clinical Psychiatry, 69*(suppl 4), 9–14.

Findling, R., McNamara, N., Branicky, L., Schluchter, M., Lemon, E., & Blumer, J. (2000). A double–blind pilot study of risperidone in the treatment of conduct disorder. *Journal of American Academy of Child and Adolescent Psychiatry, 39*(4), 509–516.

Findling, R., Reed, M., O'Riordan, M., Demeter, C., Stansbrey, R., & McNamara, N. (2006). Effectiveness, sifter and pharmacokinetics of quetiapine in aggressive children with conduct disorder. *Journal of American Academy of Child and Adolescent Psychiatry, 45*(7), 792–800.

Greene, R., & Ablon, S. (2003). *Treating explosive kids: the collaborative problem-solving approach.* New York: The Guildford Press.

Greenhill, L., Soloman, M., Pleak, R., & Ambrosini, P. (1985). Molindone hydrochloride treatment of hospitalised children with conduct disorder. *Journal of Clinical Psychiatry, 46*(8), 20–25.

Guy, W. (1976). *ECDEU. Assessment for Psychopharmacology.* Rockville: National Institute of Mental Health.

Handen, D., & Hardan, A. (2006). Open-label prospective trial of olanzapine in adolescents with sub average intelligence and disruptive behavior disorders. *Journal of American Academy of Child and Adolescent Psychiatry, 45*(8), 928–935.

Hazell, P., & Stuart, J. (2003). A randomized controlled trial of clonidine added to psychostimulant medication for hyperactive and aggressive children. *Journal of American Academy of Child and Adolescent Psychiatry, 42*(8), 886–894.

Henggeler, S. W., Schoenwald, S. K., Borduin, C. M., Rowland, M. D., & Cunningham, P. B. (1998). *Multisystemic treatment of antisocial behaviour in children and adolescents.* New York: Guildford Press.

Jefferson, J. (1982). The use of lithium in childhood and adolescence: an overview. *Journal of Clinical Psychiatry, 43*(5), 174–177.

Kafantaris, V., Campbell, M., Padron-Gayol, M., Small, A., Locascio, J., & Rosenberg, C. (1992). Carbamazepine in hospitalized aggressive conduct disordered children: an open pilot study. *Psychopharmacology Bulletin, 28*(2), 193–199.

Kaplan, S., Busner, J., Kupietz, S., Wasserman, E., & Segal, B. (1990). Effects of methylphenidate on adolescents with aggressive conduct disorder and ADHD: a preliminary report. *Journal of American Academy of Child and Adolescent Psychiatry, 29*(5), 719–723.

Kaplan, S., Heiligenstein, J., West, S., Busner, J., Harder, D., Dittman, R., et al. (2004). Efficacy and safety of atomoxetine in childhood attention-deficit/hyperactivity disorder with comorbid oppositional defiant disorder. *Journal of Attention Disorders, 8*, 45–52.

Kemph, J. P., Devane, C. L., Levin, C. M., Jarecke, M., & Millar, R. (1993). Treatment of aggressive children with clonidine, results of an open pilot study. *Journal of American Academy of Child and Adolescent Psychiatry, 32*, 577–581.

Klein, R., Abikoff, H., Klass, E., Ganeles, D., Seese, L., & Pollack, S. (1997). Clinical efficacy of methylphenidate in conduct disorder with and without attention deficit hyperactivity disorder. *Archives of General Psychiatry, 54*, 1073–1080.

Kolko, D., Bukstein, O., & Barron, J. (1999). Methylphenidate and behavior modification in children with ADHD and comorbid ODD or CD: main and incremental effects across settings. *Journal of American Academy of Child and Adolescent Psychiatry, 38*(5), 578–586.

McNair, D. M., Lorr, M., & Droppleman, L. F. (1971). *Profile of mood states manual.* San Diego: Educational Industrial Testing Service.

Malone, R. P., Luebbert, R. P., Penea-Areit, M., Biesecker, K., & Delaney, M. A. (1994). The overt aggression scale in a study of lithium in aggressive conduct disorder. *Psychopharmacology Bulletin, 30*, 215–218.

Malone, R., Delaney, M. A., Luebbert, J., Carter, J., & Campbell, M. (2000). A double blind placebo-controlled study of lithium in hospitalized aggressive children and adolescents with conduct disorder. *Archives of General Psychiatry, 57*, 649–654.

Masi, G., Milone, A., Canepa, G., Millepiedi, S., Mucci, M., & Muratari, F. (2006). Olanzapine treatment in adolescents with severe conduct disorder. *European Psychiatry, 21*, 51–57.

Monroe, R. R. (1970). *Episodic behavior disorders: a psychodynamic and neurophysiologic analysis.* Cambridge Mass: Harvard University Press.

Moretti, M., Emmrys, C., Grizenko, N., Holland, R., Moore, K., & Shamsie, J. (1997). The treatment of conduct disorder perspectives from across Canada. *Canadian Journal of Psychiatry, 42*, 637–648.

Mozes, T., Meiri, G., Ben-Amity, G., Sabbagh, M., & Weizman, A. (2005). Reboxetine as an optional treatment for hyperkinetic conduct disorder: a prospective open label trial. *Journal of Child and Adolescent Psychopharmacology, 15*(2), 259–269.

Newcorn, J., Spencer, T., Biedeman, J., Milton, D., & Michelson, D. (2005). Atomoxetine treatment in children and adolescents with attention deficit/hyperactivity disorder and comorbid oppositional defiant disorder. *Journal of American Academy of Child and Adolescent Psychiatry, 44*(3), 240–248.

Pandina, G., Aman, M., & Findling, R. (2006). Risperidone in the management of disruptive behavior disorder. *Journal of Child and Adolescent Psychopharmacology, 16*, 379–392.

Pandina, G., Bilder, R., Harvey, P., Keefe, R., Aman, M., & Gharabawi, G. (2007). Risperidone and cognitive function in children with disruptive behavior disorder. *Biological Psychiatry, 62*, 226–234.

Pappadopulos, E., Wollston, S., Chait, A., Perks, M., Connor, D., & Jensen, P. (2006). Pharmacotherapy of aggression in children and adolescents: efficacy and effect size. *Journal of Canadian Academy of Child and Adolescent Psychiatry, 15*(1), 27–39.

Petti, T. A., Fish, B., Shapiro, T., Cohen, I. L., & Campbell, M. (1982). Effects of chlordiazepoxide in disturbed children: a pilot study. *Journal of Clinical Psychopharmacology, 2*(4), 270–273.

Platt, J., Campbell, M., Green, W., & Gregan, D. (1984). Cognitive effects of lithium carbonate and haloperidol in treatment-resistant aggressive children. *Archives of General Psychiatry, 41*, 657–662.

Reyes, M., Buitelaar, J., Toran, P., Augustyns, I., & Erdekens, M. (2006). A randomized double-blind placebo controlled study of risperidone maintenance treatment in children and adolescents with disruptive behavior disorders. *American Journal of Psychiatry, 163*(3), 402–410.

Reyes, M., Croonenberghs, J., Augustyns, I., & Eerdekens, M. (2006). Long-term use of risperidone in children with disruptive behavior disorders and subaverage intelligence: efficacy, safety and tolerability. *Journal of Child and Adolescent Psychopharmacology, 16*(3), 260–272.

Rifkin, A., Karajgi, B., Dicker, R., Peri, E., Boppana, V., Hasan, N., et al. (1997). Lithium treatment of conduct disorders in adolescents. *American Journal of Psychiatry, 154*(4), 554–555.

Robins, L., Tipp, J., & McEvoy, L. (1991). Antisocial personality. In L. Robins & D. Regier (Eds.), *Psychiatric disorders in America* (pp. 258–290). New York: New York Free Press.

Snyder, R., Turgay, A., Aman, M., Binder, C., Fisman, S., Carroll, A., & the Risperidone Conduct Study Group. (2002). Effects of risperidone on conduct and disruptive behavior disorders in children with subaverage IQs. *Journal of American Academy of Child and Adolescent Psychiatry, 41*(9), 1026–1036.

Soderstrom, H., Rastam, M., & Gillberg, C. (2002). A clinical case series of six extremely aggressive youths treated with olanzapine. *European Child and Adolescent Psychiatry, 11*, 138–141.

Steiner, H., Petersen, M., Saxena, K., Ford, S., & Matthews, Z. (2003). Divalproex sodium for the treatment of conduct disorder: a randomized controlled clinical trial. *Journal of Clinical Psychiatry, 64*, 1183–1191.

Swanson, J. (1992). *School based Assessments and Interviews for ADD.* Irvine: KC Publishing.

Van Bellinghen, M., & de Troch, C. (2001). Risperidone in the treatment of behavioral disturbances in children and adolescents with borderline intellectual functioning: a double blind, placebo-controlled pilot trial. *Journal of Child and Adolescent Psychopharmacology, 11*(1), 5–13.

Weinberger, D. A. (1997). Distress and self-restraint as measures of adjustment across the life span: confirmatory factor analysis in clinical and non-clinical samples. *Psychological Assessment, 9*, 132–135.

Yudofsky, S. C., Silver, J. M., Jackson, W., Endicott, J., & Williams, D. (1986). The overt aggression scale for the objective rating of verbal and physical aggression. *American Journal of Psychiatry, 143*, 35–39.

Zubieta, J., & Alessi, N. (1992). Acute and chronic administration of trazadone in the treatment of disruptive behavior disorders in children. *Journal of Clinical Psychopharmacology, 12*(6), 346–351.

Section IV

Looking Forward: Prevention Programs and Advanced Treatment Considerations

16

The Fast Track Project: Preventing Severe Conduct Problems in School-Age Youth

Conduct Problems Prevention Research Group

This chapter is adaptated and expanded from material in CPPRG (2006) and Slough, McMahon, and CPPRG (2008).

In this chapter, we provide an overview of the Fast Track project as an illustration of one new direction in prevention science. In 1993 Coie et al. described prevention science as a new research discipline being formed at the interface of a number of professional emphases and disciplines, including psychopathology, criminology, psychiatric epidemiology, human development, and education. Prevention science represents an effort to examine risk factors, change processes and intervention effects, using rigorous methodology, thus providing an empirical basis for early prevention

---

Members of the Conduct Problems Prevention Research Group (in alphabetical order) are:

ELLEN E. PINDERHUGHES • Tufts University
JOHN D. COIE • Duke University
JOHN E. LOCHMAN • The University of Alabama
KAREN L. BIERMAN • The Pennsylvania State University
KENNETH A. DODGE • Duke University
MARK T. GREENBERG • The Pennsylvania State University
ROBERT J. McMAHON • University of Washington

R.C. Murrihy et al. (eds.), *Clinical Handbook of Assessing and Treating Conduct Problems in Youth*, DOI 10.1007/978-1-4419-6297-3_16,

efforts. Coie et al. suggested five principles integral to prevention science. Preventive interventions should: (1) address fundamental causal processes; (2) address risk factors before they become stabilized; (3) target those children who are at high risk for the negative outcome to be prevented; (4) optimally involve coordinated activities in multiple domains; and (5) incorporate developmental research.

In the arena of adolescent antisocial behavior, early age of onset has been shown to be a valid indicator of a significant developmental pathway leading to adolescent delinquency and conduct problems. "Early starters," (also described as "life-course persistent") begin their serious antisocial behavior early in childhood, as early as ages 6–8, and then continue with antisocial behavior into adulthood (Moffitt, 1993; Patterson, Reid, & Dishion, 1992). Early starters have been described as being at risk for antisocial behavior because of a combination of biological and family factors, although in some cases family dysfunction may be sufficient to initiate the sequence of escalating aggressive behaviors. Early starters represent approximately 6% of the youth population with conduct problems (Offord, Boyle, & Racine, 1991). They are likely to engage in a versatile, wide-ranging set of antisocial behaviors, including both overt and covert delinquency (Loeber et al., 1993). These youth have a poor prognosis in that they are at risk for a host of negative outcomes during adolescence and adulthood. Furthermore, they exact an extraordinary cost to society. Cohen (1998) estimated that, in the United States, a single youth who follows the early starter pathway and who persists in a criminal career as an adult will cost society at least $1.3 million. Similarly, in the DSM-IV (American Psychiatric Association, 2000), oppositional defiant disorder evident in early childhood can evolve into "childhood-onset" conduct disorder, and then into antisocial personality disorder in adulthood. Childhood-onset conduct disorder is expected to be preceded by physical aggression and poor peer relationships in the elementary school years. Because of their considerable influence on the rates of serious adolescent antisocial and criminal behavior and the high cost to society, prevention programs are particularly needed to target youth with early starting conduct problems. These preventive interventions need to be initiated early enough to impact the early stages of the developmental trajectory, and should be designed to influence the multiple causes and the chronic nature of this maladaptive process.

As we will illustrate, each of the five prevention science principles (Coie et al., 1993) is evident in the conceptual framework and intervention delivery plan for Fast Track, a prevention program designed to prevent serious adolescent problem behaviors and conduct disorder (Conduct Problems Prevention Research Group [CPPRG], 1992, 2000). We have articulated a developmental model for the prevention of adolescent antisocial behavior, and this model suggests important directions for prevention efforts (Coie, 1996; CPPRG, 1992, 2000; Dodge, Greenberg, Malone, & CPPRG, 2008). First, many children at risk for adolescent antisocial behavior can be identified as early as 6–7 years of age, based upon their display of diverse aggressive, disruptive, and noncompliant behaviors across home and school settings. Second, because high-risk children are likely to progress in a spiral of escalating and more severe behavior problems over time, early intervention is critical. As a function of these ongoing behavior problems, the child becomes enmeshed in accumulating risk factors, such as peer rejection and academic failure, clearly complicating the ease and effectiveness of intervention. Third, risk cannot be conceived as a static marker; instead, the topography of the risk markers is likely to change with age (e.g., peer group issues become more prominent in adolescence). More importantly, early risk factors influence subsequent processes within the child and the family, which mediate the child's ultimate antisocial outcomes. It is these mutable processes (e.g., parenting, academic skills, social–emotional development) that can then become the targets for well-conceived prevention programs. Fast Track, in fact, utilized the implications of these developmental patterns to design a prevention program for children. Children with high levels of behavior problems evident at home and at school were identified at school entry; intervention began early (in first grade when most children were about 6 years of age); and the focus of the intervention was adapted progressively from first grade into high school to address developmentally appropriate mediating processes within the child and the child's family and school contexts.

In the following sections, we first provide an overview of the developmental model that serves as the foundation for Fast Track. Because it is essential that the developmental model of a preventive intervention maps clearly onto the intervention research study's measurement and intervention models (Coie, 1996), we examine how the Fast Track developmental model was integrated into the corresponding intervention model. Next, the design and procedures for the Fast Track study are outlined, and findings to date of the efficacy of the program are presented. Finally, we then present a sample case illustration.

THE FAST TRACK DYNAMIC CASCADE DEVELOPMENTAL MODEL

Preschool and Elementary School Years

Environmental and contextual factors during the early preschool and grade school years contribute to children's long-term antisocial development. At the community level, living in poor, crime-ridden neighborhoods, having relatively few support services and community resources for parents, and having parents who are isolated and disconnected from helpful social supports contribute to children's risk. These community level factors contribute to parents' experience of high levels of stress. Other sources of parental stress, and risk factors for children's development, are parents' marginal employment, psychopathology, criminality, limited educational attainment, marital conflict, and single parenting (Dodge et al., 2008; McMahon, Wells, & Kotler, 2006).

These contextual difficulties in the child's family and community, often in combination with a child's unusually high level of impulsivity and irritability (Frick & Sheffield Morris, 2004), set the stage for potentially negative parent-child relations characterized by increasingly coercive interactions between a parent and child. Parents resort to harsh, but often inconsistent, discipline in response to children's oppositional behaviors, and this variability in parental response contributes to the parents' inadvertent reinforcement of their children's increasing noncompliance (Snyder, Reid, & Patterson, 2003). In this coercive cycle, both the parents and the child may then increase their rates of aversive behaviors towards each other. Coercive parent-child interactions are often accompanied by low rates of positive parental interaction with the child, and inadequate parental stimulation and support of the child's developing cognitive skills, social skills, and adaptive emotional regulation capabilities (e.g., Greenberg, Kusche, & Speltz, 1991). Thus, in addition to relying on highly aversive behaviors to control others, the high-risk child may also enter school poorly prepared for its cognitive, social, emotional, and academic demands. The deficits that evolve in children's language abilities because of an impoverished, nonstimulating environment can contribute both to poor reading readiness and to delays in the children's ability to use their cognitive processes to regulate their emotional and behavioral reactions (Greenberg et al.). The combination of parents' harsh discipline and and low involvement in parent-child interactions, in turn, may impede the development of children's adaptive social-cognitive skills. Children can become hypervigilant to hostile cues and intentions from others, and can adopt interaction styles that are overly action-oriented and that lack verbally assertive and cooperative strategies (e.g., Dodge, 2003).

During the elementary school years, the negative influence of the contextual risk factors (e.g., poor quality neighborhoods, poor parenting practices, family pathology, and parental isolation) continues to fuel child aggressive and disruptive behaviors (Greenberg, Lengua, Coie, Pinderhughes, & CPPRG, 1999). In many cases, the school context becomes an exacerbating rather than a corrective influence. Many high-risk children attend schools with a high density of other unprepared children like themselves (Rutter, Maughan, Mortimore, Ouston, & Smith, 1979), making effective teaching and school-based preventive interventions difficult (e.g., Kellam, Ling, Merisca, Brown, & Ialongo, 1998). As a result, teachers, like the parents in earlier years, can inadvertently begin to use inconsistent and punitive discipline. Finally, the parents of high-risk children often have their own history of school problems, and their discomfort in educational settings may lead to a lack of synchrony between home and school. This dysynchrony may be reflected in ineffective and acrimonious communications between parents and teachers, which further undermines the child's chance for success (Comer, 1980).

Aggressive and disruptive children over time often become rejected and stigmatized by peers (Ladd, Price, & Hart, 1990), who react to them in unusually aggressive ways (e.g., Dodge et al., 2003). The problematic children's social difficulties are often exacerbated by difficult relationships with their teachers. Teachers may provide less support to these children, in comparison to their classmates, rather than the increased support they need (e.g., Campbell, 1991). By preadolescence, parental rejection of their problematic children can become more pronounced because of increasingly aversive parent-child interactions and unpleasant confrontations with teachers and other school personnel as a result of the children's school difficulties (e.g., Patterson, DeBaryshe, & Ramsey, 1989). As a result, high-risk children, who have had histories of poor school performance and poor peer relations in elementary school, approach the transition to middle school feeling alienated from their most important sources of support and social bonding – family and school (Hawkins, Catalano, & Miller, 1992).

Middle School and High School Years

Adolescence is marked both by changes in youth characteristics and in the contextual influences affecting adjustment. Contextually, youth move from self-contained, single-teacher elementary classrooms to large, fluid middle or junior high schools (e.g., Eccles & Midgley, 1990), which lead to reductions in parent and teacher support and monitoring. Consequently, youth spend more time with and are more influenced by their peers. Four core domains are critical for their successful adaptation: (1) peer affiliation and peer influence, (2) academic achievement and academic orientation, (3) social cognition and identity development, and (4) parent and family relations.

Peer affiliation and influence. Alienation from conventional sources of social support from parents, teachers and nondeviant peers can lead high-risk youth to join with other adolescents like themselves (e.g., Cairns, Cairns, Neckerman, Gest, & Gariepy, 1988). Adolescents who associate with deviant peers have a substantially increased risk for adolescent problem behaviors. Keenan, Loeber, Zhang, Stouthamer-Loeber, and Van Kammen (1995) found that, in comparison to boys who did not have best friends who were truant or disobedient, disruptive boys who did have deviant peer associations had three to four times the odds of participating in covert and overt delinquent acts. Adolescents appear to reinforce each others' antisocial beliefs within deviant peer groups (e.g., Dishion, Patterson, & Griesler, 1994). Deviant peer influences serve both to escalate the seriousness of offending among those youth with a history of delinquency and to instigate initial delinquency among those with more marginal risk profiles (Thornberry, 1987; Vitaro, Tremblay, Kerr, Pagani-Kurz, & Bukowski, 1997). They also affect school dropout (Cairns, Cairns, & Neckerman, 1989) and early substance use (Chassin, Curran, Hussong, & Colder, 1996).

Whereas girls are at considerably lower risk than boys for overt aggression during elementary school, their risk for becoming involved in early sexual activity, substance use, and covert antisocial activity rises in adolescence, due largely to associations with older antisocial boys (Caspi, Lynam, Moffitt, & Silva, 1993). Girls who enter puberty early and who have learning problems and depressed mood are at elevated risk for associations with deviant boys who, in turn, encourage behaviors such as truancy, substance use, covert delinquency, and sexual activity. For example, girls with this early behavior problem profile are the ones at greatest risk for having babies prior to age 14 (Miller-Johnson et al., 1999).

Academic achievement and academic orientation. Children who have low commitment to school and high rates of school failure are at risk for a range of adolescent problem behaviors (Hawkins et al., 1992).

Adolescents who dislike school and spend little time on homework are frequently truant, show poor achievement, and have high rates of drug use (Hawkins et al., 1992; Hundley & Mercer, 1987). Increasing school adaptation by fostering social support in the school setting, promoting positive attitudes toward education, and supporting academic achievement may prevent adolescents' declines in school attachment and self-esteem (e.g., Hirsch & DuBois, 1991), and reduce negative outcomes such as early initiation of sexual activity (e.g., Ohannesian & Crockett, 1993).

Social cognition and identity development. Adolescents' rates of problem behaviors are heavily influenced by their deviance-prone attitudes and beliefs, such as their low motivation to attend school and achieve academically, and attraction to deviant behaviors such as stealing and lying (Wills & Filer, 1996). Adolescents who have histories of violence, delinquency, and substance use often lack effective coping skills, demonstrating impulsive behavioral reactivity, poor self-control, ineffective problem-solving skills, hostile attributional biases, and dominance-oriented social goals (Dodge, Lochman, Harnish, Bates, & Pettit, 1997; Wills & Filer, 1996).

As adolescents become increasingly autonomous and as demands for self-discipline increase in schoolwork and other areas, the importance of a positive self-identity increases. Adolescents' "possible selves," or their images of who they would strive to be, serve to guide adolescents' choices and are important motivators of their behavior (e.g., Markus & Nurias, 1986). Among high-risk youth, resilient adolescents are those who develop a positive sense of self, perceive themselves to have internal control over their environment, and have good problem-solving skills and a strong network of relationships with adults (Luthar & Zigler, 1991; Werner, 1986). The availability of a positive adult role model/mentor may serve as a protective factor promoting the development of a positive sense of self and supporting effective coping skills (e.g., Dubois & Karcher, 2006).

Parent and family relations. Poor parenting, involving weak monitoring, ineffective parental control, and low levels of parent support, contributes directly to adolescent deviant behavior (Chassin et al., 1996). Because of the greater mobility of adolescents and their increased needs for personal privacy, parents have less opportunity to monitor their adolescents' activities and their friendships. Research indicates that poor parental monitoring and discipline play a critical role in adolescents' involvement in deviant peer groups, and in early- and late-onset delinquency and drug use (e.g., Dishion & McMahon, 1998; Dishion, Nelson, & Bullock, 2004).

Strong bonds of attachment to family serve a protective function in youth otherwise at risk for delinquency and substance abuse (e.g., Johnson & Pandina, 1991). Productive parent-adolescent communication, joint problem solving, and collaborative planning are all indices of supportive family relations in adolescence; interventions focused on promoting communication and conflict resolution skills along with family problem-solving meetings reduce adolescent acting-out behaviors (Henggeler, Schoenwald, & Pickrel, 1995). Effective parental monitoring works both directly in its effects on the adolescents' behavior, and indirectly through its effects on the adolescents' involvement in certain peer groups (Fletcher, Darling, &

Steinberg, 1995). Promoting positive parent-child relationships, fostering effective parent-adolescent communications, and enhancing parental monitoring and supervision skills may all contribute to reductions in adolescent risk for deviant behaviors.

Empirical Testing of the Dynamic Cascade Model

We have recently tested a version of this dynamic cascade model of the development of serious violence in adolescence (Dodge et al. 2008). Utilizing data from the high-risk control and normative samples from the Fast Track Project (see below), we found that a variety of domains of risk factors each predicted subsequent adolescent violence. However, each succeeding domain not only mediated the effects of the preceding domain, it also provided a significant increment beyond the previous domain in enhancing the prediction of violent outcomes. To summarize, an early social context of disadvantage (i.e., neighbourhood risk, family socioeconomic status, maternal depression) predicted child social and cognitive deficits, which predicted early conduct problem behaviors, which predicted elementary school social and academic failure, which predicted parental withdrawal from supervision and monitoring, which predicted deviant peer associations, which ultimately predicted adolescent violence.

DESIGN OF THE FAST TRACK EXPERIMENT

This developmental model indicates that the dysfunctional development that is associated with the early-starting pattern of conduct problems is multiply determined and is embedded in transactions among family, peer, school, and neighborhood influences and child characteristics. Hence, prevention efforts must target both the promotion of individual competencies and the promotion of protective contextual supports. Preventive interventions must also be attentive to age-related stressors and the successive issues of risk across important developmental periods (Cicchetti, 1984). Early-starting conduct problems turn into serious and chronic problems because they divert the individual child into a sequence of experiences that intensify risk.

Data from the Rochester study (Thornberry, Huizinga, & Loeber, 1995) suggest that protective factors must be continuously present during the transition from early to late adolescence and not simply in place at a single point in childhood or adolescence. Although the negative impact of early risk factors may be buffered by the provision of protective support services during the grade school years, the risk factors themselves may continue to influence developmental trajectories during adolescence. For example, the high rates of inattention, impulsivity, and cognitive deficits that contribute to the school adjustment problems of many early-starting youth (Moffitt, 1990) may be buffered when protective support is offered during elementary school in the form of academic tutoring and effective teacher management. As the demands for focused attention and independent work completion increase with the transition to middle school, these cognitive risk factors may undermine school adaptation unless continuing support is offered at later grade levels. In addition, developmental research suggests that new risk factors emerge during adolescence and that these risk factors are associated with the escalation of antisocial and related adolescent behavior problems. Elementary-school prevention may improve child "readiness" to tackle the new challenges of adolescence. However, for high-risk children living in unstable and risky contexts, without effective protective supports the challenges of adolescence may also undermine the gains produced by early preventive efforts. Thus, a successful program for preventing serious antisocial problems requires a long-term intervention commitment.

The significance of the Fast Track Project is that it addresses the three organizing principles for the prevention of serious violent delinquency outlined by Thornberry et al. (1995): namely, it starts early, it is comprehensive, and it is carried out over the long-term of development. In Fast Track, high-risk youth were selected at school entry from poor, high-crime neighborhoods. The elementary-school intervention addressed the major risk factors implicated in the initiation of early-starting conduct problems, and used an integrated set of developmentally sensitive intervention components to promote competencies in parents (parent training and home visiting), teachers (prevention curriculum and classroom management consultation), and children (social skills training and academic tutoring), and to strengthen bonds of communication between parents and teachers.

The design of the study was a randomized trial with randomization at the level of the school as children entered first grade. The project contained two levels of preventive intervention (universal, indicated) as well as two types of participants (high risk, all students). Annual assessments using multiple sources of data for measure constructs were collected. The design permitted continuous evaluation of the developmental model, both in tests of mediation of the effects of intervention on the high-risk youth, and longer-term modeling of risk-outcomes relationships within the normative sample (see below) and the control sample of high-risk youth.

In January 1991, crime records, poverty statistics and school dropout rates were used to identify 54 high-risk schools in four geographic sites across the United States (Durham, North Carolina; Nashville, Tennessee; Seattle, Washington; and rural central Pennsylvania). Schools within the four sites were selected as high risk based on crime and poverty statistics of the neighborhoods they served. Within each site, the schools were divided into multiple paired sets matched for demographics (size, percentage free or reduced lunch, ethnic composition), and one of each pair was randomly assigned to intervention and control conditions. Using a multiple-gating screening procedure for each of three annual cohorts, all 9,594 kindergarteners in 55 schools were screened initially for classroom conduct problems by teachers. Children scoring in the top 40% within cohort and site were then solicited for the next stage of screening for home behavior problems by the parents, and 91% agreed (n=3,274) (Lochman & CPPRG, 1995). The teacher and parent screening scores were then standardized and combined into a sum score. Children were selected for inclusion into the study based on this sum score, moving from the highest score downward until desired sample sizes were reached within sites, cohorts, and conditions. Deviations were made when a child failed to matriculate in the first grade at a core school ($n=59$) or refused to participate ($n=75$), or to accommodate a rule that no child would be the only girl in an intervention group (an attempt was made to have boys and girls in each group). Ninety-five percent of the selected sample scored in the top 20% on both the parent and teacher screening measures. The outcome was that 891 children (n's = 445 for intervention and 446 for control) participated. Analyses of the initial comparability of the intervention and control groups indicated that there were no significant preintervention differences between the groups on demographic and behavioral variables. Analyses of indicated intervention effects with the high-risk group of children thus use this sample of 891 children. Across all sites, the sample was 51% African American, 47% European American, and 2% other. Boys comprised 69% of the sample. Analyses of universal intervention effects were conducted with the full populations of the intervention and control schools. The universal intervention continued throughout the elementary school years. The indicated intervention continued through Grade 10. At the time of this writing, the sample has been followed through age 20 years.

To compare improvements made by the intervention group against a normative standard, a representative sample of 387 children was selected from the control schools. Children were stratified to represent the population according to race, sex, and decile of teacher screen scores.

THE FAST TRACK INTERVENTION MODEL

The Fast Track intervention was divided into two primary phases: (a) elementary school, and (b) transition to middle and high schools, coinciding with the transition to adolescence.

Elementary School Phase[1]

Corresponding to the developmental risks associated with the early initiation of conduct problems, prevention activities during elementary school targeted the provision of: (a) positive behavioral support at school and at home; (b) fostering the home-school relationship; and (c) the promotion of parenting skills, child social skills, child social-cognitive skills, child reading skills, and mentoring for children by a same-sex, same-race community volunteer. Intervention components focused both on building the child's behavioral and cognitive skills and on changing the patterns of interaction with important people in the child's social environment (family, school, and peer) to promote healthy relationships with peers and adults.

[1]See Bierman, Greenberg, and CPPRG (1996) and McMahon, Slough, and CPPRG, (1996) for extensive descriptions of this phase of intervention. Facilitator's guides for the parent group, Parent-Child Sharing Time, and home visiting components (McMahon et al., 2010) and the Friendship Group (Bierman et al., 2010) will soon be available for the elementary-school phase of the intervention.

The intervention was organized developmentally and included three levels of prevention activities: (a) universal prevention support provided at the school level; (b) standard indicated prevention support services provided to families of children identified as high risk during the initial kindergarten screening; and (c) additional individualized indicated prevention support provided to high-risk children and families on an as-needed basis (according to criterion-referenced assessments). Prevention support was intensive with massed sessions offered at the important transition into elementary school (Grades 1–2). Sustained support was then continued through fifth grade. The content of each of the prevention services was organized developmentally, and integrated across components.

At the universal level of prevention, an adaptation of the PATHS (Promoting Alternative Thinking Strategies) Curriculum (Kusche & Greenberg, 1993) was taught by classroom teachers two to three times per week in Grades 1–5. The PATHS Curriculum model synthesizes the domains of self-control, emotional awareness and understanding, peer-related social skills, and social problem solving to increase social and emotional competence (Kusche & Greenberg, 1993). In addition to a person-oriented model that focused primarily on developmental integration, the intervention model incorporated an eco-behavioral systems orientation (Weissberg, Caplan, & Sivo, 1989), which placed primacy on the manner in which the teacher used the curriculum model. That is, program impact may be the greatest when teachers generalize support for curriculum-based skills during the day and build a healthy classroom atmosphere that supports the child's skill use and internalization of skills. It was presumed that improvements in social competence can be a function of both changes in the child, changes in the ecology, and their interaction. Fast Track staff also consulted with the school principal to bring the philosophy of PATHS to the entire school, resulting in various efforts (on a school-by-school basis) such as placing PATHS posters in school hallways, implementing new school behavior guidelines, and painting problem-solving "stop lights" on school playgrounds.

Classroom teachers were trained in the administration of this curriculum and provided individualized teacher consultation about behavioral management issues. In the early school years, targeted skills were designed to enhance adaptation to the rules and routines of school and to foster the development of positive peer relations. In later years, more advanced topics included decision-making skills, study skills, goal setting, character development, coping with peer pressure, and problem-solving skills.

At the standard indicated level of prevention, 2-h family group meetings were held regularly at local schools. Sessions were held weekly for 22 sessions in Grade 1, biweekly for 14 sessions in Grade 2, and monthly for 8 sessions each year in Grades 3–5. Each session involved separate 60-min group meetings for parents and social skill training meetings for children. Children then received 30 min of tutoring in reading skills, led by a trained paraprofessional and observed by the parent. The last 30 min of each session included a parent-child sharing session, in which parents and children participated in joint activities. Parent groups promoted the development of positive family-school relationships and taught effective communication and discipline skills (including praise and ignoring, clear instructions and rules, and time out) (McMahon, Slough, & Conduct Problems Prevention Research Group, 1996). Child social skill groups focused on friendship and play skills and self-control skills, anger-coping strategies and interpersonal problem-solving skills (Bierman, Greenberg, & Conduct Problems Prevention Research Group, 1996). Parent-child sharing sessions promoted positive relationships and offered parents an opportunity to practice new parenting skills with staff guidance. As with PATHS, the skill topics addressed in the parent and child groups followed a developmental sequence, with an increasing emphasis over time on communication skills, homework study skills, goal-setting, and negotiating parent-child conflicts. Individualized indicated services included academic tutoring, home visiting, and school-based peer pairing to promote friendships. Children and families received a standard level of these services in Grade 1. In subsequent years, criterion-referenced assessments were used to adjust the dosage of these three indicated components to match the level of functioning of each family and child. In Grade 4, a mentoring program was added, reflecting the growing significance of the child's identity development and the importance of same-gender, same-race positive role models in the identity development process.

Adolescent Phase

The adolescent phase of the intervention plan emphasized four domains associated with successful adolescent adjustment: peer affiliation and peer influence, academic orientation and achievement, social cognition and identity development, and parent and family relations. This phase of the intervention covered Grades 5–10 (CPPRG, 2000). It began with intensive prevention efforts around the transition into middle school (Grades 5–7) that were followed by continuing individualized preventive support through Grades 8–10. Due to a growing dispersion of the target sample across schools, it was not possible to serve a substantial segment of the sample with a universal prevention curriculum in adolescence.

Reflecting the developmental characteristics of adolescence, the intervention design differed in some fundamental ways from the design used in the elementary phase. Monthly group sessions involving parents and youth continued during Grades 5 and 6. As in the elementary phase, these sessions were held at the school (or other community location), were 2 h long, and included separate meetings for parents and youth, along with periods for parent-youth discussion. However, reflecting the protective role of adult supervision and monitoring in adolescence, and the corresponding importance of parent-youth communication, group sessions increasingly emphasized joint presentations to parents and youth, along with guided parent-youth discussions. Second, the emerging abstract reasoning capabilities of young adolescents, coupled with their increased independence and mobility, created an opportunity and need to focus on identity development, future goals, and decision-making around both vocational and avocational interests and activities. To meet this need, the adolescent-phase intervention included identity development workshops for youth in Grades 7 and 8, called youth forums. Third, adolescence is marked by several critical developmental changes, including puberty, the initiation of romantic relationships and sexual activity, increasing peer group affiliation, and identity development. Youth differ markedly in the age at which, and speed with which, pubertal development and these other changes occur, creating heterogeneity that has implications for risk and for preventive intervention. As adolescents become more peer-oriented, deviant peer groups also emerge in early adolescence, and can function to support and facilitate antisocial activity. Group-based interventions for high-risk adolescents can unwittingly strengthen deviant peer affiliations and thus sabotage prevention effectiveness (Dodge, Dishion, & Lansford, 2006). Given the need to respond to increasing heterogeneity within the Fast Track adolescent sample, along with the need to avoid supporting deviant affiliations, individualized criterion-referenced services (rather than group sessions) were emphasized in the later grades (Grades 7–10).

During the adolescent phase, the standard prevention activities included two kinds of curriculum-based parent and youth groups: (1) groups focused on developmental issues of adolescence, held monthly during Grades 5–6 and during the beginning of Grade 7; and (2) an additional set of group meetings that comprised a transition support program, timed around the student's transition into middle school or junior high school (Grades 5–6 or 6–7, depending upon the local school organization). The key goal of the groups was to introduce skills that could delay the onset and reduce the severity of adolescent problems. Topics for parent groups included parental positive involvement and monitoring, communication and conflict resolution skills, and parental support for student achievement. Youth group topics included coping with peer pressure, resistance and refusal skills, advanced problem solving, and goal-setting and decision-making skills. After receiving information about adolescent risks and protective skills during the family sessions, the intervention staff supported candid parent–youth discussions around issues such as middle school transition adjustment (Grades 5–6); romantic relationships and sex education (Grades 5–6); alcohol, tobacco, and drug use (Grades 6–7); and vocational goal setting (Grade 7).

The middle-school transition program was designed to provide additional support to parents and youth during the spring prior to, and the fall following, the youth's transition into middle school. This program included visits to the middle school, discussions with the school counselor, coaching in organizational and study skills, and support from middle-school student mentors. The family sessions of the transition program were directed toward helping youth and parents acquire knowledge about middle school, learn skills of adapting to middle-school life, communicate more effectively around middle-school issues, and build a positive relationship with middle-school counselors and teachers.

A new aspect of the standard intervention in adolescence involved youth forums designed as workshops for groups of 4–8 youth. In Grades 7 and 8, eight of these forums, based on Oyserman's Future Selves Program (Oyserman, Sanchez-Burks, & Harrison, 1996), encouraged youth to think about their short- and long-term life goals, to explore different life opportunities and choices, and to explore vocational opportunities, budgeting and life skills, summer employment opportunities and job interview skills.

In addition to these curriculum-based group programs, individualized prevention supports were offered to some of the high-risk youth on an "as needed" basis, according to criterion-based assessments. Given individual growth trajectories and life situations, considerable heterogeneity existed within the high-risk sample in adolescence. Individualized prevention services were designed to strengthen protective factors in areas of particular need for specific youth. The goal was to work toward equalizing the strength of protective factors across high-risk youth, rather than equalizing the amount of intervention delivered to each high-risk youth. Individualized services included: (a) academic tutoring, (b) mentoring, (c) support for positive peer-group involvement, (d) home visiting and family problem solving, and (e) liaisons with school and community agencies.

FAST TRACK OUTCOMES

Analyses of the Fast Track Program indicate that the program had significant impact on proximal outcomes that were assessed in the elementary school phase of the project, such as improvements in behavior, social skills, and parenting strategies, and some more distal outcomes assessed in adolescence, such as disruptive behavior disorder diagnoses and arrests. In this section, we briefly summarize findings to date concerning the impact of the program.

Elementary School

High-risk sample. We first examined the effects of the Fast Track program on the high-risk children at the end of the first grade (CPPRG, 1999a). In comparison to the high-risk control children, the high-risk intervention children displayed improved emotion recognition, emotion coping, abilities to generate competent solutions to social problems, and word attack skills, and higher language arts grades. In addition, the intervention children displayed improvements in independently observed positive interactions with peers at school, and had improved social preference scores on sociometric ratings.

Fast Track enhanced certain aspects of parenting. Following the first year of intervention, parents reported that they would use lower rates of physical punishment in vignettes of difficult parent-child situations; they were observed to interact in warmer, more involved ways during observed parent-child interactions in the home; they were rated by the observers as using more appropriate and consistent discipline; they were more positively involved with their children's schools; they placed more value on encouraging children's learning; and they were very satisfied with the intervention. With regards to children's actual behavior, high-risk intervention children displayed significantly greater behavioral changes during the year according to the parent and teacher ratings, and teachers rated the intervention children as having significantly lower rates of aggressive, oppositional behaviors in the school setting.

By the end of Grade 3 (CPPRG, 2002a), lower teacher ratings of conduct problems indicated that the intervention children, in comparison to the control children, were continuing to display reductions in conduct problem behavior. Parent reports of children's conduct problem behavior also indicated greater positive child behavior change (i.e., less conduct problem behavior) and lower levels of aggressive behavior in comparison to the control group. However, there was no significant main effect of intervention on formal diagnoses of oppositional defiant disorder or conduct disorder as assessed by the DISC structured interview. In contrast to the effects noted at the end of the first grade, intervention effects were no longer evident for measures of social competence or reading achievement. Intervention parents reported less use of physical punishment on vignettes about parenting situations, and rated themselves as having improved their parenting behavior to a greater degree over the previous year than did parents in the control condition.

We also employed a dichotomous measure of serious conduct problems (i.e., clinical "caseness"). Clinical caseness was based on the presence of an elevated score on at least one of the following four measures: (a) a DISC diagnosis of oppositional defiant disorder or conduct disorder, (b) existence of an individualized education plan (IEP), and (c) teacher or (d) parent reports of conduct problems in the top 15% of the distribution. Using this more person-oriented approach to data analysis revealed that 37% of the intervention sample was "case free" at the end of third grade, in contrast to 27% of the control sample. This represented a 1/3 increase in "case-free" status.

Using a similar approach to "caseness" at the end of Grades 4 and 5, we found significant intervention effects for three of four domains: (a) social competence and social cognition problems, (b) involvement with deviant peers, and (c) conduct problems in the home and community (CPPRG, 2004). There were reductions in caseness ranging from 17% to 33%. However, there were no significant intervention effects for a fourth domain that assessed school context academic and behavior problems.

Mediation of Grade 4 outcomes. We conducted an assessment of mediators for several significant outcomes for the Fast Track intervention at Grade 4 (CPPRG, 2002b). Potential mediators consisted of variables that demonstrated significant intervention effects at the end of Grade 3. The effects of these mediational analyses were largely consistent with the early starter model of conduct problems, and were decidedly domain specific. For example, improvements in parenting partially accounted for intervention effects on oppositional/aggressive behavior at home, but not at school. Improvements in children's prosocial behavior at school partially mediated intervention effects on peer social preference in the classroom. Similarly, improvement in children's social cognitions concerning their peers partially mediated intervention effects on deviant peer associations. These patterns suggest that a multifaceted intervention may be necessary in order to improve children's adjustment outcomes in the elementary years.

Universal sample. Because the PATHS program was provided to all children in the intervention schools, not just the high-risk children, and because other program components (e.g., peer pairing) included the lower-risk classmates of our target children, we also examined the universal preventive effects of Fast Track through Grades 1–3 (CPPRG, 1999b, 2010b). Analyses were conducted by removing the high-risk children from the analyses, thus permitting an examination of the effects on the remaining classmates. At the end of first grade, intervention classrooms were found to have lower peer-rated aggression and lower peer-rated hyperactive-disruptive behaviors than were the control classrooms (CPPRG, 1999b). Ratings by independent observers in the classrooms indicated that the intervention classrooms had better classroom atmosphere (e.g., better rule following, appropriate expression of feelings, greater enthusiasm and interest, and ability to stay focused and on task). In implementation analyses, teachers' rated skill in teaching the PATHS concepts emerged as a predictor of degree of improvement evident in the observers' coding of the classroom atmosphere, further indicating the role of the program in producing these positive outcome effects. This universal social and emotional learning program had important preventive effects for all students, and, thus may have increased the likelihood that intervention effects with the high-risk children would be maintained because of the improved classroom context in which the target children were embedded.

More recently, we examined the effects of the PATHS universal intervention on student behavior change (teacher ratings and peer sociometric nominations) for students who received 3 years of the intervention (CPPRG, 2010b). The longitudinal analysis involved 2,937 children who remained in the same intervention or control schools for Grades 1, 2, and 3. Modest positive effects of sustained program exposure included significant reductions in peer- and teacher-rated aggression and peer-rated hyperactive/disruptive behavior, and improvements in teacher-rated academic engagement and social competence. The effects of the teacher-rated variables were moderated by school environment, with effects stronger in less disadvantaged schools; furthermore, reductions in teacher-rated aggression were also larger in children who showed higher baseline levels of teacher-rated aggression. Gender moderated the effects of peer-nominated aggression and hyperactive-disruptive behavior, with the intervention effects noted only for boys.

Middle School

We next examined the effects of the Fast Track preventive intervention on youths' functioning in middle school in three domains: disruptive behavior problems, involvement with deviant peers, and social skills during the middle school years (CPPRG, in press). In contrast to prior findings of the effectiveness of the intervention during the elementary school years, Fast Track had little overall impact on children's functioning in these domains during middle school. There were positive intervention effects on only 2 of 17 outcomes examined. Although the intervention had positive impact on parent-rated hyperactive behaviors and youth self-reported delinquent behaviors in seventh grade, there were no intervention effects on other externalizing behavior problems or on social skills. In addition, in contrast to the findings at the end of elementary school, Fast Track children in eighth grade were more likely than control children to be involved with peers who were engaging in deviant behavior; this deviant peer involvment may have mitigated some of the earlier intervention effects.

Moderation of Intervention Effects

We have not found consistent patterns of moderation of the intervention during the elementary and middle school years. This includes demographic variables (e.g., gender, race, site, and cohort), child variables (e.g., IQ), family variables (e.g., marital status, socioeconomic status, parent mental health or substance abuse status), and neighborhood variables (e.g., poverty, instability, quality). The few scattered intervention interactions found across the elementary school analyses did not form any meaningful pattern, and did not extend beyond chance levels. This failure to find systematic evidence of moderation suggests that the modest intervention effects were generalizable during elementary and middle school, with comparable effects, for example, for boys and girls, for African American and European American children, and in urban and rural settings.

However, there is evidence of emerging moderation of intervention effects for youth's externalizing psychiatric disorders and antisocial behavior on the basis of the severity of the child's initial risk score at kindergarten (CPPRG, 2007). Significant interaction effects between intervention and initial risk level were found after Grades 3 and 6, but most strongly after Grade 9. Among the highest-risk group (top 3%) in Grade 9, intervention children showed a 75% reduction in diagnosed cases of conduct disorder, 53% reduction in cases of attention deficit hyperactivity disorder, and 43% reduction of any externalizing disorder cases, as compared to the control group. In contrast, the intervention had no impact on children who were initially at only moderate levels of risk. Similar findings were obtained with an antisocial behavior score, based on the youth's self-reported delinquency (although there was also a main effect of intervention). Youth in the highest-risk portion of the sample who participated in the Fast Track intervention reported significantly lower engagement in this measure of index crimes, interpersonal violence, and general delinquency than youth in the control group at similar levels of risk.

Effects on Youth Arrests and Delinquency

We recently examined the effects of the Fast Track preventive intervention on youth arrests and self-reported delinquent behavior through age 19 (CPPRG, 2010a). Due to the differences in how arrests for juvenile crimes are processed vs. arrests for adult crimes, we examined court records separately for arrests adjudicated as juvenile vs. adult crimes. Findings indicated that intervention influenced overall court-record juvenile arrest activity, as the odds of intervention youth being involved in court-recorded arrests was 29% lower than for control youth, the number of moderate-severity juvenile arrests was reduced by 24%, and the odds for onset of a juvenile arrest was lowered by 23% compared to the control youth. There is also evidence that intervention delayed the odds of onset of severe self-reported delinquent offenses by 18%. Intervention effects on the frequency of high-severity adult arrests (through age 19) were moderated by children's baseline levels of problem behavior. For children with the highest level of kindergarten aggression (top 13%), arrests for severe crimes were reduced by 47%. The onset of high-severity adult arrests was moderated by site – intervention effects were found for three sites, and an iatrogenic effect was found for the Nashville site.

Economic Analyses

We are conducting an ongoing extensive economic analysis of the costs and benefits of the Fast Track intervention. Analyses to date suggest that the intervention is rather costly ($58,283 per child for all 10 years of intervention; i.e., approximately $6,000/year) (Foster, Jones, & CPPRG, 2006). However, such expenditures must be evaluated relative to the other public and social costs stemming from the behavior of these youth. The costs of a life of crime include criminal justice expenditures (e.g., arrest, adjudication, and incarceration), costs to victims (e.g., medical costs, time missed from work, the value of stolen property as well as loss of life), and costs that accrue to the criminal and his or her family (e.g., lost wages). As noted earlier, Cohen (1998) estimates that the social costs of a single life of crime total at least $1.3 million. Thus, initial findings indicate that there were cost savings associated with Fast Track in areas of reduced utilization of general health and outpatient mental health services through adolescence, as well as lower arrest rates (CPPRG, in press, 2010a, 2010b; Jones et al., 2010). However, there were no cost savings associated with outcomes for special education, high school graduation, or inpatient mental health. Although such costs reductions are unlikely to fully offset the initial costs of the intensive Fast Track prevention program, some evidence for cost-effectiveness has emerged for the subgroup of youth who were at highest risk at the initial kindergarten screening in terms of conduct disorder diagnoses and self-reported index offenses (Foster et al., 2006).

CASE ILLUSTRATION[2]

Joseph (a composite of several study participants) was a 5-year-old Caucasian male who lived with his biological mother, stepfather of a few months, and his 2.5-year-old sister. Joseph's biological father had moved to another town and saw his son infrequently.

Preintervention Information

During the summer assessment prior to Joseph and his mother being invited to join Fast Track, Joseph's mother (referred to here as Ms. L.) described her biggest concerns about her son as not being able to understand what he was told, not listening well, and being always ready for a fight. On the parent screening measure (a 24-item questionnaire concerning child externalizing behavior problems drawn from existing behavior checklists), Ms. L. endorsed the following items as "often true" (the highest rating) of Joseph: easily upset, annoyed or irritated; starts fights with

[2]Identifying information in this case description has been changed. Portions of the description represent a composite of several Fast Track participants to protect the anonymity of any one child and family.

other children; stubborn; breaks rules; teases other children; whines and nags; threatens or bullies other children; sneaky; defiant toward adults; blames others for misbehavior; and temper tantrums. She also expressed concern about Joseph setting fires. His most serious incident occurred at age 4 when he burned up a tool shed; however, there had been other serious "accidents" since then. Ms. L. also stated that she and Joseph had a "personality clash," yelled at each other a lot, that it was difficult to be patient with him, and that he had "more energy than any child his age." Overall, however, Ms. L. felt that it had been "mostly pleasant" to raise him and described him as a happy child.

A behavior checklist completed by Joseph's kindergarten teacher indicated that the following behaviors occurred very frequently: stubborn; breaks rules; harms others; fights; lies; trouble accepting authority; disobedient; yells at others; and disliked by classmates. Thus, both Joseph's kindergarten teacher and his mother described him as being aggressive, oppositional, and having peer relationship difficulties. With respect to the latter, when interpreting other children's intentions of offensive actions of an ambiguous nature (e.g., being bumped or hit with a ball or being denied a request to join a group of children at play), Joseph ascribed a hostile intent to seven of eight responses to vignettes in which the child interprets an offender's intentions (e.g., "He hates me;" "Cause he is a mean kid."). Joseph's description of how he would behave in response to the offense was also aggressive, in that he responded to five of the eight situations by "punching" or by "showing who's tougher."

In addition to Joseph's social skills deficits, he struggled with learning to read and mastering basic math concepts. Ms. L. was frustrated with the teacher calling her at least once every week to complain about Joseph; and she was "no good" at helping him at home.

Attempts to recruit Ms. L. into Fast Track were initially met with refusal. Nonetheless, it was clear that she wanted Joseph to be involved, especially so that he could receive tutoring. After agreeing to participate in the program, she stated that staff should not expect her to attend parent groups but that it "might be okay" for the Family Coordinator (FC) to visit her at home.

Initial Intervention Sessions in First Grade

Home visits. Scheduling biweekly home visits with Ms. L. was generally uncomplicated as she did not work outside of the home. Once the FC arrived at her home, however, Ms. L. was habitually upset about a family (or other) incident and launched into a litany of complaints that precluded any real discussion. After several home visits, the FC ascertained that Ms. L.'s characteristic bravado was shielding a fairly anxious woman who was insecure in social situations. Over time it also became evident that some of Ms. L.'s impudence during the visits was a "test" of the commitment that Fast Track and, in particular, the FC, had to her and her family. Ms. L. held very strong opinions about parenting and did not see the necessity for discipline strategies other than her own approach of privilege removal, sending Joseph to his room, and, when necessary, using "a hand or belt" depending on the misbehavior. Ms. L. described herself as more like a single parent since she did not allow Joseph's stepfather to discipline the children. She expressed her feeling that parenting Joseph was difficult and that even after she "put her foot down," he whined and yelled until he got his way. Problem-solving sessions, centered on resolving some of their parent-child difficulties, typically resulted in Ms. L. generating only one solution, usually one with a negative focus.

Parent Group. True to her word, Ms. L. was initially resistant to Fast Track's encouragement of her attendance at parent groups, although she was pleased that Joseph was attending the first-grade Friendship Group and receiving tutoring. However, once Ms. L. was persuaded (due in part to Joseph's insistence) to visit a few of the parent groups, she attended consistently and, in time, seemed to enjoy being part of the group. She was an active participant and was particularly vocal if something was said with which she disagreed. As she gained more trust in her relationship with the FC and felt more comfortable with the group process and with other group members, the agitation and nervousness she initially demonstrated diminished.

Friendship Group. Joseph had a difficult time in Friendship Group. He played off other children's misbehavior and often spoke out of turn. He delighted in making crude jokes, throwing food at snack time, and trying to get the other children's attention with inappropriate behavior that included punching or threatening them. His behavior would improve for short periods when the Educational Coordinator (EC) attended to his appropriate behavior. His behavior also improved when he was given a task with some responsibility (e.g., setting up snacks).

Parent–Child Sharing Time. Both Ms. L. and Joseph appeared uncomfortable as they joined together for Parent-Child Sharing Time. They often teased each other maliciously and sat with their arms folded across their chests until they began an activity. Complimenting each other was a chore, especially for Ms. L., and took a good deal of coaching by the FC.

Academics and behavior at school. Joseph had a hard time with schoolwork and being attentive in class. Part of his difficulty in school could be attributed to his distractibility, inattentiveness, "constant fidgeting," and talking out of turn. He also engaged in many of the same acting-out behaviors that he demonstrated in Friendship Group.

Ms. L. had difficulty supporting Joseph in getting his homework finished and turned in on time. Additionally, Ms. L.'s relationship with school personnel was strained, at best. Her rare visits to the school usually resulted in her adamantly blaming the school for whatever incident had brought her there. In fact, Ms. L. twice threatened to quit Fast Track during the first year of the intervention because she was upset about events that occurred with Joseph at school. One such precipitating event was a school referral to Child Protective Services for a cigarette burn on Joseph's hand, which Ms. L. had employed as a disciplinary strategy to teach him not to play with matches. This incident provided an opportunity for Fast Track staff to work with Child Protective Services, and intensify the support provided to Ms. L in areas of anger management and appropriate parenting.

Intervention Strategies: Grades 1 and 2

Home visits. Home visits with Ms. L. continued on a biweekly basis throughout the first 2 years of the project. Ms. L preferred that the FC visit during school hours, but occasionally Joseph was present. During these occasions, the FC coached Joseph and his mother through problem-solving sessions on the topics of completing his homework or chores.

Recognizing that her impatience with Joseph (and others) was an impediment to their relationship, Ms. L. was eager to set goals focusing on being more patient with her son. Over the first 2 years of the project, the FC and Ms. L. agreed to concentrate on the following goals: (1) practice the methods for calming down taught in parent group and in the PATHS curriculum; (2) try to be more patient with Joseph by recognizing her own feelings and calming down; (3) let Joseph express his feelings and listen to his side of the story *before* deciding to punish him; (4) move immediately into using the time-out strategies taught in parent group for any physical aggression; (5) monitor Joseph's homework to be sure it was completed on time; and (6) make a positive comment whenever she "caught Joseph being good."

While Ms. L. eventually accepted the idea that giving praise and positive attention to Joseph was important, she found it difficult to implement. During home visits, the FC focused on finding opportunities to praise and congratulate Ms. L. on her efforts and accomplishments. This positive attention accomplished three intervention goals: (1) it allowed Ms. L. to experience how *she* felt when positively recognized; (2) it modeled an important and basic component of the parenting skills curriculum with which Joseph's mother needed to become comfortable; and (3) it reinforced Ms. L.'s efforts in attaining the goals she was working on with Joseph.

Friendship Group. The EC and cofacilitator set up a behavior plan that focused on Joseph reducing his physical aggression, using more positive and less threatening language, and behaving more seriously and in a more mature fashion during group. This included having him use calming down and "active ignoring" strategies to avoid joining in misbehavior with other group members. Joseph was rewarded with verbal praise and positive attention and received more responsibility for setting up, and sometimes leading, group activities.

Parent-Child Sharing Time. The estrangement that Joseph and his mother displayed during Parent-Child Sharing Time resulted in the decision to pair them with different partners to practice the skills that Ms. L. was learning in parent group (i.e., Ms. L. practiced with another child and Joseph practiced with another parent). Both Joseph and his mother responded well to this re-matching and the skills practices appeared rewarding for both of them.

Academics and behavior at school. Joseph continued to have difficulty behaving appropriately in the classroom. If he earned a discipline slip for his behavior, he would sometimes throw major tantrums that involved screaming, kicking, and crying. He agitated his peers with teasing, name-calling, and sometimes hitting. A similar behavior plan to the one used in Friendship Group was set up with Joseph's teacher. The plan worked particularly well during the PATHS curriculum time when Joseph recognized the same concepts being taught as in Friendship Group. Joseph also responded positively to the one-on-one reading tutoring provided by Fast Track during which he was cooperative and mostly showed good effort. Additionally, he demonstrated mature and cooperative effort during the peer-pairing sessions involving another child from the classroom and conducted by his tutor.

Progress by Third Grade

After the conclusion of the first 2 years of the intervention, Joseph's mother expressed her regret that the parent and child groups would be meeting only once a month. Her demeanor on home visits could still be antagonistic at times, but she was able to calm down and focus on parenting issues shortly after the FC arrived. Ms. L. reported that it was definitely easier to praise Joseph but noted that, "there still aren't that many opportunities to do so." Ms. L. had become skilled at the use of the time-out strategies and Joseph's aggressive behavior during arguments declined sharply. Ms. L. and the FC were able to set up long-term goals for parenting that included sharing some responsibilities with her husband. She and Joseph became much more comfortable (even animated at times) when paired together during parent–child sharing time and could make appropriate comments to each other during the complimenting exercise. Visits to the school by Ms. L., together with the FC, became more productive and much less confrontational.

Joseph continued to experience frustration and difficulty in academics early in his third grade year. His failure in reading and math prompted him to remark that it "didn't matter" because he was going to "be a bum" when he grew up. A few months into the school year, a new Fast Track tutor began meeting with Joseph four times/week for reading and math. Ms. L. had implemented the homework monitoring and reward plan and Joseph had begun turning in his homework regularly. By the end of February, Joseph was at class level in math and reading, and his attitude toward school had greatly improved. He received very few detention referrals for the remainder of that year.

Joseph made the most growth in his social skills – "a real success," as his EC remarked. He evidenced strong leadership in Friendship Group when he remembered to ignore the inappropriate behavior of others. He could also identify that he was using his ignoring skills to avoid fights and be successful in group. His ignoring of their misbehavior, in fact, often prompted more appropriate behavior by other children in the group. Importantly, he was able to generalize his Friendship Group skills and use them with his non-Fast Track schoolmates by cooperating and being a "team player." Additionally, no incidents of fire-setting had been reported since first grade.

Follow-Up Information

Joseph continued to improve (with ups and downs) in his academic and social skills throughout elementary school. Both he and his mother reported communicating and getting along better with each other. The school reported that interactions with Ms. L. were going smoothly, and Ms. L. described "trusting (her FC) more than anyone in my life."

Joseph's participation in the Fast Track intervention continued during middle school. He attended and actively participated in the youth meetings and, due to his mother's insistence, reluctantly attended the twice-weekly homework club meetings in seventh grade. The Youth Coordinator (YC) continued her involvement with Ms. L., primarily through phone calls; she also scheduled problem-solving meetings with Joseph and his mother on a monthly basis. On outings with the YC, Joseph talked openly about family, friends, school, and girls. He also developed a good relationship with his mentor who, unfortunately, moved after their first year of involvement together.

During Joseph's middle school years, his mother's and stepfather's relationship was failing and he and his mother argued "like in the old days." Following eighth grade, Joseph chose to move in with his biological father who had remarried and now had stepchildren, all younger than Joseph. Joseph had a difficult time living in the family and following their rules. Although he and his father argued loudly at times, Joseph managed to control his urges to strike out. He moved again and lived with a friend of the family for about a year. During that year, Joseph reported later, he "hung out with a bunch of losers" who were using drugs and stealing cars. Subsequently, Joseph moved back in with his mother and dropped out of high school. At age 20, Joseph was working on obtaining his GED, living with friends, and holding down a full-time job. He reported that he had given up drugs, was living with people who also did not use drugs, and felt like he was "going somewhere" with his life.

Comments

The variety and complexity of the individual children and families who participated in this intervention preclude depiction of a "typical" Fast Track family. Nonetheless, Joseph is representative of many of the children who participated in Fast Track. Joseph's behavior was causing problems at both home and school. His loud and immature behavior was disruptive in the classroom, and his negative attributions to his peers' intentions and reactive aggression caused him to be disliked by his classmates. Also, as predicted in the long-term preventive design of Fast Track, it took time for Joseph's family to become involved in the intervention process. This family did differ from many of the families participating in Fast Track in that Ms. L. was not a single parent (although her partner was often uninvolved), she did not need to work outside of the home, and she did not receive public assistance to support her family. Although Joseph did not complete high school, his involvement with Fast Track may have facilitated his decision as a young adult to pursue his education and his ability to stop using drugs and to be gainfully employed. Because data analysis is ongoing, we are as yet unable to assess the degree to which Joseph's outcomes are representative of those achieved by other participants in this comprehensive and long-term intervention. However, based on the findings to date, we are hopeful that we will continue to see intervention-related improvements for the youth at highest initial risk.

PREVENTION SCIENCE IN PRACTICE: FAST TRACK

At the beginning of this chapter, five principles for prevention science were outlined (Coie et al., 1993). Perhaps most importantly, Fast Track is an example of how a carefully articulated developmental model that accounts for the change and accumulation of risk factors and of mediating processes throughout the long developmental period starting with children at school entry and continuing through adolescence in high school can inform a complex, multicomponent intervention model. When this principle is met, as in the Fast Track model, then the remaining principles for prevention science can be readily addressed. The Fast Track intervention addresses fundamental causal processes that mediate the relation between early risk factors and later antisocial outcomes. By intervening early at the entry to school, Fast Track attempts to address risk factors before they become stabilized and relatively intransigent to intervention. Fast Track, as an indicated preventive intervention, does address high-risk children, who are screened with a multiple-gating procedure using teacher and parent ratings, but, in addition, Fast Track includes a universal preventive focus on all children in the intervention schools. Finally, because the developmental model articulates a range of factors within the child and within the child's context that contribute to children's entry and retention on the developmental trajectory leading to serious adolescent conduct problems, Fast Track has necessarily included coordinated activities in multiple domains which change over the long course of intervention.

Thus, Fast Track emerges as one exemplar of how prevention science can contribute to children's welfare and public policy. The Fast Track intervention demonstrated modest intervention effects in multiple domains throughout the 5 years of elementary school. The effects appear to have been strongest following our initial intensive preventive efforts in first grade. Small to moderate effects were maintained with sustained prevention support during this period. In contrast, there were minimal intervention effects in middle school. However, there is evidence of moderation of effects on conduct problem outcomes (especially by the end of Grade 9) based on the child's severity of initial risk as measured in kindergarten, with strong intervention effects for those youth at the highest level of initial risk. Recent analyses found a modest intervention effect for juvenile arrests. Ongoing economic analyses have indicated that although expensive, Fast Track modestly reduced utilization of general health and outpatient mental health services through adolescence, and for the highest-risk youth, with effects on conduct-problem outcomes. In terms of future directions, we plan to continue to examine the impact of the intervention through age 20, and a follow-up assessment of the sample at age 25 is ongoing.

ACKNOWLEDGMENT

This work was supported by National Institute of Mental Health (NIMH) grants R18 MH48043, R18 MH50951, R18 MH50952, and R18 MH50953. The Center for Substance Abuse Prevention and the National

Institute on Drug Abuse also has provided support for Fast Track through memoranda of agreement with the NIMH. This work was also supported in part by Department of Education grant S184U30002 and NIMH grants K05MH00797 and K05MH01027.

We are grateful for the close collaboration of the Durham Public Schools, the Metropolitan Nashville Public Schools, the Bellefonte Area Schools, the Tyrone Area Schools, the Mifflin County Schools, the Highline Public Schools, and the Seattle Public Schools. We greatly appreciate the hard work and dedication of the many staff members who implemented the project, collected the evaluation data, and assisted with data management and analyses.

REFERENCES

American Psychiatric, Association. (2000). *Diagnostic and statistical manual of mental disorders (4th ed. text rev.)*. Washington, DC: American Psychiatric Association.

Becker, J. (1994). *Mentoring high-risk kids*. Minneapolis, MN: Johnson Institute.

Bierman, K. L., Greenberg, M. T., Coie, J. D., Dodge, K. A., Lochman, J. E., & McMahon, R. J. (2010). *Fast Track peer group intervention: Facilitator's guide*. New York: Oxford University Press.

Bierman, K. L., Greenberg, M. T., & Conduct Problems Prevention Research Group, (1996). Social skills training in the Fast Track program. In R. DEV. Peters & R. J. McMahon (Eds.), *Preventing childhood disorders, substance abuse, and delinquency* (pp. 65–89). Thousand Oaks, CA: Sage.

Cairns, R. B., Cairns, B. D., & Neckerman, H. J. (1989). Early school dropout: Configurations and determinants. *Child Development, 60*, 1437–1452.

Cairns, R. B., Cairns, B. D., Neckerman, H. J., Gest, S. D., & Gariepy, J. L. (1988). Social networks and aggressive behavior: Peer support or peer rejection? *Developmental Psychology, 24*, 815–823.

Campbell, S. B. (1991). Longitudinal studies of active and aggressive preschoolers: Individual differences in early behavior and outcome. In D. Cicchetti & S. L. Toth (Eds.), *Internalizing and externalizing expressions of dysfunction: Rochester symposium on developmental psychopathology* (Vol. 2, pp. 67–90). Hillsdale, NJ: Erlbaum.

Caspi, A., Lynam, D., Moffitt, T. E., & Silva, P. (1993). Unraveling girls' delinquency: Biological, dispositional, and contextual contributions to adolescent misbehavior. *Developmental Psychology, 29*, 19–30.

Chassin, L., Curran, P. J., Hussong, A. M., & Colder, C. R. (1996). The relation of parent alcoholism to adolescent substance use: A longitudinal follow-up study. *Journal of Abnormal Psychology, 105*, 70–80.

Cicchetti, D. (1984). The emergence of developmental psychopathology. *Child Development, 55*, 1–7.

Cohen, M. A. (1998). The monetary value of saving a high-risk youth. *Journal of Quantitative Criminology, 14*, 5–33.

Coie, J. D. (1996). Prevention of violence and antisocial behavior. In R. DEV. Peters & R. J. McMahon (Eds.), *Preventing childhood disorders, substance abuse, and delinquency* (pp. 1–18). Thousand Oaks, CA: Sage.

Coie, J. D., Watt, N. F., West, S. G., Hawkins, J. D., Asarnow, J. R., Markman, H. J., et al. (1993). The science of prevention: A conceptual framework and some directions for a national research program. *American Psychologist, 48*, 1013–1022.

Comer, J. P. (1980). *School power*. New York: Free Press.

Conduct Problems Prevention Research Group. (1992). A developmental and clinical model for the prevention of conduct disorders: The FAST Track Program. *Development and Psychopathology, 4*, 505–527.

Conduct Problems Prevention Research Group. (1999a). Initial impact of the Fast Track prevention trial for conduct problems: I. The high-risk sample. *Journal of Consulting and Clinical Psychology, 67*, 631–647.

Conduct Problems Prevention Research Group. (1999b). Initial impact of the Fast Track prevention trial for conduct problems: II. Classroom effects. *Journal of Consulting and Clinical Psychology, 67*, 648–657.

Conduct Problems Prevention Research Group. (2000). Merging universal and indicated prevention programs. *Addictive Behaviors, 25*, 913–927.

Conduct Problems Prevention Research Group. (2002a). Evaluation of the first 3 years of the Fast Track prevention trial with children at high risk for adolescent conduct problems. *Journal of Abnormal Child Psychology, 30*, 19–35.

Conduct Problems Prevention Research Group. (2002b). Using the Fast Track randomized prevention trial to test the early-starter model of the development of serious conduct problems. *Development and Psychopathology, 14*, 925–943.

Conduct Problems Prevention Research Group. (2004). The effects of the Fast Track program on serious problem outcomes at the end of elementary school. *Journal of Clinical Child and Adolescent Psychology, 33*, 650–661.

Conduct Problems Prevention Research Group. (2006). The Fast Track project: Towards the prevention of severe conduct problems in school-age youth. In N. Heinrichs, K. Hahlweg, & M. Döpfner (Eds.), *Strengthening families: Evidence-based approaches to support child mental health* (pp. 439–477). Münster, Germany: Verlag für Psychotherapie.

Conduct Problems Prevention Research Group. (2007). Fast Track randomized controlled trial to prevent externalizing psychiatric disorders: Findings from grades 3 to 9. *Journal of the American Academy of Child and Adolescent Psychiatry, 46*, 1250–1262.

Conduct Problems Prevention Research Group. (2010a). Fast Track intervention effects on youth arrests and delinquency. *Journal of a Experimental Criminology 6*, 131–157.

Conduct Problems Prevention Research Group. (2010b). The effects of a multiyear universal social-emotional learning program: The role of student and school characteristics. *Journal of Consulting and Clinical Psychology, 78*, 156–168.

Conduct Problems Prevention Research Group. (in press). The difficulty of maintaining positive intervention effects: A look at disruptive behavior, deviant peer relations, and social skills during the middle school years. *Journal of Early Adolescence.*

Dishion, T. J., & McMahon, R. J. (1998). Parental monitoring and the prevention of child and adolescent problem behavior: A conceptual and empirical formulation. *Clinical Child and Family Psychology Review, 1*, 61–75.

Dishion, T. J., Nelson, S. E., & Bullock, B. M. (2004). Premature adolescent autonomy: Parent disengagement and deviant peer process in the amplification of problem behavior. *Journal of Adolescence, 27*, 515–530.

Dishion, T. J., Patterson, G. R., & Griesler, P. C. (1994). Peer adaptations in the development of antisocial behavior: A confluence model. In L. R. Huesmann (Ed.), *Aggressive behavior: Current perspectives* (pp. 61–95). New York: Plenum Press.

Dodge, K. A. (2003). Do social information-processing patterns mediate aggressive behavior? In B. B. Lahey, T. E. Moffitt, & A. Caspi (Eds.), *Causes of conduct disorder and delinquency* (pp. 254–274). New York: Guilford Press.

Dodge, K. A., Dishion, T. J., & Lansford, J. E. (Eds.). (2006). *Deviant peer influences in programs for youth: Problems and solutions.* New York: Guilford Press.

Dodge, K. A., Greenberg, M. T., Malone, P. S., & The Conduct Problems Prevention Research Group. (2008). Testing an idealized dynamic cascade model of the development of serious violence in adolescence. *Child Development, 79*, 1907–1927.

Dodge, K. A., Lansford, J. E., Burks, V. S., Bates, J. E., Pettit, G. S., Fontaine, R., et al. (2003). Peer rejection and social information-processing factors in the development of aggressive behavior problems in children. *Child Development, 74*, 374–393.

Dodge, K. A., Lochman, J. E., Harnish, J. D., Bates, J. E., & Pettit, G. S. (1997). Reactive and proactive aggression in school children and psychiatrically-impaired chronically-assaultive youth. *Journal of Abnormal Psychology, 106*, 37–51.

Dubois, D., & Karcher, M. (Eds.). (2006). *Handbook of youth mentoring.* Thousand Oaks, CA: Sage.

Eccles, J. E., & Midgley, C. M. (1990). Changes in academic motivation and self-perception during early adolescence. In R. Montemayor, G. R. Adams, & T. P. Gullotta (Eds.), *From childhood to adolescence* (pp. 134–155). Newbury Park, CA: Sage.

Fletcher, A. C., Darling, N. E., & Steinberg, L. (1995). Parental monitoring and peer influences on adolescent substance use. In J. McCord (Ed.), *Coercion and punishment in long-term perspectives* (pp. 259–271). New York: Cambridge University Press.

Foster, E.M., Jones, D.E., & Conduct Problems Prevention Research Group. (2006). Can a costly intervention be cost-effective?: An analysis of violence prevention. *Archives of General Psychiatry, 63,* 1284–1291.

Frick, P. J., & Sheffield Morris, A. (2004). Temperament and developmental pathways to conduct problems. *Journal of Clinical Child and Adolescent Psychology, 33,* 54–68.

Greenberg, M. T., Kusche, C. A., & Speltz, M. (1991). Emotional regulation, self control, and psychopathology: The role of relationships in early childhood. In D. Cicchetti & S. L. Toth (Eds.), *Internalizing and externalizing expressions of dysfunction: Rochester symposium on developmental psychopathology* (Vol. 2, pp. 21–66). Hillsdale, NJ: Erlbaum.

Greenberg, M.T., Lengua, L.J., Coie, J.D., Pinderhughes, E.E., & Conduct Problems Prevention Research Group. (1999). Predicting developmental outcomes at school entry using a multiple risk model: Four American communities. *Developmental Psychology, 35,* 403–417.

Hawkins, J. D., Catalano, R. F., & Miller, J. Y. (1992). Risk and protective factors for alcohol and other drug problems in adolescence and early adulthood: Implications for substance abuse prevention. *Psychological Bulletin, 112,* 64–105.

Henggeler, S. W., Schoenwald, S. K., & Pickrel, S. G. (1995). Multisystemic Therapy: Bridging the gap between university-and community-based treatment. *Journal of Consulting and Clinical Psychology, 63,* 709–717.

Hirsch, B. J., & DuBois, D. J. (1991). Self-esteem in adolescence: The identification and prediction of contrasting longitudinal trajectories. *Journal of Youth and Adolescence, 20,* 53–72.

Hundley, J. D., & Mercer, G. W. (1987). Family and friends as social environments and their relationship to young adolescents' use of alcohol, tobacco, and marijuana. *Journal of Clinical Psychology, 44,* 125–134.

Johnson, V., & Pandina, R. J. (1991). Effects of the family environment on adolescent substance abuse, delinquency and coping styles. *American Journal of Drug and Alcohol Abuse, 17,* 71–88.

Jones, D. E., Godwin, J., Dodge, K. A., Bierman, K. L., Coie, J. D., Greenberg, M. T., et al. (2010). The impact of the Fast Track prevention trial on health services utilization by youth at risk for conduct problems. *Pediatrics, 125,* 130–136.

Keenan, K., Loeber, R., Zhang, Q., Stouthamer-Loeber, M., & Van Kammen, W. B. (1995). The influence of deviant peers on the development of boys' disruptive and delinquent behavior: a temporal analysis. *Development and Psychopathology, 7,* 715–726.

Kellam, S. G., Ling, X., Merisca, R., Brown, C. H., & Ialongo, N. (1998). The effect of the level of aggression in the first grade classroom on the course and malleability of aggressive behavior into middle school. *Development and Psychopathology, 10,* 165–185.

Kusche, C. A., & Greenberg, M. T. (1993). *The PATHS (promoting alternative thinking strategies) Curriculum.* Deerfield, MA: Channing-Bete Co.

Ladd, G. W., Price, J. M., & Hart, C. H. (1990). Preschoolers' behavioral orientations and patterns of peer contact: Predictive of peer status? In S. R. Asher & J. D. Coie (Eds.), *Peer rejection in childhood* (pp. 90–115). Cambridge, UK: Cambridge University Press.

Lochman, J.E., & Conduct Problems Prevention Research Group. (1995). Screening of child behavior problems for prevention programs at school entry. *Journal of Consulting and Clinical Psychology, 63,* 549–559.

Loeber, R., Wung, P., Keenan, K., Giroux, B., Stouthamer-Loeber, M., Van Kammen, W. B., et al. (1993). Developmental pathways in disruptive child behavior. *Development and Psychopathology, 5,* 103–133.

Luthar, S. S., & Zigler, E. (1991). Vulnerability and competence: A review of research on resilience in childhood. *American Journal of Orthopsychiatry, 61,* 6–22.

Markus, H., & Nurius, P. (1986). Possible selves. *American Psychologist, 41,* 954–969.

McMahon, R. J., Slough, N., & Conduct Problems Prevention Research Group. (1996). Family-based intervention in the Fast Track program. In R. DEV. Peters & R. J. McMahon (Eds.), *Preventing childhood disorders, substance abuse, and delinquency* (pp. 90–110)). Thousand Oaks, CA: Sage.

McMahon, R. J., Slough, N. M., Lochman, J. E., Dodge, K. A., Coie, J. D., Bierman, K. L., et al. (2010). *Fast Track parent group intervention: Facilitator's guide*. New York: Oxford University Press.

McMahon, R. J., Wells, K. C., & Kotler, J. S. (2006). Conduct problems. In E. J. Mash & R. A. Barkley (Eds.), *Treatment of childhood disorders* (3rd ed., pp. 137–268). New York: Guilford Press.

Miller-Johnson, S., Winn, D., Coie, J., Maumary-Gremaud, A., Hyman, C., Terry, R., et al. (1999). Motherhood during the teen years: A developmental perspective on risk factors for child-bearing. *Development and Psychopathology, 11*, 85–100.

Moffitt, T. E. (1990). Juvenile delinquency and attention deficit disorder: Boys' developmental trajectories from age 3 to age 15. *Child Development, 61*, 893–910.

Moffitt, T. E. (1993). Adolescence-limited and life-course-persistent antisocial behavior: A developmental taxonomy. *Psychological Review, 100*, 674–701.

Offord, D. R., Boyle, M. H., & Racine, Y. A. (1991). The epidemiology of antisocial behavior in childhood and adolescence. In D. J. Pepler & K. H. Rubin (Eds.), *The development and treatment of childhood aggression* (pp. 31–54). Hillsdale, NJ: Erlbaum.

Ohannesian, C., & Crockett, L. J. (1993). A longitudinal investigation of the relationship between educational investment and adolescent sexual activity. *Journal of Adolescent Research, 8*, 167–182.

Oyserman, D., Sanchez-Burks, J., & Harrison, K. (1996). *Social identity and possible selves in adolescence*. Unpublished manuscript, University of Michigan.

Patterson, G. R. (1982). *Coercive family process*. Eugene, OR: Castalia.

Patterson, G. R., DeBaryshe, B. D., & Ramsey, E. (1989). A developmental perspective on antisocial behavior. *American Psychologist, 44*, 329–335.

Patterson, G. R., Reid, J. B., & Dishion, T. J. (1992). *Antisocial boys*. Eugene, OR: Castalia.

Rutter, M., Maughan, B., Mortimore, P., Ouston, J., & Smith, A. (1979). *Fifteen thousand hours: Secondary schools and their effects on children*. Cambridge, MA: Harvard University Press.

Slough, N.M., McMahon, R.J., & the Conduct Problems Prevention Research Group. (2008). Preventing serious conduct problems in school-age youth: The Fast Track program. *Cognitive and Behavioral Practice, 15*, 3–17.

Snyder, J., Reid, J., & Patterson, G. (2003). A social learning model of child and adolescent antisocial behavior. In B. B. Lahey, T. E. Moffitt, & A. Caspi (Eds.), *Causes of conduct disorder and juvenile delinquency* (pp. 27–48). New York: Guilford Press.

Thornberry, T. P. (1987). Toward an interactional theory of delinquency. *Criminology, 25*, 863–891.

Thornberry, T. P., Huizinga, D., & Loeber, R. (1995). The prevention of serious delinquency and violence: Implications from the program of research on the causes and correlates of delinquency. In J. C. Howell, B. Krisberg, J. D. Hawkins, & J. Wilson (Eds.), *Sourcebook on serious violent and chronic juvenile offenders* (pp. 213–237). Thousand Oaks, CA: Sage.

Vitaro, F., Tremblay, R. E., Kerr, M., Pagani-Kurtz, L., & Bukowski, W. M. (1997). Disruptiveness, friends' characteristics, and delinquency: A test of two competing models of development. *Child Development, 68*, 676–689.

Weissberg, R. P., Caplan, M. Z., & Sivo, P. J. (1989). A new conceptual framework for establishing school-based social competence promotion programs. In L. A. Bond & B. E. Compas (Eds.), *Primary prevention and promotion in the schools* (pp. 255–296). Newbury Park, CA: Sage.

Werner, E. E. (1986). Resilient offspring of alcoholics: A longitudinal study from birth to age 18. *Journal of Studies on Alcohol, 47*, 34–40.

Wills, T. A., & Filer, M. (1996). Stress-coping model of adolescent substance use. In T. H. Ollendick & R. J. Prinz (Eds.), *Advances in clinical child psychology* (Vol. 18, pp. 91–132). New York: Plenum Press.

17

Prevention: The Role of Early Universal and Targeted Interventions

MATTHEW R. SANDERS and ALINA MORAWSKA

Preventive interventions for children and adolescents with conduct problems are designed to forestall the development of subsequent mental health problems. Mrazek and Haggerty (1994) differentiated among three types of preventive interventions: universal (targeting an entire population irrespective of risk), selective (targeting individuals or subgroups with elevated risk), and indicated (targeting high-risk individuals who are identified as having minimal but detectable problems foreshadowing disorder). Prevention programs can include narrowly targeted programs that focus on vulnerable children or high-risk families, universal programs offered to all families, or blended models that combine universal and indicated interventions (Prinz & Sanders, 2007; Sanders, 1999, 2008; Sanders & Woolley, 2005).

Preventive interventions target potentially modifiable risk and protective factors known to be associated with the development of conduct and other mental health problems. In the case of early onset conduct problems, there are multiple factors to consider. First, parenting factors such as inadequate or dysfunctional parenting including inconsistent, harsh, and coercive parenting, poor communication, and inadequate monitoring or supervision need to be considered (Sanders, Bor, & Morawska, 2007; Sanders & Markie-Dadds, 1996; Sanders, Markie-Dadds, Tully, & Bor, 2000). Second, interventions could also potentially target family factors such as low parenting self-efficacy, high parental stress, depression, anger, and interparental conflict (Behrens & Sanders, 1994; Plant &

MATTHEW R. SANDERS • The University of Queensland
ALINA MORAWSKA • The University of Queensland

R.C. Murrihy et al. (eds.), *Clinical Handbook of Assessing and Treating Conduct Problems in Youth*, DOI 10.1007/978-1-4419-6297-3_17,

Sanders, 2007; Sanders & McFarland, 2000; Sanders & Woolley, 2005). Third, potentially modifiable child-related risk factors such as attention difficulties, poor impulse control, learning or academic difficulties, peer relationship problems, including peer rejection, and exposure to antisocial peer models are worthy of investigation. And, finally, broader environmental factors such as conditions of living including overcrowding, unsafe neighborhoods, and inadequate recreational spaces or age-appropriate activities for children all need to be examined.

Given the wide range of potential targets for intervention that have been shown in longitudinal studies to be associated with the development of conduct problems, it is tempting to argue that interventions that target as many of these factors as possible are superior to those that target only a few of the factors. However, not all factors are amenable to intervention or are able to produce change in child conduct problems. Further, despite its conceptual appeal, there is limited evidence showing that the concurrent targeting of multiple child, parent, family, school, and neighborhood risk factors is effective in preventing conduct problems. Family-based preventive interventions hold the most promise and have the strongest empirical support in reducing conduct problems, particularly so in younger children (see Sanders, Bor, & Morawska, 2007).

The case for prevention for conduct problems is compelling. Childhood conduct problems are widespread, yet treatment services reach only a small number of parents who might benefit (Sanders, Markie-Dadds, Rinaldis, Firman, & Baig, 2007). Of those accessing mental health services only a minority receive evidence-based interventions. Furthermore, many high-risk families are reluctant to participate in treatment services and of those who do access these services high dropout rates are common (Morawska & Sanders, 2006). Unfortunately, participation in mental health services can still be associated with social stigma, and treatment services once a child has developed a severe conduct problem are expensive. In this chapter, we make the case for the value of combining universal and indicated preventive interventions in reducing conduct problems in children. There are promising signs that preventive interventions, particularly those focusing on parenting and family relationships, can be effective in both treating and preventing conduct problems (Mihalopoulos, Sanders, Turner, Murphy-Brennan, & Carter, 2007; Sanders et al., 2007). Hence, we focus primarily on the role of universal and indicated parenting interventions in the prevention of conduct problems. We make the case that both universal and indicated interventions are required to reduce the prevalence rates of conduct problems. We begin by examining the prevalence of dysfunctional parenting practices to set the context for the adoption of a public health approach to parenting intervention. Next, we discuss three examples of large-scale universal prevention efforts to illustrate principles and challenges involved in delivering large-scale prevention programs. Finally, we make the case for complementing universal programs with more targeted parenting services for high-risk children and families. We conclude that a multilevel suite of evidence-based parenting interventions targeting entire populations of parents provides a promising basis for achieving population level effects on rates of serious conduct problems in children and adolescents.

PREVALENCE OF PARENTING AND FAMILY RISK FACTORS

In a household survey of Australian parents, Sanders and colleagues found that a large number of parents from diverse socioeconomic backgrounds reported that their children had significant behavioral and emotional problems (Sanders et al., 2007). Twenty-nine percent (29%) of parents of 2–12-year-old children had significant conduct problems and 9% of children met diagnostic criteria for oppositional defiant disorder (ODD). More concerning was the high prevalence of coercive or ineffective parenting practices with over half of parents reporting use of practices such as hitting/smacking and 70% reporting shouting and becoming angry with their children. Similarly, reports of the use of corporal punishment in the USA indicate that the majority of parents have used some form of physical punishment (Straus & Stewart, 1999).

ROLE OF PARENTING INTERVENTIONS IN PREVENTION

Given the demonstrated importance of parenting to children's development, it is not surprising that interventions that change dysfunctional or inadequate parenting practices improve children's behavior and adjustment. Substantial evidence shows that parenting programs based on social learning models (e.g., Patterson, 1982; Taylor & Biglan, 1998) are effective in the management of early onset conduct problems (Serketich & Dumas, 1996). Several meta-analyses show that group and individually administered programs that improve parenting skills lead to sustained reduction in the disruptive behavior of children with ODD, conduct disorders (CD), and attention-deficit hyperactive disorder (ADHD; de Graaf, Speetjens, Smit, de Wolff, & Tavecchio, 2008a; de Graaf, Speetjens, Smit, de Wolff, & Tavecchio, 2008b; Nowak & Heinrichs, 2008; Thomas & Zimmer-Gembeck, 2007). There is also evidence that parenting programs can be used as early preventive interventions with families of difficult-to-manage toddlers and preschool-aged children to forestall the development of serious conduct problems (Morawska & Sanders, 2006; Sanders et al., 2000). Despite the demonstrated efficacy of parenting interventions, few parents access these programs and consequently many children continue to develop potentially preventable problems (Biglan, 1995).

A more comprehensive model of parenting intervention is required and is essential to prevent conduct problems in children. The Triple P-Positive Parenting Program developed by Sanders and colleagues at the University of Queensland (see Sanders, 2008) is discussed below as an example of a multilevel system of parenting support to illustrate the fundamental principles of how to develop prevention programs and services. This model is used to highlight the potential advantages of blending universal and indicated intervention components within the same integrated multilevel system of evidence-based parenting interventions, to reduce the prevalence of behavioral and emotional problems in children and adolescents.

MAKING THE POPULATION APPROACH REALLY WORK

Prevention programming using a public health model requires a series of interrelated tasks and activities to be accomplished (Sanders, 2008). The completion of these tasks and activities increases the likelihood of successful outcomes being achieved. These principles include (a) establishing the baseline prevalence rates of target child problems and of the targeted risk or protective factors affected by the intervention, (b) ensuring evidence exists that changing the targeted risk and protective factor leads to an improvement in the targeted child factors, (c) having well developed and culturally appropriate interventions available, (d) developing an effective training and dissemination system, (e) making the program widely available, and (f) tracking outcomes at a population level. These steps and associated tasks are summarized in Table 17.1. We now turn to the design of an intervention system that incorporates universal and indicated elements.

Universal and Indicated Preventive Approaches to Parenting

This approach is premised on an assumption that greater support for parents in general in the task of raising their children will benefit parents, children, and society at large. The primary goal of universal parenting support programs is to normalize and destigmatize preparation for parenthood. At the outset, it should be noted that although universal parenting programs have been in existence for many years there is relatively little empirical evidence concerning the efficacy of these programs. We will focus our discussion on universal parenting interventions made available to all parents that have been subjected to empirical validation.

Evidence-based programs can be differentiated from the massive increase in publicly accessible information on parenting through a plethora of government and commercially sponsored Web sites. The popularity of the Web as a means of accessing parenting advice is partly a reflection of the widespread concern of parents, and society in general, regarding how children are raised. The Web is being used increasingly by government agencies to relatively cheaply disseminate parenting information and advice. The current generation of parents has widespread access to parenting advice with information widely available on the Web and through self-help books on a range of topics. Apart from basic parenting advice on managing common behavioral, emotional, and developmental problems in children, a vast array of health, educational, mental health, social welfare, legal, and financial advice is also available.

However, the proliferation of parenting information and advice that has been accelerated further by the advent of reality television programs on parenting has been criticized. For example, journalists have labeled some government initiatives aimed at increasing parenting support as an example of the "Nanny State" interfering with family life. The variable quality of the parenting advice provided, lack of quality control mechanisms, and the lack of evaluation work to decrease parental and professional confidence in many parenting Web sites and to increase parent confusion. Although parenting television shows and Web-based delivery of parenting

Table 17.1. Principles of positive parenting: tasks, brief descriptions, activities, and outcomes

Task	Brief description	Activities	Outcomes
Task 1			
Establishing baseline prevalence rates of target child problems	Information is required concerning the base rates of targeted behavioral and emotional problems in the areas targeted before the intervention begins	Collation of statutory archival data on factors such as substantiated cases of child maltreatment; hospitalisation; emergency room data on child maltreatment; number of out-of-home placements; household survey data on parenting practices; and number of child behavioral and emotional difficulties	Base rates per 100,000 of child population as an index of the targeted problem prior to intervention
Task 2			
Establishing the baseline prevalence rates of the targeted risk or protective factors affected by the intervention	Example risk factors are exposure to a harsh, inconsistent parenting style and mental health problems in parents. Example protective factors: access to professional support, high levels of social and emotional support	Household survey data or computer-assisted telephone surveys of parents within target age range to establish base rates on parenting problems expected to shift as a function of the intervention	Base rates per 100,000 of child population as an index of the targeted problem prior to intervention
Task 3			
Establishing evidence that changing the targeted risk and protective factor leads to an improvement in the targeted child factor/s	Before an intervention is implemented widely, programs are required that have been demonstrated to be effective in changing risk and protective factors	The compilation of evidence from randomized clinical trials establishing the efficacy and effectiveness of intervention components to be used in the population level activity	Clear data indicating the expected effect size related to interventions; estimated numbers of parents needed to participate to achieve prevalence rate reductions in child behavior outcomes
Task 4			
Having well-developed culturally appropriate interventions available	Parents from quite diverse cultural, linguistic, and religious backgrounds may seek support with parenting issues.	Conducting consumer preference surveys and focus groups of parents from diverse	A set of programs for the engagement and implementation in the

(continued)

Table 17.1. (continued)

Task	Brief description	Activities	Outcomes
	A program needs to be both effective and culturally acceptable to all parents	communities living in different catchment areas to determine cultural acceptability of the parenting skills, methods of engagement, and the mode of delivery. Includes an analysis of gender differences.	community. May mean multiple concurrent engagement strategies for different population groups
Task 5 Development of an effective training and dissemination system	A multidisciplinary training program is needed that equips service providers with the content and process knowledge and skills they require to deliver different levels of the program with fidelity.	Conducting evaluations of training programs to determine the extent to which training procedures change in parent consultation skills, service providers, confidence, or self-efficacy, and program satisfaction	Having an efficient and effective training and dissemination process that builds in quality assurance to promote program fidelity
Task 6 Making the program widely available	Quality materials are needed that can can be made readily available to service providers	Ensuring that policy and funding initiatives are available to widely disseminate the training program to multiple agencies, organizations, and service providers in the catchment area	Having a trained and accredited workforce, ready to deliver the program to families
Task 7 Tracking outcomes at a population level	This focus requires some form of population-level auditing, community surveillance, or surveying of parents to assess whether parental concerns about children's behavioral and emotional problems have decreased and whether there has been an increase in parent use of positive parenting methods and a decrease in dysfunctional parenting practices	The administration of the baseline survey measures to determine whether there have been changes in the prevalence rates of targeted child and parent problems	Quantitative data being available to determine whether statistically meaningful changes in prevalence rates have occurred and hence, whether the population strategy has been effective

information such as fact sheets are popular, little is known about the efficacy of these modalities for the delivery of universal parenting advice.

Research evaluating the effectiveness of the Triple P system has been at the forefront of international efforts to examine the efficacy of universal parenting programs. Within the five-level Triple P system, *Universal Triple P* is the first level of intervention. It involves the development of a comprehensive media and communication strategy tailored to local needs. A series of studies using randomized designs have examined the effects of the mass media, including an observational documentary-style reality television series on parenting *Driving Mum and Dad Mad* (Calam, Sanders, Miller, Sadhnani, & Carmont, 2008), and a lifestyle television program on parenting, *Families* (Sanders, Montgomery, & Brechman-Touissant, 2000).

As experience in delivering public health parenting interventions increases, several studies have begun to document the processes involved in implementing evidence-based parenting programs on a large scale and to report the outcomes achieved at a whole of population level. The Great Parenting Experiment (Calam et al., 2008), the Every Family Initiative (Sanders et al., 2008), and the Triple P System Population Trial (Prinz, Sanders, Shapiro, Whitaker, & Lutzker, 2009) are used as examples of large-scale universal interventions to illustrate factors that determine the effectiveness of universal interventions.

The Great Parenting Experiment: Effects of Media and Self-Help Interventions on Parenting. In one of the few evaluations of a media intervention on parenting using a randomized design (Calam et al., 2008), it was shown that simply watching a six episode television series on parenting that documented five families with disruptive children undergoing an 8-week Group Triple P intervention was associated with significant improvements in the behavior of viewers' children and parental adjustment. This popular ITV television series in the UK, "Driving Mum and Dad Mad," was presented in a highly accessible and entertaining observational documentary format. Television viewing figures demonstrated that it was the most popular show in its time slot, attracting 4.2 million viewers. In the evaluation study that ran concurrently with the series, 454 parents with children aged 2–9 years were randomized to a standard condition (simply viewing the series) or an enhanced condition where, in addition to viewing, parents received a self-directed workbook and had access to Web-based materials and e-mail support.

Parents in both conditions reported significant improvements in their children's disruptive behavior and improvements in their dysfunctional parenting practices, and their own affect (anger, depression, and stress). Effects were greatest for the enhanced condition, who in addition reported decreased partner conflict over parenting and higher overall levels of program satisfaction. The level of improvement was related to dosage, with greatest changes occurring in families who watched all episodes. Improvements achieved at postintervention by parents in both groups were maintained at 6-month follow-up.

The success of this media intervention is consistent with an increasing literature showing that brief, low-cost, self-directed parenting programs can be effective in teaching parenting skills. A self-directed version of a ten-session Triple P program either when delivered alone (Markie-Dadds

& Sanders, 2006) or in association with brief weekly telephone consultations (Morawska & Sanders, 2007) can be effective in reducing child conduct problems. Parenting self-help interventions have been shown to be effective in reducing conduct problems for toddlers (Morawska & Sanders, 2006, 2007), preschoolers (Sanders et al., 2007; Markie-Dadds & Sanders, 2006), and teenagers (Stallman & Ralph, 2007). Short-term effects have been either maintained or shown further improvement over time in these studies (Sanders et al., 2007).

These findings are promising and point to the potential usefulness of quality television programs documenting evidence-based parenting programs. However, little is known about the characteristics of families that do well in a media intervention and if such factors are identified whether they are consistent with the predictors of outcomes found in studies of face-to-face interventions. In the Sanders et al. (2008) study, although 40% of parents who completed the intervention showed significant improvements on measures of dysfunctional parenting and significant improvements in their children's behavior, not all parents benefited. In fact, those parents with the highest levels of dysfunctional parenting and lowest self-efficacy at preintervention were at greater risk of not completing the intervention program. This suggests that further research is needed to study these and other potential predictors of both outcomes and the persistence or maintenance of engagement over time.

Every Family Initiative. The *Every Family* initiative was a large-scale intervention targeting parents of 4–7-year-old children making the transition to primary school. All five levels of Triple P were delivered by a range of practitioners, across a variety of settings, to families in the *Every Family* catchment areas. The Triple P system was adopted as the parenting program in *Every Family* because it met essential criteria considered important for a public health approach to parenting to be effective. These features included the following:

1. *A Clearly Articulated Public Health Theoretical Framework.* The Triple P system of intervention comprises five levels of intervention of increasing intensity and narrowing population reach including, a media and communication strategy, a large group positive parenting seminar series, brief primary care interventions, more intensive small group and individual programs, and enhanced family intervention for parents who require more intensive intervention services.
2. *A substantial Evidence Base* concerning the efficacy and effectiveness of the parenting advice used and for the different levels and delivery modalities used in the program (see Nowak & Heinrichs, 2008).
3. *The Use of a Self-Regulation Framework For Working with Parents* (Karoly, 1993), which encourages parents, in consultation with service providers, to determine their own goals and the kinds of behaviors, skills, and values they are seeking to promote in their children. The self-regulation approach is particularly relevant to population level applications in cross culturally diverse communities because goals can be developed in line with parents' cultural beliefs. Parents differ in their self-regulatory capabilities due to many factors such as mental health problems, drug and alcohol

problems, and relationship conflict. However, an empowerment model that promotes parental self-regulation encourages all parents to take responsibility for their own parenting decisions and has the advantage of being able to be used in universal as well as more tailored and targeted interventions.

4. *The Use of an Existing Multidisciplinary Workforce* and established networks and referral pathways to deliver the program (e.g., GPs, psychologists, nurses, social workers, guidance officers, counselors, teachers) as well as different delivery formats (e.g., media, groups, seminars, individual face-to-face or phone consultation) to ensure that sufficient numbers of local service providers are trained and able to deliver the program.
5. *The Use of a Variety of Service Delivery Contexts*, including GP practices, schools, preschools, childcare centers and mental health services. The rationale for using many different settings to deliver parenting advice is that parents often report that the advice they receive from different services is confusing and sometimes contradictory.
6. *Evidence Concerning Cross-Cultural Acceptability and Effectiveness of Triple P*. Several trials have documented the beneficial effects of Triple P with culturally and linguistically diverse parents including Indigenous parents (Turner, Richards, & Sanders, 2007), Chinese and Japanese parents (e.g., Leung, Sanders, Leung, Mak, & Lau, 2003; Matzumoto, Sofronoff, & Sanders, 2007), and African American parents and service providers (Prinz et al, 2009).

Program outcomes were assessed through a computer-assisted telephone interview of a random sample of 3,000 households in each community at pre-intervention and then again after 2 years of intervention (Sanders et al., 2008). At postintervention significantly more parents in the Triple P communities were aware of the program and had participated than in the comparison communities. Compared to care-as-usual (CAU), there were significantly greater reductions in the Triple P communities in the number of children with clinically elevated and borderline behavioral and emotional problems as measured by the Strengths and Difficulties Questionnaire. Similarly, parents reported a greater reduction in the prevalence of depression, stress, and coercive parenting. This study showed that parenting risk factors and children's psychosocial problems could be reduced at a population level through a large-scale universal parenting intervention.

Triple P South Carolina Population Trial. A third large-scale demonstration of the potential benefits of making parenting programs widely available is the *Triple P System Population Trial* (TPSPT). Although this trial did not specifically focus on conduct problems, it did focus on coercive parenting that is often associated with child maltreatment and is often considered a risk factor for conduct problems. The TPSPT randomized 18 moderate-sized South Carolina counties to two intervention conditions (nine counties each) and assessed the effects at a population level on indices of child abuse and neglect. The intervention condition involved county-wide implementation of all levels of the Triple P System vs. a CAU comparison. The selected counties, ranging in population size from 50,000 to 175,000, were matched in pairs based on child maltreatment prevalence rate, approximate size (population), and poverty level (proportion of households below the poverty line), and then assigned to condition. The referent population in the 18 counties for the TPSPT consists of the parents/caregivers in all households with one or more children in the birth to 7-year-old range.

A key facet of the intervention involved the engagement, training, and support of a broad array of service providers (practitioners) from several disciplines and settings, including health centers (primary healthcare providers), family support services (social workers, psychologists, and therapists affiliated with county health centers, mental health centers, and schools), social services (prevention workers, social workers), preschool and childcare settings (directors, teachers), kindergartens (teachers, guidance counselors, parent educators), private-sector practitioners, and other community organizations having direct contact with parents and families.

As part of the population approach, the TPSPT involved several media and informational strategies: (a) local newspaper coverage of Triple P programming in each county; (b) positive parenting articles in local newspapers; (c) public service radio spots about positive parenting and Triple P programming; (d) informational flyers and brochures distributed to community centers, advocacy organizations, and other entities having frequent contact with large numbers of parents; and, (e) informational mailings to family households in the nine Triple P System counties.

The evaluation showed that after 3 years of implementation there were significantly lower rates of substantiated child maltreatment cases, hospitalization, emergency room visits (due to maltreatment-related injuries), and out-of-home placements than in CAU counties. This is the first study to document population level effects on child maltreatment due to a large-scale parenting intervention.

KEY LEARNINGS FROM UNIVERSAL APPROACHES

The adoption of a population approach to parenting intervention represents a clear paradigm shift (Prinz & Sanders, 2007). The approach is very different to the delivery of a clinical treatment model. Parental motivation to engage in a preventive intervention is reliant upon the active engagement of a larger number of people often working in diverse agencies. There are several key findings that have resulted from our experience with large scale interventions.

1. *Ecological Approach to Training And Ongoing Support of Providers.* A survey of over 1,000 professionals following training in Primary Care Triple P, which involves three to four brief sessions delivered in a primary care context (Turner & Sanders, 2006), identified a number of barriers for primary care staff in delivering the program following training. Many of the common barriers were related to the posttraining work environment, such as integration of the program with their usual caseload or responsibilities, access to supervision, and ability to schedule afterhours appointments. To circumvent such issues, and maximize agency support for the introduction of Triple P, the following strategies have been employed.

2. *Information and Administrative/Clinical Support.* The Triple P team endeavors to provide information and support specific to the needs of each agency adopting the program. Support is provided at a number of levels. We provide an orientation for administrators, supervisors, or managers with clear information about both the program being introduced (e.g., its evidence base, format, and target populations), and the training and accreditation procedures, as well as providing a forum for the discussion of expectations of agency staff members involved in implementing the program (e.g., flexible work hours to allow for late appointments and evening groups). Further supportive mechanisms include the development of procedural guidelines and performance targets, regular updates and reviews of these targets, and assisting sites in identifying and overcoming barriers to implementation. We also aim to support practitioners implementing the program by ensuring that staff have access to adequate training, supervision (see below) and resources, and that they are equipped with strategies and materials for program promotion (e.g., brochures and posters, signup sheets displayed at schools and community centers, press releases). Moreover, we provide regular updates on Triple P research and disseminate these to agencies and practitioners via a biannual newsletter and Web pages (e.g., http://www.triplep.net). On another level, as advocates for agencies, we have provided briefings to policy advisers and ministers, and regular updates to key stakeholders.
3. *Promotion of Supervision Networks.* Research has identified the importance of ongoing supervision in psychological practice (Holloway & Neufeldt, 1995) for promoting greater utilization of the training undertaken by a practitioner and as a means of maintaining program fidelity in a dissemination strategy (e.g., Henggeler, Schoenwald, Liao, Letourneau, & Edwards, 2007). Effective supervision of agency staff includes peer support and mentoring of practitioners who are new to the program (Webster-Stratton & Taylor, 1998). In the dissemination of Triple P, we encourage establishment of peer support networks and the adoption of a self-regulatory approach to supervision. The self-regulatory perspective involves training practitioners to use self-directed learning strategies such as self-monitoring and self-evaluation, personal goal setting, and self-reward for goal attainment (Halford, Sanders, & Behrens, 1994). Self-regulatory skills enable practitioners to direct their own learning, skill acquisition, and problem solving subsequent to participating in skills training workshops. As noted earlier, we propose that practitioners will be more receptive and motivated to use self-regulatory skills in organizational environments that support and encourage staff to do so. Thus, strategies employed to support the establishment of supervision networks include the provision of supervision guidelines, identification of a coordinator, and ongoing assistance to overcome administrative obstacles and process issues.
4. *Availability of Ongoing Consultation.* Backer and colleagues proposed that ongoing contact with program inventors impacts positively on

program implementation in dissemination efforts (Backer, Lieberman, & Kuehnel, 1986). The Triple P team has encouraged practitioners to access ongoing back-up consultative advice post-training. Triple P staff have also had ongoing e-mail contact, held teleconferences, attended staff meetings and arranged update days to address administrative issues (e.g., data management, performance indicators), logistical issues (e.g., avoidance of accreditation workshops due to anxiety; referral strategies), and clinical issues (e.g., dealing with specific populations, clinical process problems) identified by practitioners. These contacts actively engage agency staff in "troubleshooting."

5. *Strategies to Maintain Intervention Quality.* In any large-scale early intervention effort, maintenance of program integrity is crucial to ensure that the implementation does not drift too far from validated methodology. We have endeavored to develop high-quality training materials, practitioner manuals (e.g., Sanders, Markie-Dadds & Turner, 2001), and parent resources (e.g., Sanders, Markie-Dadds, & Turner, 1996) to ensure that the program is standardized, easy to follow, accessible, and culturally sensitive. Strategies to further support program integrity include practitioner attendance at structured training courses and the demonstration of core competencies through the accreditation process, and the provision of protocol adherence checklists to guide practitioners through the session content. The supervision and ongoing back-up consultation outlined earlier also serve to enhance program integrity and implementation quality over time.
6. *Self-Regulatory Approach/Framework to Practice.* All evidence-based programs face the challenge of how to promote good fidelity in the delivery of the program once initial training has been provided. Two contrasting approaches can be described: one argues for the importance of close supervision and external monitoring of fidelity in a manner akin to that used in clinical trials where interventions were first tested. The alternative approach, which we favor, is the adoption of a self-regulatory framework. This latter approach encourages organizations to use a self-regulatory approach so that organizational support strategies are used to promote program adherence through the adoption of workforce development strategies. This includes ensuring that program delivery becomes part of an individual's workload, is supported through ensuring that resources and staff are available to deliver the program, and through encouraging reflective practice via peer supervision and professional development groups using a self-regulation framework.
7. *Targeted Approach with High-Need Populations.* While large scale, population level approaches are critical to the success of prevention efforts aimed at reducing the prevalence of parenting and family risk factors for conduct problems, it is also essential to consider the needs of specific populations. It is widely recognized that within a public health approach, population level strategies need to be blended with targeted approaches (Prinz & Sanders, 2007). While a brief intervention is likely to be adequate for many families, some parents require more intensive, tailored support. A targeted approach

involves more intensive support for families (e.g., additional sessions and individual clinician support); it may target specific groups of parents based on identified risk factors (e.g., socioeconomic status) or it may tailor interventions to the needs of specific population groups (e.g., parents of children with disabilities). The guiding assumption is that evidence-based parenting interventions need to be flexible in meeting the needs of diverse parents.

Low socioeconomic status (SES) is a commonly recognized risk factor for ineffective parenting and the development of conduct problems (Bradely, Corwyn, McAdoo, & Coll, 2001; Grant et al., 2003; Mangusson & Duncan, 2002). However, it is noteworthy that the effect of low SES on the development of conduct problems is an indirect one and the role of mediating variables is important to pursue. For example, parents from a low SES may have less job stability leading to psychological stress that can impact negatively on the parent–child relationship. Psychological stress of this kind can result in increased marital conflict and more dysfunctional parenting (Whitbeck et al., 1997). It is these suboptimal parenting behaviors that are associated with negative developmental outcomes (Conger & Elder, 1994; Conger et al., 1992, 1993).

Socioeconomic disadvantage therefore serves as an indicator for a range of risk factors and serves as a common criterion for selected interventions. The evidence to date indicates that parents from socioeconomically disadvantaged backgrounds benefit from Triple P (e.g., Sanders et al., 2000) and that the addition of more intervention does not necessarily provide better outcomes. For example, Sanders et al. (2000) examined the effects of various intensities of Triple P (Self-help Triple P vs. Standard Triple P vs. Enhanced Triple P) for socioeconomically disadvantaged parents of preschool children and found that while the more intensive interventions led to greater changes at post-intervention, these differences were less evident at 1-year and 3-year follow-up (Sanders et al., 2007). Zubrick et al. (2005) reported that Group Triple P delivered in socioeconomically disadvantaged areas also led to sustained positive effects over a period of 2 years. Finally, McTaggart and Sanders (2007) found that irrespective of their sociodemographic background, parents who completed Triple P were equally likely to succeed in changing their parenting practices. The results of the study examining Group Triple P showed that parents' capacity to change dysfunctional parenting practices was not moderated by the child's gender, family income, family type, or pre-intervention level of parental stress, but was partially mediated by changes in parental satisfaction and parenting efficacy.

Despite these positive findings, parents from disadvantaged backgrounds may be less likely to access intervention in the first place (Heinrichs, Bertram, Kuschel, & Hahlweg, 2005) and may have some difficulties attending programs (Zubrick et al., 2005). Thus, the issues of appropriate engagement strategies and support need to be carefully addressed and planned in any population approach.

The poor health status of Indigenous children in Australia in comparison to the wider population has been well documented (Ring & Brown, 2003). Indigenous children and youth are extremely disadvantaged on most indices of health and well-being: they have higher rates of health risk behaviors, early school dropout, suicide, involvement with the juvenile justice system, family fragmentation, and forced removal of children and are overrepresented in abuse and neglect cases (Human Rights and Equal Opportunities Commission (HREOC), 1997; Trewin & Madden, 2003; Zubrick et al., 2004). Mainstream parenting programs have had difficulty in recruiting and maintaining the involvement of Indigenous parents, suggesting the need for more culturally appropriate parenting programs tailored to the needs of Indigenous parents.

Turner, Richards and Sanders (2007) investigated the effects of a culturally tailored version of Triple P for Indigenous parents in a randomized trial. The assumption taken in tailoring the program was that while positive parenting principles and strategies can cut across cultures, what may vary according to culture are the goals and target behaviors, practical implementation of strategies, and ways of sharing information. Extensive community consultation occurred in the development of the tailored program. While program content was seen as appropriate, changes were made to the language and images used in program resources, and to the examples used to depict parenting strategies (e.g., culturally tailored video, workbook, and presentation aids were developed). The structure of group sessions was altered to allow more time to discuss the social and political context for parenting, develop trust, slow the pace of presentation, and share personal stories. Indigenous parents attending Group Triple P reported significant decreases in rates of problem child behavior in comparison to those in the waitlist condition, as well as a significant decrease in reliance on some dysfunctional parenting practices, and these gains were maintained at 6-month follow-up. The program resulted in high rates of consumer satisfaction; moreover, there were generally positive comments about the cultural acceptability of the program content, resources, and format. The results of this study provided empirical support for the effectiveness and acceptability of a culturally tailored approach to Group Triple P conducted in a community setting. The outcomes are a significant step toward increasing appropriate service provision for Indigenous families and reducing barriers to accessing available services in the community. Further they affirm that only minor modifications to delivery format and resources are needed to produce a culturally sensitive intervention.

While the role of the family environment and parenting as a contributing factor to children's physical health and illness is increasingly acknowledged, to date there has been limited research investigating the efficacy of targeted parenting interventions for these groups. Chronic illness and disability deserve attention in their own right, but they are also associated with higher levels of both internalizing and externalizing problems (Einfeld & Tonge, 1996; McQuaid, Kopel, & Nassau, 2001). There is now increasing evidence that tailored parenting interventions for these populations can assist in not only reducing child conduct problems, and the risk factors associated with the development and maintenance of such problems, but also in helping families to better manage their child's disability or illness. Three examples relating to childhood disability, childhood obesity, and childhood asthma are presented below to illustrate the range of populations to which parenting interventions can be adapted.

Stepping Stones Triple P is a variant of Triple P, which has been developed for parents of children with a disability. It focuses on the additional needs of families of children with disabilities, such as adapting to having a child with a disability and being a part of the community. Additional strategies to address the specific developmental needs of children are also included. Research to date has supported the efficacy of this tailored version for parents of children with various disabilities including cerebral palsy and nonspecified developmental delays (Plant & Sanders, 2007; Roberts, Mazzucchelli, Studman, & Sanders, 2006), chromosomal disorders (Plant & Sanders, 2007), and more recently autistic spectrum disorders (Whittingham, Sofronoff, Sheffield, & Sanders, 2009).

Childhood obesity is increasingly identified as a crisis in relation to children's current health and well-being and their future outcomes (World Health Organization, 2000). Being overweight or obese in childhood is associated with both substantial medical comorbidity, including respiratory, orthopedic, endocrine, gastrointestinal, and cardiovascular problems (e.g., Redline et al., 1999; von Mutius, Schwartz, Neas, Dockery, & Weiss, 2001), as well as psychosocial comorbidity, with weight-related teasing, physical bullying, and social exclusion commonly experienced (Griffiths, Wolke, Page, Horwood, & ALSPAC Study Team, 2006; Hayden-Wade et al., 2005; Hesketh, Wake, & Waters, 2004; Storch et al., 2007). While parents play a critical role in children's weight and obesity, they often do not have the skills to change children's behavior or to make family lifestyle changes and lack confidence in their ability to manage their child's behavior (Borra, Kelly, Shirreffs, Neville, & Geiger, 2003; Walsh & Wardle, 1997). Lifestyle Triple P is a variant specifically tailored to meet the needs of parents of overweight and obese children. Lifestyle Triple P aims to prevent chronic weight problems by improving children's nutritional intake and activity levels and increasing parents' skills and confidence in managing children's lifestyle behavior. Through a 6-month series of group sessions and individual telephone consultations, parents are trained how to facilitate gradual changes in family lifestyle and how to maintain those changes over the long term. Outcomes 1 year after participating in Lifestyle Triple P have indicated that nearly half the sample had achieved reliable decreases in body mass and body fat (West, Sanders, Cleghorn, & Davies, in press).

Finally, the management of a range of chronic childhood illnesses such as asthma can present difficulties for parents and increase the risk of not only ongoing illness-related morbidity but also conduct problems. Childhood asthma is the most common chronic illness suffered by children (Australian Bureau of Statistics, 2002), yet adherence to asthma management plans is generally poor (AIHW Australian Centre for Asthma Monitoring, 2005). A link between child behavior problems, parenting and asthma morbidity, and adherence to management plans has been documented (DeMore, Adams, Wilson, & Hogan, 2005; Kaugars, Klinnert, & Bender, 2004; McQuaid et al., 2001). In a recent study of reasons for difficulties with adherence to medication, parents reported simply "forgetting to give medication" and their child's "reaction to being given medication" as the primary barriers to optimal adherence (Burgess, Sly, Morawska, Cooper, & Devadason, 2008). Parents also encounter a range of difficulties associated with managing their child's asthma including communication with school and other caregivers about their child's asthma management, identifying unique symptoms, and avoiding asthma-inducing triggers, as well as broader concerns about their child's behavior (Morawska, Stelzer, & Burgess, 2008). Based on the literature to date, it would appear that an appropriate parenting intervention program would target basic behavioral management skills, in addition to applying these behavior management principles to asthma management. A current trial is evaluating the efficacy of such an intervention.

POLICY IMPLICATIONS

Although the prevention of conduct problems has been recognized as an important priority for many governments including Australia, New Zealand, the United Kingdom, Canada, the USA, and various European governments, the approach typically advocated is to screen and target high-risk children or vulnerable families and restrict parenting interventions to this group. We contend that failure to view the prevention of conduct problems from a public health perspective that requires a blend of universal and indicated elements targeting parenting will continue to ensure that most children whose parents engage in parenting practices that contribute to the development of antisocial behavior will fail to access these interventions. Further research investment is needed to examine the effectiveness of public health approaches in the prevention of conduct problems.

CONCLUSIONS

Child conduct problems are common and pose a significant public health concern that needs to be addressed in a strategic fashion. Population level approaches to the prevention of conduct problems have the potential to make significant inroads into reducing the burden of child behavioral and emotional problems for families and communities; however, these universal programs need to be backed up by targeted interventions to assist families who require a more intensive or tailored approach. Triple P is an example of a population health approach that combines universal and selected approaches to most effectively and efficiently target child behavioral and emotional problems. There is now a solid evidence base for the universal approach embodied within Triple P, as well as a range of selected Triple P interventions based on this approach. The self-regulatory framework, flexible delivery, individual tailoring, and range of options available in the Triple P system, supported by an extensive and expanding evidence base, provide an effective approach to reducing the population prevalence of conduct problems.

REFERENCES

AIHW Australian Centre for Asthma Monitoring. (2005). *Asthma in Australia.* Canberra: AIHW.

Australian Bureau of Statistics. (2002). *National health survey.* Canberra: ABS.

Backer, T. E., Lieberman, R. P., & Kuehnel, T. G. (1986). Dissemination and adoption of innovative psychosocial interventions. *Journal of Consulting and Clinical Psychology, 54,* 111–118.

Behrens, B. C., & Sanders, M. R. (1994). Prevention of marital distress: Current issues in programming and research. *Behaviour Change, 11*(2), 82–93.

Biglan, A. (1995). Translating what we know about the context of antisocial behavior into a lower prevalence of such behavior. *Journal of Applied Behavior Analysis, 28,* 479–492.

Borra, S. T., Kelly, L., Shirreffs, M. B., Neville, K., & Geiger, C. J. (2003). Developing health messages: Qualitative studies with children, parents, and teachers help identify communications opportunities for healthful lifestyles and the prevention of obesity. *Journal of the American Dietitians Association, 103,* 721–728.

Bradely, R. H., Corwyn, R. F., McAdoo, H., & Coll, C. (2001). The home environments of children in the United States: Part I. Variations by age, ethnicity and poverty status. *Child Development, 72,* 1844–1867.

Burgess, S. W., Sly, P. D., Morawska, A., Cooper, D. M., & Devadason, S. G. (2008). Assessing adherence and factors associated with adherence in young children with asthma. *Respirology, 13,* 559–563.

Calam, R., Sanders, M. R., Miller, C., Sadhnani, V., & Carmont, S. (2008). Can technology and the media help reduce dysfunctional parenting and increase engagement with preventative parenting interventions? *Child Maltreatment, 13,* 347–361.

Conger, R. D., Conger, K. J., Elder, G. H., Jr., Lorenz, F. O., Simons, R. L., & Whitbeck, L. B. (1992). A family process model of hardship and adjustment of early adolescent boys. *Child Development, 63,* 526–541.

Conger, R. D., Conger, K. J., Elder, G. H., Jr., Lorenz, F. O., Simons, R. L., & Whitbeck, L. B. (1993). Family economic status and adjustment of early adolescent girls. *Developmental Psychology, 29,* 206–219.

Conger, K. J., & Elder, G. H., Jr. (1994). *Families in troubled timed.* New York: Aldine de Gruyter.

de Graaf, I., Speetjens, P., Smit, F., de Wolff, M., & Tavecchio, L. (2008a). Effectiveness of the Triple P Positive Parenting Program on behavioral problems in children: A meta-analysis. *Behavior Modification, 32*(5), 714–735.

de Graaf, I., Speetjens, P., Smit, F., de Wolff, M., & Tavecchio, L. (2008b). Effectiveness of the Triple P Positive Parenting Program on Parenting: A meta-analysis. *Family Relations, 57,* 553–566.

DeMore, M., Adams, C., Wilson, N., & Hogan, M. B. (2005). Parenting stress, difficult child behavior, and use of routines in relation to adherence in pediatric asthma. *Children's Health Care, 34*(4), 245–259.

Einfeld, S. L., & Tonge, B. J. (1996). Population prevalence of psychopathology in children and adolescents with intellectual disability: II epidemiological findings. *Journal of Intellectual Disability Research, 40,* 99–109.

Grant, K. E., Compas, B. E., Stuhlmacher, A. F., Thurm, A. E., McMahon, S. D., & Halpert, J. A. (2003). Stressors and child and adolescent psychopathology: Moving from markers to mechanisms of risk. *Psychological Bulletin, 129,* 447–466.

Griffiths, L. J., Wolke, D., Page, A. S., Horwood, J. P., & ALSPAC Study Team. (2006). Obesity and bullying: Different effects for boys and girls. *Archives of Disease in Childhood, 91,* 121–125.

Halford, W. K., Sanders, M. R., & Behrens, B. C. (1994). Self regulation in behavioral couples therapy. *Behavior Therapy, 25*(3), 431–452.

Hayden-Wade, H. A., Stein, R. I., Ghaderi, A., Saelens, B. E., Zabinski, M. F., & Wilfley, D. E. (2005). Prevalence, characteristics, and correlates of teasing experiences among overweight children vs. non-overweight peers. *Obesity Research, 13,* 1381–1392.

Heinrichs, N., Bertram, H., Kuschel, A., & Hahlweg, K. (2005). Parent recruitment and retention in a universal prevention program for child behavior and emotional

problems: Barriers to research and program participation. *Prevention Science, 6,* 275–286.
Henggeler, S. W., Schoenwald, S. K., Liao, J. G., Letourneau, E. J., & Edwards, D. L. (2007). Transporting efficacious treatments to field settings: The link between supervisory practices and therapist fidelity in MST programs. *Journal of Clinical Child and Adolescent Psychology, 31*(2), 155–167.
Hesketh, K., Wake, M., & Waters, E. (2004). Body mass index and parent-reported self-esteem in elementary school children: evidence for a causal relationship. *International Journal of Obesity, 28,* 1233–1237.
Holloway, E. L., & Neufeldt, S. A. (1995). Supervision: Its contribution to treatment efficacy. *Journal of Consulting and Clinical Psychology, 63,* 207–213.
Human Rights and Equal Opportunities Commission (HREOC). (1997). *Bringing them home: Report of the National inquiry into the separation of Aboriginal and Torres Strait islander children their familiesfrom.* Canberra, ACT: HREOC.
Karoly, P. (1993). Mechanisms of self-regulation: A systems view. *Annual Review of Psychology, 44,* 23–52.
Kaugars, A. S., Klinnert, M. D., & Bender, B. G. (2004). Family influences on pediatric asthma. *Journal of Pediatric Psychology, 29*(7), 475–491.
Leung, C., Sanders, M. R., Leung, S., Mak, R., & Lau, J. (2003). An outcome evaluation of the implementation of the triple P-Positive Parenting Program in Hong Kong. *Family Process, 42,* 531–544.
Mangusson, K. A., & Duncan, G. J. (2002). Parents in poverty. In M. H. Bornstein (Ed.), *Handbook of parenting* (2nd ed., pp. 95–121). Mahwah, NJ: Erlbaum.
Markie-Dadds, C., & Sanders, M. R. (2006). Self-directed Triple P (Positive Parenting Program) for mothers with children at-risk of developing conduct problems. *Behavioral and Cognitive Psychotherapy, 34*(3), 259–275.
Matsumoto, Y., Sofronoff, K., & Sanders, M. (2007). The efficacy and acceptability of the Triple P parenting program in a cross-cultural context: Results of an efficacy trial. *Behavior Change, 24,* 205–218.
McQuaid, E. L., Kopel, S. J., & Nassau, J. H. (2001). Behavioral adjustment in children with asthma: A meta-analysis. *Journal of Developmental & Behavioral Pediatrics, 22*(6), 430–439.
McTaggart, P., & Sanders, M. (2007). Mediators and moderators of change in dysfunctional parenting in a school-based universal application of the Triple-P Positive Parenting Programme. *Journal of Children's Services, 2*(1), 4–17.
Mihalopoulos, C., Sanders, M. R., Turner, C. M., Murphy-Brennan, M., & Carter, R. (2007). Does the Triple P-Positive Parenting Program provide value for money? *Australian and New Zealand Journal of Psychiatry, 41,* 239–246.
Morawska, A., & Sanders, M. R. (2006). Self-administered behavioral family intervention for parents of toddlers: Part I – Efficacy. *Journal of Consulting and Clinical Psychology, 74,* 10–19.
Morawska, A., & Sanders, M. R. (2007). Are parent-reported outcomes for self-directed or telephone-assisted behavioral family intervention enhanced if parents are observed? *Behavior Modification, 31,* 279–297.
Morawska, A., Stelzer, J., & Burgess, S. W. (2008). Parenting asthmatic children: Identification of parenting challenges. *Journal of Asthma, 45,* 465–472.
Mrazek, P. J., & Haggerty, R. J. (1994). *Reducing risks for mental disorders.* Washington: National Academy Press.
Nowak, C., & Heinrichs, N. (2008). A comprehensive meta-analysis of Triple P-Positive Parenting Program using hierarchical linear modeling: Effectiveness and moderating variables. *Clinical Child and Family Psychology Review, 11,* 114–144.
Patterson, G. R. (1982). *Coercive family process.* Eugene, OR: Castalia Press.
Plant, K. M., & Sanders, M. R. (2007). Reducing problem behavior during care-giving in families of preschool-aged children with developmental disabilities. *Research in Developmental Disabilities, 28,* 362–385.
Prinz, R. J., & Sanders, M. R. (2007). Adopting a population-level approach to parenting and family support interventions. *Clinical Psychology Review, 27,* 739–749.
Prinz, R. J., Sanders, M. R., Shapiro, C. J., Whitaker, D. J., & Lutzker, J. R. (2009). Population-based prevention of child maltreatment: The US Triple P system population trial. *Prevention Science, 10*(1), 1–12.

Redline, S., Tishler, P. V., Schluchter, M., Aylor, J., Clark, K., & Graham, G. (1999). Risk factors for sleep-disordered breathing in children. Associations with obesity, race, and respiratory problems. *American Journal of Respiratory and Critical Care Medicine, 159*, 1527–1532.

Ring, I., & Brown, N. (2003). The health status of indigenous peoples and others. *BMJ, 327*, 404–405.

Roberts, C., Mazzucchelli, T., Studman, L., & Sanders, M. R. (2006). Behavioral family intervention for children with developmental disabilities and behavioral problems. *Journal of Clinical Child and Adolescent Psychology., 35*, 180–193.

Sanders, M. R. (1999). Triple P-Positive Parenting Program: Towards an empirically validated multilevel parenting and family support strategy for the prevention of behavior and emotional problems in children. *Clinical Child and Family Psychology Review, 2*, 71–90.

Sanders, M. R. (2008). Triple P-Positive Parenting Program as a public health approach to strengthening parenting. *Journal of Family Psychology, 22*(4), 506–517.

Sanders, M. R., Bor, W., & Morawska, A. (2007). Maintenance of treatment gains: A comparison of enhanced, standard, and self-directed Triple P-Positive Parenting Program. *Journal of Abnormal Child Psychology, 35*(6), 983–998.

Sanders, M. R., & Markie-Dadds, C. (1996). Triple P: A multilevel family intervention program for children with disruptive behavior disorders. In P. Cotton & H. Jackson (Eds.), *Early intervention & prevention in mental health* (pp. 59–85). Carlton South VIC: Australian Psychological Society.

Sanders, M. R., Markie-Dadds, C., Rinaldis, M., Firman, D., & Baig, N. (2007). Using epidemiological household survey data on parenting practices to inform policy and planning decisions regarding implementation of evidence-based parenting interventions. *Child: Care, Health and Development, 33*(6), 768–783.

Sanders, M. R., Markie-Dadds, C., Tully, L. A., & Bor, W. (2000). The Triple P-Positive Parenting Program: A comparison of enhanced, standard, and self-directed behavioral family intervention for parents of children with early onset conduct problems. *Journal of Consulting and Clinical Psychology, 68*(4), 624–640.

Sanders, M. R., Markie-Dadds, C., & Turner, K. M. T. (1996). *Every parent's survival guide [Video]*. Brisbane: Families International.

Sanders, M. R., Markie-Dadds, C., & Turner, K. M. T. (2001). *Standard Triple P: Practitioner manual: Brisbane*. Australia: Families International.

Sanders, M. R., & McFarland, M. (2000). Treatment of depressed mothers with disruptive children: A controlled evaluation of cognitive behavioral family intervention. *Behavior Therapy, 31*, 89–112.

Sanders, M. R., Montgomery, D. T., & Brechman-Touissant, M. L. (2000). The mass media and the prevention of child behavior problems: The evaluation of a television series to promote positive outcomes for parents and their children. *Journal of Child Psychology and Psychiatry, 41*, 939–948.

Sanders, M. R., Ralph, A., Sofronoff, K., Gardiner, P., Thompson, R., Dwyer, S., et al. (2008). Every family: a population approach to reducing behavioral and emotional problems in children making the transition to school. *Journal of Primary Prevention, 29*, 197–222.

Sanders, M. R., & Woolley, M. L. (2005). The relationship between global, domain and task-specific self-efficacy and parenting practices: Implications for parent training. *Child: Care, Health and Development, 31*, 65–73.

Serketich, W. J., & Dumas, J. E. (1996). The effectiveness of behavioral parent training to modify antisocial behavior in children: A meta-analysis. *Behavior Therapy, 27*, 171–186.

Stallman, H. M., & Ralph, A. (2007). Reducing risk factors for adolescent behavioral and emotional problems: A pilot randomised controlled trial of a self-administered parenting intervention. *Australian e-Journal for the Advancement of Mental Health, 6*(2), 1–13.

Storch, E. A., Milsom, V. A., DeBraganza, N., Lewin, A. B., Geffken, G. R., & Silverstein, J. H. (2007). Peer victimization, psychosocial adjustment, and physical activity in overweight and at-risk for overweight youth. *Journal of Pediatric Psychology, 32*, 80–89.

Straus, M. A., & Stewart, J. H. (1999). Corporal punishment by American parents: National data on prevalence, chronicity, severity, and duration, in relation to child, and family characteristics. *Clinical Child and Family Psychology Review, 2*(2), 55–70.

Taylor, T. K., & Biglan, A. (1998). Behavioral family interventions for improving child-rearing: A review of literature for clinicians and policy makers. *Clinical Child and Family Psychology Review, 1*, 41–60.

Thomas, R., & Zimmer-Gembeck, M. J. (2007). Behavioral outcomes of parent–child interaction therapy and Triple P-Positive Parenting Program: A review and meta-analysis. *Journal of Abnormal Child Psychology, 35*, 475–495.

Trewin, D., & Madden, R. (2003). *The health and welfare of Australia's Aboriginal and Torres Strait islander peoples*. Canberra, ACT: Australian Bureau of Statistics and the Australian Institute of Health and Welfare.

Turner, K. M. T., Richards, M., & Sanders, M. R. (2007). Randomised clinical trial of a group parent education programme for Australian Indigenous families. *Journal of Paediatrics and Child Health, 43*, 429–437.

Turner, K. M. T., & Sanders, M. R. (2006). Help when it's needed first: A controlled evaluation of a brief, preventive behavioral family intervention in a primary care setting. *Behavior Therapy, 37*, 131–142.

von Mutius, E., Schwartz, J., Neas, L. M., Dockery, D., & Weiss, S. T. (2001). Relation of body mass index to asthma and atopy in children: The National Health and Nutrition Examination Study III. *Thorax, 56*, 835–838.

Walsh, P. J., & Wardle, J. (1997). Cause and effect beliefs and self-esteem of overweight children. *Journal of Child Psychology and Psychiatry, 38*, 645–650.

Webster-Stratton, C., & Taylor, T. K. (1998). Adopting and implementing empirically supported interventions: A recipe for success. In A. Buchanan & B. L. Hudson (Eds.), *Parenting, schooling and children's behavior: Interdisciplinary approaches* (pp. 127–160). Aldershort: Ashgate.

West, F., Sanders, M., Cleghorn, G., & Davies, P. S. W. (in press). Randomised clinical trial of a family-based lifestyle intervention for childhood obesity. *Behavior Research and Therapy.*

Whitbeck, L. B., Simons, R. L., Conger, R. D., Wickrama, K. A. S., Ackley, K. A., & Elder, G. H., Jr. (1997). The effects of parents' working conditions and family economic hardship on parenting behaviors and children's self efficacy. *Social Psychology Quarterly, 60*, 291–303.

Whittingham, K., Sofronoff, K., Sheffield, J., & Sanders, M. R. (2009). Stepping Stones Triple P: An RCT of a parenting program with parents of a child diagnosed with an Autism Spectrum Disorder. *Journal of Abnormal Child Psychology, 37*, 469–480.

World Health Organization. (2000). *Obesity: Preventing and managing the global epidemic: Report of a WHO consultation*. Geneva, Switzerland: Report No. 894 WHO Technical Report Series.

Zubrick, S. R., Lawrence, D. M., Silburn, S. R., Blair, E., Milroy, H., Wilkes, T., Eades, S., D'Antoine, H., Read, A., Ishiguchi, P., & Doyle, S. (2004). *The Western Australian Aboriginal child health survey: The health of Aboriginal children and young people. Available at:* www.ichr.uwa.edu.au. Perth: Telethon Institute for Child Health Research.

Zubrick, S. R., Ward, K. A., Silburn, S. R., Lawrence, D., Williams, A. A., Blair, E., et al. (2005). Prevention of child behavior problems through universal implementation of a group behavioral family intervention. *Prevention Science, 6*(4), 287–304.

18

Evidence-Based Treatments for Conduct Problems Among Ethnic Minorities

JUDY K. HO, KRISTEN M. McCABE, MAY YEH, and ANNA S. LAU

Effective treatment of conduct problems for ethnic minority youth is an urgent public health priority (Loeber, Burke, Lahey, Winters, & Zera, 2000). Ethnic minority populations are rapidly increasing, with current estimates indicating that 48% of US children are from ethnic minority backgrounds. This figure is projected to increase to 62% by 2050 (U.S. Department of Commerce, 2008). Disruptive behavior is the most common reason for referral for youth mental health treatment in the USA (Lavigne et al., 1998), and oppositional defiant disorder (ODD) and conduct disorder (CD) are the predominant youth disorders seen in community mental health clinics (Frick, 1998; Kazdin, 1995). Without adequate treatment, disruptive behavior in early childhood is associated with a high degree of impairment and poor long-term prognosis (Lahey, Loeber, Quay, Frick, & Grimm, 1997).

Rates of disruptive behavior disorders (DBDs) are especially high among low-income, ethnic minority children. Studies have found higher rates of

JUDY K. HO • University of California
KRISTEN M. McCABE • University of San Diego
MAY YEH • San Diego State University
ANNA S. LAU • University of California

R.C. Murrihy et al. (eds.), *Clinical Handbook of Assessing and Treating Conduct Problems in Youth*, DOI 10.1007/978-1-4419-6297-3_18,

CD for African Americans (Costello et al., 1988; Costello, Farmer, Angold, Burns, & Erkanli, 1997), Mexican Americans (Vaszonyi & Flannery, 1997), and Native Americans (Beals et al., 1997) compared to Caucasian Americans. Higher incidences of official juvenile delinquency have also been found for Latino American and African American adolescents (Farrington, 1987; Rutter & Giller, 1983). Occurrences of early-onset conduct problems are as high as 35% in ethnically diverse, low-income families (Chambless & Hollon, 1998; Proctor, Vosler, & Murty, 1992), as compared with 4–16% in the general population (Cohen et al., 1993). CD and ODD more frequently occur among youth from families of low socioeconomic status, and CD, ODD, and delinquency more frequently occur in neighborhoods with high crime rates where large numbers of ethnic minority families reside (Lahey, Miller, Gordon, & Riley, 1999; Loeber & Farrington, 1998; Sampson & Laub, 1997). Even more troubling, research indicates that ethnic minority youth with conduct problems suffer from more significant associated impairments than Caucasian American youth. Ethnic minority children and adolescents in the USA with disruptive behavior problems are more vulnerable to impairment in several key domains, including family, peer, and school functioning, than Caucasian American children with similar behavior problems (Ezpeleta, Keeler, Erkanli, Costello, & Angold, 2001). Further, ethnic minority boys from low socioeconomic families are more likely to be diagnosed with persistent and pervasive associated problems relating to conduct functioning compared to their Caucasian American, higher socioeconomic status counterparts (Proctor et al., 1992). Therefore, effective treatment of conduct problems for ethnic minority youth is especially imperative.

TREATING ETHNIC MINORITY YOUTH WITH CONDUCT PROBLEMS

Given the disproportionate impact of conduct problems in ethnic minority youth, and the particularly high burden associated with these problems among ethnic minority families, identifying effective treatments for conduct problems for ethnic minority youth is crucial. An expanding array of evidence-based treatments (EBTs) is available, and clinicians are faced with the task of selecting an appropriate intervention for a particular child's presenting problem, developmental stage, family composition, and treatment preferences. In addition, clinicians must determine whether that EBT is culturally appropriate for the family and whether it may need to be adapted to be effective within the family's cultural context.

This task has been made difficult by the historical underrepresentation of ethnic minorities in clinical trials (USDHHS, 2001). Unfortunately, despite the large number of African American and Latino American youth with conduct problems, most efficacious interventions have been developed and tested with Caucasian American samples (Eyberg, Nelson, & Boggs, 2008).

When ethnic minorities have been included in clinical trials, they have rarely been present in sufficient numbers to examine the impact of care for different ethnic groups (USDHHS). Encouragingly, there has been a significant expansion in the research base on EBTs for minority youth and families over the past decade (Huey & Polo, 2008). Several recent randomized controlled trials (RCTs) include significant proportions of ethnic minority youth, many studies have enrolled ethnic-specific samples, and several multigroup trials have examined race/ethnicity as an organizing variable of interest in outcomes analyses (Huey & Polo). Along with this new wave of research, an influx of efficacy and effectiveness studies that specifically address the treatments of conduct problems for ethnically diverse youth have surfaced.

Despite the expanding research base, there are still significant gaps in our knowledge of how EBTs work for minority youth with conduct problems. Although ethnic minority youth are increasingly represented in trials, some racial/ethnic groups are rarely included in substantial numbers (e.g., Asian American, American Indian, Alaskan Native). As yet, relatively few studies have examined whether EBTs validated on predominantly Caucasian American samples achieve similar benefits in minority groups by evaluating ethnicity as a treatment moderator or predictor of change. As such, some have argued that the current evidence-base is still not strong enough to warrant large-scale dissemination of EBTs to particular ethnic minority communities (Bernal & Scharrón-del Río, 2001). These researchers caution against widespread use of standard EBTs in diverse populations because many EBTs have not established "ethnic invariance" (i.e., standard treatments are equally powerful when applied to ethnic minorities; Huey & Polo, 2008), and point to the comparatively poorer outcomes from community-based effectiveness studies that include greater ethnic diversity than most clinical trials (e.g., Chambless & Ollendick, 2001). Some have argued that "ethnic disparities" (i.e., standard EBTs are less powerful when applied to ethnic minorities; Huey & Polo) are plausible, if not probable, and recommend making significant adaptations to EBTs before employing them with ethnic minority families (Bernal, Bonilla, & Bellido, 1995; Hall, 2001; Huey & Polo; Lau, 2006). The Surgeon General's Report on *Mental Health, Culture, Race, and Ethnicity* (USDHHS, 2001) concludes that in general, EBTs still represent the best treatments available to ethnic minorities, and what is needed is an understanding of when these EBTs should be used with minority groups in standard form, when they require significant cultural modifications to be effective, and when they may be contraindicated for specific cultural groups.

The main goal of this chapter is to synthesize the existing literature to provide an overview of a culturally specific evidence-base for ethnic minority youth with conduct problems. We hope that the information presented here will be helpful in guiding clinician decisions for providing effective and culturally sensitive care to their client in light of a research base that is still in development and aid investigators in planning future studies to expand research efforts in this area.

RESEARCH BASE ON EBTs FOR ETHNIC MINORITY YOUTH WITH CONDUCT PROBLEMS

Identifying EBTs for Ethnic Minority Youth with Conduct Problems

- We reviewed published controlled clinical trials to select examples of evidence-based psychosocial treatments for conduct problems that have been evaluated with ethnic minority youth. Conduct problems were defined broadly, based on the symptoms of ODD and CD as specified in the Diagnostic and Statistical Manual of Mental Disorders (4th ed., DSM-IV: American Psychiatric Association, 1994), such as noncompliance, aggression, disruptive classroom behavior, delinquent behavior, or general disruptive behavior. Similar to the approach used by Huey and Polo (2008), we excluded interventions involving (a) medication only, (b) reading only, (c) teaching/tutoring focus only, and (d) relocation only (e.g., moving child to a foster placement). However, different from the Huey and Polo review, we incorporated examples of treatments intended to prevent conduct problems in at-risk youth (i.e., primary or universal prevention programs). For this review, we prioritized treatments for conduct problems that, based on the existing evidence, most likely met criteria for either "well-established," "probably efficacious," or "possibly efficacious" treatments for at least one ethnic minority group (e.g., African American, Latino American, Asian American, Native American, or American Indian), using criteria outlined by Chambless et al. (1996) (Chambless & Hollon, 1998; Chambless & Ollendick, 2001). Well-established treatments require at least two high-quality between-group trials by different groups of investigators that show the treatment is superior to placebo or another treatment, or equivalent to an established treatment (Chambless et al.). Probably efficacious treatments require only one high-quality trial comparing treatment to a placebo condition or alternative treatment, or two trials comparing the treatment to a no-treatment control (Chambless et al.). Finally, possibly efficacious treatments require at least one study showing the treatment to be efficacious in the absence of conflicting evidence (Chambless & Hollon, 1998).

We primarily described trials that included a substantial proportion of at least one ethnic minority group in their sample (i.e., one of the major racial/ethnic minority groups comprises at least 20% of the total sample). However, due to the paucity of literature for certain minority groups (e.g., Native Americans, American Indians, and Asian Americans), we included a handful of studies that utilized these cultural groups in their sample, even if their proportion to the total sample was not substantial (i.e., less than 20%). Finally, the treatments reviewed have been evaluated with "well-conducted" trials with clear inclusion/exclusion criteria, appropriate control or comparison conditions, random assignment, reliable measures to assess outcomes, and clearly described statistical procedures (Brestan & Eyberg, 1998).

Broad Typology of EBTs for Ethnic Minority Youth with Conduct Problems

In the extant literature on treatments for youth conduct problems, evidence regarding their applicability to minority youth can be found from a range of approaches. Interventionists have varied in the extent to which cultural considerations have driven the design, tailoring, or evaluation of their treatments. To organize our review, we have broadly categorized these approaches as follows:

1. *Developing a treatment protocol to meet the needs of a specific ethnic minority group(s), and evaluating the treatment with a sample including a large proportion of ethnic minority families.* This category encompasses the development of novel "culturally sensitive therapies" (Hall, 2001) that are built bottom-up for a particular ethnic minority group, guided by a theoretical framework and techniques that are grounded in the cultural and ecological context of the target group. These interventions are typically tested in clinical trials largely or solely populated by members of the specific cultural group for which the treatment was developed.
2. *Developing a treatment protocol without a particular ethnic minority group in mind, then evaluating the effects of the treatment with a sample that includes a substantial proportion of ethnic minority youth and their families.* This sampling of minority youth and their families may be a product of happenstance or convenience (i.e., access to recruitment sites heavily populated by minority youth), or by design (i.e., specific efforts to recruit underrepresented groups to increase the likelihood of generalizability). In the latter case, the aim may be to examine whether an EBT established as efficacious in trials with largely Caucasian American samples is similarly effective for different ethnic groups. In some trials, the inclusion of significant proportions of at least two racial/ethnic groups (e.g., Caucasian Americans and African Americans) affords the examination of treatment by ethnicity interactions to explore potential differential effects of care. If adequately powered, these moderation analyses provide one way to demonstrate that a treatment shows "ethnic invariance" vs. "ethnic disparity" (Huey & Polo, 2008).
3. *Developing a treatment protocol without a particular ethnic minority group in mind, and then examining a culturally adapted version of the treatment protocol with a sample that includes a substantial proportion of ethnic minority youth and families.* This approach takes a well-established or probably efficacious EBT protocol, which was originally developed and tested with largely Caucasian American samples, and modifies it with particular cultural elements to address the needs, values, attitudes, and beliefs of a specific cultural group. Two types of treatment adaptations may be considered to ensure fit with the needs of the target population, while assuring fidelity to the original EBT protocol (Lau, 2006). The first adaptation strategy involves *contextualizing content.* This may involve adding novel treatment components to target group-specific risk or protective processes,

designed to accommodate the specific cultural factors and utilize particular cultural strengths of the target community. The second adaptation strategy involves *enhancing engagement* in effective EBT strategies that have demonstrated low social validity in certain populations; that is, when members of a community (e.g., racial/ethnic, or geographic region) view certain treatment strategies as irrelevant, unhelpful, or unacceptable (Lau). Both of these interventions are usually tested in clinical trials largely or solely composed of ethnic minority subjects, often the specific cultural group for which the treatment adaptations were tailored.

Each of these approaches makes an important contribution to our knowledge of how to provide culturally responsive services to ethnic minority youth with conduct problems. In the subsequent sections, we review examples of each of these approaches, provide a summary of the current state of the science on treating conduct problems in ethnic minority youth, note implications for clinical work with ethnic minority families, and offer recommendations for future cultural adaptations of EBTs for minority youth.

EBTs DEVELOPED FOR AND TESTED WITH SPECIFIC ETHNIC MINORITY GROUPS

Overview

In this section, we describe several treatments for conduct problems that have been developed for specific ethnic minority group(s), and then tested in these cultural groups to evaluate the treatment's efficacy and/or effectiveness. These treatments were usually pioneered to address the specific needs of a particular cultural group in order to improve engagement, treatment utilization and adherence, and treatment outcomes for the target population. Before and/or during treatment development, researchers gather information on culture-specific attitudes, values, and beliefs regarding pertinent issues such as child development, family dynamics, development of mental health problems, and use of professional mental health treatment. In many of these interventions, theoretical culture-specific models of developmental trajectories, family relationships, and risk or resiliency factors for conduct problems serve as the basis for the construction of treatment strategies. Below, we offer several examples of these types of treatments utilizing diverse modalities (e.g., family therapy, parent management training (PMT), cognitive-behavioral therapy) in varying stages of empirical validation (e.g., well-established, probably efficacious; clinical trials, effectiveness studies) for different cultural groups (e.g., African American, Latino American).

Family Therapy

The University of Miami Center for Family Studies has been designing and implementing family-based interventions for minority families in the Miami area for the past several decades (Muir, Schwartz, & Szapocznik, 2004).

Their work has focused primarily on Hispanic immigrant families with drug-using, conduct-problem adolescents. Treatments range from universal prevention to indicated intervention, and within-family protocols as well as ecological protocols that involve working with both family systems and related systems outside of the family (e.g., school, living environment).

Brief Strategic Family Therapy (BSFT) (Santisteban et al., 2003) is a family-based intervention that was developed in response to the findings of a cross-cultural survey given to Cuban immigrants and Caucasian Americans in Miami (Szapocznik, Scopetta, Aranalde, & Kurtines, 1978). BSFT was designed to be syntonic with predominant Cuban values, and integrated structural family therapy conditions (Minuchin, Rosman, & Baker, 1978) with strategic family therapy approaches (Haley, 1976; Szapocznik et al.) that were specifically tailored to the needs of Cuban immigrant families with adolescents at risk for conduct problems and substance abuse. Risk factors specific to the Cuban population that were addressed in this approach include stress and family disruption due to immigration, acculturation, and inner-city living conditions. Additionally, BSFT draws on particular strengths of this community, including strong extended family networks and familial focus. The efficacy of BSFT in reducing behavior problems and drug abuse in youth has been tested in two randomized, controlled NIDA Stage-II studies, which are efficacy trials of promising interventions identified in NIDA Stage-I investigations. In the first study with 69 (80% Cuban, 20% other – mostly Colombian) Hispanic 6–12-year-old boys with behavioral problems, Szapocznik et al. (1989) found that BSFT and psychodynamic child therapy were both superior to a recreation control condition in reducing child behavioral and emotional problems, but that BSFT was superior to both of the other conditions in improving observer-rated family functioning at 1-year follow-up. In a second study, Santisteban et al. randomly assigned 126 Hispanic adolescents (64 Cuban, 18 Nicaraguan, 12 Colombian, 8 Puerto Rican, 4 Peruvian, 2 Mexican, 19 other Hispanics) referred for disruptive behavior problems to receive either BSFT or a group counseling (GC) program that did not enlist family functioning as a mechanism of change. The GC condition consisted of a participatory-learning group intervention in which adolescents were led by a facilitator and were encouraged to discuss and solve problems amongst themselves. This control condition did not represent an empirically validated group intervention, but was designed to represent groups conducted in school settings, and used to control for factors common in any therapeutic intervention targeting problem behaviors (i.e., attention, support, drug abuse information, and problem-solving). BSFT was significantly more efficacious in reducing conduct problems, associations with antisocial peers, and marijuana use, while simultaneously improving observer-rated family functioning compared to the group counseling program (Santisteban et al.).

The prevailing belief in traditional family systems work was that therapy had to be delivered to the entire family conjointly. However, given the difficulties of engaging entire families of adolescents with conduct problems, Szapocznik, Foote, Perez-Vidal, Hervis, & Kurtines (1985) explored whether *One-Person BSFT* could achieve similar beneficial outcomes to

BSFT. One-Person BSFT utilizes the systemic concept of complementarity, which suggests that behaviors of other family members may change in response to changes in one family member. The efficacy of One-Person BSFT was examined in a sample of 35 predominantly low-income Hispanic (77% Cuban) drug-abusing adolescents who were randomized to receive either one-person or whole-family BSFT (Szapocznik, Kurtines, Foote, Perez-Vidal, & Hervis, 1983, 1986). Both types of BSFT showed significant improvements in conduct problems, adolescent drug use, and family functioning. Overall, the efficacy of One-Person BSFT was not significantly different from conjoint BSFT (Szapocznik et al.).

A family-based prevention program, *Bicultural Effectiveness Training (BET)* (Szapocznik, Santisteban, Kurtines, Perez-Vidal, & Hervis, 1984) was conceived based on observations that families of Cuban adolescents with behavior problems were often characterized by acculturation discrepancies between parents and children, with parents tending toward an orientation to Hispanic culture, and youth tending toward an orientation to mainstream American culture. Sharing goals with BSFT but aiming to achieve them through a psychoeducational prevention program for youth at-risk for conduct problems, BET focused on reframing family conflicts as intercultural (i.e., American vs. Hispanic) instead of intergenerational (i.e., parent vs. adolescent) to facilitate problem-solving and collaboration among family members. A small RCT with 31 Cuban adolescents indicated that BET was as effective as Structural Family Therapy (Szapocznik et al., 1986) in reducing conduct problems and improving family interactions, and that BET was effective in facilitating family members' awareness of different cultural systems. Next, *Family Effectiveness Training (FET)* (Szapocznik et al., 1989) was developed to combine the preventive and psychoeducational focus of BET for at-risk Hispanic youth and families with the concrete restructuring intervention techniques used in BSFT with Hispanic preadolescents who were already evidencing significant conduct problems. A randomized trial of 79 Hispanic families with conduct disordered adolescents aged 6–12 (76% Cuban, 24% other Hispanic groups) comparing FET to a no-contact control, found that FET was significantly more efficacious than the control condition in reducing children's problem behaviors and improving family functioning (Szapocznik et al., 1989).

To address extrafamilial risk factors and problems as well as within-family issues, *Structural Ecosystem Therapy (SET)* (Robbins, Schwartz, & Szapocznik, 2004) was developed as an ecological extension of BSFT. In SET, BSFT techniques are utilized in working with the family–peer, family–school, and family–juvenile justice mesosystems. Similarly, *Familias Unidas* (United Families; Coatsworth, Pantin, & Szapocznik, 2002) was developed as a prevention program that extends BET and FET concepts to reduce risk and build resilience at multiple eco-development levels for Hispanic adolescents at risk for conduct problems. Familias Unidas engages Hispanic immigrant families into an empowerment process in which they build a strong parent-support network used to increase knowledge of culturally relevant parenting. Intervention activities proceed from parents' support networks, where parent groups meet with a facilitator to discuss the worlds of the child, including family, school, and peers.

Home visits are also provided where parents enact the intervention skills learned in session with their own adolescents in the naturalistic family setting. Within the family microsystem, activities are conducted to encourage effective behavior management techniques and increase parent–adolescent bonding. In the family–peer and family–school mesosystems, activities are conducted to encourage parents to manage their youths' peer activities and to develop collaborations with the school system. Parent-support groups are used to help connect Hispanic immigrant parents with each other to reduce the social isolation and daily stressors of moving to a new country with unfamiliar cultural practices (Coatsworth, Pantin, & Szapocznik, 2002). The efficacy of Familias Unidas was evaluated in a randomized trial by Pantin et al. (2003). One hundred and sixty-seven Hispanic adolescents in 6th and 7th grade (39% Cuban, 27% Central American, 17% South American, 5% Puerto Ricans, 10% other Hispanic) and their parents/families were assigned to Familias Unidas or a no-intervention control, and results indicated that Familias Unidas was significantly more efficacious than the control condition in increasing parental investment and decreasing adolescent behavior problems (Pantin et al., 2003).

Multicomponent Treatment Programs

The *Bridges to High School Program (Bridges/Puentes)* (Gonzales, Dumka, Deardorff, Carter, & McCray, 2004) is a universal prevention program designed to prevent school disengagement and negative mental health trajectories of Mexican American youth during the transition to junior high school. The program was developed using culturally specific empirical research with Mexican Americans to identify the most salient predictors of mental health as target variables for change. Focus groups and individual interviews were also used to determine intervention needs, preferences, and barriers to participating in services for low-income families (Dumka, Gonzales, Woods, & Formoso, 1998). Intervention consisted of group sessions and an individualized home visit (10 weeks total), and includes an adolescent stress coping skills intervention, a parenting skills intervention, and a family strengthening intervention. A Spanish-language version of the intervention was also developed. The program was initially evaluated in an uncontrolled trial of 22 families (13 assigned to a Spanish-language group, 9 assigned to an English-language group) with 19 Mexican Americans, 1 African American, 1 Caucasian American, and 1 other race/ethnicity, which examined pre- and postintervention measures of adolescent and parent functioning. Results showed that parents reported an increase in supportive parenting and decrease in inconsistent discipline, and fewer problem behaviors exhibited by their adolescents. In addition, adolescents reported increased use of coping strategies and decreased depressive symptoms. They also reported significant changes in their mothers' parenting skills, including increased parental monitoring and decreased inconsistent discipline (Gonzales et al., 2004).

Currently, a field trial is in progress consisting of 480 adolescents from inner-city schools, who have been randomly assigned to participate in either the Bridges/Puentes Program or a low-dose workshop condition, with equal numbers of Spanish-dominant and English-dominant Hispanic families assigned to participate in separate language-based programs. The two intervention conditions were implemented for three consecutive years beginning in 2003. The results of this clinical trial will provide information on the efficacy of the Bridges/Puentes Program compared to a workshop condition and any differential effect of the program as a function of adolescent gender, high initial levels of symptomatology, and language of program delivery (Information available at http://www.asu.edu/clas/asuprc/bridges.html).

Summary

A growing number of investigators have dedicated research programs to developing and testing treatments for conduct problems in specific groups of ethnic minority youth, and we have highlighted several examples of these treatments in this section. Although much headway has been made in particular for Latino American youth and their families, virtually all of the studies highlighted are in the very early stages of empirical validation. Most of the studies appear to be at the "possibly efficacious" stage of validation. These treatments include: (a) FET for the treatment of conduct problems in mostly Cuban, Hispanic families; (b) BET with Cuban families; (c) Familias Unidas in the prevention of conduct problems in mostly Cuban, Hispanic families, and (d) Bridges/Puentes in the prevention of conduct problems in Mexican American families. Only two treatment protocols, the one-person BSFT and the BET, meet criteria for "probably efficacious" interventions for predominantly Cuban families (BSFT) and Cuban families only (BET). Finally, of the studies reviewed in this section, only one treatment protocol, the original BSFT, meets criteria for a "well-established" treatment for predominantly Cuban, Hispanic families. Although these studies were conducted in ethnic-specific samples (e.g., predominantly Cuban American or Mexican American), it is possible that treatment benefits may also generalize to other Latino American populations that were included in the samples in insufficient numbers (e.g., Colombians for BSFT, Central and South Americans for Familias Unidas). For most of these treatments, additional RCTs need to be conducted to establish their efficacy for treating conduct problems at the "well-established" level for a particular cultural group (e.g., Cubans or Mexican Americans). Further research should also evaluate the efficacy of well-established treatment protocols with samples of families from other countries of origin (e.g., Venezuela, Spain) that are likely to share similar cultural values to groups for which interventions have been validated (e.g., Cuban Americans) to determine the treatments' applicability to other Latino American and Hispanic populations. As BSFT has demonstrated well-established efficaciousness, next steps may include effectiveness studies that evaluate outcomes for youth with comorbid problems in different types of community settings. These real-world studies may greatly aid implementation and dissemination efforts of BSFT and other EBTs for conduct problems in ethnic minority families.

TREATMENTS DEVELOPED WITHOUT SPECIFIC CULTURAL CONSIDERATIONS, THEN TESTED UNADAPTED WITH ETHNIC MINORITY FAMILIES

Overview

In this section, we describe treatments for conduct problems that were pioneered without a specific ethnic minority group in mind, but were developed to assist individuals with a specific constellation of risk factors or clinical problems (e.g., inner-city, low-income juvenile delinquent adolescents). Similar to treatments described in the previous section, these treatments have also been grounded in strong theoretical models of development and psychopathology, although they may not be culturally specific. Although these treatments did not address cultural issues relative to ethnic minorities as a main aim in the development phase, they were subsequently evaluated in efficacy and/or effectiveness studies that included a large proportion of ethnic minority families. In a few of these studies, treatment by ethnicity interactions were examined for two or more racial/ethnic groups (e.g., African American vs. Caucasian American) in order to directly compare whether treatment outcomes differed between different cultural groups. Next, we provide an overview of interventions that are most likely efficacious for particular cultural groups, as these groups have been represented in substantial numbers in RCTs that achieved positive outcomes. These types of treatments utilize various modalities (e.g., family therapy, PMT, cognitive-behavioral therapy) and are in varying stages of empirical validation (e.g., well-established, probably efficacious; clinical trials, effectiveness studies) for different cultural groups (e.g., African American, Latino American).

Multisystemic Therapy (See Also Chap. 11)

Multisystemic Therapy (MST) (Henggeler, Melton, & Smith, 1992) is a family-based, individualized intervention that draws on a systems and social-ecological framework to intervene with adolescents with severe conduct problems. MST therapists are trained in diverse evidence-based strategies (e.g., behavioral parent training, contingency contracting) and work intensively (sometimes on a daily basis) with families in their natural environment (e.g., home, school) for a relatively short period of time (3–6 months). Their work is guided by treatment principles that (a) emphasize the relation between behavior problems and their broader systemic context; (b) utilize systematic strengths, to promote responsible family behavior; (c) use present and action-oriented interventions to target behaviors that maintain the problem; and (d) promote developmentally appropriate strategies that involve family participation.

MST may be the only efficacious treatment for African American chronic and violent juvenile offenders, as evidenced by outcomes from four RCTs (Borduin et al., 1995; Henggeler et al., 1992; Henggeler, Melton, Brondino, Scherer, & Hanley, 1997; Henggeler, Clingempeel, Brondino, & Pickrel, 2002). Each of these studies included a significant proportion of African American youth and families in the study samples (e.g., 56% of 96 participants were African American in Henggeler et al.; 30% of 200 participants in Borduin et al.; 81% of 155 participants in Henggeler et al.; and 50% of 118 in Henggeler et al). Compared to usual community services, MST resulted in greater reductions in criminal offending, re-arrests, and time incarcerated (Henggeler et al., 1992; Henggeler, Melton, Brondino, Scherer, & Hanley, 1997; Henggeler, Clingempeel, Brondino, & Pickrel, 2002). In the longest follow-up study to date of a MST clinical trial (Borduin et al.), results showed that MST participants had significantly lower recidivism rates (50% for MST participants vs. 81% for individual therapy participants) 13.7 years post clinical trial (Schaeffer & Borduin, 2005). Further, MST participants had 54% fewer arrests and 57% fewer days of confinement in adult detention facilities than individual therapy participants (Schaeffer & Borduin, 2005).

Several studies have extended the application of MST to other disruptive, externalizing problems in community samples. Henggeler et al. (1999) examined the effectiveness of home-based MST as an inpatient hospitalization alternative for youth in serious psychiatric crises. One hundred and sixteen youth approved for emergency psychiatric hospitalization was assigned to either home-based MST or inpatient hospitalization. This sample consisted of 64% African American, 34% Caucasian American, 1% Asian American, and 1% Hispanic American youth. Results showed that MST was more effective than emergency hospitalization in decreasing youth externalizing symptoms, improving family functioning, and improving school attendance. On a related note, (Huey et al., 2004) examined the effectiveness of MST in reducing attempted suicide among predominantly African American youths (65% of 156 participants) referred for emergency psychiatric hospitalization. Results showed that MST was significantly more effective than hospitalization at decreasing rates of attempted suicide at 1-year follow-up, and the rate of symptom reduction over time was also greater for youth receiving MST. MST effectiveness was also examined in an ethnically diverse sample of 118 juvenile offenders (50% African American, 47% Caucasian American, 1% Asian American, 1% Latino American, 1% Native American) who met DSM-III-R criteria for substance abuse or dependence. Participants were randomly assigned to MST or usual community services, and outcomes showed that MST reduced alcohol, marijuana, and other drug use at posttreatment, and reduced total days in out-of-home placements by 50% at 6-month follow-up (Henggeler, Pickrel, & Brondino, 1999).

Recently, the first RCT of MST with juvenile offenders in the USA conducted without direct oversight by the treatment developers was completed by (Timmons-Mitchell, Bender, Kishna, & Mitchell 2006). Ninety-three youth (77.5% Caucasian American, 15.5% African American, 4.2% Latino American, 2.8% Biracial) were randomly assigned to MST or treatment as usual (TAU) conditions. Results showed that recidivism at 18-month follow-up was reduced for MST participants compared to TAU participants (66.7% and 86.7%, respectively); however, lower effect sizes were reported compared to previous effectiveness and efficacy trials that included oversight by the treatment developers. These results indicate that strategies to improve real-world implementation and outcomes of MST for culturally diverse families should be investigated.

Race/ethnicity was examined as a moderator in four efficacy and effectiveness studies of MST, and race/ethnicity was not found to moderate treatment effects in any of these studies for the included groups. These included: (a) an investigation that examined the efficacy of MST on juvenile offenders (56% African Americans, 42% Caucasian Americans, 2% Latino American; Henggler, Melton, & Smith, 1992); and (b) a long-term follow-up of the sample 13.7 years posttreatment (76% Caucasian Americans, 22% African Americans, 1% Asian American, 1% Latino American; Schaeffer & Borduin, 2005); (c) an efficacy study investigating MST for attempted suicides (65% African Americans, 33% Caucasian Americans, 2 % Latino American; Huey et al., 2004); and (d) an effectiveness study examining MST for substance-abusing and dependent delinquents (50% African Americans, 47% Caucasian Americans, 1% Asian American, 1% Native American; Henggeler et al., 1999). In all of these studies, outcomes were similar across the various groups. However, it should be noted that some of these studies included some racial/ethnic groups in small proportions to the general sample and relatively few participants in each cell. Thus, any conclusions about race/ethnicity as a moderator of MST effectiveness should be considered tentative.

Parent Management Training (PMT; See Also Chaps. 5, 6, 8, and 16)

PMT focuses on teaching parents behavioral strategies to reduce behavioral problems such as aggression, defiance, temper tantrums, noncompliance, and property destruction. PMT uses didactic instruction, modeling, role playing, and home practice to teach parenting skills in problem-solving, monitoring, discipline, and positive encouragement, and is considered one of the most efficacious outpatient treatments for childhood conduct problems (Miranda et al., 2005). Various versions of PMT programs have been designed to prevent or reduce the incidence of conduct problems and related problem behaviors, delinquency, early substance use, and association with deviant peers (Miranda et al. 2005).

The *Incredible Years (IY) Parent Program* is an empirically validated program used successfully for children with conduct problems (Taylor & Biglan, 1998; Webster-Stratton, Hollinsworth, & Kolpacoff, 1989; Webster-Stratton & Hammond, 1997) and as a school-based prevention program for low-income, ethnically diverse (N=426, 17% African American, 6% Hispanic, 4% Asian American, 4% Native American, and 6% Multiracial) families enrolled in Head Start (Webster-Stratton, 1998). The Head Start is a national program that provides grants to local public and private nonprofit and for-profit agencies to provide comprehensive child development services to economically disadvantaged children and families. The program has a special focus on helping preschoolers develop the early reading and math skills they need to be successful in school and promotes school readiness by enhancing the social and cognitive development of children through the provision of educational, health, nutritional, and social services (USDHHS, 2009). This study is unusual in that it contained two of the most understudied racial/ethnic groups in the research base, Asian Americans and Native Americans. The program focuses on teaching parenting competencies, fostering parents' involvement with school, decreasing children's problem behaviors, and improving children's social and academic competencies. It is delivered in a group-format by a trained leader who facilitates discussion among parents, educates through videotaped vignettes, promotes collaborative skills, and encourages individualization by allowing group members to select their own goals and examples (Reid, Webster-Stratton, & Beauchaine, 2001). Incredible Years children were observed to exhibit significantly higher social competence, fewer conduct problems, less noncompliance, and less negative affect than control children. In addition, teachers reported that IY mothers were more involved in their children's education (Webster-Stratton, 1998).

Incredible Years Program Response was compared among a low-income sample of African American, Asian American, Caucasian Americans, and Hispanic mothers whose children were enrolled in Head Start (Reid et al., 2001). This study was unusual in that it included sufficient numbers of four ethnic groups (370 Caucasian American, 120 African American, 71 Latino American, and 73 Asian American mothers). Head Start centers were randomly assigned to IY groups or a control condition (Head Start program without IY). Posttreatment, IY mothers were observed to be more positive, less critical, more competent, and more consistent in their parenting than control mothers. Children of IY parents were observed to exhibit fewer behavior problems than control children. At 1-year follow-up, 52% of IY children exhibited a 30% increase in positive affect from baseline, whereas only 37% of control children exhibited this difference. Differences in treatment response across ethnic groups were few (only 3 of 51 effects examined), and did not exceed the number expected by chance and was thus not further interpreted by the authors. Also noteworthy, parents from all study groups reported high satisfaction levels following the parenting program, and minority parents were as likely as Caucasian American parents to continue attending groups and complete research assessments, which suggests that IY is accepted by and effective with low-income, ethnically diverse families. However, there was statistically significant differential enrollment for minorities vs. Caucasian American families (28% and 17% chose not to enroll in the program, respectively), suggesting that initial recruitment to the treatment program may be more difficult in minority families (Reid et al., 2001), similar to findings from other literature on recruitment (Harachi, Catalano, & Hawkins, 1997).

Cognitive Behavioral Therapy and Skills Training (See Also Chap. 9)

Some support has been found for the use of *Cognitive Behavioral Therapy* (CBT) interventions aimed at reducing anger, aggression, and antisocial behavior in youth. Larkin and Thyer (1999) evaluated the effectiveness of a Cognitive-Behavioral Group Counseling Program provided to 52 ethnically diverse (32% African Americans, 19% Caucasian Americans, 5%

Asian American, 2% Latino American, 2% Multiracial) behaviorally disruptive elementary school children.

The program consisted of several CBT approaches that have been previously shown to be useful in treating behavioral problems in young children, including problem-solving strategies, self-instruction, modeling, role play, social skills training, and covert imagery. The group intervention provided an arena for providing positive support, peer assistance, and group approval to students who aim to change problematic behaviors into prosocial ones (Semrud-Clikeman, 1995). Compared to youth assigned to a delayed treatment (DT) condition, youth in the immediate group (IT) condition showed significant improvements in perceived self-control and self-esteem, and these gains were maintained at 5 month follow-up. Youth in the DT condition received the same treatment 3 months after the IT group, and after the program was completed, the DT group reported improvements similar to those obtained by the IT group (Larkin & Thyer, 1999).

Three studies examined social-cognitive interventions specifically with African American adolescents. (Lochman, Coie, Underwood, & Terry 1993) evaluated the efficacy of a *Social Relations Intervention Program* for aggressive, rejected children, whom often exhibit social-cognitive difficulties that may be particularly suited to CBT intervention. The training program consisted of four components: (a) social problem-solving, (b) positive play training, (c) group skill training; and (d) dealing effectively with strong negative feelings. These components were based on prior successful skills training programs, and were designed to change rejected children's low peer acceptance (Lochman et al.). A sample of 52 African American aggressive, rejected and nonaggressive, rejected children was randomly assigned to the intervention or control condition. Results revealed that at both posttreatment and 1-year follow-up, the social relations intervention was effective, but only for the aggressive, rejected children (evidenced by significant reduction in aggression and social rejection, and improvement in peer prosocial behavior) and not the nonaggressive, rejected children. These findings are important because the aggressive, rejected group of children were at the greatest risk for negative adolescent outcomes such as conduct problems and drug use.

Hudley and Graham (1993) investigated an *Attributional Intervention* designed to reduce aggressive males' tendency to attribute hostile interventions to peers following ambiguously caused peer provocations. The authors became interested in examining treatments for aggressive minority youth because findings suggest that aggressive minority youth made more attributions of biased intent on the part of a hypothetical peer provocateur, they reported more anger, and were more likely to endorse aggressive behavior than a comparable group of nonaggressive children. The intervention consisted of a 12-session cognitive intervention designed specifically for this study, with a primary goal of training aggressive boys not to infer hostile intent in negative social encounters of ambiguous causes. One hundred and one African American boys (aggressive and nonaggressive) were randomly assigned to the attributional intervention, an attention training program (to control for possible effects of participating in a special program), or an assessment-only control. Results suggested that participants in the attributional intervention were less likely to presume hostile intent by peers of ambiguous provocation, less likely to endorse hostile retaliation, and less likely to engage in verbally hostile behaviors posttreatment. Also, boys in the attribution treatment group were rated as less aggressive by their teachers posttreatment (Hudley & Graham).

Huey and Rank (1984) examined the effects of *Group Assertiveness Training* in 48 African American male adolescents who were selected for their aggressive classroom behavior. The assertiveness training focused on teaching appropriate alternative responses in conflictual situations using concepts from the Verbal Response Model of Assertiveness (Winship & Kelley, 1976). Boys were randomly assigned to assertive training groups, discussion groups which utilized a reflective approach, and a no-treatment control group. Results indicate that participants in the assertive training groups exhibited significantly less aggressive behavior compared to the two other groups posttreatment, establishing the treatment as possibly efficacious (Huey & Rank).

Barrera et al. (2002) examined the efficacy of the *Schools and Homes in Partnership (SHIP) program*, a comprehensive intervention designed to reduce conduct problems among early elementary school children. The program draws from research on social behavior interventions (Taylor, Eddy, & Biglan, 1999) to modify children's cognitions and social behaviors associated with aggression. In addition, the SHIP program includes parent training (McNeil, Eyberg, Eisenstadt, Newcomb, & Funderburk, McNeil, Eyberg, Eisenstadt, Newcomb, & Funderburk, 1991; Taylor & Biglan, 1998) to improve parenting effectiveness, and academic instruction (Francis, Shaywitz, Stuebing, Shaywitz, & Fletcher, 1996; Kellam, Mayer, Rebok, & Hawkins, 1998) to ensure academic success of children through effective teaching techniques. The authors noted the importance of determining the validity of interventions for different cultural groups and included a significant number of Latino American (study sample consisted of 168 Latino American and 116 Caucasian American families), for which a subsample of parents were primarily Spanish-speaking. To deliver the intervention to Latino American families, the authors adapted the standard treatment by creating Spanish-language intervention materials, translating measures into Spanish, and training bilingual-bicultural staff. Families were randomly assigned to SHIP or an assessment-only control. At 1-year follow-up, SHIP participants showed improvements on observed negative social behavior and parent-reported antisocial behavior. Overall, SHIP was equally successful in decreasing conduct problems for Latino American and Caucasian American children. Although the protocol itself was not significantly adapted for the Latino American participants, it should be noted that the researchers did attend to the needs of the Spanish-speaking participants by creating Spanish-language treatment materials, and training bilingual-bicultural staff. Thus, this study took substantial steps toward strengthening cultural responsiveness of the intervention.

Multicomponent Treatments

Kazdin, Siegel, and Bass (1992) also examined multicomponent interventions by evaluating the effects of *Problem-Solving Skills Training (PSST)* alone, *Parent Management Training (PMT)* alone, and PSST and PMT combined in a randomized trial with 97 African American (31% of sample) and Caucasian American (69% of sample) children referred for severe antisocial behavior. PSST is a research-based treatment that combines cognitive and behavioral techniques to teach problem-solving skills (e.g., generating alternative solutions, and teaching means-end thinking) to manage interpersonal conflicts. Within the PSST sessions, practice, modeling, role playing, corrective feedback, and reinforcement strategies were used to develop problem-solving skills. The PMT program used in this investigation drew on procedures described by (Patterson, Reid, Jones, & Conger 1975) and Fleishman and Conger (1978). PMT sessions included teaching positive reinforcement, shaping, negotiating and contracting, providing time out, and appropriate reprimands. Didactic instruction, modeling, and role play were used to develop specific skills. Children and families were randomly assigned to 1 of 3 conditions: PSST, PMT, or a combination of the two interventions. Results showed that while all three conditions evidenced significant improvements in overall child dysfunction, prosocial behaviors, and aggressive, antisocial, and delinquent behaviors, the PSST and PMT combined condition led to more significant changes in antisocial behavior, delinquency, and symptoms of parent dysfunction than either treatment alone. Further, the combined condition also placed a greater proportion of youth within the range of nonclinical levels of functioning by the end of treatment (Kazdin et al., 1992), demonstrating the utility of this multicomponent intervention over the separate evidence-based protocols.

Coping Power (see Chap. 9) is a multicomponent prevention program designed to prevent adolescent substance use, a clinical problem that commonly co-occurs with CD and delinquency. The Coping Power program consists of a child component (Lochman, Lenhart, & Wells, 1996) which was derived from an earlier Anger Coping Program (Lochman et al., 1987) focused on teaching skills in contingency reinforcement, generating alternative solutions, problem-solving, planning, and coping with anxiety and anger arousal. Coping Power also consists of a parent component (Wells, Lenhart, & Lochman, 1996) largely drawn from social learning theory-based parenting programs developed by researchers in the field of child aggression (e.g., Patterson et al., 1975), and focused on teaching skills for identifying prosocial and disruptive child behaviors, rewarding appropriate behaviors, giving effective instructions and setting rules and expectations, and applying effective consequences. In an initial efficacy study of the Coping Power program, Lochman & Wells (2002a) randomly assigned 193 aggressive boys (60% African American, 40% Caucasian American) to one of three conditions: (a) cognitive-behavioral Coping Power child component, (b) combined Coping Power child and behavioral parent training components, and (c) no-treatment control. Results indicated that Coping Power had positive effects on boys' social informational processing (e.g., attributions), temperament, and their perceptions of parents' consistency in parenting. One-year follow-up revealed that the two intervention cells produced reductions in youth's self-reported delinquent behavior, in parent-reported alcohol and marijuana use by youth, and improvements in teacher-rated functioning at school compared to the control condition. Further, results indicated that intervention effects on lower rates of parent-rated substance use in youth and youth delinquent behavior were most apparent for youth and parents who received the full Coping Power program with both child and parent components (Lochman & Wells, 2002a).

More recently, the full Coping Power program was offered within both a broader universal intervention (named Coping with the Middle School Transition Program) designed to impact a community population as well as within an indicated intervention (Coping Power) that provides more intensive programming to higher risk groups who already show some symptoms (e.g., high aggression) that predict later disorder (substance use, conduct disorder). In Lochman and Well's (2002b) study, 245 children identified as being aggressive and/or disruptive were randomly assigned to 1 of 4 cells: the Coping Power indicated intervention, the universal intervention, the combined Coping Power plus universal intervention, or a no-treatment control condition. The sample was predominantly African American and Caucasian American, and the distribution of African American children across cells was similar (Coping Power + universal = 75%, Coping Power only = 78%, Universal only = 78%, Control = 81%). Results showed that all three intervention cells demonstrated lower rates of substance use at posttreatment than did the control cell, and evidenced significant improvements in social competence, self-regulation, and parenting. Social competence and social behavior were especially improved for participants in the combined treatment condition.

The long-term effectiveness of the Coping Power program in preventing substance use, delinquency, and school-based aggressive behavior outcomes for at-risk children was examined at 1-year follow-up (Lochman & Wells, 2003). Results indicate that prior findings of posttreatment improvement for this sample (Lochman and Wells, 2002b) has led to preventive effects on delinquency and substance use at 1-year follow-up, and moderation analyses demonstrated that Coping Power had equally positive effects on African American and Caucasian American children. In addition, the program had equally positive effects on children who came from high crime neighborhoods where a disproportionate number of ethnic minority families reside, or children who came from nonproblematic neighborhoods (Lochman & Wells, 2003).

The Fast Track Project (Conduct Problems Prevention Research Group (CPPRG), 1992, see Chap. 16) is a universal prevention program based on developmental theory and longitudinal research suggesting that persistent and serious antisocial behavior develops from child, family, and community risk factors that interact across the period of time from early childhood through adolescence. The prevention program includes components that address classroom/school risk factors including youth cognitive-behavioral training and social skills building (Bierman, Greenber, & CPPRG, 1996), family risk factors such as problematic parent–school communications (McMahon, Slough, & CPPRG, 1996), and extends from first grade through 10th grade for youth, with heavier program elements in the first 2 years of elementary school and at the transition to middle school. The program posits that improvements in child competencies, parenting effectiveness, school context, and home–school communication will help to reduce the development of conduct problems for youth (CPPRG, 2002b, c).

A randomized trial was conducted with a predominantly African American and Caucasian American sample (N=891, 51% African American, 47% Caucasian American, 2% other) in 1st grade which compared a multi-year Fast Track Program to a no-intervention control condition. At 3-years posttreatment, teachers reported significantly lower rates of child aggressive, disruptive, and disobedient behaviors for Fast Track participants, with 37% of intervention children rated as being free of serious conduct problems compared with 27% of control children (CPPRG, 2002a).

Summary

Several treatments, although originally pioneered without specific cultural groups in mind, have been demonstrated to reduce conduct problems and produce other positive long-term outcomes for ethnic minority youth. Compared to treatments described in the first section, more of these treatments have surpassed the "possibly efficacious" classification to meet the more rigorous criteria for "probably efficacious" interventions, and thus are at somewhat more advanced stages of empirical validation. In the group of treatments described in this section, four protocols appear to meet criteria for "possibly efficacious": (a) Cognitive-Behavioral Group therapy for African Americans and Latino American, (b) Social Relations Intervention for African Americans, (c) SHIP Intervention Program for Latino American, and (d) Fast Track Prevention Program for African Americans. Further research with larger samples of these cultural groups should be conducted to confirm these results.

Encouragingly, five of the treatments described in this section appear to meet the more rigorous criteria for "probably efficacious" interventions. These include parent management-based protocols (IY for African Americans, Latino American, and Asian American), two cognitive-behavioral-based protocols (Attributional Treatment and Group Assertiveness Training for African Americans), and two multicomponent treatments (the Coping Power Program and Combined PSST + PMT for African Americans). Finally, only one treatment reviewed in this section warrants the "well-established" classification and has been evaluated for effectiveness in community settings: MST for African Americans.

The interventions in this category have already been empirically validated for children with conduct problems, albeit in predominantly Caucasian American samples. Although the majority of treatments described in this section will require additional RCTs to classify as "well-established" treatments for particular ethnic minority groups, results thus far are very promising and provide evidence that these protocols can indeed achieve positive outcomes for ethnic minority individuals. Importantly, none of these treatments have been found to be harmful for ethnic minority groups, and in the absence of conflicting evidence, this may suggest that they are safe to use in treating disruptive problems in various cultural populations. As MST has already reached the highest level of empirical validation for African Americans, next steps may be to test this effective intervention in large proportions of other cultural groups that may share a similar constellation of risk factors as inner-city African American youth. Preliminary evidence from studies with MST and IY suggest that implementation of these protocols in real-world settings may be met with specific challenges such as reduction in the magnitude of treatment effects (Timmons-Mitchell et al., 2006) and engagement of minority families in initial enrollment (Reid et al., 2001). Thus, real-world effectiveness trials will become increasingly important as researchers and clinicians prepare for the implementation and widespread dissemination of these EBTs into community clinics.

TREATMENTS DEVELOPED WITHOUT SPECIFIC CULTURAL CONSIDERATIONS, THEN CULTURALLY ADAPTED AND TESTED WITH ETHNIC MINORITY FAMILIES

Overview

Miranda et al. (2005) stated that many EBTs tested with minority youth appear to be effective even without significant structural adaptation, and several of the treatments we have outlined in the previous section seem to support this view. The EBTs described signify the possibility that some EBTs originally developed without specific cultural considerations may be ready for use with some ethnic groups in their original unadapted form.

However, most studies to date cannot answer the question of whether standard, unadapted treatments achieve a similar magnitude of effects in ethnic minority groups as they do in Caucasian American samples. Only a small handful of studies have tackled the question of whether race/ethnicity moderates treatment outcomes, and of these studies, ethnic minority participants are usually present in small proportions to the total sample, presenting challenges to reaching definitive conclusions about ethnic disparity or equivalence. Some multicultural health scholars theorize that ethnic disparity for some EBTs are very likely, especially when cultural considerations are not addressed (de Anda, 1997). Moreover, these investigators maintain that culture-responsive treatments do offer unique benefits to ethnic minority populations (Bernal et al., 1995; Sue & Zane, 1987; Tharp, 1991), and that EBTs not specifically designed for particular ethnic minority populations may suffer from lower enrollment, higher dropout of immigrant and minority parents (Holden, LaVigne & Cameron, 1990; Kazdin & Whitley, 2003), poor engagement, client discomfort, and subsequent treatment failure (Huey & Polo, 2008). Indeed, Reid et al. (2001) found that initial enrollment was significantly lower for ethnic minority families compared to Caucasian American families in a study of the IY program.

In response to these concerns, some clinical researchers have recently taken existing EBTs and culturally tailored these protocols to increase their appeal and fit for diverse cultural groups. Unlike the first category of treatments described in this review in which novel treatments are built bottom-up for a particular cultural group, this approach starts from an existing empirically validated treatment manual that was tested in predominantly Caucasian American samples and developed without culture-specific considerations, and builds on its core components by adding culture-specific elements and enhancements for a particular ethnic group.

Researchers that have adopted a cultural modification approach have drawn on the qualitative and quantitative research available on ethnic minority mental health and culture, as well as input from cultural stakeholders, to develop culturally adapted versions of EBTs which are then tested with ethnic minority families. Two types of adaptation approaches, contextualizing content and/or enhancing engagement, are typically used to ensure the adapted intervention accommodates the distinctive cultural factors present in the target community (Lau, 2006). The aim of these culturally adapted EBTs has generally been to increase acceptability to ethnic minority families, and to focus on presentation of therapeutic techniques to increase cultural relevance and engagement, rather than altering the core components of the EBTs. The small but gradually accumulating body of evidence suggests that culturally adapted EBTs also hold great promise in the treatment of conduct problems in ethnic minority youth. Below, we describe a few of these approaches.

Family Therapy

The *Strengthening Families Program (SFP)* (Kumpfer, Alvarado, Whiteside, & Tait, 2005) is a multicomponent, 14 session family-skills intervention developed in 1982 on a NIDA grant. The program has three components: parent, child, and family-skills training courses. SFP has been found to be effective in reducing substance use and other problem behavior (Spoth, Redmond, & Shin, 2001), but was not necessarily developed with a particular cultural group in mind. Subsequently, the *Strong African American Families Program (SAAF)* (Brody et al., 2004), a preventive intervention for rural African American mothers and their preadolescents, was adapted from the original SFP. SAAF was adapted from SFP using focus group data from rural African American parents, longitudinal, developmental research with rural African American families (Brody, Murry, Jim, & Brown, 2002), as well as Gibbon and Gerrard's cognitive model of adolescent health risk behavior (Gibbons & Gerrard, 1997; Gibbons, Gerrard, & Lane, 2003), which has been evaluated with rural African American families. This program specifically identified family-based protective processes for alcohol use among rural African American families (e.g., Brody, Flor, Hollett-Wright, & McCoy, 1998; Brody et al., 2004, 2006), and is grounded in previous family centered and universal prevention models (e.g., Bank, Patterson, & Reid, 1987; Dishion & Kavanaugh, 2000). Brody et al. (2006) describe these protective processes as "regulated-communicative" parenting, which includes limit setting, monitoring, racial socialization, clear expectations about alcohol use, and inductive discipline.

Although this prevention program was developed to specifically target alcohol use, the parenting processes targeted are also implicated in the prevention of conduct problems. Thus, to examine the efficacy of SAAF in the prevention of conduct problems, a randomized trial with 667 African American 11-year olds and their primary caregivers was conducted. Families were randomly assigned to receive SAAF or to a control condition. Results showed that youth receiving SAAF had significantly reduced rates of both alcohol use and conduct problems compared with control youth (who were mailed informational pamphlets regarding early adolescent development) over a 29-month period (Brody, Kogan, Chen, & Murry, 2008), demonstrating that SAAF is possibly efficacious in preventing conduct problems.

Parent Management Training

The *Nuestras Familias* intervention (Our Families; Martinez & Eddy, 2005) is a parent management-based protocol grounded in a conceptual framework that integrates two related theories of development; social interaction learning theory (Reid, Patterson, & Snyder, 2002) and ecodevelopmental theory (Szapocznik & Coatsworth, 1999), then further informed by recent studies on the acculturation process in Latino American families. The program was designed to impact parenting practices and family environmental variables through the development of a number of parenting skills (e.g., encouragement, monitoring, discipline, problem-solving) that exert direct effects on youth conduct related problems. The efficacy of Nuestras Familias was examined in a sample of 73 Spanish-speaking Latino American (90% ancestry from Mexico, 10% ancestry from Peru or Central American countries) parents with middle-school-aged youth at risk for problem behaviors (Martinez & Eddy, 2005). Families were randomly assigned to Nuestras Familias or a control (no-intervention) condition, and results posttreatment showed that Nuestras Familias produced benefits in parenting outcomes (general parenting, skills encouragement, and overall effective parenting skills) and youth outcomes (aggression, externalizing problems, likelihood of smoking and use of alcohol, marijuana, and other drugs). However, interaction analyses by youth nativity status showed that the intervention was more effective for parents of US born youth than for parents of foreign-born youth. Authors noted that future interventions should be developed to address the unique contexts of immigrant families.

Parent–Child Interaction Therapy (PCIT) (See Also Chap. 5)

PCIT (Eyberg & Robinson, 1982) is an empirically supported behavioral parenting skills program for treating young children with disruptive behavior based on Baumrind's (1966) developmental theory. Parent–Child Interaction Therapy teaches authoritative parenting – a combination of nurturance, good communication and firm control. Authoritative parenting style has been linked to fewer child behavior problems in multiple studies (Linver, Brooks-Gunn, & Kohen, 2002) including ethnic minority children (Querido, Warner, & Eyberg, 2002). Parent–Child Interaction Therapy is delivered in two phases of treatment: (a) Child-directed Interaction (CDI), in which parents learn skills to strengthen the parent–child bond, increase child prosocial behavior, and decrease negative child behavior; (b) Parent-directed Interaction (PDI), in which parents learn additional skills to reduce child noncompliance and other negative behaviors. The efficacy of PCIT has been established in studies with predominantly Caucasian American samples demonstrating its superiority to wait-list control (Nixon, Sweeny,

Erickson, & Touyz, 2003) and to parent group didactic training (Eyberg & Matarazzo, 1980).

The need for studies that directly evaluate the incremental value of cultural adaptations led to the development of *Guiando a Ninos Activos* (Guiding Active Children; GANA; McCabe, Yeh, Garland, Lau, & Chavez, 2005), a culturally adapted version of PCIT for Mexican Americans. The purpose of the study was to combine data from quantitative and qualitative studies to inform the development of a culturally modified version of PCIT, with the ultimate goal of developing a methodology that could be transferable to the adaptation of other treatment approaches and for other cultural groups. A critical step in the development of this program was a randomized trial comparing the culturally modified version (GANA) to standard PCIT and Treatment as Usual (TAU) to evaluate the unique contribution of the cultural modifications.

An Approach to Cultural Modification

Because the empirical literature provides limited guidance on how to adapt treatments for ethnic minority families, McCabe et al. (2005) developed a modification process that included gathering information regarding potential cultural adaptations to PCIT from the clinical literature, the empirical literature, expert opinion, and qualitative data collected from Mexican American parents and therapists. Next, the treatment developers used this information to arrive at a set of proposed modifications to PCIT. Finally, the proposed modifications were reviewed by a group of researchers with expertise in the adaptation of mental health treatments, a panel of Mexican American therapists that work clinically with Mexican American families, and Dr. Sheila Eyberg, the creator of PCIT. Final decisions were made about the acceptability of the full package of proposed modifications both from a practical and theoretical perspective.

The GANA Program

The resulting GANA program adopts a public health approach to mental health problems (Bruce, Smith, Miranda, Hoagwood, & Wells, 2002; USDHHS, 2001), in which the program provider plays an active role in engaging families in the program, addressing barriers to participation, and preventing treatment dropout. In addition, the GANA program recognizes that Mexican Americans are heterogeneous, such that adaptations that might enhance the program for one family would actually decrease to fit for another. To ensure that parenting experts are able to tailor the GANA program to the needs of individual families, a detailed assessment of a number of culturally influenced concepts that may have an important effect on how parents respond to the program is conducted in the first session. For example, parents are asked to provide information on their conceptualization of their child's problems, beliefs about the causes of their child's problems, the role of extended family members in raising the child, beliefs about discipline, attitudes and expectations for the program, and use of alternative treatments (a complete list can be found in McCabe et al., 2005). These concepts are referenced throughout treatment so that the program can be presented in ways congruent with the parents' belief system about the causes of their children's problems and the types of intervention that they believe will be helpful. In addition, some constructs are assessed continuously throughout treatment because they may change, such as the degree to which an extended family member is supportive or unsupportive of the child's participation in the program, so that the therapist will be able to address changes as they occur and before a family drops out. Other adaptations to the program include: (a) framing the program as an educational/skill-building intervention to reduce the stigma associated with seeking "mental health services," (b) showing families two 15-min videotape presentations that describe the phases of the program and show examples of families in PCIT sessions (Zebell & Urquiza, 2002a, b) before treatment to reduce unrealistic expectations that have been found to predict treatment dropout for Mexican American families (McCabe, 2002), (c) increasing therapist training about Mexican American culture, (d) giving GANA therapists extra time during each session to focus on rapport building and training in establishing rapport with Mexican Americans, (e) eliciting complaints during each session to ensure that respect for authority does not prevent the parent from voicing complaints that, left unaddressed, might lead to treatment dropout, (f) translating and simplifying written handouts used in each session of PCIT-as well as including pictures of Mexican American families engaged in PCIT so that parents could more readily identify with the examples, and (g) implementing a comprehensive engagement protocol based on (McKay, Stoewe, McCadam, & Gonzalez 1998) approach that explicitly targets mothers, fathers, and grandparents.

Finally, a RCT was conducted in which 50 Mexican American families whose 3–7-year-old child suffered from clinically significant behavior problems were randomly assigned to receive either GANA, standard PCIT, or Treatment as Usual (TAU). Ninety-three percent (N=54) of families completed a posttreatment assessment. All three treatment approaches produced significant pre–post improvement in conduct problems across a wide variety of parent-report measures. GANA produced results that were significantly superior to TAU across a wide variety of both parent report and observational indices; however, GANA and PCIT did not differ significantly from one another. PCIT was superior to TAU on two of the parent report indices and almost all of the observational indices. There were no significant differences between the three groups on treatment dropout, and families were more satisfied with both GANA and PCIT than with TAU. These data suggest that both PCIT and GANA are "probably efficacious" with Mexican American youth.

Summary of Culturally Adapted/Culturally Modified Interventions

The work of culturally adapted EBTs is just beginning, although this approach has garnered increasing interest recently among the research community. SAAF is possibly efficacious for African American youth with conduct problems, and Nuestras Familias is possibly efficacious for the treatment of conduct problems in predominantly Mexican American, Hispanic families. GANA, as well as the unadapted version of PCIT, are probably efficacious for Mexican American families. The limited evidence suggests that culturally adapted EBTs, similar to culture-specific interventions built bottom-up, may be better equipped to address issues such as enrollment, engagement, and retention of ethnic minority families through their focus on cultural processes in treatment development/adaptation. However, the jury is still out on whether culturally adapted treatment programs are more effective than unadapted versions, as very few studies to date have conducted RCTs to compare outcomes achieved by culturally adapted EBTs to unadapted EBTs for ethnic minority families.

SUMMARY OF THE LITERATURE BASE

The research base on EBTs for ethnic minority youth with conduct problems is still in its infancy. In contrast to a substantial number of treatments that have been deemed well-established or probably efficacious for treating conduct problems in predominantly Caucasian American samples, only two treatments described thus far meet the highest standard of empirically validation as "well-established" interventions for ethnic minority populations (MST for African Americans, and BSFT for predominantly Cuban, Hispanic Americans). Also, compared to the effectiveness research base with predominantly Caucasian American samples, almost all of the existing studies with ethnic minorities are RCTs, and studies investigating treatment effectiveness in community settings are necessary to evaluate the applicability of these intervention protocols to real-world community participants. Nevertheless, it is encouraging that several treatments described are quite promising and "possibly efficacious" for ethnic minority youth, and a smaller handful have reached the more stringent "probably efficacious" classification. Further, research in this area is continuing to grow, with a number of studies currently underway to examine treatments for conduct problems in ethnic minority youth.

Although several unadapted EBTs appear to produce positive outcomes for ethnic minority youth with conduct problems, the question of whether treatment effects of these protocols vary as a function of ethnicity remain largely unanswered. Very few EBT studies thus far have examined race/ethnicity as a moderator of treatment outcomes, and of those that have, usually very small numbers of ethnic minority participants were present in each of the treatment or control conditions. Further, only a very limited number of racial/ethnic comparisons have been conducted in these studies (with the most common comparison examining differential effects for African Americans vs. Caucasian Americans) due to small sample sizes of particular minority groups such as Native Americans and Asian Americans. Because of these issues, no definitive conclusions about differential treatment effects can be drawn. The very limited literature to date seems to point toward "ethnic invariance," suggesting that these treatments were not more efficacious or effective for the ethnic groups examined.

Based on the limited data available that support ethnic invariance and scant evidence to the contrary, several investigators (Kazdin, 1993) have argued there is little empirical support for the superiority of culturally adapted programs, which are usually time consuming and costly to develop. Indeed, researchers intending to culturally adapt a treatment protocol must balance a variety of considerations in developing and testing the modified intervention. These considerations include a detailed examination of the literature to determine how outcomes achieved by ethnic minority families compare to outcomes achieved by Caucasian American families using the standard protocol, a thorough evaluation of findings regarding risks and resiliency factors for the development of conduct problems in the selected cultural population, a careful analysis regarding fidelity to empirically established strategies within the standard intervention, and the design of a rigorous methodology for testing the efficacy of the adapted intervention. As one may have surmised, the development of a culturally adapted EBT is no small task.

However, as discussed earlier, there are researchers who argue that cultural adaptations are necessary and worthwhile in certain circumstances. For example, concerns are growing about the fit of unadapted PMT and other parent-focused treatments for ethnically diverse families of youth with conduct problems (Forehand & Kotchick, 2002). Ethnic minority families may not readily accept the parenting strategies taught in PMT, as there are wide variations in parenting practice and family values across cultural groups (Lau, 2006). This can greatly affect parents' receptivity to and level of comfort with the intervention, the therapeutic process (e.g., engagement and fidelity), and subsequent outcomes in real-world, community settings, for which very little is known due to the paucity of PMT effectiveness studies with different cultural groups. Proponents of cultural adaptation of PMTs and other EBTs offer preliminary evidence which suggests that culturally adapted versions of PMT that address culture-specific issues result in significant improvement in enrollment and retention of African American, Latino American, Asian/Pacific Islander American, and American Indian families (Kumpfer, Alvarado, Smith, & Bellamy, 2002).

TO ADAPT OR NOT TO ADAPT: THAT IS THE QUESTION

Faced with these conflicting schools of thought and limited substantiation for either argument, how does one answer the question: To adapt or not to adapt?

A useful framework for identifying circumstances where cultural adaptations of EBTs may be most indicated was proposed by Lau (2006). Specifically, Lau stated that ethnic-specific treatment adaptation may be warranted when evidence points to significant variability across cultural groups in (a) contextual processes influencing vulnerability and protection from the target problem and/or (b) response to standard EBT strategies for the target problems (Lau). Regarding the first element in this framework, the considerably higher prevalence of conduct problems (Proctor et al., 1992) and higher vulnerability to impairments in key life domains (school, peer, family) in certain ethnic minority groups (Ezpeleta et al., 2001; Proctor et al.) may call for a consideration of culturally adapted EBTs for some minority groups. Regarding the second element, the growing concerns about the fit of PMT and other parent-focused treatments for ethnically diverse families (Lau) and preliminary evidence of differential enrollment of minority families in parent-based protocols (Reid, Webster-Stratton, & Beauchaine, 2001) may also warrant consideration of culturally adapted versions to be used with ethnic minority families.

Once a culturally adapted version has been developed, it should be tested with a research design that will evaluate its outcomes in comparison to the original, unadapted protocol. In order to determine whether cultural adaptations can incrementally improve outcomes and engagement for specific cultural groups, research studies must compare standard versions of EBTs with ethnic minority families to culturally modified versions of those interventions. Such a comparative design allows us to determine whether the investment made in cultural adaptations is worthwhile, unnecessary, or even harmful. However, very few studies in the literature have taken such a comparative approach.

As described earlier, McCabe et al. (2005) implemented this comparative approach to examine the incremental validity of adapted PCIT (i.e., GANA) by conducting a RCT in which they compared it to standard PCIT for Mexican Americans. This research design represents a standard for developing culturally sensitive applications of PCIT that retain the effectiveness (i.e., retention, outcome, and satisfaction) of the empirically established treatment (Butler & Eyberg, 2006). Adherence to this standard for the testing and application of PCIT and other EBTs to diverse cultural groups will assure that efficacy is maintained and enhanced (Eyberg, 2005).

McCabe et al. (2005) found that outcomes achieved by GANA and original PCIT were not significantly different from each other. This supports the growing body of research suggesting that EBTs, even in unmodified form, can be highly effective for Latino American families, and extends it by demonstrating that a culturally modified version can also be at least as effective. Cultural adaptations, such as those incorporated in GANA, may offer therapists specific options for adapting existing EBT models to the cultural characteristics of families in their practice. This flexibility may increase the appeal of EBTs such as PCIT to therapists with large numbers of ethnic minority families in their caseload.

RECOMMENDATIONS FOR CLINICAL PRACTICE AND FUTURE RESEARCH DIRECTIONS

The evidence-base for treatments of conduct problems in ethnic minority youth, albeit in its infancy, provides some initial guidelines for how best to treat ethnic minority youth with conduct problems. Foremost, we endorse Huey and Polo's (2008) recommendation to use EBTs as first-line interventions for minority youth. Although the research base is still in development, evidence thus far supports the use of EBTs when treating youth from minority populations, especially those identified as well-established, probably efficacious, or possibly efficacious with particular cultural groups. Research efforts investigating the utility of culturally specific and culturally adapted protocols compared to standard, unadapted EBTs should be prioritized to increase our knowledge about specific effects of culturally responsive practices. The results of these investigations will assist both researchers and clinicians in deciding when the use of a culturally adapted protocol may be warranted and appropriate. Several EBTs that have been empirically established for predominantly Caucasian American samples appear to hold great promise for treating minority youth with conduct problems, such as *Multidimensional Treatment Foster Care* (Chamberlain & Reid, 1998), *Parent Management Training Oregon* (Bernal, Klinnert, & Schultz, 1980), and the *Triple P* Standard and Enhanced Protocols (Sanders, Markie-Dadds, Tully, & Bor, 2000; see Chap. 17). Future studies may consider evaluating these empirically validated standard treatment protocols for use in minority youth, and/or developing and testing culturally adapted protocols if deemed appropriate for particular ethnic groups.

REFERENCES

American Psychiatric Association. (1994). *Diagnostic and statistical manual of mental disorders*. Arlington: American Psychiatric Publishing.

Bank, L., Patterson, G. R., & Reid, J. B. (1987). Delinquency prevention through training parents in family management. *Behavior Analyst, 10*, 75–82.

Barrera, M., Jr., Biglan, A., Taylor, T. K., Gunn, B. K., Smolkowski, K., et al. (2002). Early elementary school intervention to reduce conduct problems: a randomized trial with Hispanic and non-Hispanic children. *Prevention Science, 3*, 83–94.

Baumrind, D. (1966). Effects of authoritative control on child behavior. *Child Development, 37*, 887–907.

Beals, J., Piasecki, J., Nelson, S., Jones, M., Keane, E., Dauphinais, P. R., et al. (1997). Psychiatric disorder among American Indian adolescents: prevalence in Northern Plains youth. *Journal of the American Academy of Child and Adolescent Psychiatry, 36*, 1252–1259.

Bernal, G., Bonilla, J., & Bellido, C. (1995). Ecological validity and cultural sensitivity for outcome research: Issues for the cultural adaptation and development of psychosocial treatments with Hispanics. *Journal of Abnormal Child Psychology, 23*, 67–82.

Bernal, G., & Scharrón-del Río, M. R. (2001). Are empirically supported treatments (EST) valid for ethnic minorities? *Cultural Diversity and Ethnic Minority Psychology, 7*, 328–342.

Bernal, M. E., Klinnert, M. D., & Schultz, L. A. (1980). Outcome evaluation of behavioral parent training and client-centered parent counseling for children with conduct problems. *Journal of Applied Behavior Analysis, 13*, 677–691.

Bierman, K. L., Greenberg, M. T., & Conduct Problems Prevention Research Group (CPPRG). (1996). Social skills training in the Fast Track Program. In R. D. Peters & R. J. McMahon (Eds.), *Preventing childhood disorders, substance use, and delinquency* (pp. 65–89). Thousand Oaks: Sage.

Borduin, C. M., Mann, B. J., Cone, L. T., Henggeler, S. M., Fucci, B. R., Blaske, D. M., et al. (1995). Multisystemic treatment of serious juvenile offenders: long-term prevention of criminality and violence. *Journal of Consulting and Clinical Psychology, 63*, 569–578.

Brestan, E. V., & Eyberg, S. M. (1998). Effective psychosocial treatments of conduct-disordered children and adolescents: 29 years, 82 studies, and 5, 272 kids. *Journal of Clinical Child Psychology, 27*, 180–189.

Brody, G. H., Flor, D. L., Hollett-Wright, N., & McCoy, J. K. (1998). Children's development of alcohol use norms: contributions of parent and sibling norms, children's temperaments, and parent – child discussions. *Journal of Family Psychology, 12*, 209–219.

Brody, G. H., Dorsey, S., Forehand, R., & Armistead, L. (2002). Unique and protective contributions of parenting and classroom processes to the adjustment of African American children living in single-parent families. *Child Development, 73*, 274–286.

Brody, G. H., Murry, V. M., Gerrard, M., Gibbons, F. X., Molgaard, V., McNair, L., et al. (2004). The strong African American families program: translating research into prevention programming. *Child Development, 75*, 900–917.

Brody, G. H., Murry, V. M., Gerrard, M., Gibbons, F. X., McNair, L., Brown, A. C., et al. (2006). The Strong African American families program: prevention of youths' high-risk behavior and a test of a model of change. *Journal of Family Psychology, 20*, 1–11.

Brody, G., Kogan, S., Chen, Y., & Murry, V. M. (2008). Long-term effects of the Strong African American Families Program on youth conduct problems. *Journal of Adolescent Health, 43*, 474–481.

Bruce, M. L., Smith, W., Miranda, J., Hoagwood, K., & Wells, K. B. (2002). Community-based interventions. *Mental Health Services Research, 4*, 205–214.

Butler, A. M., & Eyberg, S. M. (2006). Parent-child interaction therapy and ethnic minority youth. *Vulnerable Children and Youth Studies, 1*, 246–255.

Chamberlain, P., & Reid, J. B. (1998). Comparison of two community alternatives to incarceration for chronic juvenile offenders. *Journal of Consulting and Clinical Psychology, 66*, 624–633.

Chambless, D. L., & Ollendick, T. H. (2001). Empirically supported psychological interventions: controversies and evidence. *Annual Review of Psychology, 52*, 685–716.

Chambless, D. L., Baker, M. J., Baucom, D. H., Beutler, L. E., Calhoun, K. S., Crits-Christoph, P., et al. (1998). Update on empirically validated therapies, II. *The Clinical Psychologist, 51*, 3–16.

Chambless, D. L., Sanderson, W. C., Shoham, V., Bennett Johnson, S., Pope, K. S., Crits-Cristoph, P., et al. (1996). An update on empirically validated therapies. *The Clinical Psychologist, 49*, 5–18.

Coatsworth, J. D., Pantin, H., & Szapocznik, J. (2002). Familias Unidas: a family-centered ecodevelopmental intervention to reduce risk for problem behavior among Hispanic adolescents. *Clinical Child and Family Psychology Review, 5*, 113–132.

Cohen, P., Cohen, J., Kasen, S., Velez, C. N., Hartmark, C., Johnson, J., et al. (1993). An epidemiological study of disorders in late childhood and adolescence – I. Age- and Gender-Specific prevalence. *Journal of Child Psychology and Psychiatry, 34*, 851–867.

Conduct Problems Prevention Research Group. (1992). A developmental and clinical model for the prevention of conduct disorder: the FAST Track Program. *Development and Psychopathology, 4*, 509–527.

Conduct Problems Prevention Research Group. (2002a). Evaluation of the first three years of the Fast Track Prevention Trial with children at high risk for adolescent conduct problems. *Journal of Abnormal Child Psychology, 30*, 19–35.

Conduct Problems Prevention Research Group. (2002b). Implementation of the Fast Track Program: an example of a large-scale prevention science efficacy trial. *Journal of Abnormal Child Psychology, 30*, 1–17.

Conduct Problems Prevention Research Group. (2002c). Predictor variables associated with positive Fast Track outcomes at the end of the third grade. *Journal of Abnormal Child Psychology, 30*, 37–52.

Costello, E. J., Costello, A. J., Edelbrock, C., Burns, B. J., Ducan, M. K., Brent, D., et al. (1988). Psychiatric disorders in primary care: Prevalence and risk factors. *Archives of General Psychiatry, 45*, 1107–1116.

Costello, E. J., Farmer, E. M., Angold, A., Burns, B. J., & Erkanli, A. (1997). Psychiatric disorders among American Indian and white youth in Appalachia: the Great Smoky Mountains Study. *American Journal of Public Health, 87*, 827–832.

De Anda, D. (1997). *Controversial issues in multiculturalism.* Boston: Allyn & Bacon.

Dishion, T. J., & Kavanaugh, K. (2000). A multilevel approach to family-centered prevention in schools: Process and outcome. *Addictive Behaviors, 25*, 899–911.

Dumka, L. E., Gonzales, N., Woods, J., & Formoso, D. (1998). Using qualitative methods for develop contextually relevant measures and preventive interventions: an illustration. *American Journal of Community Psychology, 26*, 600–633.

Eyberg, S. M. (2005). Tailoring and adapting parent-child interaction therapy to new populations. *Education and Treatment of Children, 28*, 197–201.

Eyberg, S. M., & Matarazzo, R. G. (1980). Training parents as therapists: a comparison between individual parent child interaction training and parent group didactic training. *Journal of Clinical Psychology, 36*, 492–499.

Eyberg, S. M., & Robinson, E. A. (1982). Parent-child interaction training: effects on family functioning. *Journal of Clinical Child Psychology, 11*, 130–137.

Eyberg, S. M., Nelson, M. M., & Boggs, S. R. (2008). Evidence-based psychosocial treatments for children and adolescents with disruptive behavior. *Journal of Clinical Child & Adolescent Psychology, 37*, 215–237.

Ezpeleta, L., Keeler, G., Erkanli, A., Costello, E. J., & Angold, A. (2001). Epidemiology of psychiatric disability in childhood and adolescence. *Journal of Child Psychology and Psychiatry, 42*, 901–914.

Farrington, D. P. (1987). Early precursors of frequent offending. In J. Q. Wilson & G. C. Loury (Eds.), *From children to citizens* (Families, schools, and delinquency prevention, Vol. III, pp. 27–49). New York: Springer.

Fleischman, M. J., & Conger, R. E. (1978). An approach to families of aggressive children: procedures for didactic parent training groups. Unpublished manuscript, Family Research Associates.

Forehand, R., & Kotchick, B. A. (2002). Behavioral parent training: current challenges and potential solutions. *Journal of Child and Family Studies, 11*, 377–384.

Francis, D. J., Shaywitz, S. E., Stuebing, K. K., Shaywitz, B. A., & Fletcher, J. M. (1996). Developmental lag versus deficit models of reading disability: a longitudinal, individual growth curves analysis. *Journal of Educational Psychology, 88*, 3–17.

Frick, P. J. (1998). *Conduct disorders and severe antisocial behavior.* New York: Plenum.

Gibbons, F. X., & Gerrard, M. (1997). Health images and their effects on health behavior. In B. P. Buunk & F. X. Gibbons (Eds.), *Health, coping, and well-being: perspectives from social comparison theory* (pp. 63–94). Mahwah: Erlbaum.

Gibbons, F. X., Gerrard, M., & Lane, D. (2003). A social reaction model of adolescent health risk. In J. M. Suls & K. Wallston (Eds.), *Social psychological foundations of health and illness* (pp. 107–136). Malden: Blackwell.

Gonzales, N. A., Dumka, L. E., Deardorff, J., Carter, S. J., & McCray, A. (2004). Preventing poor mental health and school dropout of Mexican American Adolescents following the transition to junior high school. *Journal of Adolescent Research, 19*, 113–131.

Haley, J. (1976). *Problem-solving therapy.* San Francisco: Jossey-Bass.

Hall, G. C. N. (2001). Psychotherapy with ethnic minorities: empirical, ethical, and conceptual issues. *Journal of Consulting and Clinical Psychology, 69*, 502–510.

Harachi, T. W., Catalano, R. F., & Hawkins, J. D. (1997). Effective recruitment for parenting programs within ethnic minority communities. *Child and Adolescent Social Work Journal, 14*, 23–29.

Henggeler, S. W., Melton, G. B., & Smith, L. A. (1992). Family preservation using multisystemic therapy: an effective alternative to incarcerating serious juvenile offenders. *Journal of Consulting Clinical Psychology, 60*, 953–961.

Henggeler, S. W., Melton, G. B., Brondino, M. J., Scherer, D. G., & Hanley, J. H. (1997). Multisystemic Therapy with violent and chronic juvenile offenders and their families: the role of treatment fidelity in successful dissemination. *Journal of Consulting and Clinical Psychology, 65*, 821–833.

Henggeler, S. W., Pickrel, S. G., & Brondino, M. J. (1999). Multisystemic treatment of substance abusing and dependent delinquents: outcomes, treatment fidelity, and transportability. *Mental Health Services Research, 1*, 171–184.

Henggeler, S. W., Rowland, M. D., Randall, J., Ward, D. M., Cunningham, P. B., et al. (1999). Home-based Multisystemic Therapy as an alternative to the hospitalization of youths in psychiatric crisis: clinical outcomes. *Journal of American Academy of Child and Adolescent Psychiatry, 38*, 1331–1339.

Henggeler, S. W., Clingempeel, W. G., Brondino, M. J., & Pickrel, S. G. (2002). Four-year follow-up of Multisystemic Therapy with substance-abusing and substance-dependent juvenile offenders. *Journal of the American Academy of Child & Adolescent Psychiatry, 41*, 868–874.

Holden, G. W., Lavigne, V. V., & Cameron, A. M. (1990). Probing the continuum of effectiveness of parent training: characteristics of parents and preschoolers. *Journal of Clinical Child Psychology, 19*, 2–8.

Hudley, C., & Graham, S. (1993). An attributional intervention to reduce peer-directed aggression among African-American boys. *Child Development, 64*, 124–138.

Huey, S. J., Jr., & Polo, A. J. (2008). Evidence-based psychosocial treatments for ethnic minority youth. *Journal of Clinical Child & Adolescent Psychology, 37*, 1262–1301.

Huey, S. J., Henggeler, S. W., Rowland, M. D., Halliday-Boykins, C. A., Cunningham, P. B., et al. (2004). Multisystemic therapy effects on attempted suicide by youths presenting psychiatric emergencies. *Journal of American Academy of Child and Adolescent Psychiatry, 43*, 183–190.

Huey, W. C., & Rank, R. C. (1984). Effects of counselor and peer-led assertive training on Black adolescent aggression. *Journal of Counseling Psychology, 31*, 95–98.

Kazdin, A. E. (1993). Adolescent mental health prevention and treatment programs. *American Psychologist, 48*, 127–141.

Kazdin, A. E. (1995). *Conduct disorders in childhood and adolescence* (2nd ed.). Thousand Oaks: Sage.

Kazdin, A. E., Siegel, T., & Bass, D. (1992). Cognitive problem-solving skills training and parent management training in the treatment of antisocial behavior in children. *Journal of Consulting and Clinical Psychology, 60*, 733–747.

Kazdin, A. E., & Whitley, M. K. (2003). Treatment of parental stress to enhance therapeutic change among children referred for aggressive and antisocial behavior. *Evidence Based Mental Health, 6*, 120.

Kellam, S. G., Mayer, L. S., Rebok, G. W., & Hawkins, W. E. (1998). Effects of improving achievement on aggressive behavior and of improving aggressive behavior on achievement through two preventive interventions: an investigation of causal paths. In B. P. Dohrenwend (Ed.), *Adversity, stress, and psychopathology* (pp. 486–505). New York: Oxford University Press.

Kumpfer, K. L., Alvarado, R., Smith, P., & Bellamy, N. (2002). Cultural sensitivity and adaptation in family-based prevention intervention. *Prevention Science, 3*, 241–246.

Kumpfer, K. L., Alvarado, R., Whiteside, H. O., & Tait, C. (2005). The Strengthening Families Program (SFP): an Evidence-Based, Multicultural Family Skills Training Program. In J. Szapocznik, P. H. Tolan, & S. Sambrano (Eds.), *Preventing substance abuse* (pp. 3–14). Washington, DC: American Psychological Association Books.

Lahey, B. B., Loeber, R., Quay, H. C., Frick, P. J., & Grimm, J. (1997). Oppositional defiant disorder and conduct disorder. In T. A. Widiger, A. J. Frances, H. A. Pincus, R. Ross, M. B. First, & W. Davis (Eds.), *DSM-IV Sourcebook* (Vol. 3, pp. 189–209). Washington DC: American Psychiatric Association.

Lahey, B. B., Miller, T. L., Gordon, R. A., & Riley, A. W. (1999). Developmental epidemiology of the disruptive behaviour disorders. In H. C. Quay & A. E. Hogan (Eds.), *Handbook of disruptive behavior disorders* (pp. 23–48). New York: Kluwer/Plenum.

Larkin, R., & Thyer, B. A. (1999). Evaluating cognitive-behavioral group counseling to improve elementary school students' self-esteem, self-control, and classroom behavior. *Behavioral Interventions, 14*, 147–161.

Lau, A. (2006). Making the case for selective and directed cultural adaptations of evidence-based treatments: examples from parent training. *Clinical Psychology: Science and Practice, 13*, 295–310.

Lavigne, J. V., Arend, R., Rosenbaum, D., Binns, H. J., Christoffel, K. K., & Gibbons, R. D. (1998). Psychiatric disorders with onset in the preschool years: I Stability of Diagnoses. *Journal of American Academy of Child and Adolescent Psychiatry, 37*, 1246–1254.

Linver, M. R., Brooks-Gunn, J., & Kohen, D. E. (2002). Family processes as pathways from income to young children's development. *Developmental Psychology, 38*, 719–739.

Lochman, J. E., & Wells, K. C. (2002a). Contextual social-cognitive mediators and child outcome: a test of the theoretical model in the Coping Power Program. *Development and Psychopathology, 14*, 971–993.

Lochman, J. E., & Wells, K. C. (2002b). The Coping Power Program at the middle school transition: universal and indicated prevention effects. *Psychology of Addictive Behaviors, 16*, S40–S54.

Lochman, J. E., & Wells, K. C. (2003). Effectiveness of the Coping Power Program and of classroom intervention with aggressive children: outcomes at a 1-year follow-up. *Behavior Therapy, 34*, 493–515.

Lochman, J. E., Lampron, L. B., Gemmer, T. C., & Harris, S. R. (1987). Anger-coping interventions for aggressive children: guide to implementation in school settings. In P. A. Keller & S. Heyman (Eds.), *Innovations in clinical practice: A source book* (Vol. 6, pp. 339–356). Sarasota, FL: Professional Resource Exchange.

Lochman, J. E., Coie, J. D., Underwood, M. K., & Terry, R. (1993). Effectiveness of a social relations intervention program for aggressive and nonaggressive, rejected children. *Journal of Consulting Clinical Psychology, 61*, 1053–1058.

Lochman, L. E., Lenhart, L. A., & Wells, K. C. (1996). *Coping Power program: child component.* Duke University Medical Center, Durham, NC: Unpublished manual.

Loeber, R., & Farrington, D. (1998). *Serious and violent juvenile offenders: risk factors and successful interventions.* Thousand Oaks, CA: Sage.

Loeber, R., Jeffrey, D., Lahey, B. B., Winters, A., & Zera, M. (2000). Oppositional defiant and conduct disorder: a review of the past 10 years, Part I. *Journal of American Academy of Child and Adolescent Psychiatry, 41*, 1275–1293.

Martinez, C. R., Jr., & Eddy, J. M. (2005). Effects of culturally adapted parent management training on Latino youth behavioral health outcomes. *Journal of Consulting and Clinical Psychology, 73*, 841–851.

McCabe, K. M., Yeh, M., Garland, A. F., Lau, A. S., & Chavez, G. (2005). The GANA program: A tailoring approach to adapting parent–child interaction therapy for Mexican Americans. *Education and Treatment of Children, 28*, 111–129.

McCabe, K. M. (2002). Factors that predict premature termination among Mexican-American children in outpatient psychotherapy. *Journal of Child and Family Studies, 11*, 347–359.

McKay, M., Stoewe, J., McCadam, K., & Gonzalez, J. (1998). Increasing access to child mental health services for urban children and their caregivers. *Health and Social Work, 23*, 9–16.

McMahon, R. J., Slough, N. M., & Conduct Problems Prevention Research Group (CPPRG). (1996). Family-based intervention in the FAST Track Program. In R. D. Peters & R. J. McMahon (Eds.), *Preventing childhood disorders, substance abuse and delinquency* (pp. 90–110). Thousand Oaks: Sage.

McNeil, C. B., Eyberg, S., Eisenstadt, T. H., Newcomb, K., & Funderburk, B. (1991). Parent–child interaction therapy with behavior problem children: Generalization of treatment effects. *Journal of Clinical Child Psychology, 20*, 140–151.

Minuchin, S., Rosman, B. L., & Baker, L. (1978). *Psychosomatic families: anorexia nervosa in context.* Cambridge: Harvard University Press.

Miranda, J., Bernal, G., Lau, A., Kohn, L., Hwang, W. C., & LaFromboise, T. (2005). State of the science on psychosocial interventions for ethnic minorities. *Annual Review of Clinical Psychology, 1*, 113–142.

Muir, J. A., Schwartz, S. J., & Szapocznik, J. (2004). A program of research with Hispanic and African American families: three decades of intervention development and testing influenced by the changing cultural context of Miami. *Journal of Marital and Family Therapy, 30*, 285–303.

Nixon, R. D. V., Sweeny, L., Erickson, D. B., & Touyz, S. W. (2003). Parent–child interaction therapy: a comparison of standard and abbreviated treatments for oppositional defiant pre-schoolers. *Journal of Consulting and Clinical Psychology, 71*, 251–260.

Pantin, H., Coatsworth, D., Feaster, D. J., Newman, F. L., Briones, E., Prado, G., et al. (2003). Familias Unidas: the efficacy of an intervention to increase parental investment in Hispanic immigrant families. *Prevention Science, 4*, 189–201.

Patterson, G. R., Reid, J. B., Jones, R. R., & Conger, R. E. (1975). *A social learning approach to family intervention: Families with aggressive children (vol 1).* Eugene: Castalia.

Proctor, E. K., Vosler, N. R., & Murty, S. (1992). Child demographics and DSM diagnosis: a Multi-Axis Study. *Child Psychiatry and Human Development, 22*, 165–183.

Querido, J. G., Warner, T. D., & Eyberg, S. M. (2002). The cultural context of parenting: an assessment of parenting styles in African American families. *Journal of Clinical Child and Adolescent Psychology, 31*, 272–277.

Reid, M. J., Webster-Stratton, C., & Beauchaine, T. P. (2001). Parent training in Head Start: a comparison of program response among African American, Asian American, Caucasian, and Hispanic mothers. *Prevention Science, 2*, 209–227.

Reid, J. B., Patterson, G. R., & Snyder, J. (2002). *Antisocial behavior in children and adolescents: a developmental analysis and model for intervention.* Washington, DC: American Psychological Association.

Robbins, M. S., Schwartz, S. J., & Szapocznik, J. (2004). Structural ecosystems therapy with adolescent exhibiting disruptive behavior disorders. In J. Ancis (Ed.), *Culturally based interventions: alternative approaches to working with diverse populations and culture bound syndromes* (pp. 71–99). New York: Brunner-Routledge.

Rutter, M., & Giller, H. (1983). *Juvenile delinquency: trends and perspectives.* Harmondsworth: Penguin.

Sampson, R. J., & Laub, J. H. (1997). A life-course theory of cumulative disadvantage and the stability of deliquency. *Advances in Criminological Theory, 7*, 133–161.

Sanders, M. R., Markie-Dadds, C., Tully, L. A., & Bor, W. (2000). The triple p-positive parenting program: a comparison of enhanced, standard, and self-directed behavioral family intervention for parents of children with early onset conduct problems. *Journal of Consulting and Clinical Psychology, 68*, 624–640.

Santisteban, D. A., Coatsworth, J. D., Perez-Vidal, A., Kurtines, W. M., Schwartz, S. J., et al. (2003). Efficacy of brief strategic family therapy in modifying Hispanic adolescent behavior problems and substance use. *Journal of Family Psychology, 17*, 121–133.

Schaeffer, C. M., & Borduin, C. M. (2005). Long-term follow-up to a randomized clinical trial of Multisystemic Therapy with serious and violent juvenile offenders. *Journal of Consulting and Clinical Psychology, 73*, 445–453.

Semrud-Clikeman, M. (1995). *Child and adolescent therapy.* Boston, MA: Allyn and Bacon.

Spoth, R. L., Redmond, C., & Shin, C. (2001). Randomized trial of brief family interventions for general populations: adolescent substance use outcomes 4 years following baseline. *Journal of Consulting and Clinical Psychology, 69*, 627–642.

Sue, S., & Zane, N. (1987). The role of culture and cultural techniques in psychotherapy: a critique and reformulation. *American Psychologist, 42*, 37–45.

Szapocznik, J., Scopetta, M. A., Arandalde, M. A., & Kurtines, W. M. (1978). Cuban value structure: clinical implications. *Journal of Consulting and Clinical Psychology, 46*, 961–970.

Szapocznik, J., Kurtines, W. M., Foote, F., Perez-Vidal, A., & Hervis, O. E. (1983). Conjoint versus one-personal family therapy: some evidence for the effectiveness of conducting family therapy through one person. *Journal of Consulting and Clinical Psychology, 54*, 395–397.

Szapocznik, J., Santisteban, D., Kurtines, W. M., Perez-Vidal, A., & Hervis, O. E. (1984). Bicultural effectiveness training: a treatment intervention for enhancing intercultural adjustment. *Hispanic Journal of Behavioral Sciences, 6*, 317–344.

Szapocznik, J., Foote, F., Perez-Vidal, A., Hervis, O. E., & Kurtines, W. M. (1985). *One-person family therapy.* Miami: Miami World Health Organization Collaborating Center for Research and Training in Mental Health, Alcohol and Drug Dependence, Department of Psychiatry, University of Miami.

Szapocznik, J., Kurtines, W. M., Foote, F., Perez-Vidal, A., & Hervis, O. E. (1986). Conjoint versus one-personal family therapy: further evidence for the effectiveness of conducting family therapy through one person. *Journal of Consulting and Clinical Psychology, 54*, 395–397.

Szapocznik, J., Rio, A., Murray, E., Cohen, R., Scopetta, M. A., Rivas-Vasquez, A., et al. (1989). Structural family versus psychodynamic child therapy for problematic Hispanic boys. *Journal of Consulting and Clinical Psychology, 57*, 571–578.

Szapocznik, J., Santisteban, D., Rio, A., Perez-Vidal, A., Santisteban, D. A., & Kurtines, W. M. (1989). Family effectiveness training: an intervention to prevent drug abuse and problem behavior in Hispanic adolescents. *Hispanic Journal of Behavioral Sciences, 11*, 3–27.

Szapocznik, J., & Coatsworth, J. D. (1999). An ecodevelopmental framework for organizing the influences on drug abuse: a developmental model of risk and protection. In M. D. Glantz & C. R. Hartel (Eds.), *Drug abuse: Origins & interventions* (pp. 331–366). Washington, DC: American Psychological Association.

Taylor, T. K., & Biglan, A. (1998). Behavioral family interventions for improving childrearing: a review of the literature for clinicians and policy makers. *Clinical Child and Family Psychology Review, 1*, 41–60.

Taylor, T. K., Eddy, J. M., & Biglan, A. (1999). Interpersonal skills training to reduce aggression and delinquent behavior: limited evidence and the need for an evidence-based system of care. *Clinical Child and Family Psychology Review, 2*, 169–182.

Tharp, R. G. (1991). Cultural diversity and treatment of children. *Journal of Consulting and Clinical Psychology, 59*, 799–812.

Timmons-Mitchell, J., Bender, M. B., Kishna, M. A., & Mitchell, C. C. (2006). An independent effectiveness trial of multisystemic therapy with juvenile justice youth. *Journal of Clinical Child and Adolescent Psychology, 35*, 227–236.

United States Department of Commerce. (2008). *An older and more diverse nation by midcentury*. Washington, D. C.: United States Department of Commerce.

United States Department of Health and Human Services. (2001). *Mental health: Culture, race, and ethnicity – a supplement to mental health: A report of the Surgeon General.* Rockville: U.S. Department of Health and Human Services, Office of the Surgeon General.

United States Department of Health and Human Services (2009). *About the office of head start.* http://www.acf.hhs.gov/programs/ohs/index.html. Accessed 19 April 2009.

Vazsonyi, A. T., & Flannery, D. (1997). Early adolescent delinquent behaviors: associations with family and school domains. *Journal of Early Adolescence, 17*, 271–293.

Webster-Stratton, C., Hollinsworth, T., & Kolpacoff, M. (1989). The long-term effectiveness and clinical significance of three cost-effective training programs for families with conduct problem children. *Journal of Consulting and Clinical Psychology, 57*, 550–553.

Webster-Stratton, C. (1998). Preventing conduct problems in Head Start children: strengthening parenting competencies. *Journal of Consulting and Clinical Psychology, 66*, 715–730.

Webster-Stratton, C., & Hammond, M. (1997). Treating children with early-onset conduct problems: a comparison of child and parent training interventions. *Journal of Consulting and Clinical Psychology, 65*, 93–109.

Wells, K. C., Lenhart, L. A., & Lochman, J. E. (1996). *Coping Power program: parent component*. Durham, NC: Unpublished manual, Duke University Medical Center.

Winship, B. J., & Kelley, J. D. (1976). A verbal response model of assertiveness. *Journal of Counseling Psychology, 23*, 215–220.

Zebell, N. (Producer), & Urquiza, A.J. (Producer) (2002a). *Compliance Video/Dando Ordenes Efectivas – SER DIRECTO – (Spanish Language Version) [Video]*. (Available from UCDMC CAARE Center, PCIT Training Services, 3300 Stockton Blvd. Sacramento, CA 95812).

Zebell, N. (Producer), & Urquiza, A.J. (Producer), (2002b). *Relationship Enhancement "Fortaleciendo la Relacion Familiar – "A DIARIO" (Spanish Language Version). [Video]*. (Available from UCDMC CAARE Center, PCIT Training Services, 3300 Stockton Blvd. Sacrmaneto, CA 95812).

19

Evidence-Based Treatment Programs for Conduct Problems: Are They Cost Effective?

E. MICHAEL FOSTER

INTRODUCTION

Over the last decade and a half, interest in the economic analysis of interventions and services to prevent or treat behavioral health problems among children and youth has grown (Aos, Lieb, Mayfield, Miller, & Pennucci, 2004; Foster, Jonnes, & Dodge, 2003). The need for such research has been recognized by the National Institutes of Health. For example, the National Institute of Mental Health's (NIMH) 1996 plan for prevention research recognized this gap and stated: "Too little attention, however, has been focused on conducting cost–benefit or cost-effectiveness analyses that can reliably demonstrate whether preventive interventions indeed save money and improve health." Such information is of great importance to policy makers: "cost benefit or cost-effectiveness analyses need to become an integral part of NIMH-supported prevention effectiveness trials" (p. 17–18) (National Advisory Mental Health Council, 1996). However, the growth of interest has outstripped that of progress. For example, of the 23 programs in the National Institute on Drug Abuse (NIDA), "Preventing Drug Use Among Children and Adolescents: A Research-Based Guide for Parents, Educators and Community Leaders," only one has been subjected to economic analysis – the Strengthening Families Program (Spoth, Guyll, & Day, 2002).

E. MICHAEL FOSTER • University of North Carolina

R.C. Murrihy et al. (eds.), *Clinical Handbook of Assessing and Treating Conduct Problems in Youth*, DOI 10.1007/978-1-4419-6297-3_19,

This chapter reviews existing evidence on the cost-effectiveness of evidence-based treatments for aggressive problems in youth. We limit our attention to conduct cisorder (CD) and its precursor, oppositional defiant disorder (ODD). There are economic analyses of other interventions that seek to improve children's development such as that of Perry Preschool (Steven Barnett, 1985, 1996; Belfield, Nores, Barnett, & Schweinhart, 2006; Schweitzer, 2003), the Abcederian project (Barnett & Masse, 2007), and the Chicago Child–Parent Centers (Reynolds, Temple, Robertson, & Mann, 2002).

Our focus here is on targeted interventions designed to reduce conduct problems in children and youth. Within this narrow scope, the number of economic analyses of any sort is rather limited. While we review studies that are available, our focus here is more on what one might do rather than what has been done to date. However, we begin by reaffirming the importance of economic analysis to the treatment of problem behaviors.

Aggression is expensive, but prevention is not necessarily cost-effective. The argument that economic analysis is a critical component of research on the treatment of aggression and conduct problems is a strong one. Particularly problematic are "early starters," children or youth whose conduct problems emerge early in life; moreover, such problems often lead to personal and social costs later (Foster, Jones, & Conduct Problems Prevention Research Group, 2005). Those costs include criminal activities, substance use and abuse, and problems associated with early sexual debut, such as unwanted pregnancies and sexually transmitted diseases. The costs of a life of crime include government expenditures for criminal justice investigation, arrest, adjudication, and incarceration; costs to victims, such as medical costs, time missed from work, the value of stolen property, as well as loss of life; and costs that accrue to the criminal and his or her family, such as lost wages. In the most comprehensive analysis of its kind, Cohen (1998, 2005) estimates that high-risk youth may generate lifetime social costs approaching US$2 million (current dollar value). This value is averaged across a range of likely values and based on the costs to society of three categories of individuals: the career criminal ($1.3–1.5 million per person), heavy drug user ($370,000–970,000), and high-school dropout ($243,000–388,000). The high costs of conduct problems – and the fact that a small proportion of children and youth account for a disproportionate share of crime and delinquency – suggest that society should consider devoting considerable resources to targeted prevention.

Perhaps the relative dearth of economic analyses of prevention studies is due to the fact that one might perceive the answer as obvious. As Russell argues, however, several features of prevention work against cost-effectiveness, even for effective programs (Russell, 1986). First, by its very nature, prevention expenditures often occur long before the resulting benefits. Because money now is worth more than money later, a dollar spent today has to generate more than a dollar's worth of benefits in the future. Second, because of imperfect targeting, prevention programs often expend resources on those who may not have developed the problem or illness. No screening measure has a perfect positive predictive value. Those expenditures raise the costs of the program but generate little or perhaps no return.

(Furthermore, for mental disorders, incorrectly labeling a young person as disordered can create still other costs, perhaps further offsetting any savings from serving those who actually benefit.)

These challenges are especially relevant for conduct problems. As noted, research suggests that intervention for those at risk for conduct problems should begin early in life, before a series of self-reinforcing mechanisms become entrenched (Carolyn Webster-Stratton & Taylor, 2001). Starting early may be necessary, but at the same time, doing so raises the bar for cost-effectiveness. Many of the costs of problem behaviors are realized during adolescence, so intervening early lengthens the time between when expenditures are made and their payoff is realized. Moreover, screening for behavioral disorders is an uncertain enterprise. An added problem, discussed in more detail below, is that many interventions were designed to maximize the likelihood of efficacy, not cost-effectiveness.

BACKGROUND ON THE INCREDIBLE YEARS SERIES AND THE FAST TRACK INTERVENTION

The illustrations of economic analyses presented below focus on the Incredible Years Series and the Fast Track Intervention. In this section, we present background information on the two programs.

The Incredible Years Series

The Program

Developed by Carolyn Webster-Stratton and evaluated by colleagues at the University of Washington's Parenting Clinic, The Incredible Years Parents, Teachers, and Children Training Series (IYS) is a multicomponent program designed to treat young children with or at risk of developing early-onset conduct problems (see Chap. 6). The program has been adapted to serve as a cost-effective, community-based prevention program for children at risk for the development of CD. Over the past 20 years, this intervention has been widely implemented in both clinical and natural environment contexts such as mental health settings and schools.

Ultimately, the IY Series strives to prevent delinquency, drug abuse, and violent acts among high-risk children. However, immediate goals of the program include the reduction of conduct problems in children; the enhancement of social, emotional, and academic capabilities of children; the promotion of parental competence and positive discipline strategies; the strengthening of families as well as the school–home connection; and the enhancement of teacher classroom management skills (Webster-Stratton, 2000).

The IY Series comprises three components each focusing on different contexts for and types of children's social interactions. The three treatment components include (1) a child-based program (referred to as Child Training or CT), (2) a parent-based program (referred to as Parent Training or PT), and (3) a teacher-based program (referred to as Teacher Training or TT). (Since our focus is on the psychological and psychiatric sectors, this chapter does not discuss the last of these in any detail.) CT and PT leaders initially learn program curricula from certified IY trainers. Following training, CT and PT leaders deliver program curricula to child and parent participants, respectively, during weekly small group sessions. For a detailed description of treatment component goals, curriculum, and implementation methods, please see Webster-Stratton (2000) and Chap. 6.

Webster-Stratton and colleagues have implemented the IY Series using the three single treatment components either alone (i.e., CT program alone) or stacked in various combinations (i.e., CT plus TT and/or PT). Different combinations of the IY components are recommended depending on the targeted child population.

The IY Series has been effective in reducing the frequency of children's conduct problems regardless of treatment locale. Service agencies (mental health agencies, child welfare systems, and schools) continue to implement the IY Series with large-scale diffusion of the program occurring across the USA, Canada, United Kingdom, and Norway. Agencies adopting the IY Series are responsible for budgeting for initial training from certified IY trainers, program materials (videotapes, group leader manuals, parent and child materials, and handouts), program implementation, and ongoing consultation with IY trained staff. Following the initial materials and training fees, the IY Series may be offered to participants from successive cohorts at minimal cost to the service agency.

Past literature has assessed the impact of participant characteristics, individual component intensity, and multicomponent delivery methods on the effectiveness of the IY Series. Numerous randomized control group studies by the developer (e.g., Webster-Stratton, 1990; Webster-Stratton & Hammond, 1997; Webster-Stratton et al., 2001) and independent investigators (Barrera et al., 2002; Miller & Rojas-Flores, 1999; Scott, Spender, Doolan, Jacobs, & Aspland, 2001; Taylor, Schmidt, Pepler, & Hodgins, 1998) demonstrate that the IY Series consistently improves child behavior across a range of outcome indicators. The Incredible Years Series has been identified as an effective CD/ODD treatment and prevention program for young children by the Office of Juvenile Justice and Delinquency Prevention (Webster-Stratton, 2000). Additionally, when an independent review committee of the American Psychological Association reviewed findings from over 82 studies of CD interventions, the Incredible Years Series was identified as only one of two behavioral intervention strategies that met the criteria for well-established efficacious CD treatments (Brestan & Eyberg, 1998). With strong client outcomes, the IY Series was a prime candidate for economic evaluation to determine the actual costs of the benefits.

Evaluation Data

Outcome data from 21 separate cohorts of children taking part in six IY Series clinical trials were combined (Webster-Stratton, 1982, 1984, 1994; Webster-Stratton & Hammond, 1997; Webster-Stratton, Hollinsworth, & Kolpacoff, 1989; Webster-Stratton, Reid, & Hammond, 2004). All clinical trials were performed in Seattle; participants resided within a 60 mi radius of the Seattle metropolitan area. Data collection took place over a span of nearly 20 years (between the early 1980s and late 1990s). The final combined sample involved 459 children, between the ages of 3 and 8, who had been randomized to treatment and control groups. Outcome data from separate cohorts could be combined because of common program implementation and data collection procedures.

The following criteria were required for entry into the IY trials: (1) the child was between 3 and 8 years of age, (2) the child had no debilitating physical impairment, intellectual impairment, or history of psychosis and was not already receiving psychological treatment, (3) the primary clinic referral reason was for conduct problems such as noncompliance, aggression, and oppositional behavior that continued for more than 6 months, (4) parent-report symptoms on the Eyberg Child Behavior Inventory (ECBI) were more than two standard deviations above the mean, and (5) the child met criteria for ODD and/or CD according to either the Diagnostic and Statistical Manual of Mental Disorders, Third Edition, Revised (DSM-III-R) or the DSM-IV (APA, 1994), depending on the child's study entry date (Webster-Stratton & Reid, 2003)

Families were assigned to one of seven treatment conditions: (1) Child Training only (CT), (2) Parent Training only (PT), (3) Child Training and Parent Training (CT+PT), (4) Parent Training and Teacher Training (PT+TT), (5) Child Training and Teacher Training (CT+TT), (6) Child Training, Parent Training, and Teacher Training (CT+PT+TT), and (7) a control condition (CON). The number of participants in each group ranged from 11 to 54 and is described in more detail in the original paper (Foster, Olchowski, & Webster-Stratton, 2007).

Fast Track Intervention

The Intervention

The Fast Track project is a randomized trial designed to evaluate a comprehensive intervention (See Chap. 16). Intervention components are delivered in grades 1–10 and target multiple critical determinants of development: parenting, peer relations, and social-cognitive and cognitive skills. During the elementary school phase of the intervention, all at-risk families were offered parent training with home visits, academic tutoring, and social-skill training. Parent and child group interventions were conducted during a 2-h "enrichment program" held at the school building on Saturdays or weekday evenings. During the first 60–90 min of this enrichment program, at-risk target children met in groups of five or six called "friendship groups" led by Educational Coordinators and co-leaders, while parents met in a group led by Family Coordinators to discuss parenting strategies that would support child school adjustment and improve behavior. In the following 30 min, parent–child pairs participated in positive cooperative activities and parents practiced positive parenting skills with staff support, called Parent–Child Sharing Time. Academic tutoring to promote reading skills was provided by paraprofessional tutors in the last 30 min of the group meeting and twice more each week during school hours to all children in grade 1.

Group meetings were held weekly during grade 1 for 22 sessions, biweekly during grade 2 for 14 sessions, monthly during grades 3 through 5 for nine sessions each year, and four times during grade 6. In addition to the group meetings, individual support was provided through peer pairing and home visits to children and parents to help them generalize the skills presented in the group setting and to address individual needs. Tutors provided a weekly session for pairing with popular peers to enhance friendships. Children and families received a standard level of services in grade 1, to the extent that they could be delivered. In subsequent years, criterion-referenced assessments were used to adjust the dosage of some of these components to match the level of functioning of each family and child. In grade 2 and beyond, each child was assessed by the teacher for reading performance in the classroom. Children who scored in the lowest one-third of the classroom were targeted for reading tutoring. Similar assessments and individualized services were completed for other types of tutoring, home visits, peer coaching, mentoring, and after-school programming. A mentoring program was added in grade 4 to provide same-gender, same-race role models to promote children's positive identity development, if indicated by criterion-referenced assessments. Monthly group sessions for parents and youth continued in grades 5 and 6 to deal with the challenges of transitioning into middle school, resistance to drug use, and sexual development. In grades 7 and 8, workshops were held relating to identity and vocational goal setting.

In addition to indicated interventions, a universal intervention was provided to the class rooms in which targeted youth were located. This curriculum, which was an adaptation of the PATHS Curriculum (Kusche & Greenberg, 1993), was designed to promote a more competent and less aggressive social ecology, focusing on social and emotional development. The curriculum started by raising awareness of emotion words and knowledge; moved to teaching social problem-solving, impulse control, and reflective thought; and grew to address student-specific social dilemmas in later grades. Teachers implemented this classroom-level program throughout grades 1–5, teaching an average of two to three lessons per week. In addition, the universal intervention included weekly consultation with teachers, during which classroom behavior management issues were addressed. From grades 7 through 10, individualized intervention plans were developed and implemented with each youth, based on triannual assessments of risk and protective factors. Further details on intervention components are provided elsewhere. (See citations above.)

Evaluation Data

The intervention is being evaluated through a multicohort, multisite, multiyear study of program participants and comparable children and youth in similar schools, and that study provides the data for these analyses. In particular, schools within four sites (Durham, NC, Nashville, TN, Seattle, WA, and rural central Pennsylvania) were selected as high-risk based on crime and poverty statistics of the neighborhoods they served.

Within each site, the schools were divided into nine multiple paired sets, matched for demographics (geographic site, within-site location, size of school, percentage of free or reduced lunch, ethnic composition), and the sets were randomly assigned to intervention and control conditions. (There were two matched sets of schools at three sites, and three at the fourth.)

Within participating schools, subjects were identified using a multiple-gating procedure. For each of three annual cohorts, all kindergarteners in 54 schools (9,594 in total) were screened for classroom conduct problems by teachers. Those children scoring in the top 40% within cohort and site were then solicited for the next stage of screening for home behavior problems by the parents. Data collected from parents revealed that they were in agreement with teachers in over 90% of cases (n=3,274) (Lochman & Conduct Problems Prevention Research, 1995). The teacher and parent screening scores were then standardized and combined into a sum score, based on the screening of a representative sample of about 100 children within each site (which also served as a normative comparison). These summed scores represented a total severity-of-risk screen score. Children were selected for inclusion into the study based on this screen score, moving from the highest score downward until desired sample sizes were reached within sites, cohorts, and conditions. Deviations were made when (a) a child failed to matriculate in the first grade at a core school (n=59), (b) a child refused to participate (n=75), (c) or a school did not heed the rule that more than one girl must be in an intervention classroom. Ninety-five percent of the selected sample scored in the top 20% on both the parent and teacher screening measures. The outcome was that 891 children (Ns=445 for intervention and 446 for control) participated. Note that these levels of problems are defined relative to other children in these high-risk schools. On the kindergarten Teacher's Report Form of the Child Behavior Checklist, which provides national norms, the average Externalizing T-score (available for 88% of the high-risk sample) was 66.4, and 76% of these children scored in the clinical range (T-scores of 60 or higher).

The study has collected data from a range of informants – the youth themselves, care givers, teachers, and peers – and has obtained key archival data as well (such as school records). Over time, rates of attrition have been modest: 83% of subjects continued to provide data at the year-10 follow-up.

Participation was defined as attendance at one or more group sessions. Ninety-six percent of parents and 98% of children participated during grade 1 (or year 2 of the project). Of these families, 79% of parents and 90% of children attended at least 50% of all sessions. In grade 2, 88% of parents and 92% of children participated, with 79% of parents and 87% of children attending at least 50% of all sessions. In grade 3, 80% of parents and 86% of children participated, with 78% of parents and 84% of children attending at least 50% of all sessions. The proportion of families unable to participate in the intervention increased modestly across the years, primarily due to moves out of the area. In the last year of the group sessions (grade 6), 43 of the 445 intervention families (10%) did not participate but had still received the majority of the services in previous years.

BACKGROUND ON ECONOMIC ANALYSIS

In performing economic evaluation, economists have a primary goal in mind. That goal is to assess the impact of the intervention or program on the "efficiency" of society's resource allocation. An allocation is efficient if changing the allocation of resources would actually reduce societal well-being. In other words, the use of resources in the treatment or intervention must be preferred to their value in alternative uses. As we discuss below, any economic evaluation has a perspective – a position from which costs and benefits of the program are measured. For economists, the societal perspective takes precedence over the alternatives. Note that in measuring a program's societal impact, economists count all individuals as equals. This assumption is critical to economic analysis and the source of a great deal of criticism of economic evaluation. Within this framework, a dollar transferred from a poor person to a rich one leaves society no better or worse off. (More specifically, the only net effect involves the resources used to collect that dollar.)

The formal tools of economic evaluation may take one of several forms: benefit–cost analysis, cost-effectiveness analysis, and cost-utility analysis. Perhaps best known is benefit–cost analysis. A benefit–cost analysis (BCA) provides a full accounting of the resource implications of an intervention, policy, or program. One measures both the costs and benefits of the intervention and then calculates net benefits – that is, the benefits of the intervention less its costs. If the net benefits are positive, then the intervention or treatment is desirable. A key feature of benefit–cost analysis is that the benefits should reflect societal willingness to pay for the resource or outcome involved. In this case, the contribution of each individual to societal well-being depends on his or her willingness to pay for the program's outcome. Individuals may have greater willingness to pay (because they have more income, for example), and those individuals have more influence on policy decisions.

A second form of economic evaluation is cost-effectiveness analysis (CEA). Although the term cost-effectiveness is often used as a synonym for economic evaluation, CEA actually refers to a specific form of such an evaluation. Unlike benefit–cost analysis, cost-effectiveness analysis does not require one to measure outcomes in dollar terms. Rather, the outcome measures remain in their natural metric (e.g., a 1-point difference on a symptom checklist or a percentage point reduction in the number of teenagers giving birth). The analyst then compares interventions or programs in terms of their added (or incremental) costs per added unit of the outcome measure (Zerbe & Dively, 1994). The incremental cost-effectiveness ratio (ICER) is calculated as

$$\frac{C_{\mathrm{N}} - C_{\mathrm{O}}}{E_{\mathrm{N}} - E_{\mathrm{O}}} < \lambda. \tag{19.1}$$

E_{N} and E_{O} represent the effect of the new and old treatments, respectively, and C_{N} and C_{O}, the corresponding costs. One could calculate such ratios for a variety of outcome measures.

The key question in cost-effectiveness analysis is whether the ICER of a new treatment relative to an existing one exceeds a policy maker's or society's willingness to pay (λ) for the outcome of interest. For these analyses, λ can be interpreted as society's (or a policy maker's) willingness to pay for a one standard deviation improvement in the measures of behavior problems used as outcomes. If the ICER is less than λ the new technology or treatment is desirable (or preferred to treatment O, the old treatment).

Because the ICER is an estimate, however, one cannot say for certain whether the ICER is larger than λ. Rather, the best one can do is to estimate the probability that the inequality is true. Calculating this probability is complicated by the unique statistical properties of ratios. A variety of solutions have been proposed involving the delta method, Feiler's method, and bootstrapping among others (Briggs & Fenn, 1998; Briggs, 2000; O'Brien & Briggs, 2002; Sendi & Briggs, 2001).

None of these methods have proven to be entirely satisfactory. Even if appropriate confidence intervals were developed for ICERs, conceptual problems remain. Specifically, negative regions of the confidence interval are ambiguous. A negative ICER may indicate either that a new treatment is more costly and less effective or that the new treatment is less costly and more effective. Under these two scenarios, decision-makers would make completely opposite decisions; however, a negative ICER value offers no insight into which of the two decisions is appropriate.

As a result, until recently, analysts skirted these issues by not reporting confidence intervals. This solution is hardly satisfactory, and for that reason, two related alternatives have been proposed: (a) net benefits (NB) and (b) the closely related net health benefits. While both involve manipulating the familiar cost-effectiveness ratio (19.1), we employ the former here because we judge it easier to interpret (Hoch, Briggs, & Willan, 2002; Lothgren & Zethraues, 2000; Sendi & Briggs, 2001). We can express net benefits as follows:

$$\widehat{\mathrm{NB}} = \lambda(\hat{E}_{\mathrm{N}} - \hat{E}_{\mathrm{O}}) - (\hat{C}_{\mathrm{N}} - \hat{C}_{\mathrm{O}}) \tag{19.2}$$

NB values greater than zero indicate that the new treatment is preferred relative to the old treatment. Policy makers and researchers are able to calculate the probability of a positive NB value (i.e., P(NB>0)) across a range of values of λ; to generate cost-effectiveness acceptability curves (CEACs), these probability values are plotted. The CEAC is a useful tool for policy makers since different stakeholders may have varying tolerance for uncertainty. As a result, the CEAC provides policy makers with the ability to make informed decisions under uncertainty (Claxton, Lacey, & Walkter, 2000).

A third form of economic evaluation, cost-utility analysis, is actually a specific form of cost-effectiveness analysis. The outcome or measure of effectiveness is a measure of overall well-being based on respondent ratings of several dimensions of well-being. The scores on the different dimensions are then combined using weights that reflect the relative desirability of different combinations of the attributes. Those weights capture caregiver or other stake holder preferences for the attributes involved. A familiar measure of this sort is the quality-adjusted life year (QALY) (Drummond,

O'Brien, Stoddart, & Torrance, 1997). QALYs play an especially important role in the British National Health System (NHS) as discussed below.

Finally, a related form of economic analysis involves costs of illness studies. Those studies involve estimating the broader societal costs of illness, such as alcoholism or cigarette smoking and many others (Rice, Hodgson, & Kopstein, 1985; Rice, Kelman, & Miller, 1991; Sobocki, Lekander, Borgstrom, Strom, & Runeson, 2007). A cost of illness study generally includes the costs of treatment as well as effects on employment (Gold, Russell, Siegel, & Weinstein, 1996). Because willingness to pay is difficult to measure, economists may use the reduction in costs of illness as the measure of the benefits of an intervention. This measure understates the full benefits of the intervention. Costs of illness, for example, generally do not capture pain and suffering. (Kenkel, 1994).

Note that each of these studies can be conducted from any of several perspectives – participants, taxpayers, funding agencies or other payors, victims of crime, and society (the sum of the other perspectives). As noted, economists emphasize the societal perspective, but the other perspectives may be quite informative. For example, the relative costs and benefits for participants may affect their willingness to participate in the program or the level of engagement.

Regardless of the form and perspective of economic evaluation chosen, the foundation for each is a good estimate of a program's costs. The next subsection outlines economist's view of costs and their measurement.

Measuring the Costs of an Intervention

In this subsection, we begin by discussing the broad principles of cost estimation and then turn to the direct costs of the program. We then consider the morbidity-related costs and the impact of the intervention on those costs. Finally, we examine the direct costs of the IYS.

How Do Economists Think About Costs?

Economists' efforts to define and measure costs are guided by four principles. As mentioned above, the first is that the costs of a program or intervention vary depending on the perspective from which they are assessed. Economists emphasize the societal perspective, which encompasses impact of the program on all groups, such as intervention participants and taxpayors. By that standard, they assess whether a program is "efficient." By efficient, economists mean an allocation of resources such that further reallocation could not improve societal well-being.

As noted, the societal perspective includes other relevant perspectives, such as those of patients, the insurer or other payor, the provider, and other citizens (such as taxpayers). Some costs may drive the decision-making of one party but be completely irrelevant for another. For example, the travel or time costs for participants may be quite high. Unless an agency is reimbursing families, these costs may be ignored. The agency would consider them only indirectly and to the extent the costs manifest themselves on their budget sheet – for example, large travel costs might mean high rates of no-shows, which create costs for the agency.

As noted, the effects of a program on different groups offset each other. In the case of reduced use of cash transfers (such as the Temporary Assistance to Needy Families program), the only (net) societal cost involves program administration: The gain to taxpayors offsets the losses borne by the former recipients. There are other instances where the societal perspective diverges from that of other perspectives. For example, payments made for mental health service may not equal the costs of producing that service (Hargreaves, Shumway, Hu, & Cuffel, 1998). Those charges are the "costs" for the agency or program that pays for the services. These payments, however, may be a poor proxy for societal costs. This divergence exists for several reasons. As a result of market imperfections, payments made by some clients may implicitly subsidize other clients. The privately insured, for example, may subsidize the uninsured. As a result, payments made on behalf of the latter may understate the costs of society for the services involved.

The second through fourth principles involve this broader, societal perspective. A second principle is that economists measure costs in terms of opportunity costs: the value of a resource in its next best use (Gold, Russell, Siegel, & Weinstein, 1996). In many ways, this emphasis on foregone uses is what distinguishes an economist's approach from that of an accountant. This difference is most apparent in instances where a cost (or resource use) generates no bookkeeping entry. As an example, volunteer time requires no payment by the agency sponsoring an intervention. The time involved, however, has a value in alternative uses – the volunteer could spend that time at work or in leisure activities (or even volunteering at another program). These implicit time costs also might involve the time of program participants. Although economists may disagree somewhat as to how that time should be valued, they generally agree that such costs should be included.

A third principle shaping economists' reckoning of costs is that some costs are morbidity related. In a prevention program targeted to the mental health of children, these costs are particularly important. Children with emotional and behavioral problems are frequently involved in many child-serving sectors, and the costs of the services involved are potentially enormous. In many cases, these costs are actually reduced by a prevention program and so represent areas of so-called cost offset. For example, improvements in a child's mental health may reduce his or her use of health services or the use of mental health services by his or her parents (Foster & Bickman, 2000) or expenditures in the child-welfare sector (Foster & Connor, 2005). On the other hand, a preventive program may link families to these services and so increase their use (and related expenditures) as a result (e.g., the Starting Early, Starting Smart program (Cannon, Karoly, & Kilburn, 2001)). In some cases, these indirect costs may not be immediately apparent. For example, an intervention may reduce school dropout. Although this effect has obvious benefits, it also creates costs related to resources used while the individuals remain in school (Barnett, 1985).

A fourth feature of an economist's view of costs is that marginal costs are the costs that matter (Warner & Luce, 1982). By "marginal" an economist means costs incremental or costs that change as a result of the activity involved. Consider, for example, an intervention that affects the use of special education. The relevant costs are those above and beyond the costs of education in a regular classroom – after all, the latter would be incurred even if the child were not in special education (unless the intervention affects the likelihood that a child leaves school altogether).

Costs seem rather concrete to the noneconomist, but the attentive reader will note the hypothetical nature of some of these costs – for example, the value of resources in alternative (i.e., hypothetical) uses. For that reason, even in estimating costs, economists often have to make assumptions about markets or the behavior of economic agents. It is important that the resulting estimates be subject to sensitivity analyses – that is, calculations based on alternative assumptions about the value of key parameters.

Before turning to the details of cost estimation, a key point about efficacy studies is worth making. In those studies, the delivery of services may differ from that anticipated in the real world. An interventionist, for example, may receive more supervision than is possible in an actual clinical setting. No doubt that researchers should consider this possibility in advance of the study (whether it involves a cost analysis or not), but the relevant point here is that the cost estimate must describe the resources used to generate outcomes. High levels of supervision may be responsible for the improved outcomes; in that case, that supervision must be included in the corresponding cost estimates. Alternative costs estimates (such as those for lower levels of supervision) can be calculated when the corresponding outcomes become available through future studies.

In the next subsection, we consider how these principles would be applied to estimating the direct costs of an intervention in an efficacy trial. We illustrate this discussion with our work evaluating the Incredible Years Series in a clinical setting.

Measuring and Valuing Direct Costs

With the broad principles outlined above, estimating costs involves a set of practical steps required to collect the necessary information and to perform the necessary calculations. Gold et al. (1996) identified three steps in measuring the costs of an intervention or service: identifying the resources involved, measuring their use, and valuing the resources used in dollar terms. We examine each of these for the direct costs of the CT and PT components of the IYS. Note that the following discussion presumes that evaluation and service delivery are conducted by the same unit. As a result, the two activities share space and administration; furthermore, some individuals work on both tasks. Although common, this sharing of tasks not only raises issues about blinding the individuals involved to the intervention status of participants but also complicates estimating the costs of the intervention. These personnel must track their allocation of time to intervention and research. This task might involve time sheets that relevant personnel complete weekly. Ideally, because retrospective reports may be unreliable, these sheets would be completed prospectively. For other shared resources, such as the costs of space, one can either track the use of space or divide the costs between the two activities based on other information (as discussed later).

Consistent with the economic principles identified previously, we want to capture all of the resources involved in delivering an intervention. This accounting includes implicit costs (those resources for which no explicit payments are made), such as parental time and donated space. Time contributed by volunteers also would be included.

Table 19.1 enumerates the different resources used in delivering the Incredible Years CT and PT Programs. The explicit costs of the intervention involve both fixed and variable costs. Fixed costs are those costs that do not change as the number of participants expands. In this case, fixed costs include the costs of facilities. Variable costs, on the other hand, depend on the number of participants.

Some costs are quasi-fixed, such as staff training. For a given child, those costs are fixed – the training has occurred and will not increase as an additional child is treated. However, over time, one can anticipate that trained staff (e.g., a nurse) will turnover, and new training will be required. For that reason, to maintain the services over time, one would have to spread the costs of training over the anticipated tenure of the provider. In that case, the training is best viewed like a piece of equipment that will depreciate over time. From that perspective, a sensible practice would be to spread the costs of training over the expected number of children the provider could be expected to treat. An interventionist's tenure is not likely to be observed during the course of the study or in fact the study's funding may end, truncating tenure below that level that would be observed in the real world. For that reason, the analyst may perform calculations using a reasonable estimate.

Information on the resources involved could be determined from several sources. Principal among these are project budgets, which identify the resources used as well as costs to the project of those resources. In the case of some resources (particularly implicit costs), additional information would be needed from other sources, such as parental reports of time use.

In the case of explicit costs, these costs are naturally expressed in dollar terms. The challenge here is to allocate these costs between intervention delivery and other activities, such as research. In the case of implicit costs, measuring the resources involved in dollar terms often requires additional information.

For many interventions, labor costs are a primary component of explicit costs and are included in the fixed costs allocated subsequently. These costs can be calculated by using budget information on wages and salaries and on fringe benefits. Total labor costs would be allocated to the intervention based on the division of time use reported on the time sheets (discussed previously). Individuals devoting their time exclusively to research could be ignored or, if one were interested in the total costs of research, included in a separate tabulation.

Next, one would estimate other variable costs, such as supplies and materials. To the extent these resources could be related directly to intervention delivery, expenditures would be included in the costs of the intervention.

Table 19.1. Total per-child cost by IY treatment category

	CT	PT	CT+PT	PT+TT	CT+TT	CT+PT+TT
Treatment combination	Child training only	Parent training only	Both child & parent training	Both parent & teacher training	Both child & teacher training	All three
Training fees						
CT leader training by Cert. IY trainer (three 8-h days)	$3,600		$3,600		$3,600	$3,600
PT leader training by Cert. IY trainer (three 8-h days)		$3,600	$3,600	$3,600		$3,600
TT teacher training by Cert. IY trainer (four 8-h days)				$4,800	$4,800	$4,800
CT leader-in-training's time (three 8-h days)	$480		$480		$480	$480
PT leader-in-training's time (three 8-h days)		$480	$480	$480		$480
TT teacher-in-training's time (four 8-h days)				$400	$400	$400
Material fees (training and small group session)						
CT small group session materials	$1,244		$1,244		$1,244	$1,244
CT leader lesson plans	$150		$150		$150	$150
CT small group session handouts (for 6 children)	$14		$14		$14	$14
PT training materials		$15	$15	$15		$15
PT small group session materials		$1,390	$1,390	$1,390		$1,390
CT and PT parent manuals (for 12 parents)	$179	$179	$179	$179	$179	$179
TT teacher handbook and classroom handouts				$35	$35	$35
Additional fees – staff time						
CT leader's time in sessions	$880		$880		$880	$880
CT weekly supervision	$440		$440		$440	$440
PT leader's time in sessions		$720	$720	$720		$720
PT leader additional time		$480	$480	$480		$480

TT consultation costs				$390	$390	$390
Additional fees – IY implementation						
PT small group session meals		$1,000	$1,000	$1,000		$1,000
PT small group session babysitting fees		$1,080	$1,080	$1,080		$1,080
PT small group session cab vouchers		$240	$240	$240		$240
PT small group session day care costs		$288	$288	$288		$288
TT training session snacks				$160	$160	$160
Total cost (TC)	$6,987	$9,472	$16,280	$15,257	$12,772	$22,065
Total per-child cost (TC/number of children served)[a]	$1,164	$1,579	$2,713	$1,868	$1,454	$3,003

[a]Total per-child costs were calculated under the assumption that CT and PT small group sessions served six children (e.g., total per-child cost of CT ($1,164)=($6,987)/6). Total per-child costs for stacked treatment categories involving TT (i.e., PT+TT, CT+TT, and CT+TT+PT) were computed using two assumptions regarding the number of children served. For each teacher participating in TT, it was assumed that, on average, 20 classroom students were exposed to the program. Thus, the total cost of TT ($5,785) was divided by 20 to yield a total per-child TT cost of $289; this per-child cost was added to per-child costs of PT and CT to form the total per-child costs for the three stacked treatment categories involving TT; thus, total per-child costs for PT+TT, CT+TT, and CT+TT+PT were calculated using two different treatments

Expenditures on items that could not be linked to either the intervention or research (e.g., photocopying costs that were not tracked) could be included in (joint) fixed costs that are allocated as described later. Next, one would allocate fixed costs, including those costs that could not be divided between the intervention and research. Principal among these are space costs, including utilities and telecommunication costs. One could potentially include the costs of space used by specific personnel in the same proportion as they use their time. However, this would leave other space used by intervention and project personnel (such as conference rooms and meeting space) unallocated.

For that reason, following Hargreaves et al. (1998), we recommend that all space and similar shared costs are allocated based on the overall distribution of personnel time (and resulting costs) between the intervention and evaluation. Note that some costs involve resources that are purchased in a given year but that are used by project staff over several years. These costs include equipment costs, such as computers. These costs can be amortized over time by using standard accounting principles. Also included in this category are training costs. Project staff may be trained in a given year but work with program participants over time. As a result, some portion of their training should be attributed to future years. Using an estimate of the average amount of time personnel remain with a project, one could amortize those costs as well.

As discussed previously, not all explicit costs can be tracked on project budgets. These costs include out-of-pocket costs of participation borne by families. Included here are transportation costs as well as baby-sitting costs for a participant's siblings. One could estimate those costs by having parents complete a short questionnaire at a few intervention sessions. These explicit costs represent the costs of the intervention to taxpayors (or other funding source) and participants. They also are part of the costs of the intervention to society.

Implicit costs are primarily of two types – time and space. The latter involves space used by an intervention for which no payments are made, such as classrooms used for evening parent training. One could argue that the opportunity cost for this space is often zero as well: These groups are conducted after the normal business day or at a time when the space would not otherwise be used. This point is debatable, however, and one might consider the sensitivity of one's conclusions to this assumption. Estimates of the opportunity cost include the costs of similar space one might rent in the community.

Time costs represent a second type of implicit costs. A treatment may require substantial amounts of a parents' time. Parents receive incentive payments in a research study, but those payments may not fully compensate them for their time. Although family groups were scheduled at convenient times, parental participation reduces leisure time. Such time, however, is not without value. Because they conceivably could work during those hours, parents pay an implicit price for their leisure (in terms of reduced wages). This suggests that their leisure time is worth at least as much as their wage rate. For that reason, following Gorsky, Haddix, and Shaffer (1996), we recommend that one value parental time using parents' wage rate (Gorsky, Haddix, & Schaffer, 1996). One could calculate these costs using the results of a brief survey of parents concerning time spent on intervention-related activities and their wage rate. (To avoid double-counting costs, one would only include the amount by which these costs exceed any incentive payments made.)

Measuring and Valuing Morbidity-Related Costs

As discussed previously, a second type of cost involves morbidity-related costs – namely, the costs of alternative services used by children engaged in the intervention. The first step in measuring these costs is identifying the resources (or services) involved. Having done that, we consider the means for measuring and valuing each service.

The list of potential services and resources one might include is nearly endless. Children use many types of resources, and changes in their mental health likely will stimulate ripple effects through a range of child-serving sectors. Because research resources are not limitless, one has to prioritize based on what one knows about the prevention program and the population it targets. Possible criteria include the potential magnitude of costs associated with the alternative service as well as whether one would expect any relation between the service and the intervention. In the case of the Incredible Years, one system likely affected includes the educational system.

Increased use of school services likely includes disciplinary referrals as well as special education. Potential sources of information include parental reports or, for older children, self-reports. Because of concerns about the accuracy of such reports, school records may prove more reliable if available. School records can report a level of detail of service use of which parents are unaware or unreliable, such as the percentage of time spent in a special classroom.

For each type of service, one can convert measures of service use into dollar values using per-unit costs. A full discussion of the methods for valuing special education is beyond the scope of this chapter. However, at least in the USA, schools do not determine special education costs at the child level. Rather, schools know what they spend on the "inputs" – teachers and other resources – but generally do not translate this figure into a per-child estimate. Even under the best of circumstances, therefore, obtaining per-unit costs for special education is challenging. As an alternative, one might turn to special studies of the costs of special education (Chambers, Parrish, & Harr, 2002; Chambers, Parrish, Lieberman, & Wolman, 1998). Those studies generally involve a district or a state, and whether and how well they would apply in another location is unknown.

Placing a dollar value on other uses of school services is difficult. For example, the marginal cost of one trip to the principal's office is likely small or zero for an individual child. The school will not have a principal devoted to just that child, no matter how poorly behaved. (Issues of additional costs arise if one were to think of large groups of children being treated or a universal program. In that situation, one might divert an assistant principal from disciplinary issues to other functions.)

ILLUSTRATIVE ANALYSIS

In this section we present economic analyses for each of the two programs. We present a cost-effectiveness analysis and an analysis of the intervention's effect on costly outcomes.

Cost-Effectiveness of the Incredible Years

As discussed above, cost-effectiveness analysis focuses on the incremental costs and benefits of one program vs. alternative uses of the resources involved. The cost-effectiveness analysis of the IYS focused on the cost-effectiveness of the alternative combinations of the intervention's components. As noted above, the data for these analyses were provided by clinical evaluations of the intervention over a series of cohorts. We estimated the costs of the intervention following the principles of economics. A key consideration is that the costs were measured from the perspective of a potential provider of the program. We estimated the costs of actually delivering the services rather than what a payor might pay for the intervention. We also did not include participants' costs which are essential for a societal perspective. (For more details on cost estimation, see (Foster, Olchowski and Webster-Stratton, 2007).)

The full analyses considered several outcome measures, but in our illustration here, we present data on the Behar Problem Behavior Questionnaire, a teacher-reported measure of problem behaviors.

Figure 19.1 presents the CEAC for this outcome. There is one CEAC line for each of the treatments considered. At each level of willingness to pay (WTP), the highest line corresponds to the treatment most likely cost-effective. In general, parent and teacher training is most cost-effective across a range

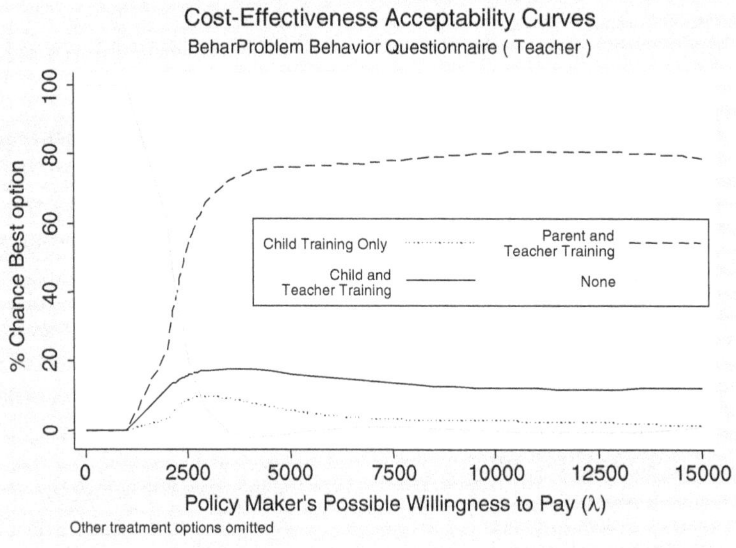

Fig. 19.1. Illustrative cost-effectiveness acceptability curves.

of possible values for WTP. AT low levels of willingness to pay, no treatment is most cost-effective – this finding is quite sensible if not informative. If one does not value treatment outcomes, then treatment cannot be cost-effective.

Ideally, at every willingness to pay, one of the lines would achieve 100% certainty. As one can see, for most of the range of WTP, the line hovers in the range of 80%. This position corresponds to a type-I error of roughly 20% – that is, if we pick parent and teacher training, there is a 20% chance that that treatment was not cost-effective.

Of course, the major issue with a figure such as Fig. 19.1 is locating *the* appropriate value of λ. A policy maker might assess his or her own WTP based on other information, such as the link between aggression and costly outcomes. In the next section, we consider the effect of an intervention on costly outcomes, such as involvement in special education.

EFFECT OF THE FAST TRACK INTERVENTION ON COSTLY OUTCOMES

Cost-effectiveness analyses have been conducted using study data (Foster & Jones, 2007; Foster, Jones, & Conduct Problems Prevention Research Group, 2006), but our focus here is on recently conducted analyses of the effect of the intervention on costly problem behaviors, such as the use of health and mental health services, arrests and involvement in the juvenile justice system, substance use, special education services, grade retention, and high-school graduation. These analyses focused on data collected from parents, youth, and from court and medical records.

The analysis dealt with key features of the study design such as variation across the four sites in the intervention's impact. The analysis also allowed for variation across key subgroups, such as those defined by initial risk status and gender. Prior research had suggested that the intervention's effect was moderated by initial severity (Conduct Problems Prevention Research Group, 2007). However, obtaining separate estimates for the various subgroups defined by site, gender, and risk status would lead to numerous underpowered analyses and potential chance findings resulting from multiple testing.

For that reason, the study employs a meta-analytic approach to combining estimated intervention effects across subgroups. Such an approach is similar to multilevel modeling in the sense that the structure of the sample (e.g., region) is incorporated in the estimation process. As indicated, 16 subgroups were defined by site, gender, and initial risk status (4 × 2 × 2). A key feature of these analytic methods is they allow the test of the null hypothesis that intervention effects are uniform across the subgroups.

The analytical models generally were regression-based with the specific model reflecting the distribution of each outcome. For example, many of the outcomes involved counts (e.g., number of arrests), so we employed negative binomial models given their appropriateness for the highly dispersed count variables seen in this study. In other instances, the outcome involved the timing of an event (such as first arrest), and for those outcomes we employed hazard modeling.

The analytical model employed a range of other covariates to capture baseline differences between the treatment and the comparison groups. At the beginning of the study, the Fast Track principal investigators identified 25 covariates that represent key characteristics of the participating subjects/families, and these have been used consistently in various analyses of intervention impact (Conduct Problems Prevention Research Group, 2007). For these analyses, we added four background variables representing parent and household characteristics: whether the biological father was in the household, whether the mother had been a teenager at first childbirth, maternal education, and number of children in the household. Collectively, when analyzing study outcomes, this set of variables controlled for preexisting intervention group differences. Because sample sizes for some of the 16 subgroups were small, including all of the covariates as regressors was impractical. For that reason, we calculated the propensity score from these 29 control variables and included that score in statistical models to represent the likelihood of study participation. As demonstrated by Rubin and Rosenbaum, the propensity score captures all information in the covariates related to intervention status (Rosenbaum, 1983, 2002, 2004).

The good news about having multiple sources of data is that some information is available for nearly all youth in the study at each point in time. However, the bad news is that with so many sources, an individual is likely missing data from one or more. Overall, *by* year 13 of the project, missing data rates for the entire sample reached 25–30% (these rates vary across measures and data sources).

As a result, the handling of missing data is quite important. We employed multiple imputation (MI) as implemented in the SAS package IVEware (Raghunathan, Lepkowski, Van Hoewyk, & Solenberger, 2001). This program provides data imputation most appropriate when the full data include outcomes that are distributed as unordered categorical, ordered categorical, count, and continuous variables. As is typical with MI estimation routines, IVEware methods rely on the assumption that data are missing at random (MAR), and we assume that our models satisfy this assumption given the inclusion of multiple measures of baseline and follow-up participant characteristics. All outcomes used in the primary analyses were included in the MI models, and analyses were based on five imputed datasets. MI estimation was performed separately by intervention status. Doing so maintained important interactions between intervention status and other key constructs (and thus, interaction terms did not need to be included in the MI models). Separation of imputation models by intervention status also is important if the pattern of missingness differs between groups. We did not impute separately by site because of sample size. In that sense, our imputation model is more restrictive than our analytical model.

Overall, the findings generally indicate lower rates and costs for health and mental health services and lower antisocial behavior and justice system involvement for intervention-group youth than control-group youth. However, no differences were consistently found in other domains of substance use, special education services, school dropout, or grade retention.

The parent and youth reports of health services were consistent: At older ages (project years 11 through 13), both parents and youth in the intervention group reported lower use of outpatient mental health services. Analyses of medical records supported these findings and documented lower associated costs. We also detected consistency between parent report of general health use and the costs indicated in the medical records. Both sources showed that the control group made greater use of general health services for mental health purposes as well as for any reason, than the intervention group. For inpatient mental health services use across the ages examined, youth and parent reports were consistently nonsignificant. Overall, the assessment of health services is generally consistent across parent report, youth report, and medical records.

The various sources of information on delinquency were somewhat consistent. Intervention youth indicated fewer arrests than control youth, but the same result was not found with parent report (considering the same time frame) nor were there significant differences in the number of crimes documented in the court records. However, consistent with the youth reports, parents in the intervention group (compared with control group) reported lower levels of youth antisocial behavior. Additionally, our models indicated a trend ($p<0.10$) for a lower likelihood of jail time served by the intervention group as documented in the court records.

Other Studies

Other economic analyses can be found in the literature. Most prominent of these is that of Multisystemic Therapy (MST, see Chap. 11). Shoenwald et al. (1996) consider the effect of the program as an alternative to out-of-home placements of substance-abusing juvenile offenders. The analysis falls within the category of a cost of illness impact study.

Within a randomized trial with 118 participants, the authors considered the incremental costs of the program relative to observed reductions in days of incarceration, hospitalization, and residential treatment at approximately 1 year post-referral. They find that the program incremental costs were nearly offset by the reductions in days of out-of-home placement during the year.

The Washington State Institute for Public Policy has conducted a more extensive (and current) reanalysis. Their analyses suggest that the program costs $4,264 and generates net benefits of $18,213 (Drake, 2007) per treated youth. The difference between the two studies reflects a variety of technical issues, such as difference in the way specific outcomes were valued.

CONCLUSIONS

These analyses illustrate the potential usefulness of economic analysis of treatment of conduct problems in youth. One can see from the field of early childhood education that the impact of such analyses can be enormous. Advocates have referred repeatedly to the return generated by early childhood education as justification for their programs, and policy makers often find their arguments persuasive. At this point, this potential is not yet realized. At best, there are only a handful of interventions for youth with conduct problems for which economic analyses are available. Even if one includes somewhat related studies (e.g., treatment foster care), the number of studies involved is modest.

Further limiting our ability to assess the economic merits of treatment is inconsistency across studies. As noted, economic evaluations of social programs frequently differ in the way program costs are calculated (Foster, Porter, Ayers, Kaplan, & Sandler, 2007). While not sufficient, such consistency is certainly necessary for between-study comparisons. A much cited report conveys the relative benefits of alternative approaches to reducing delinquency (Aos et al., 2004). However, the authors are well aware that these comparisons potentially overlook real differences in the programs with regards to the way information was calculated and reported by the original evaluators.

Another problem is that such analyses are inherently interdisciplinary. An economic evaluation of treatment requires those with a substantive knowledge of the outcome measures (at the very least) as well as someone with the necessary background in health economics. Assembling a team with the required expertise poses the usual challenges to interdisciplinary research, but the problem is not insurmountable. After all, the literature is filled with many cost-effectiveness studies of interventions and treatments for physical disorders.

Include Economic Analysis at the Start of the Study

The literature on the cost-effectiveness of treatment for physical disorders offers other lessons. One of those is that economic analyses need to be included in the original study design. Some advantages of including the economic analysis at the start of the study are practical. For example, it is quite a bit easier to estimate the costs of a treatment or service as it is delivered than retrospectively. For example, input may be needed from staff concerning their allocation of time, but as time passes, those individuals may take other positions. Other issues are more scientific. For example, statistical power needs to be set with economic analysis in mind. As cost-effectiveness involves a ratio that is the function of two estimates, the standard error of the ratio will be larger than that for either individual. This issue is amplified by the tendency for costs to be highly right-skewed.

But more fundamentally, the interventions themselves – and not just the evaluations – need to be designed with economic efficiency. Interventions like Fast Track were designed to maximize the chance of efficacy. This decision made sense at the time: the intervention targeted a group of individuals for whom few if any interventions had proven effective. And, developmental theory suggested that intervening in multiple domains was mostly likely to change outcomes. For better or worse, it is not clear how an intervention like Fast Track could ever have been funded on a large scale even if it had reduced costly outcomes.

Fortunately, a new generation of interventions are being designed and evaluated that are much less costly. These interventions include the Incredible Years Series as well as the Triple P Positive Parenting Program (Bor, Sanders, & Markie-Dadds, 2002; Sanders, 1999; Sanders, Markie-Dadds,

Tully, & Bor, 2000; Sanders, Turner, & Markie-Dadds, 2002). Designing interventions with an eye toward cost-effectiveness has other broad-ranging implications. For example, many interventions not only overuse limited resources of a payor (like the Medicaid program), but also the resources of the participants, notably their time costs (Foster, Taylor, & Shelton-Johnson, 2007). As an economist would expect, psychologists (like any economic agent) over-use a resource for which they bear no costs (participants' time). Reductions in the length of interventions will reduce the costs to society. (In fact, they may even improve efficiency by reducing absenteeism.) Similarly, psychologists may be on the wrong side of other tradeoffs between effectiveness and costs. Group therapy, for example, may be less effective than individual therapy, but much more cost-effective.

Better Integration with Research on Health Policy

Research in this area would be improved by other extensions and changes in the way psychologists and psychiatrists conduct research. Namely, if effective treatment is to be eventually delivered, it likely will have to be integrated with existing public health infrastructure.

The first change would be a broader consideration of the health policy context of research on the effectiveness and economic analysis of treatments. It is well known among health services researchers that the delivery of health services varies enormously across communities. In many studies of effectiveness, the comparison group receives treatment as usual which means treatment in the community – and that treatment can vary a lot within and between studies. This issue is relevant even for a study in one community – the nature of service delivery in that community shapes how the results of that study might be interpreted in a community where health service delivery differs. And as one considers the broader use of services (e.g., involvement in special education), the importance of policy context only grows. Service delivery within schools varies enormously across districts and states. This variation has enormous implications for understanding the costs of illness.

Most studies of the effect of treatments treat site (i.e., community) as a nuisance. Fast Track, for example, includes four sites, but the investigators have done very little to assess between site variation and even less to understand that variation. This problem does not affect Fast Track alone. Large clinical trials have ignored site as well. The Multimodal Treatment Study of Children With Attention Deficit and Hyperactivity (MTA) generally ignores site even though one of the sites is outside the USA (Arnold et al., 1997; Richters et al., 1995). As these studies better reflect the context in which they occur, health economists may prove of more use than just conducting economic analyses.

A More Open Research Process

Finally, research on costs and benefits is only as good as the evidence of effectiveness on which it is based. For that reason, independent replication is essential to effectiveness research in general and economic evaluation in particular. Currently, many studies in the field do not involve publicly available data. The Fast Track data, for example, while available to select researchers who apply, have only been examined by a relatively small group of researchers: those who developed the intervention. Such limitations represent a natural conflict of interest. Some of these processes are likely to be quite subtle. Any analysis of a mental health intervention is likely to involve issues of judgment (e.g., about the scaling of an outcome measure). Those judgments and broader questions of design and analysis need to be made without regard to the treatment outcomes.

Economic analysis also raises broader issues associated with the replication of cost-effectiveness data between countries. The Incredible Years Series has been replicated by investigators in Canada (Taylor et al., 1998). Such work may provide insights on clinical outcomes, but given the dramatic differences in the health care systems, the intervention's impact on participant involvement in school or other health services may very well differ substantially to the USA.

REFERENCES

American Psychiatric Association. (1994). Diagnostic criteria from DSM-IV. Washington, D.C.: The American Psychiatric Association.

Aos, S., Lieb, R., Mayfield, J., Miller, M., & Pennucci, A. (2004). *Benefits and costs of prevention and early intervention programs for youth.* Seattle, WA: Washington State Public Policy Institute.

Arnold, L. E., Abikoff, H. B., Cantwell, D. P., Conners, C. K., Elliott, G., Greenhill, L. L., et al. (1997). National institute of mental health collaborative multimodal treatment study of children with ADHD (the MTA). Design challenges and choices. *Arch Gen Psychiatry, 54*(9), 865–870.

Barnett, W. S. (1985). *The Perry preschool program and its long-term effects: A benefit-cost analysis.* Ypsilanti, MI: High/Scope Educational Research Foundation.

Barnett, W. S. (1996). *Lives in the balance: Age-27 benefit–cost analysis of the High/Scope Perry Preschool Program.* Ypsilanti, MI: High/Scope.

Barnett, W. S., & Masse, L. N. (2007). Comparative benefit–cost analysis of the Abecedarian program and its policy implications. *Economics of Education Review, 26*(1), 113–125.

Barrera, M., Jr., Biglan, A., Taylor, T. K., Gunn, B. K., Smolkowski, K., Black, C., et al. (2002). Early elementary school intervention to reduce conduct problems: A randomized trial with Hispanic and non-Hispanic children. *Prevention Science, 3,* 83–94.

Belfield, C. R., Nores, M., Barnett, S., & Schweinhart, L. (2006). The High/Scope Perry Preschool Program: Cost–benefit analysis using data from the age-40 followup. *Journal of Human Resources, 41*(1), 162–190.

Bor, W., Sanders, M. R., & Markie-Dadds, C. (2002). The effects of the Triple P-Positive Parenting Program on preschool children with co-occurring disruptive behavior and attentional/hyperactive difficulties. *Journal of Abnormal Child Psychology, 30*(6), 571–587.

Brestan, E. V., & Eyberg, S. M. (1998). Effective psychosocial treatments of conduct-disordered children and adolescents: 29 years, 82 studies, and 5,272 kids. *Journal of Clinical Child Psychology, 27*(2), 180–189.

Briggs, A. H. (2000). Handling uncertainty in cost-effectiveness models. *Pharmacoeconomics, 17,* 479–500.

Briggs, A., & Fenn, P. (1998). Confidence intervals or surfaces? Uncertainty on the cost-effectiveness plane. *Health Economics, 7,* 723–740.

Cannon, J. S., Karoly, L. A., & Kilburn, M. R. (2001). *Directions for costs and outcome analysis of starting early, staring smart: Summary of a cost expert meeting.* Santa Monica, CA: Rand.

Chambers, J., Parrish, T., Lieberman, J., & Wolman, J. (1998). What are we spending on special education in the US? CSEF brief, *8*, 1–4.

Chambers, J., Parrish, T., & Harr, J. J. (2002). What are we spending on special education in the US? 1999-2000. CSEF brief, *8*, 1–4.

Claxton, K., Lacey, L. F., & Walkter, S. G. (2000). Selecting treatments: A decision theoretic approach. *Journal of the Royal Statistical Society: Series A (Statistics in Society), 163*(Part 2), 211–225.

Cohen, M. A. (1998). The monetary value of saving a high-risk youth. *Journal of Quantitative Criminology, 14*, 5–33.

Cohen, M. A. (2005). *The costs of crime and justice.* New York: London.

Conduct Problems Prevention Research Group. (2007). Fast track randomized controlled trial to prevent externalizing psychiatric disorders: Findings from grades 3 to 9. *Journal of the American Academy of Child and Adolescent Psychiatry, 46*(10), 1250–1262.

Drake, E. (2007). *Evidence-based juvenile offender programs: Program description, quality assurance, and cost.* Olympia, WA: Washington State Institute for Public Policy.

Drummond, M. F., O'Brien, B., Stoddart, G. L., & Torrance, G. W. (1997). Methods for the Economic Evaluation of Health Care Programmes (2nd ed.). New York, NY: Oxford Univeristy Press.

Foster, E. M., & Bickman, L. (2000). Refining the costs analyses of the Fort Bragg Evaluation: The impact of cost offset and cost shifting. *Mental Health Services Research, 2*(1), 13–25.

Foster, E. M., & Connor, T. (2005). The public costs of better mental health services for children and adolescents. *Psychiatric Services, 56*, 50–55.

Foster, E. M., Jones, D. E., & Conduct Problems Prevention Research Group. (2005). The high costs of aggression: Public expenditures resulting from conduct disorder. *American Journal of Public Health, 95*(10), 1767–1772.

Foster, E. M., Jones, D., & Conduct Problems Prevention Research Group. (2006). Can a costly intervention be cost-effective?: An analysis of violence prevention. *Archives of General Psychiatry, 63*, 1284–1291.

Foster, E. M., & Jones, D. (2007). The economic analysis of prevention: An illustration involving the fast track project. *Journal of Mental Health Policy and Economics, 10*(4), 165–175.

Foster, E. M., Jones, D., & Dodge, K. A. (2003). Issues in the economic evaluation of prevention programs. *Applied Developmental Science, 7*(2), 74–84.

Foster, E. M., Olchowski, A. E., & Webster-Stratton, C. H. (2007). Is stacking intervention components cost-effective? An analysis of the Incredible Years program. *Journal of the American Academy of Child and Adolescent Psychiatry, 46*(11), 1414–1424.

Foster, E. M., Porter, M. M., Ayers, T. S., Kaplan, D. L., & Sandler, I. (2007). Estimating the costs of preventive interventions. *Evaluation Review, 31*(3), 261 286.

Foster, E. M., Taylor, T., & Shelton-Johnson, D. (2007). Measuring time costs in psychosocial interventions: How and Why. *American Journal of Community Psychology, 40*(1–2), 64–81.

Gold, M. R., Russell, L. B., Siegel, J. E., & Weinstein, M. C. (Eds.). (1996). *Cost-effectiveness in health and medicine.* New York: Oxford University Press.

Gorsky, R. D., Haddix, A. C., & Schaffer, P. A. (1996). Cost of an Intervention. In A. C. Haddix, S. M. Teutsch, P. A. Shaffer & D. O. Dunet (Eds.), Prevention Effectivness: A Guide to Decision Analysis and Economic Evaluation (pp. 57–75). New York: Oxford University Press.

Hargreaves, W. A., Shumway, M., Hu, T. W., & Cuffel, B. (1998). *Cost-outcome methods for mental health.* New York: Academic Press.

Hoch, J. S., Briggs, A. H., & Willan, A. R. (2002). Something old, something new, something borrowed, something blue: A framework for the marriage of health econometrics and cost-effectiveness analysis. *Health Economics, 11*, 415–430.

Kenkel, D. (1994). Cost of illness approach. In D. Kenkel & R. Fabian (Eds.), *Valuing Health for Policy: An Economic Approach,* (pp. 42–71) Chicago.

Kusche, C., & Greenberg, M. (1993). *The PATHS Curriculum.* Unpublished manuscript, Seattle, WA: Developmental Research and Programs.

Lochman, J. E., & Conduct Problems Prevention Research, G. (1995). Screening of child behavior problems for prevention programs at school entry. *Journal of Consulting and Clinical Psychology, 63*(4), 549–559.

Lothgren, M., & Zethraues, N. (2000). Definition, interpretation, and calculation of cost-effectiveness acceptability curves. *Health Economics, 9*, 623–630.

Miller, L. S., & Rojas-Flores, L. (1999). *Preventing conduct problems in urban, latino preschoolers through parent training: A pilot study.* New York: New York University Child Study Center.

National Advisory Mental Health Council. (1996). *A plan for prevention research for the National Institute of Mental Health.* Washington, DC: National Institutes of Health, National Institute of Mental Health.

O'Brien, B. J., & Briggs, A. H. (2002). Analysis of uncertainty in health care cost-effectiveness studies: An introduction to statistical issues and methods. *Statistical Methods in Medical Research, 11*, 455–468.

Raghunathan, T. E., Lepkowski, J. M., Van Hoewyk, J., & Solenberger, P. (2001). A multivariate technique for multiply imputing missing values using a sequence of regression models. *Survey Methodology, 27*(1), 85–95.

Reynolds, A. J., Temple, J. A., Robertson, D. L., & Mann, E. A. (2002). Age 21 cost-benefit analysis of the Title I Chicago child–parent centers. *Educational Evaluation and Policy Analysis, 24*(4), 267–303.

Rice, D. P., Hodgson, T. A., & Kopstein, A. N. (1985). The economic costs of illness: a replication and update. Health Care Financ Rev, *7*(1), 61–80.

Rice, D. P., Kelman, S., & Miller, L. S. (1991). Estimates of economic costs of alcohol and drug abuse and mental illness, 1985 and 1988. Public Health Rep, *106*(3), 280–292.

Richters, J. E., Arnold, L. E., Jensen, P. S., Abikoff, H., Conners, C. K., Greenhill, L. L., et al. (1995). NIMH collaborative multisite multimodal treatment study of children with ADHD: I. Background and rationale. *Journal of the Amercian Academy of Child and Adolescent Psychiatry, 34*(8), 987–1000.

Rosenbaum, P. R., & Rubin, D. B. (1983). The Central role of the propensity score in observational studies for causal effects. Biometrika, *70*(1), 41–55.

Rosenbaum, P. R. (2002). Observational Studies. New York: Springer-Verlag.

Rosenbaum, P. R. (2004). Design sensitivity in observational studies. Biometrika, *91*(1), 153–164.

Russell, S. (1986). *Is prevention better than the cure?* Washington, DC: The Brookings Institution.

Sanders, M. R. (1999). Triple P-Positive Parenting Program: Towards an empirically validated multilevel parenting and family support strategy for the prevention of behavior and emotional problems in children. *Clinical Child and Family Psychology Review, 2*(2), 71–90.

Sanders, M. R., Markie-Dadds, C., Tully, L. A., & Bor, W. (2000). The triple P-positive parenting program: A comparison of enhanced, standard, and self-directed behavioral family intervention for parents of children with early onset conduct problems. *Journal of Consulting and Clinical Psychology, 68*(4), 624–640.

Sanders, M. R., Turner, K. M., & Markie-Dadds, C. (2002). The development and dissemination of the Triple P-Positive Parenting Program: A multilevel, evidence-based system of parenting and family support. *Prevention Science, 3*(3), 173–189.

Scott, S., Spender, Q., Doolan, M., Jacobs, B., & Aspland, H. (2001). Multicentre controlled trial of parenting groups for child antisocial behaviour in clinical practice. *British Medical Journal, 323*, 194–198.

Sendi, P. P., & Briggs, A. H. (2001). Affordability and cost-effectiveness: Decision-making on the cost-effectiveness plane. *Health Economics, 10*(7), 675–680.

Shoenwald, S. K., Ward, D. M., Henggeler, S. W., Pickrel, S. G., & Patel, H. (1996). Multisystemic therapy treatment of substance abusing or dependent adolescent offenders: Costs of reducing incarceration, inpatient and residential placement. *Journal of Child and Family Studies, 5*(4), 431–444.

Sobocki, P., Lekander, I., Borgstrom, F., Strom, O., & Runeson, B. (2007). The economic burden of depression in Sweden from 1997 to 2005. Eur Psychiatry, *22*(3), 146–152.

Spoth, R. L., Guyll, M., & Day, S. X. (2002). Universal family-focused interventions in alcohol-use disorder prevention: Cost-effectiveness and cost–benefit analyses of two interventions. *Journal of Studies on Alcohol, 63*, 219–228.

Taylor, T. K., Schmidt, F., Pepler, D., & Hodgins, H. (1998). A comparison of eclectic treatment with Webster-Stratton's Parents and Children Series in a children's mental health center. *Behavior Therapy, 29*, 221–240.

Warner, K. E., & Luce, B. R. (1982). *Cost–benefit and cost-effectiveness analysis in health care.* Ann Arbor, MI: Health Administration Press.

Webster-Stratton, C. (1982). The long-term effects of a videotape modeling parent-training program: Comparison of immediate and one-year follow-up results. *Behavior Therapy, 13*, 702–704.

Webster-Stratton, C. (1984). A randomized trial of two parent-training programs for families with conduct-disordered children. *Journal of Consulting and Clinical Psychology, 52*, 666–678.

Webster-Stratton, C. (1990). Enhancing the effectiveness of self-administered videotape parent training for families with conduct-problem children. *Journal of Abnormal Child Psychology, 18*, 479–492.

Webster-Stratton, C. (1994). Advancing videotape parent training: A comparison study. *Journal of Consulting and Clinical Psychology, 62*, 583–593.

Webster-Stratton, C. (2000). The incredible years training series. *Juvenile Justice Bulletin*, 1–23.

Webster-Stratton, C., & Hammond, M. (1997). Treating children with early onset-conduct problems: A comparison of child and parent training interventions. *Journal of Consulting and Clinical Psychology, 65*, 93–109.

Webster-Stratton, C., Hollinsworth, T., & Kolpacoff, M. (1989). The long-term effectiveness and clinical significance of three cost-effective training programs for families with conduct-problem children. *Journal of Consulting and Clinical Psychology, 57*, 550–553.

Webster-Stratton, C., Mihalic, S., Fagan, A., Arnold, D., Taylor, T., & Tingley, C. (2001). *Blueprints for violence, book eleven: The Incredible Years Parent, Teacher, and Training Series.* Boulder, CO: Center for the Study and Prevention of Violence.

Webster-Stratton, C., & Reid, M. J. (2003). Treating conduct problems and strengthening social and emotional competence in young children: The Dina Dinosaur Treatment Program. *Journal of Emotional and Behavioral Disorders, 11*, 130–143.

Webster-Stratton, C., Reid, M. J., & Hammond, M. (2004). Treating children with early-onset conduct problems: Intervention outcomes for parent, child, and teacher training. *Journal of Clinical Child and Adolescent Psychology, 33*, 105–124.

Webster-Stratton, C., & Taylor, T. (2001). Nipping early risk factors in the bud: Preventing substance abuse, delinquency, and violence in adolescence through interventions targeted at young children (0–8 years). *Prevention Science, 2*(3), 165–192.

Zerbe, R. O., Jr., & Dively, D. D. (1994). Benefit-cost analysis in theory and practice. New York: Harper Collins College Publishers.

20

Epilogue: Future Directions in Research and Practice

RACHAEL C. MURRIHY, THOMAS H. OLLENDICK, and ANTONY D. KIDMAN

This volume brings together leading researchers in the field of child and adolescent conduct problems to deliver an integrated representation of the latest knowledge with regard to phenomenology, etiology, assessment, and evidence-based treatment (EBT). Trends and commonalities, evidenced across the chapters, are identified and discussed in this section. So too are the significant advances that have propelled forward our understanding of conduct problems, along with a consideration of questions that remain unanswered. Finally, we will contemplate future directions for research and treatment in this field.

Foremost, this volume draws attention to the cornucopia of comprehensive psychosocial treatments for youth with conduct problems that are available to practitioners today (see Parts 2 and 3). These treatments have been subject to extensive, high-quality evaluation including efficacy, effectiveness, and transportability studies. Further, they have been endorsed by Division 53 of the American Psychological Association, the Society of Clinical Child and Adolescent Psychology, as "well established" and "probably efficacious" for conduct problems in preschool and school-aged children, and to a lesser extent, in adolescents.

Practitioners are unquestionably spoilt for choice with regard to EBT of conduct problems in youth: nine psychosocial treatment protocols are listed in this book alone. However, despite substantial progress in the number of

RACHAEL C. MURRIHY • University of Technology, Sydney
ANTONY D. KIDMAN • University of Technology, Sydney
THOMAS H. OLLENDICK • Virginia Tech

R.C. Murrihy et al. (eds.), *Clinical Handbook of Assessing and Treating Conduct Problems in Youth*, DOI 10.1007/978-1-4419-6297-3_20,

EBTs on offer, researchers are still working toward a full understanding of the underlying etiological nature of conduct problems. While extensive risk factors across multiple domains – the child, parent, school, peers, and neighborhood – have been identified, how those factors interact, which factors weigh more heavily, and how protective factors influence the development of conduct problems are all issues that are far from understood.

In a major step toward understanding these important etiological factors, researchers have commenced the complex task of identifying homogenous groups of youth with conduct disorder (CD), for the purpose of elucidating distinct developmental pathways, determining prognoses, streamlining treatment, and maximizing outcomes for different populations. Unraveling more information about these homogenous groups and determining, through an understanding of etiological mechanisms, components of treatment best suited to these subtypes stands as the greatest challenge facing the field today.

TRENDS ACROSS TREATMENT APPROACHES

Early Intervention and Population Level Approaches

Program developers in this book adamantly assert that the earlier interventions can be implemented with youth experiencing conduct problems, the more likely they are to avoid the negative trajectory often associated with this stable and persistent disorder. Early intervention, prior to starting school, can prevent conduct problems from snowballing into academic underperformance and poor relationships – problems that require more resource-intensive interventions down the track (Eyberg and Bussing, Chap. 6). Moreover, this time period represents an important window of opportunity, as families of young children are more likely to complete treatment than families of older children.

Historically, early intervention preventive programs have targeted a high-risk group of individuals or families (e.g., see Webster-Stratton and Reid, Chap. 5) and provided treatments such as parent management training. Sanders and Morawska (Triple P, Chap. 17) argue however, that alone, this approach will never make significant inroads into lowering the prevalence of conduct problems because most parents who would benefit from the modification of their parenting practices do not have access to such treatment (Triple P; Chap. 17). Instead, they advocate that large-scale, population level strategies are needed because they enable widespread access to parenting support without the associated stigma of clinical treatment. These universal population level strategies (e.g., documentary style television series) need to be blended with targeted parenting approaches for those at high risk who may need additional support. (See Fast Track, Chap. 16 and Triple P, Chap. 17 for examples of multilevel interventions with strong empirical support.)

Sanders and Morawska contend that the movement away from a clinical treatment focus toward a population level approach, combining universal and indicated treatments, represents a major "paradigm shift" in the approach to preventing and treating conduct problems. It is expected that future approaches to the preventive treatment of conduct problems will concentrate heavily on such blended approaches.

Emphasis on Treatment Engagement

High attrition rates, strongly associated with low treatment readiness and poor engagement, are widely recognized by the experts in this book as a major barrier to the treatment of conduct problems in youth. Typically, children and adolescents are ambivalent about therapy as they see no need to change their behaviors and may even hold positive beliefs about the social value of aggression. Parents, on the other hand, may be ambivalent for a range of reasons including learned helplessness, disillusionment with psychological care, psychopathology (including an aggressive response set), and chaotic lifestyles. Both youth and parents may also struggle with the logistical side of fitting therapy into a busy life, beset with competing demands (Murrihy, Chap. 12).

To overcome these barriers to successful engagement, Rhodes and Dadds (Chap. 4) argue that therapists must be aware of and continually monitor both therapeutic issues (factors influenced by therapist) and familial process issues (factors that exist within the child's system) that can impact upon and occur within therapy. Indeed, this focus on process issues is common to all treatment protocols reviewed in Part 2. Case study reports, in particular, highlight the importance that is attached to process issues in enhancing treatment engagement and therapeutic rapport. They illustrate that practitioners, across modalities, need to be constantly mindful of a wide range of similar process issues, and then use this knowledge to facilitate engagement and adherence to therapy, and to overcome therapeutic blocks. For example, Alexander and Robbins draw attention to the "engagement and motivation phases" of Functional Family Therapy (FFT) and they advocate, among other strategies, "therapist-matching," or the pairing of clients to therapists with regard to ethnicity, gender, and even clothing (Chap. 10). Schaeffer, McCart, Henggeler, and Cunningham (Multisystemic Therapy, MST, Chap. 11) also employ process-related strategies to optimize engagement, such as ensuring that all members of a family are able to express their perspective of the treatment problem within a respectful environment. Murrihy (Chap. 12) underscores the importance of addressing therapy-interfering beliefs held by the parent (e.g., "the child's behavior is intentional") and/or the child (e.g., "anger is an effective way of getting what I want"), and aligning therapist/family goals. As a final illustration, Greene (Collaborative Problem Solving, CPS, Chap. 8), demonstrates an awareness of process issues when advising therapists to avoid challenging parents who view the child as "having the problem" too early. He recommends that notions of reciprocity in child–parent interactions are introduced later with a view to ultimately arriving at a shared perspective of the case formulation.

Ho, McCabe, Yeh, and Lau (Chap. 18) express concern that youth and families from ethnic minority groups are particularly susceptible to poor engagement because of process issues that arise from the cultural gap between these populations and Caucasian-American based therapies. They suggest that culturally modified EBTs (either standard EBTs that are culturally modified or culturally specific therapies built from the ground) may be better suited to minority groups and point to preliminary research that has shown improved enrolment and retention rates.

Multifaceted Assessment Process

Youth with conduct problems are a broadly heterogeneous group and thus, effective case formulation and treatment relies heavily on information derived from a comprehensive assessment process. Indeed, few disorders require such a complex and wide-ranging assessment. Each treatment approach in this book, regardless of which model/s is ascribed to, captures information from multiple domains and informants, using multiple methodologies. Practitioners assess a broad array of risk factors including child characteristics, familial characteristics, and contextual social factors. They also acquire information about certain characteristics – age, gender, type of aggression, temperament, and comorbid conditions – that inform about the onset, presentation, and course of CDs (Wolff & Ollendick, Chap. 1). Methods used to assess oppositional defiant disorder (ODD) and CD are wide ranging; however, behavioral observation (either in the clinic or at home) is particularly important for assessing family relational patterns and process issues (as illustrated by the structured toy-play situation in the Helping the Noncompliant Child intervention, HNC, Chap. 7).

The goal of assessment, according to Kimonis and Frick (Chap. 3), goes beyond the simple matching of behaviors to Diagnostic and Statistical Manual of Mental Disorders-IV criteria. Through the assessment process, practitioners must generate an understanding of the child's unique pattern of risk factors that are responsible for perpetuating conduct problems. Once identified, these risk factors are integrated into a functional analysis that guides the "best fit" treatment intervention for each family (Rhodes and Dadds, Chap. 4).

Integrative Treatment Models

Once assessment is complete, and rapport between the practitioner and youth is established (an ongoing process), the therapist develops a plan to target designated risk factors (e.g., inconsistent parenting, poor supervision, peer conflict, poor school–home bond), through multiple change agents (child, parent, family members, teachers), across multiple domains (both home and school). To implement this multifaceted and complex approach to treatment, most approaches have relied upon more than one therapeutic framework, instead of adopting a thoughtful integration of therapeutic approaches.

Multisystemic therapy (Chap. 11) provides a good example of an integrative model, employing strategies from structural/strategic and behavioral family therapy, behavioral parent training, cognitive behavioral therapy, and motivational interviewing. FFT (Chap. 10), another theoretically integrative approach, is described by the authors as a "relational, family based, ecosystemic, communication therapy, and cognitive-behavioral based model." In a similar vein, Greene describes CPS (Chap. 8) as a "hybrid" model embracing transactional, systemic, and social learning theories. Other therapies, including Parent Child Interaction Therapy (PCIT; Chap. 6), Incredible Years (IY; Chap. 5), and HNC (Chap. 7), all utilize structured play therapy alongside the more widely researched behavioral therapies. In short, although parent management training, based on behavioral principles, represents the core feature of most therapies (particularly those with children), treatment interventions can include a fusion of models that range widely from systemic therapies to motivational interviewing to parent-assisted academic support (IY) to collaborative problem solving (CPS) to social skills training for parents.

Focus on Generalization and Maintenance of Gains

In the past, criticism has been leveled at the lack of skill generalization from the therapy session to the wider environment (both at home and outside home) and the maintenance of new skills beyond therapy termination. In response, program developers have met these criticisms directly by (a) placing a strong focus on employing strategies that enhance generalization and maintenance and (b) comprehensively evaluating the treatments and providing confirmation of both setting generalization and maintenance of these skills over the long term. A number of common strategies, employed across interventions outlined in Part 2, are thought to be responsible for strengthening skills generalization and the consolidation of therapeutic gains over time. These include the use of instructional techniques that optimize learning and enable repeated skills practice in the "real world," and a focus on the reinforcing role undertaken by parents/caregivers.

Instructional techniques. The instructional techniques used to enhance skills generalization and maintenance of gains are similar across treatment interventions. Most interventions demonstrate modeling of challenging situations (on video or in vivo), followed by role-plays (with family members) in which corrective feedback from the therapist is used to "fine tune" skills. These role-plays approximate real life scenarios for the individual and/or parents as much as possible to aid setting generalization. An example of these instructional techniques can be evidenced in the IY series (Chap. 5) of programs, which use video-modeling of skills, employing a wide range of models, settings, and situations to increase skill generalizability. After watching the videos, the child or parent discusses the content of the video before role-playing the skills themselves, with live feedback from the therapist and other group members. Other therapies, such as HNC (Chap. 7) and PCIT (Chap. 6), often use "bug in the ear" approaches giving live feedback to the parent in one-on-one training sessions with their child to optimize learning.

The provision of regular homework is also commonplace across interventions to encourage the repeated practice of new skills outside sessions and to overcome any barriers that may arise in the implementation of strategies. At the start of each session, a discussion of how homework went over the last week takes place, and the therapist provides coaching on any adjustments needed. An example of a homework task to encourage skills generalization, taken from the Coping Power program (Chap. 9), is the use of a weekly goal sheet. Each week the students write down an operationally defined goal they wish to achieve, work on the goal during the week, and rewards are given for successful goal attainment.

In therapies such as PCIT (Chap. 6) and HNC (Chap. 7), the therapist progressively hands over responsibility for problem solving to the parent/s or caregiver as therapy progresses. In this way, the parents improve their confidence and gain valuable experience in problem solving difficult issues prior to having to "go it alone." Finally, the last sessions of therapy are devoted to reviewing skills and teaching family members how to manage situations that are likely to be problematic in the future. This strategy heightens the likelihood that gains will be maintained in the future, at least in the short term.

Parent-focused approach. Parent or caregiver involvement is integral to the wider generalization and maintenance of skills in both child and adolescent interventions. According to the social ecological theory guiding MST (an adolescent-based therapy, Chap. 11), conduct problems are a result of poorly functioning systems (or the interplay between these systems), and therefore problems are best addressed within this naturally occurring context by key members of this ecology. Parents, therefore, as central figures in a child's ecology, undertake training in the change process and receive the therapeutic support necessary to ensure that gains are maintained in the absence of the therapist. It is thought that by conducting therapy in the natural environment, the therapist can avoid barriers that often emerge when the skill is transferred from the therapy session to the external environment.

In reality, skills generalization and maintenance in MST is assisted by a wide range of parent-focused strategies. For example, parents might agree to access instrumental and emotional support structures (e.g., grandmother) when they are struggling to deliver parent management techniques following the cessation of therapy. After hearing about an argument between his son and a teacher, a father may coach his son in social problem solving, or, in a further example, parents might take responsibility for investigating local after-school groups to facilitate healthy peer associations.

Parents clearly play a crucial role in the generalization and maintenance of skills in both children and adolescents. Because of this, it is also vital to consider any barriers that may exist within the parent, which would prevent them from carrying out this role effectively. Specifically, Greene (Chap. 8), taking a transactional perspective, cautions that parents (like their children) may have "lagging skills" (e.g., communication skills deficits, poor impulse control, disorganization), which can affect how well skills are practiced outside therapy. Addressing these gaps is hence crucial in ensuring that parents are capable of assisting their children in successfully generalizing and maintaining their new skills.

Parental beliefs may also stand in the way of the successful generalization and maintenance of skills. Greene explains "...adults may bring very rigid definitions regarding adult 'authority' to parent-child interactions, leaving little room for discussion, processing, (or) working toward mutually satisfactory solutions." In a second example of unhelpful beliefs, a parent with an aggressive response style may not support the use of the anger management techniques their teenager learns in individual or group therapy. Anticipating such a possibility, Lochman (Group-Based Treatment, Chap. 9) added parent training sessions to his original child anger control training groups, in recognition of the importance of parents as reinforcers of program material. Interestingly, the maintenance of gains over time, with regard to youth delinquency, improved after this addition was made.

ADVANCES, UNRESOLVED ISSUES, AND FUTURE DIRECTIONS

Subtypes of Conduct Disorder

As was touched upon in the introduction to this chapter, one of the key advances in this field over the last decade has been the identification of homogenous groups of youth with CD (Kimonis & Frick, Chap. 3; Wolff and Ollendick, Chap. 1). Driven by the need to understand more about the etiological nature of the disorder and to simplify the complex process of assessment and treatment selection, subtypes have been identified that categorize youth with CD. These subtypes have unique causal factors, developmental pathways, and trajectories (Kimonis & Frick, Chap. 3). Consequently, it is expected that they would also benefit from different treatment regimes (though further research is required in this area).

Four subtypes have been identified to date, and the distinction between these subtypes is clearly supported by research (Kimonis & Frick, Chap. 3). The four subtypes identified thus far include (a) childhood-onset limited CD (conduct problems that diminish before adolescence), (b) life-course-persistent childhood-onset CD with callous-unemotional (CU) traits (low affective response, proactive and reactive aggression, lack of guilt/remorse), (c) life-course persistent childhood-onset CD without CU traits (emotional dysregulation, angry reactivity, characterized by remorse), and (d) adolescent-onset CD (problems onset at puberty, often abate by adulthood). In addition to the identification of further subtypes, the next challenge for researchers is to add to the few existing studies investigating which specific treatment components are most effective for each subtype. Kimonis and Frick assert that research of this kind will streamline the treatment process in place today and ultimately improve outcomes.

Critically, in what represents a major advancement in this field, developmental pathways associated with each of these subtypes have been identified. The implications of this breakthrough are vast. If, for example, a practitioner determines through assessment that a youth has the adolescent-onset subtype of CD, he will be cognizant of the strong probability that problems are related to an overreaction to the natural rebellion process associated with identity formation. He will also be aware that relationships with delinquent peers are likely to play a causal role in this presentation, as the adolescent tries to gain status with friends through engaging in antisocial behaviors. Furthermore, the practitioner knows that in the absence of other lasting vulnerabilities – neurocognitive deficits, temperamental problems, academic and peer difficulties, family dysfunction (more likely found in the childhood-onset subtype) – the prognosis for his client is good. Generally speaking, problems for youth with adolescent-onset CD are much less likely to persist until adulthood compared to their childhood-onset counterparts.

Two further subtypes of CD that have received much research attention are the life-course-persistent childhood-onset CD, with and without CU traits. The identification of these subtypes, and associated developmental pathways, represents exciting progress in this area, mostly because of the treatment implications they bring. If a practitioner determines the presence of CU traits in a child with conduct problems, she is aware that temperamental factors, such as low emotional responsivity and fearlessness (believed to be largely a result of genetics), may be impacting on how the child perceives punishment. In the absence of sufficient arousal to punishment cues, normal development of conscience can be compromised. By contrast, had it been determined at assessment that the child did not have CU traits, the practitioner would consider the likelihood that emotional dysregulation was playing a causative role in the child's impulsive reactivity. That is to say, high arousal may be interfering with the child's ability to understand parental messages when disciplined. Furthermore, she would also consider the likely role of ineffective family practices (inconsistent and noncontingent family practices, coercion cycles) and physical abuse, often causal factors in the non-CU subtype. Lastly, the practitioner understands that prognosis differs for the two subtypes. The course for children with CU traits tends to be more severe, stable, and chronic than for those without CU traits, with greater long-term risk of developing antisocial personality disorder including psychopathy.

Assessment of CD subtypes. Although there have been some problems concerning the reliability of instruments used to identify youth with CU traits (perhaps due to a limited item pool), Kimonis and Frick highlight that progress is occurring with the emergence of new questionnaires that have larger item pools and demonstrated validity. Unfortunately, no method is yet available to assist in establishing whether children under 10 years of age with conduct problems *without CU traits* are likely to have the childhood-onset limited or life-persisting subtype. Knowledge of this kind is vitally important, as it would help to identify which youth to target for preventive treatment.

Matching treatment to ODD and CD subtypes. Kimonis and Frick (Chap. 3) assert that treatment could be better streamlined if treatment components could be matched directly to subtype. For example, anger control training and parent management training may be more relevant for childhood-onset CD without CU traits, due to the role of emotional dysregulation and ineffective parenting practices in this subtype. Likewise, it has been tentatively suggested that those with CU traits may be more likely to respond to positive parenting approaches (positive reinforcement) and a warm parent–child relationship, as opposed to punishment-oriented behavior modification strategies.

It is of critical importance that effective treatments for children with CU traits be identified to avoid the possibility of these children being labeled as "untreatable." Having said this, research is in the very early stages with regard to validating components of treatment that are effective for each subtype. Moreover, there is still more to be understood about the developmental mechanisms of the four subtypes identified, as well as other possible developmental pathways to CD. Once determined, the key targets for each subtype can be elucidated and effective treatments for these targets matched to subtype. We look forward to similar developments in the treatment of ODD. Treatment matching may well lead to advances in the successful management of these youth as well.

Treatment and Protective Factors

Shoemaker's chapter (Sociological Perspectives; Chap. 2) reminds practitioners of the importance of the role played by protective factors in preventing youth delinquency. Shoemaker considers why it is that people do not offend more often than they do and relays the answer of control theorists that "...some type of control prevents a person from offending." This might be an external control such as the social bond formed with representatives of institutions (e.g., ties to teachers, ministers, family members), a personal, internal control (e.g., self-control or self-concept), or a mixture of the two. Shoemaker's chapter highlights the importance of ensuring that adolescents have robust social bonds with family and school, healthy peer associations, sufficient self-control (determined by parenting), and a positive self-concept.

Multisystemic therapists (Chap. 11) are strongly oriented toward optimizing protective factors in the therapeutic process to buffer against targeted risk factors. They build on the existing strengths of the adolescent, family, and extended network to establish powerful protective factors. For example, an extended family member with after school availability is enlisted to provide after-school supervision, or in another example, a cooperative teacher is asked to maintain regular correspondence with parents to improve the home–school bond.

Moreover, McMahon (Fast Track; Chap. 16) highlights that protective factors should be continually present during the transition from childhood to early to late adolescence as opposed to being present in one developmental period only. For example, cognitive deficits and impulsivity, typically buffered by protective support (academic tutoring, effective teacher management) in elementary school, may continue to impact upon adaptive school functioning in adolescence where focused attention and autonomous work is required. Thus, protective services must be incorporated into treatment interventions at this later developmental stage as well. According to McMahon, this focus on addressing changing risk and protective factors throughout the long developmental period necessitates a "long-term intervention commitment" from clinicians working with this "early-starter" population (McMahon, Chap. 16).

Gender and Expression of Conduct Problems

Prevalence rates for ODD and CD clearly favor boys over girls, though this gender gap narrows in adolescence. There has been some criticism, however, that these figures are reflective of a diagnostic system with greater relevance to boys (overt physical aggression and delinquent behavior), as it fails to capture the behavioral expression of aggression more typical of girls.

Research has shown that while girls can act in an overtly aggressive and delinquent manner, more commonly they demonstrate antisocial behavior through relational aggression. This form of aggression takes place when girls engage in destructive gossip and rumor-mongering with the express purpose of socially alienating another girl. Recent efforts aside, Wolff and Ollendick (Chap. 1) highlight that research in this area is sparse and more remains to be discovered about the differences between genders as it relates to the risk for, and the manifestation of, conduct problems. Inclusion of relational aggression, and other female-specific criteria, in the current diagnostic nomenclature certainly warrants further consideration.

Comorbidity and Treatment Impact

The high level of comorbidity of both externalizing and internalizing disorders in youth with conduct problems is clear. Over 90% of youth with ODD and CD will be diagnosed with at least one other disorder and this "tends to be the rule rather than the exception" (Wolff & Ollendick, Chap. 1). Indeed, comorbidity can affect symptom onset [e.g., in youth with comorbid attention deficit hyperactivity disorder (ADHD), problem behaviors tend to have an earlier onset], expression, and course of the disorder. Thus, practitioners need to know more about the impact of comorbity on the child or adolescent, when determining appropriate treatment.

For youth diagnosed with ADHD in addition to ODD or CD, studies have shown that the co-occurrence of these disorders tends to exacerbate symptoms such as aggression; however, results are not as straightforward concerning comorbid ODD or CD and internalizing disorders. Depending on which study is examined, the presence of anxiety or depression with comorbid ODD or CD either worsens or improves the therapeutic picture. It may be that certain features of anxiety work in an opposing fashion – for example, inhibition may serve as a protective factor while withdrawal may act as an exacerbating factor in the development of conduct problems. However, not enough is known to reach a conclusion, and further research investigating the expression of comorbid ODD or CD and internalizing disorders is required.

Knowledge of the temporal ordering of comorbid disorders is also an important consideration for treatment planning. While some research does exist in this area, typically, studies only span a brief period of time. Thus, longitudinal investigations are imperative. Furthermore, while it is established that CD increases the risk of developing a second diagnosis, more research is needed to identify the moderators of this relationship (e.g., the severity of the primary disorder may predict the development of a second disorder; Wolff & Ollendick, Chap. 1).

Evidence-Based Treatments and Ethnic Minority Populations

Almost 50% of the youth in the USA are from ethnic minority backgrounds, a figure predicted to be on the increase. Interestingly, this growing population includes a disproportionate number of youths with conduct problems. Shoemaker (Chap. 2) attributes this overrepresentation of ethnic youth to a number of possible factors. First, immigrants, particularly second generation youth, may experience tension as a result of conflict between their host culture and immigrant country – this tension may be expressed as delinquency. Second, areas with a high turnover of ethnic populations can lack community integration and stability, resulting in weaker social controls and associated difficulties in problem solving conduct issues.

Given the high rates of conduct problems in ethnic minority populations in the USA and elsewhere around the world, research into effective treatments for this population represents an urgent public health priority (Ho, McCabe, Yeh & Lau, Chap. 18). Currently, research into EBTs for ethnic minorities is in its infancy, and it is not yet clear whether (a) established EBTs tested mainly on Caucasian Americans are effective for ethnic minority groups, and (b) if they are effective, are they superior to culturally modified treatments?

A limited number of randomized controlled trials (RCTs), evaluating ethnic invariance in established EBTs (i.e., "standard treatments are equally powerful when applied to ethnic minorities") have found promising results. Standard treatments have been identified as either possibly or probably efficacious in certain minority populations (using Chambless and colleagues' criteria). However, with the exception of MST for African Americans, which has already met the well-established criterion, more RCTs with larger samples are needed for standard EBTs to reach the well-established criterion for minority populations. Magnitude of effect is also an issue; research has not yet provided an answer as to whether minority youth fare as well as Caucasian Americans receiving standard EBTs. Future studies should focus on ethnicity as a moderator of treatment outcomes.

While these results are encouraging, "real world" effectiveness studies of standard EBTs must follow to determine (a) if results are as impressive with comorbid samples in community settings, and (b) whether specific issues related to engagement and adherence arise. Criticisms launched at standard EBTs are that they result in fewer enrolments, poorer engagement, and higher drop out in ethnic minorities compared with the sample they were designed to treat. In particular, parent management training has received considerable attention because the cultural variation inherent in parenting practices is thought to impact on treatment engagement and retention. Interestingly, in line with these criticisms, the preliminary evidence available to date suggests better engagement and retention outcomes for minority populations using culturally adapted treatment protocols.

That said, Ho, McCabe, Yeh and Lau conclude that the "jury is out" as to whether culturally specific (protocols designed from scratch) or culturally adapted (adapted versions of standard EBTs) treatment protocols are superior to standard EBTs. Research should be urgently undertaken to compare the effectiveness of standard unadapted EBTs with that of culturally adapted EBTs. Finally, researchers should also include a wider range of ethnic minorities in their studies when examining ethnicity as a predictor of change, rather than just African Americans and Hispanic Americans.

Group Treatment and Deviancy Training

The ability to service a greater number of mental health clients has made group treatment an attractive option for service providers operating on limited resources. For some time now, intervention groups for the treatment of conduct problems have been operating in both schools and community health settings. In the last decade, however, concerns have grown over the iatrogenic effects identified in some studies aggregating deviant youth.

Although this research raises some cause for concern, it is clear from the limited studies available that the relationship between group treatment and deviancy training is not straightforward. In fact, one study has shown higher levels of deviancy training in "mixed" groups of adolescents than in "pure" CD groups. Certainly, a wide range of group characteristics (e.g., cohesiveness) and individual characteristics (e.g., age) influence youth susceptibility and vulnerability to deviancy training and peer contagion (Murrihy, Chap. 12).

Not surprisingly, given the lack of empirical knowledge about risk factors for deviancy training, little psychological research exists (see Chap. 12) regarding strategies to minimize deviancy training. Nonetheless, program developers from the Coping Power program have relied on their combined group experience to recommend the use of both intervention strategies (e.g., two facilitators, group rules) and behavioral management strategies (e.g., changing students' seating arrangements, "buddying" systems) to minimize deviancy training. Building on this clinical wisdom, further research to investigate the mechanisms underlying deviancy training, as well as to confirm strategies that can be used to minimize the occurrence of iatrogenic outcomes, should be a priority.

Residential Treatments

Youth with conduct problems at the severe end of the spectrum often receive treatment in residential settings for their own protection and that of the community. Questions have been raised, however, as to the effectiveness of these diverse therapeutic interventions. Clearly, the provision of effective treatments at this juncture is of vital importance given the severity of these presentations and the possibility that this may represent the "last chance" treatment for many youth. Shedding light on this issue, Coventry and Swanson (Chap. 14) reviewed the effectiveness of boot camps, an intensive military-style treatment of 90–120 days duration, commonly adopted by governments as a cheaper alternative to incarceration. The authors concluded that the use of hard labor, strict discipline, and degradation to break down individualism and bring about conformity does not reduce long-term recidivism rates. Rather than improve youth outcomes, boot camps can be physically and psychologically dangerous, even lethal in some instances.

In place of this military-style approach, Coventry and Swanson recommend that boot camps shift to a rehabilitative focus. Such a focus aims to successfully reintegrate boot camp attendees into the community through the provision of training in social competencies, educational and vocational skills, coupled with follow-up care. Once established (and some uniformity is needed across these programs), these rehabilitative programs need to be assessed in an empirical fashion.

Another variant of the "camping" treatment interventions is wilderness camps (Coventry & Swanson, Chap. 14). These camps adopt a therapeutic agenda, teaching problem solving skills and improving self-esteem through challenging outdoor adventure activities. Unfortunately, research has shown that, similar to boot camps, attendance at wilderness camps does not result in reductions in delinquency over the long term (despite some immediate improvements in self-confidence). This is not an entirely surprising finding given the disconnection between the training setting and the child's usual environment.

By contrast, LeBuffe, Robison, and Chamberlin-Elliott, reviewing residential treatment centers in Chap. 13, found evaluation outcomes to be encouraging. They concluded that research in the last decade "suggest(s) the positive value of residential treatment for youth, families and society," while simultaneously stressing that results are not conclusive and more needs to be done in this area. They argue that efficacy research, generally avoided because of the unethical nature of waitlists and complexity of presentations, needs to be replaced by clinical quality improvement methodologies.

Cost Effectiveness Analyses

Foster (Chap. 19) alerts program developers that the National Institute of Mental Health (USA) is dissatisfied with the current number of cost-effectiveness analyses attached to treatment studies. They are pushing for these analyses to become a compulsory part of future prevention trials. This information, they state, is important for government policy makers in determining the allocation of limited resources.

Specifically, few cost-effectiveness analyses have been undertaken for programs treating children with conduct problems (with the exception of Fast Track, Incredible Years, and Triple P). Foster expects this is because clinicians obviously think that prevention would be cost-effective – especially given the lifetime social cost of US $2 million for each youth – but this is not necessarily the case.

Foster highlights that there are problems associated with measuring cost, specific to conduct problems that work against cost-effectiveness. The first difficulty is that early intervention is recommended, yet every dollar invested in childhood is worth significantly less by the time treatment succeeds in adolescence: "A dollar spent today has to generate more than a dollar's worth of benefits in the future" (Foster, Chap. 19). Second, indicated and selected treatments service a significant number of youth who would not have gone on to develop the disorder (i.e., the false positives receive unnecessary treatment).

Practitioners, in determining cost-effectiveness or the cost of illness (a number of approaches to determining cost benefit are outlined in Chap. 19), need to take cost-effectiveness into account when they first design their program. This is advisable for practical reasons, such as keeping accurate records for time allocated to treatment, and for statistical reasons so that power can be set accordingly. Efficiency should be a consideration, rather than just a sole focus on maximizing the efficacy of a program. Recruiting a team member with expertise in health economics is also important, as is the independent replication of cost-effectiveness analyses. Finally, programs need to be more consistent in the way intervention costs are calculated, so that between-program comparisons can be made.

SUMMARY

This volume highlights that a great deal has been achieved over the last quarter of a century in the field of youth-related conduct problems. The plethora of EBTs available, supported by high-quality research, represents an outstanding achievement for the field of clinical psychology. Moreover, treatment approaches will continue to benefit from (a) ongoing research into ODD and CD subtypes and developmental pathways, which will hopefully allow further streamlining of treatment, and (b) a better understanding of other factors, such as gender, ethnicity, and comorbidity, that also impact on the course and expression of ODD and CD. In short, this knowledge will enable program developers to "fine tune" existing treatment protocols or, in the case of treatment for ethnic minorities where standard EBTs will not suffice, treatments may need to be culturally adapted.

Early intervention in children with conduct problems is widely advocated, yet the standard approach for delivering preventive interventions is changing. A "paradigm shift" is underway in this area – rather than employing a clinical treatment approach exclusively as has been done in the past (e.g., targeting a selected population for participation in a treatment intervention), a population level approach is indicated instead. Universal interventions that reach a wide audience (e.g., documentaries) are blended with selected approaches for those needing additional assistance. We expect to see more of this population level blended approach in the coming years.

Preventive programs must also demonstrate their cost-effectiveness. A perceived lack of expertise among mental health clinicians, or perhaps a lack of interest in these analyses, has resulted in clinicians generally steering clear of undertaking cost-effectiveness analyses on their research trials. This avoidance, however, is a risky practice to continue with large funding bodies such as the National Institute of Mental Health putting the onus on clinicians to demonstrate that their preventive treatments are cost effective.

Conduct problems are the most commonly presenting and costly problems facing youth mental health today, and therefore, identification of EBTs is of the utmost importance. The good news is that research in this area is progressing at a rapid rate and we have seen a proliferation of EBTs for both children and adolescents. Having identified a multitude of risk factors already, researchers are now poised to further unravel the multiple developmental pathways that lead to the development of ODD and CD. With such a solid research grounding in place, we look forward to seeing what the next 25 years will bring.

Index

R

www.ingramcontent.com/pod-product-compliance
Lightning Source LLC
Chambersburg PA
CBHW080735150926
51501CB00005B/170
* 9 7 8 1 4 4 1 9 6 2 9 5 9 *